Prehospital Trauma Care

Prehospital Trauma Care

edited by

Eldar Søreide

University of Bergen and Rogaland Central Hospital
Stavanger, Norway

Norwegian Air Ambulance Ltd.
Høvik, Norway

Christopher M. Grande

International Trauma Anesthesia and Critical Care Society (ITACCS)
Baltimore, Maryland

Harvard Medical School and
Brigham and Women's Hospital
Boston, Massachusetts

West Virginia University School of Medicine
Morgantown, West Virginia

SUNY Buffalo School of Medicine
Buffalo, New York

MARCEL DEKKER, INC. NEW YORK • BASEL

ISBN: 0-8247-0537-8

Cover photo by Bo Eklund

This book is printed on acid-free paper.

Headquarters
Marcel Dekker, Inc.
270 Madison Avenue, New York, NY 10016
tel: 212-696-9000; fax: 212-685-4540

Eastern Hemisphere Distribution
Marcel Dekker AG
Hutgasse 4, Postfach 812, CH-4001 Basel, Switzerland
tel: 41-61-261-8482; fax: 41-61-261-8896

World Wide Web
http://www.dekker.com

The publisher offers discounts on this book when ordered in bulk quantities. For more information, write to Special Sales/Professional Marketing at the headquarters address above.

Current printing (last digit):
10 9 8 7 6 5 4 3 2 1

PRINTED IN THE UNITED STATES OF AMERICA

To all the trauma patients whose future depends on the care given before they reach the hospital, and to all the men and women worldwide who strive to provide high quality prehospital trauma care.

To my children, Lina, Christian and Eidbjorg, and to my wife Elise: Without your joyful presence, love, and understanding, nothing would be the same.

Eldar Søreide

To my lovely wife, Dr. Lesley K. Wong, who has supported me in all ways, and who is my source of strength.

To my colleagues at the Harvard Medical School and the Brigham and Women's Hospital in Boston, the Jon Michael Moore Trauma Center at West Virginia University in Morgantown, and the Trauma Team at Erie County Medical Center, SUNY Buffalo School of Medicine in Buffalo, for their support.

To the Directors and Executives of ITACCS, whose continued dedication has allowed many wonderful programs dedicated to the advancement of education and science in trauma care to achieve fruition.

Christopher M. Grande

Preface

On behalf of the International Trauma Anesthesia and Critical Care Society (ITACCS), we are pleased and honored to present *Prehospital Trauma Care*.

Each of the predominant fields in the care of the injured—anesthesiology, critical care, emergency medicine, and surgery—has an idiosyncratic bias regarding management of the trauma patient. Some of these biases are based on traditional teachings, and others stem from differences reflected in the body of literature accumulated in each specialty. Often, what is well known and accepted in one specialty must be "rediscovered" independently by another before becoming part of practice standards (perhaps the most obvious example is the variety of approaches to management of the difficult airway). For these reasons, to the extent possible, we have paired contributors from different specialty backgrounds as author teams, e.g., a surgeon with an anesthesiologist or an emergency medicine physician with a surgeon.

The second aspect that has a profound impact on the way trauma is practiced is geography and culture. Although electronics have made the world a much smaller place, medical practitioners are still largely held to a standard of care that is provincial in nature. A great deal of time and scientific evidence is required to break down the barriers that keep local groups doing things the way the previous generation did, despite the fact that a group elsewhere has developed a better approach to the same issue.

Evidence-based medicine has entered modern medicine at full speed. Hence, we have aimed to include and discuss evidence-based recommendations for clinical care whenever present and feasible. Randomized controlled trials are few, and we know more about what is not useful and may be harmful to the patient than what has been proven *beyond doubt* to improve survival. Being realistic, we know that in most situations the actual care given to a patient will be based on sound judgment and the experience of the traumatologist involved. Therefore, as editors, one of our goals has been to recruit authors from different parts of the world. In this way, we hope to present various geographic and cultural perspectives within the same context.

Finally, the approach to management of any given clinical problem within the realm of trauma care will differ as a function of the locations in which treatment is undertaken.

Trauma care is often viewed as a ''chain of survival,'' stretching from the site of injury in the field to the emergency department, to the operating room, to the intensive care unit, and beyond to the rehabilitation center. How one manages the same problem will vary depending on the point of care. Factors active in this decision-making process include the prevailing environment (lighting, temperature, climate), equipment, distance, and clinical competence. The prehospital arena is considered by many to be the most challenging because of its propensity for adverse factors.

We have attempted to cover the topics within a framework of the highest quality of care and then to qualify this framework within the context of the prehospital environment. Our editorial protocol has been to subject each chapter to two cycles of peer review: the first undertaken by the respective Part editors and the second by each of us as general editors.

The book is divided into four parts. Part A covers the general aspects of prehospital trauma care. It starts with a historic view on scope and practice, then moves to demographics and mechanism of injury. The chapters in this part also focus on the organization of prehospital trauma care in developed societies worldwide. The role of the physician in different systems varies from that of a hospital-based medical director to actually providing care at the scene. The chapters present different configurations of the prehospital trauma team around the world and explain why crew-resource management (CRM), research, and continuous quality improvement are so important.

Part B covers the initial care of the patient; with in-depth discussion on everything from advanced airway management to state-of-the art fluid resuscitation and prevention of hypothermia. A frequently forgotten aspect of high-quality trauma care is the provision of adequate analgesia. This topic is also covered.

Trauma is not a generic disease. Hence, therapy will differ according to the anatomical disruption and physiological consequences of the injury. In Part C, the individual approach is taken one step further. Each chapter presents the clinical challenges and treatment modalities of the different injuries the reader is likely to encounter in his or her practice. The first two chapters of this section explain why blunt and penetrating trauma should be dealt with differently. The following chapters focus on special groups of patients—for example, the traumatized child and the entrapped patient—and special trauma situations—such as chemical injuries and accidental hypothermia.

Part D covers transport issues and special problems, e.g., how to provide high-quality care in rural areas and how to ensure the interactions upon the arrival in the emergency department work to the benefit of the patient. In our experience, both topics present major challenges to a trauma system.

Since improving the trauma chain of survival and securing a continuum of care is the ultimate goal for us all, we felt it was as important to focus on human factors as on specific therapies. Hence, Chapter 40 covers prevention issues, not only how to reduce the number of fatalities caused by car crashes and the use of guns for the wrong purposes, but also how to learn from our own errors and thus improve what we teach the next generation of prehospital care providers. That way, they can do an even better job for the severely injured patient.

In the course of this work, we have learned a great deal and have come to appreciate new methods for dealing with old problems. In an effort to meet the expectations of the broad audience for the book, we have endeavored to fuse the perspectives of a variety of medical specialties as well as geographic and cultural perspectives regarding trauma care. We expect *Prehospital Trauma Care* to have broad appeal, not only to the range of physicians involved in trauma care but also to the flight nurses and paramedics providing prehospital care to injured patients worldwide. We offer this work to the trauma care community in the spirit of international collegiality, with the hope that the readers will benefit as we have.

Eldar Søreide
Christopher M. Grande

Foreword

This substantial work brings together a distinguished, multinational authorship to address the subject of prehospital trauma care. The subject does not lend itself easily to evidence-based scientific study and the authors stand out in medical society as leaders in this difficult field.

The fate of the seriously injured is often sealed in the first hour or so after injury. Management during this prehospital period may make the difference not only between life and death but also between quality survival and the depressing, frustrating misery of long-term disability. Thus, an authoritative and comprehensive book on the subject, which will certainly be a most valuable resource for consultation and reference searches, is extremely timely and will surely be appreciated by the prehospital tyro.

Where evidence-based science is available, this book has it. Where it is not, common sense, sound advice, the pros and cons, and honest opinion are given by experienced practitioners. The balance between delay on site for interventions and forgoing these in favor of immediate transfer to definitive care in the hospital is carefully outlined and guidance is given for specific conditions that may benefit from a particular strategy.

Prehospital Trauma Care adds to the already considerable list of volumes that have been published as a result of initiatives emanating from the members of the International Trauma Anesthesia and Critical Care Society (ITACCS). This Society, which is now multidisciplinary, is devoted to the study and enhancement of trauma care. It is the only truly international society to have taken on this role. The chapter authors are members of the Society and forgo their royalties in favor of the furtherance of improvement in the standards of trauma care.

Originally the concept of John Schou and Christopher Grande, Executive Director of ITACCS, the book has now come to fruition thanks to the special talents and energy of Eldar Søreide and members of the ITACCS Prehospital Care Committee. The editors and the contributors are to be congratulated on a splendid contribution to the literature.

Peter Baskett, F.R.C.A., F.R.C.P., F.F.A.E.M.
Department of Anesthesia
Frenchay Hospital
Bristol, United Kingdom

Foreword

An international prehospital trauma care textbook for health care providers, under the auspices of anesthesiologists, is long overdue. Why? (1) Because the weakest link in the emergency medical services (EMS) life support chain (trauma chain of survival) is the prehospital phase of management by lay bystanders, emergency medical technicians, paramedics, nurses, and physicians. (2) Because anesthesiologists pioneered the change from ''scoop-and-run'' in the 1950s, when the victim was rushed without life support (in a hearse or station wagon) to the nearest hospital—to ''resuscitate while moving fast'' to the most appropriate hospital, using a mobile ICU or helicopter. (3) Because the majority of potentially salvageable trauma victims who die or become crippled need resuscitation for coma or shock, conditions requiring anesthesiologists' expertise in titrated cardiovascular-pulmonary-cerebral life support. In addition to an anticipated increase in the use of simulators to acquire knowledge, skills, and judgment, the operating room anesthesiology environment will remain essential for training in titrated life support. Anesthesiologists, surgeons, and emergency physicians with experience in the management of severe polytrauma should jointly make prehospital trauma care increasingly more effective. They stand on the shoulders of the Anglo-American anesthesiologists and surgeons who pioneered modern traumatologic resuscitation during World War II.

In the 1960s, when I served on the U.S. National Research Council Committee on EMS (chaired by the visionary Sam Seeley), my push away from bandaging wounds and splinting fractures to resuscitation and life support was received by nonanesthesiologists as a revolution. To us it seemed logical to have innovations in basic and advanced trauma life support based on facts of pathophysiology and therapeutics, as documented with clinically realistic models in large animals and by physiological observations in patients. Epidemiological randomized clinical outcome studies in resuscitation medicine have limitations. *Whom* and *how* to teach should be based on the results of education research. Survival without brain damage often depends on lay bystanders providing life-supporting first aid (LSFA). Well-designed self-training systems can be more effective than instructor courses.

The prevention of accidents is, of course, most important. As we move into the twenty-first century, however, we must also appreciate the fact that some traumatism will always be with us. Researchers should seek results that are clinically important. For *basic* trauma life support we can expect innovation in positioning, and in control of airway, temperature, and external hemorrhage. For *advanced* trauma life support, most important are the prehospital arena, time factors (not hours, but seconds to minutes), and cerebral preservation and resuscitation. Rigid ''cookbook'' protocols should be replaced by titrated life support. Current research is clarifying optimal resuscitation fluids and strategies, differences between dangerous accidental hypothermia and beneficial therapeutic hypothermia, hibernation strategies for prolonged transport of rural and military casualties, and exciting potentials for the immediate prehospital mitigation of secondary derangements in patients with severe brain trauma. The search for an ideal blood substitute needs openness, not secrecy because of patent considerations. Better use should be made of emergency thoracotomy. For exsanguinations cardiac arrest, ''suspended animation'' is not science fiction but ready for clinical feasibility trials—for the immediate induction of profound hypothermic preservation of the organism, to buy time for transport and repair, followed by delayed resuscitation. Traumatologic resuscitation can be the greatest gift of modern anesthesiology to society.

Peter Safar, M.D., Ph.D.
Safar Resuscitation Center
University of Pittsburgh
Pittsburgh, Pennsylvania

Introduction

The impetus for the development of modern emergency medicine has come from a variety of concerns. Among the major forces has been the realization that traumatic injuries have often been neglected and that modern management of their care has been much better for wartime combatants than for civilians. Second, has been the recognition that cardiac arrest is capable of resuscitation, and need not be an automatic death sentence. Third has been the development of the specialty of emergency medicine promulgated by the concept that the principles and practice of emergency medicine are capable of being taught.

While there is much international variation in who will conduct the practice of emergency medicine, and how it will be organized economically as well as academically, it is interesting how common are the prehospital care approaches to emergencies.

Prehospital Trauma Care is a clear example of how it is possible to draw across international boundaries to find the principles of management, with contributors from many countries in Europe, North America, Asia, and the Middle East.

Whether the care is rendered on ground or in the air, whether one utilizes physicians, nurses, or paramedics, the initial principles are fairly constant. One can argue about acts allowed but much less frequently about responsibilities. Thus, the book is aimed more toward a discussion of those common responsibilities and less toward the individual disciplines of the practice specialty of the chapters authors who come from a variety of backgrounds, including emergency medicine, anesthesia, and surgery.

It has become evident in trauma that previously well patients who become injured will often be able to compensate for their injuries, and can therefore often *look* well enough to initially mask some very serious injuries. It is therefore imperative to have rules of management that will acknowledge the importance of mechanism of injury. To do that requires not only adequate training of the prehospital personnel but subsequent communication to the subsequent treating physicians.

There is evidence that the way patients are treated within a trauma unit or emergency department (ED) is strongly guided by the way in which the field personnel present the case. For example, if the victim of an automobile accident arrives at the hospital in backboard and spinal immobilization, and with an IV line running, it is quite probable that he will receive a full trauma workup. On the other hand, if the victim arrives walking into the ED he will probably receive a much more cursory workup.

While there has been debate about whether more patients are being immobilized than is necessary, we must pay attention to the downstream effects of our initial patient perception. Moreover, it is very easy for field personnel to be fooled by the compensatory powers of the otherwise healthy patient who may have already self-extricated from the accident and is walking around at the scene.

Two cases are presented here. Case 1 involves a 32-year-old man whose truck rolled after it had slid on ice in a single-vehicle accident in a rural community. He extricated himself from the wreck and realized he needed some help. Unfortunately, he was on a remote rural highway and had to walk two miles to the nearest farmhouse to obtain help. Because he had walked that far, he was not immobilized by the prehospital personnel who thought he had only minor injuries. He was found to have a pelvic fracture, a main shaft femur fracture, and a ruptured spleen. He later bled to death from the undetected ruptured spleen. It is highly probable that if he had been picked up at the site of the accident and treated aggressively in the field, he would have had a more aggressive workup at the hospital and his ruptured spleen would have been found in time for surgical intervention.

Case 2 involves a 59-year-old woman who was riding in the back seat of a Jeep. While the car was stopped in bad traffic, another vehicle came around a curve and plowed into the rear of the Jeep at high speed. The woman crawled out of the back of the Jeep and was standing on the highway when the paramedics arrived. She complained of a knee injury. She was transported to the hospital by ambulance along with her daughter, who complained of an ankle injury. Although the Jeep was totally destroyed in the accident, the accident was deemed minor and was communicated as such to the hospital personnel. The patient was discharged after a cursory workup that included no imaging studies other than that of the knee. Eight hours later the patient expired from exsanguination, again from a ruptured spleen. It is again highly probable that a major mechanism of injury, perceived and acted upon by the field personnel, would have guided a more objective workup of the patient at the hospital, with an objective evaluation of the patient's abdomen with ultrasound or a CT scan. This, in turn, would have enabled surgical intervention in a timely and lifesaving fashion.

The reality is that emergency care is in great need of highly organized, well-constructed, and efficient prehospital care. One simply cannot isolate a small piece of that care and expect to have good outcomes.

This book describes the principles of trauma and prehospital care that have been derived from multiple international experiences. It does not reveal an infinite possibility of responses, but rather a unified, coordinated approach that will be effective in many countries and in many circumstances, from rural to urban.

It is very exciting to perceive that emergency medicine is international in its uniformity, and as well, that there is a growing international collegiality of education and academics that will serve all our nations.

Peter Rosen, M.D.
Department of Emergency Medicine
University of California San Diego
Medical Center
San Diego, California

Contents

PART D. Transportation and Specific Problems (Part Editors: Christian Lackner and Daniel Scheidegger)

Contributors

Allysan Armstrong-Brown, M.D. Department of Anesthesia, Sunnybrook and Women's College Health Sciences Centre, Toronto, Ontario, Canada

Paul S. Auerbach, M.D., M.S., F.A.C.E.P. Division of Emergency Medicine, Department of Surgery, Stanford University School of Medicine, Stanford, California

Tim Auger Parks Canada Rescue, Parks Canada, Banff National Park, Banff, Canada

David J. Baker, M. Phil, D.M., F.R.C.A. SAMU de Paris, Hôpital-Necker Enfants Malades, Paris, France

Paul Barach, M.D., M.P.H. Department of Anesthesia and Critical Care, Center for Patient Safety, Pritzker School of Medicine, University of Chicago, Chicago, Illinois

Paul Berlin, M.S., NREMT-P Pierce County Fire District 5, Gig Harbor, Washington

Guttorm Bratteboe, M.D. Department of Anesthesia and Intensive Care and Hyperbaric Medicine Unit, Department of Occupational Medicine, Haukeland University Hospital, Bergen, Norway

Enrico M. Camporesi, M.D. Department of Anesthesiology and Physiology, State University of New York Upstate Medical University, Syracuse, New York

Richard Carmona, M.D., M.P.H., F.A.C.S. Department of Surgery, Public Health and Family and Community Medicine, University of Arizona, Tucson, Arizona

Charles D. Deakin, M.A., M.D., M.R.C.P., F.R.C.A. Department of Anaesthetics, Southampton General Hospital, Southampton, United Kingdom

Jan De Boer Free University of Amsterdam, Amsterdam, The Netherlands

Stefano Di Bartolomeo, M.D. Friuli Venezia Giulia Regional Emergency Helicopter Medical Service, Udine, Italy

Wolfgang F. Dick, M.D., Ph.D., F.R.C. A. Clinic of Anesthesiology, University Hospital, Mainz, Germany

Richard P. Dutton, M.D. Division of Trauma Anesthesiology, R Adams Cowley Shock Trauma Center, University of Maryland Medical System, Baltimore, Maryland

Anders Ersson, M.D. Department of Anesthesiology, Intensive Care Unit, Malmo University Hospital, Malmo, Sweden

William F. Fallon, Jr., M.D., F.A.C.S. Division of Trauma, Critical Care, Burns and Metro Life Flight, MetroHealth Medical Center, Cleveland, Ohio

Craig Geis Geis-Alvarado & Associates, Inc., Novato, California

Dario Gonzalez, M.D., F.A.C.E.P. Fire Department of the City of New York/Emergency Medical Services, New York, New York

Christopher M. Grande, M.D., M.P.H. International Trauma Anesthesia and Critical Care Society (ITACCS), Baltimore, Maryland; Department of Anesthaesiology, Harvard Medical School and Department of Anesthesiology, Perioperative and Pain Medicine, Brigham and Women's Hospital, Boston, Massachusetts; Department of Anesthesiology, Jon C. Moore Trauma Center, Robert C. Byrd Health Sciences Center, West Virginia University School of Medicine, Morgantown, West Virginia; and Department of Anesthesiology, Erie County Medical Center, SUNY Buffalo School of Medicine, Buffalo, New York

Kim J. Gupta, M.B.C.h.B., F.R.C.A. Department of Anesthesia, Royal United Hospital, Bath, United Kingdom

Hengo Haljamäe, M.D., Ph.D. Department of Anesthesiology and Intensive Care, Sahlgrenska University Hospital, Göteborg, Sweden

Daniel G. Hankins, M.D., F.A.C.E.P. Department of Emergency Medicine, Mayo Clinic; and Mayo Medical Transport, Rochester, Minnesota

Walter Hasibeder, M.D. Division of General and Surgical Intensive Care Medicine, Department of Anaesthesia and General Critical Care Medicine, The Leopold Franzens University of Innsbruck, Innsbruck, Austria

Jens Hauke, M.D. Department of Anesthesiology and Intensive Care Medicine, Federal Armed Forces Medical Center Ulm, Ulm, Germany

Stephen R. Hayden, M.D., F.A.C.E.P., F.A.A.E.M. Department of Emergency Medicine, University of California San Diego Medical Center, San Diego, California

Matthias Helm, M.D. Department of Anesthesiology and Intensive Care Medicine, Federal Armed Forces Medical Center Ulm, Ulm, Germany

Ken Hillman, M.B.B.S., F.F.I.C.A.N.Z.C.A., F.R.C.A. Department of Anesthetics, Emergency Medicine, and Intensive Care, The University of New South Wales, Sydney, Australia

Susan Kaplan, M.D. Department of Anesthesiology, MCP-Hahnemann University, Philadelphia, Pennsylvania

Judith R. Klein, M.D. Division of Emergency Medicine, UCSF–San Francisco General Hospital, San Francisco, California

Herbert Kuhnigk, M.D., D.E.A.A. Department of Anesthesiology, University of Wuerzburg, Wuerzburg, Germany

Asgeir M. Kvam, M.D. Department of Emergency Medical Services, EMS Dispatch Center, Ullevaal University Hospital, Oslo, Norway

Lorenz A. Lampl, M.D., Ph.D. Department of Anesthesiology and Intensive Care Medicine, Federal Armed Forces Medical Center Ulm, Ulm, Germany

Markus D. W. Lipp, M.D. Anesthesiology Clinic, Johannes Gutenberg University of Mainz, Mainz, Germany

Freddy K. Lippert, M.D. Department of Anesthesiology and Intensive Care Medicine, Trauma Center, Mobile Intensive Care Unit, and Major Incident Command Center, Rigshospitalet, Copenhagen University Hospital, Copenhagen, Denmark

David Lockey, F.R.C.A., F.I.M.C., R.C.S. (Ed) Intensive Care Unit, Frenchay Hospital, Bristol, United Kingdom

Pål Madsen, M.D. Norwegian Air Ambulance Ltd., Høvik, Norway

Peter Mair, M.D. Department of Anesthesia and Intensive Care, The Leopold Franzens University School of Medicine, Innsbruck, Austria

Charlene Mancuso, R.N., B.S.N., M.P.A., C.E.N. Division of Trauma, Critical Care, Burns and Metro Life Flight, MetroHealth Medical Center, Cleveland, Ohio

Gregg S. Margolis, M.S., NREMT-P Emergency Health Services Programs, The George Washington University, Washington, D.C.

Antonio Marques, M.D. Emergency Department, Hospital Geral de Santo Antonio, Porto, Portugal

Jeremy Mauger, B.Sc., M.B., B.S., F.R.C.A. Department of Anaesthetics, St. George's Hospital, London, United Kingdom

Kimball I. Maull, M.D. The Trauma Center at Carraway and Carraway Methodist Medical Center, Birmingham, Alabama

Aleksandra J. Mazurek, M.D. Department of Anesthesiology, Children's Memorial Hospital; and Northwestern University Medical School, Chicago, Illinois

Maureen McCunn, M.D. Departments of Anesthesiology and Critical Care, R Adams Cowley Shock Trauma Center, University of Maryland Medical System, Baltimore, Maryland

Philippe-Gabriel Meyer, M.D. Department of Anesthesiology, Hôpital-Necker Enfants Malades, Paris, France

Moshe Michaelson, M.D. Trauma Unit, Rambam Medical Center, Technion Institute, Haifa, Israel

Giuseppe Nardi, M.D. Friuli Venezia Giulia Regional Emergency Helicopter Medical Service, Udine, Italy; and Intensive Care Unit, Emergency Department, S. Camillo Hospital, Rome, Italy

Søren Loumann Nielsen, M.D. Department of Anesthesiology and Intensive Care Medicine, Trauma Center, Mobile Intensive Care Unit, and Major Incident Command Center, Rigshospitalet, Copenhagen University Hospital, Copenhagen, Denmark

Jerry P. Nolan, F.R.C.A. Department of Anesthesia and Intensive Care, Royal United Hospital, Bath, United Kingdom

Peter Oakley Trauma Research Department, North Staffordshire Hospital, Stoke-on-Trent, United Kingdom

Michael J. A. Parr, M.B., B.S., M.R.C.P., F.R.C.A., F.A.N.Z.C.A. Intensive Care Unit, Liverpool Hospital, University of New South Wales, Sydney, Australia

Hans-R. Paschen, M.D. Department of Anesthesiology and Intensive Care Medicine, Amalie Sieveking-Krankenhaus, Hamburg, Germany

Paul E. Pepe, M.D. Department of Medicine, University of Texas Southwestern Medical School; and Department of Emergency Medical Services, Parkland Memorial Health System, Dallas, Texas

J. D. Polk, D.O. Metro Life Flight, MetroHealth Medical Center, Cleveland, Ohio

Gail E. Rasmussen, M.D. The Meridian Anesthesiology Group, Meridian, Mississippi

Agnès Ricard-Hibon, M.D. Department of Anesthesia and Intensive Care Medicine, Hôpital Beaujon, Clichy, France

Frans Rutten, M.D., F.D.S.A. Trauma Center, HEMS Program Netherlands South–West/Rotterdam, Oosterhout, The Netherlands

Birgit Schober, M.D. Department of Anesthesia and Intensive Care, Rogaland Central and University Hospital, Stavanger, Norway

Wolfgang Schobersberger, M.D. Division of General and Surgical Intensive Care Medicine, Department of Anaesthesia and General Critical Care Medicine, The Leopold Franzens University of Innsbruck, Innsbruck, Austria

John Schou, M.D. Department of Anesthesiology, Kreiskrankenhaus Lörrach, Lörrach, Germany

Lance Shepherd, M.D., C.C.F.P.-EM University of Calgary and Shock Trauma Air Rescue Service, Calgary; Banff Prehospital EMS and Banff Emergency Department, Banff, Canada

Tom Silfvast, M.D., Ph.D. Department of Anesthesia and Intensive Care, Helsinki University Hospital; and Helsinki Area HEMS, Helsinki, Finland

Charles E. Smith, M.D., F.R.C.P.C. Case Western Reserve University Medical School and Department of Anesthesiology, MetroHealth Medical Center, Cleveland, Ohio

Eldar Søreide, M.D., Ph.D. University of Bergen; Department of Anesthesia and Intensive Care, Rogaland Central Hospital, Stavanger, Norway; and Norwegian Air Ambulance Ltd., Høvik, Norway

Michael Sugrue, M.B., B.Ch., B.A.O., F.R.A.C.S., F.R.C.S.I. Trauma Department, The Liverpool Hospital, Sydney, Australia

Thomas A. Sweeney, M.D., F.A.C.E.P. Department of Emergency Medicine, Christiana Care Health Systems, Wilmington, Delaware

Eran Tal-Or, M.D. Trauma Unit, Rambam Medical Center, Technion Institute, Haifa, Israel

Nelson Tang, M.D., F.A.C.E.P. Department of Emergency Medicine, The Johns Hopkins University School of Medicine, Baltimore, Maryland

Koichi Tanigawa, M.D. Department of Emergency and Critical Care Medicine, Fukuoka University Hospital, Fukuoka, Japan

Andreas Thierbach, M.D. Department of Anesthesiology, University Hospital, Mainz, Germany

Stephen H. Thomas, M.D., M.P.H. Department of Emergency Medicine, Massachusetts General Hospital; and Harvard Medical School, Boston, Massachusetts

Wolfgang Ummenhofer, M.D. Department of Anesthesia, University of Basel/Kantonsspital, Basel, Switzerland

Luc Van Camp, R.N., M.S.N., M.P.H., M.T.Q.M. Ziekenhuis Oost-Limburg, Genk, Belgium

Gary M. Vilke, M.D. F.A.C.E.P. Department of Emergency Medicine, University of California San Diego Medical Center, San Diego, California

Ron M. Walls, M.D., F.A.C.E.P., F.R.C.P.C. Department of Emergency Medicine, Brigham and Women's Hospital; and Division of Emergency Medicine, Harvard Medical School, Boston, Massachusetts

Marvin Wayne, M.D., F.A.C.E.P. Emergency Medical Services, City of Bellingham and Whatcom County, Bellingham, Washington; University of Washington, Seattle, Washington; and Yale University, New Haven, Connecticut

Suzanne K. Wedel Boston Medical Center/Boston University of Medicine, and Boston MedFlight, Boston, Massachusetts

Janet Williams, M.D., F.A.C.E.P. Center for Rural Emergency Medicine and Department of Emergency Medicine, West Virginia University, Morgantown, West Virginia

Torben Wisborg, M.D., D.E.A.A. Department of Anesthesiology and Intensive Care, Hammerfest Hospital; and Royal Norwegian Rescue Helicopter Service, Hammerfest, Norway

David W. Yates, M.D. University of Manchester and Hope Hospital, Salford, United Kingdom

Doreen Yee, M.D. Department of Anesthesia, Sunnybrook and Women's College Health Sciences Centre, Toronto, Ontario, Canada

Richard D. Zane, M.D. Department of Emergency Medicine, Brigham and Women's Hospital; and Harvard Medical School, Boston, Massachusetts

1

Prehospital Trauma Care: Scope and Practice

WOLFGANG UMMENHOFER

University of Basel/Kantonsspital, Basel, Switzerland

KOICHI TANIGAWA

Fukuoka University Hospital, Fukuoka, Japan

I. WHAT HAVE WE LEARNED FROM THE PAST?

A. The Importance of Military Influence

The nature of trauma and the care of the wounded is essentially independent of the circumstances under which injuries occur. Initial resuscitation, triage, transport (evacuation), and definitive care for the injured demand basic strategic and organizational systems. Unfortunately, major advances in trauma care can be greatly attributed to experiences gained in wars, and thus we can benefit from the lessons compiled in the history of military medicine.

Before the nineteenth century, medical care for war-wounded casualties was essentially nonexistent. There was no organized evacuation of the wounded and no hospitals available to handle extensive casualties. In the beginning of the nineteenth century, however, Baron Dominique-Jean Larrey, Napoleon's surgeon, developed the concept of a medical corps that included surgeons, stretcher bearers, medical aids, and ambulances to provide war casualties with immediate care in the field. Also, during the late phase of the American Civil War, the U.S. Army Medical Corps was set up. This organization was capable of dealing with the mass casualties encountered, and included medical staff, ambulances, and hospital systems consisting of aid stations, field hospitals, and rear general hospitals. In a series of reforms, this system contributed to the basis for the future development of care for war-wounded casualties, and became the model for U.S. conflicts up to the Vietnamese War [1].

1. World War I

It was estimated that 1,850,000 soldiers were killed in World War I (WWI). The main cause of early death on the battlefield was shock and hemorrhage [1]. No field hospitals were initially planned for nontransportable patients who needed immediate life-saving surgery. Surgeons were plagued by the delay in getting injured soldiers to surgery. Most of the emergency surgery was done in the casualty clearing station with little opportunity to select patients. Early in the war, 20% of the soldiers who reached the casualty clearing station were considered moribund and inoperable. Later, because of the improvement in methods of resuscitation, more of the moribund patients were operated on; however, the death rate was still high. The high morbidity and mortality could be attributed largely to problems of evacuation and limited resuscitation.

2. World War II

Advances in the care of soldiers during World War II (WWII) included the improvement of organized approaches to the wounded and advances in fluid resuscitation. An effective triage system was introduced, and the hospital facilities were organized in the combat zone area. These facilities were situated as far forward as possible to administer earlier care. They consisted of several stations with different functions, including an aid station, collecting and sorting stations, a casualty clearing station or field ambulance, and a mobile surgical hospital. All patients coming from the front were screened and triaged, and life-saving measures were instituted. The need for blood transfusion was recognized and blood banks were rapidly set up during the war. Blood-volume deficits were thus rapidly restored if possible with whole blood, plasma, and electrolyte solutions.

3. Korean War

Napoleon's surgeon, Baron Larrey, had also pointed out the importance of shortening the interval between injury and definitive surgical care at the hospital. By WWI the time was 12 to 18 hr, and by WWII, about 6 to 12 hr. In the Korean War, during which a limited helicopter service was introduced, the time was reduced to between 2 and 4 hr. The lower mortality in the Korean conflict was thus achieved because of the shorter, smoother evacuation. Other advances, which also contributed to better survival rates in casualties, included the administration of large quantities of resuscitative fluids perioperatively, the introduction of new antibiotics to combat gram negative organisms, better monitoring of electrolytes, and the establishment of a renal center behind the mobile army surgical hospital (MASH), where soldiers who had oliguria were evacuated by helicopter. Of the early deaths, the majority were caused by irreversible shock or uncontrolled hemorrhage. Late causes of death were sepsis, secondary hemorrhage, chest complications, and other associated injuries with or without acute renal insufficiency.

4. Vietnam

Most soldiers wounded in Vietnam were brought to fixed army hospitals directly by helicopter from or near the site of injury. A helicopter could carry up to nine patients, depending on the number of stretchers [2]. This eliminated the multiple stops and transfers of previous wars. The seriously wounded reached the operating room 1 to 2 hr after injury, the average evacuation time being 35 min. Resuscitation was initiated by medical corpsmen, taken over by helicopter evacuation medics, and finally handled by the receiving medical personnel. In hospitals, supplies and equipment were comparable to those of a modern city in North America, and there was sufficient surgical, medical, and anesthetic potential at each hospital to deal with all types of wounds. With these advances, the latter stages of the Vietnam War saw an unprecedented reduction in mortality, to 2.3% for those wounded in action.

5. Recent Conflicts

The battle conditions prevalent during the Vietnam conflict were so well suited for the implementation of these advances that the evacuation helicopters and forward surgical hospitals epitomized that war. Overshadowed by this dramatic combination of the helicopter and MASH units, advances in the immediate care of the wounded and in prehospital resuscitation were also taking place. These advances, coupled with a high-intensity battlefield, which precludes easy and rapid evacuation from the combat zone, led to reconsidering the forward surgery practices. Emphasis was put on early treatment of casualties in the field by vigorous replacement of blood volume, advanced respiratory management, and surgical resuscitation. Evacuation from the battlefield proceeded only after hemodynamic stabilization of the casualty and after the initiation of all required resuscitative steps. This type of approach was already used in the North African campaign against Rommel, as well as during the landing of the Allied Forces at Normandy. It was reintroduced in a modernized style in recent conflicts, such as the Arab–Israeli War [3], Desert Storm [4], and Yugoslavia [5].

B. Evolution of Resuscitation

Exsanguination and shock have been the major causes of morbidity and mortality in trauma patients. In the beginning of the nineteenth century, Baron Larrey first described the use of compressive bandages to arrest hemorrhage. Later, in the U.S. Civil War, initial resuscitation at the edge of the battlefield included controlling bleeding, bandaging wounds, and administering opiates and whisky for pain and shock. Friedrich von Esmarch introduced the first-aid bandage to the battlefield in 1869. By the turn of the twentieth century, many ingenious causes of shock were advanced, but unfortunately no successful treatment resulted. In 1918, Canon et al. detailed their understanding of wound shock and resuscitation [6]. They stated that everything should be done to promote factors favorable to the restoration of a normal and stable blood flow, and anything unfavorable to such restoration should be scrupulously avoided. There are certain practices, such as the prompt arrest of hemorrhage, the lessening of sepsis by appropriate dressings, and the reduction of pain by suitable splints, the judicious use of morphine, and careful transport, that are generally recognized as important measures in the care of a wounded man who is in shock or liable to shock.

Canon et al. [6] extended the views to the two aspects of trauma management, the prevention of hypothermia and the development of metabolic acidosis. In 1919, Keith confirmed Henderson's statement that the cause of shock was hypovolemia, which could be corrected by blood-volume replacement [7]. As a result, Bayliss advocated intravenous infusion of normal saline and later gum acacia with saline as replacement fluids [8]. Unfortunately there was a limited amount of intravenous fluid that could be administered safely during WWI. With the discovery of blood typing, attention turned to the use of blood transfusion. Blood transfusion did not become commonplace until after 1917, however. Circulatory failure from hemorrhage and shock were thus unsuccessfully treated during WWI.

The period between the world wars saw a common use of intravenous therapy using colloids, plasma, blood, and crystalloids. During WWII, blood-volume deficiency was rapidly restored if possible with whole blood, plasma, and electrolyte solutions before surgery. The successful treatment of shock in WWII, however, led to kidney failure in some instances, which almost always resulted in death. In the Korean War, the patient with posttraumatic renal failure was dealt with successfully by the establishment of a renal center in which dialysis could be carried out. In Vietnam, where moribund patients were rapidly evacuated to hospitals, the serious problems of acute pulmonary insufficiency and multiple organ damage arose, which at the same time were also the most common sequelae in civilian practice.

Over the last three decades, the availability and capability of new medical technologies have profoundly affected the standard and quality of care. The basic principles of trauma care remain unchanged, however. In recent years, the introduction of the protocols and philosophy of Advanced Trauma Life Support (ATLS®) has been a major advance in the improvement of the standard of care available to trauma patients. This relatively simple system provides a safe, reliable method for immediate management of the injured patient. It is now generally accepted that ATLS® reduces morbidity and mortality rates. Battlefield Advanced Trauma Life Support (BATLS), a military variant of the civilian ATLS®, was introduced to deal with the second peak of death in the battlefield [9].

In cases of ongoing hemorrhage, however, a failure of ATLS®/BATLS principles will also be anticipated, particularly among those injured who are suffering from a major leak in the vascular tree. Bickell et al. demonstrated that in penetrating torso injuries the mortality of patients who had not received fluid resuscitation was lower than those who received intravenous fluid at the scene or on arrival in the emergency room [10]. Certainly there are some patients who eventually succumb to hemodilution and exsanguination, and their hypovolemic shock cannot simply be treated by constant administration of intravenous fluids. Accordingly, emphasis on early aggressive volume restoration was replaced with a new approach in ATLS®; that is, stop the bleeding and then restore the volume. In the case of internal hemorrhage, immediate surgical resuscitation will be required to save the injured. The aim of such surgical resuscitation is to give an opportunity for the individuals to receive more specific treatment. The concept of damage control surgery thus emerged [11]. Examples of this approach would be the packing of the hepatic bed to stem hemorrhage. Closure can be accompanied by towel clip or Opsite®. When resources become available, a more extensive surgical procedure can be performed. In the battlefield, this concept demands the forward deployment of field surgical teams.

Trauma care has adhered to the basic principles of traumatology that have been painfully learned from the long history of wars. For the last 40 years, the approach to the trauma patient has been relatively standard and unchanged. During the past decade, however, debates concerning the type, volume, and timing of fluid resuscitation have been the focus of basic and clinical research in trauma. What are the objectives of the initial resuscitation? Does aggressive fluid resuscitation do good or harm? Can we apply the same strategy toward penetrating and blunt trauma? We need to seek answers to these very important questions. We can no longer afford to have evolutionary steps provide answers. Evidence-based trauma and emergency care must now dictate appropriate treatment.

II. CONTEMPORARY PROBLEMS: FINDING THE WAY

A. Prehospital Treatment: Paramedic- or Physician-Based?

Evolving emergency medical services (EMS) have increased the possibilities for prehospital treatment and stabilization of emergency patients. But, invasive diagnostic and therapeutic procedures at the emergency site are not always lifesaving as they present new risks that can potentially further harm the trauma victim, and most important, are time-consuming. Amazingly, except for cases of nontraumatic, out-of-hospital cardiac arrest, there is almost no convincing scientific evidence to prove that prehospital care has had an impact on morbidity or mortality [12]. In an American outcome study, Demetriades et al. have compared paramedic versus private transportation (performed by bystanders or police) of trauma patients and demonstrated a higher mortality, even in severely injured patients (ISS $>$ 15), for professional EMS transportation [13]. A positive influence of ATLS® on the survival of severely injured patients at the scene is thus still unproven and the subject of an ongoing discussion between ''scoop-and-run'' or ''stay-and-play'' protagonists.

On the other hand, for the in-hospital environment, safe procedures for airway management, spinal cord control, and circulation surveillance have been established by the American College of Surgeons ATLS® program during the past two decades, and it has been adopted by more than 30 countries worldwide. It is therefore puzzling why these safe procedures are not immediately applied at the accident site during the hazardous period of extrication and transportation [14].

Field rescue personnel in the United States are paramedic-based, whereas in many European countries emergency physicians are part of the prehospital team. In the Franco-German model, physicians and technology are sent to the scene in the hope of providing a higher level of emergency care before the patient's arrival at the hospital. Emergency medicine is practiced exclusively in the prehospital setting, where physicians (usually anesthesiologists) provide most of the care. Emergency departments are often rudimentary because patients are triaged in the field and admitted directly to inpatient specialty services. In this model, emergency medicine is not an officially recognized specialty and is usually controlled by anesthesiologists [15] who receive special education and training for their prehospital work. It has been shown that invasive procedures are more often and more successfully performed by trained physicians compared with paramedic-only teams [16]. In contrast, Sampalis et al. found no advantage for the prehospital use of physicians with regard to patient outcome: ''Although we do not have any reason to believe that the care provided by physicians is inferior to that provided by paramedics, the care provided by paramedics is more consistent and standardized'' [17]. A comparison between a German and an American air rescue system evaluating prehospital procedures and outcome of patients with multiple injuries found that although invasive techniques were more often performed in the physician-staffed German system, overall mortality of patients did not differ between the two countries [18].

A conclusion as to whether the skills of physicians or paramedics are superior for field purposes is beyond the scope of this chapter. It is crucial that both groups are well trained and prepared for the extremely uncontrolled and dynamic prehospital environment. Compared with physicians, paramedics with years of prehospital experience may be better adapted to the effects of witnessing violence, making urgent decisions, and trying to deliver optimum care with only limited resources. Paramedics are more familiar with the influences of weather, noise, lightning, hazardous conditions, communicable disease, and interactions with hostile or upset citizens at the accident scene [19].

Occasionally cooperation between experienced EMS personnel and young clinicians, who are unaccustomed to coping with a complex situation at the accident scene, is impaired by a feeling of superiority on the part of the paramedics and an unconscious attitude of hierarchical superiority on the part of the physician, thus ideally, long-term teams for prehospital treatment should be established. A high frequency of personnel changes will handicap prehospital performance, and physicians who work primarily in-hospital will experience difficulty in reliably cooperating during their occasional fieldwork (see Sec. III.A.).

On the other hand, with regard to relevant prehospital techniques, clinicians—mainly those with such specialties as anesthesiology—are well trained in methods of airway management, venous access, and pain control. In times of sufficient supply of qualified physicians, even those motivated for prehospital work, it is not easy to understand the rationale for attempting to educate paramedics in the performance of invasive procedures without the opportunity for them to participate in the daily routine of a busy operating or emergency room.

Furthermore, the situation is complicated by medicolegal aspects at accident scenes, at which there are hazards for the occurrence of errors such as failed tracheal intubation or drug-dosing problems. An outcome study utilizing ''mortality'' as the endpoint will not reflect the goal quality of skills rendered to the injured patient if she or he fails to survive a hazardous invasive procedure. For example, even when an endotracheal tube is later demonstrated to have been placed in the correct anatomical position at the accident scene, one cannot be certain that proper technique was used; a two-minute attempt to place the tube without intermittent oxygenation is not a successful intubation [19].

In the United States, physician involvement is considered to be more of a supervisory and backup role than a primary care, first-responder role [20]. Pepe recommended that emergency medicine curricula should reflect the growing need to provide proper role models and train physicians to become ''streetwise'' and to assume leadership in EMS. In order to do so, however, emergency systems must be designed accordingly and offer possibilities for young physicians to establish proper skills and knowledge in field trauma management.

Whereas the American system does not offer many possibilities to physicians for prehospital experiences, the Franco–German model sometimes has in-hospital inconsistency of care due to the missing specialty of emergency medicine. Critics have noted that emergency physicians are not subject to the same supervision and quality assurance controls as physicians in Anglo-American systems. Because career prospects are poor, talented physicians are lost to other specialties [15].

B. Scoop-and-Run Versus Stay-and-Play

One source of the still ongoing discussion of what constitutes the ''gold standard'' of prehospital performance is the different evolutionary development in rescue systems, mainly in the United States and continental Europe (see Sec. II.A.). The mainly hospital-based ATLS® in the United States often regards prehospital procedures elsewhere as mere time-consuming efforts. On the other hand, the prehospital presence of emergency physicians as exists in continental Europe often gives rise to the illusion of being able to stabilize a severely injured trauma victim even in cases when only hospital-based resources guarantee adequate treatment. Furthermore, physicians tend to disregard time consumption in the prehospital setting, but time has been shown to be the only variable predictor of outcome in the multiply injured patient [17,21,22].

Spaite et al. reviewed and compared the literature that currently exists on the use of advanced life support (ALS) procedures by prehospital personnel. They found no objective proof that the primary determinant of outcome for the trauma patient is the time interval from injury to the operating room. The ''studies'' that supported this relationship were flawed and nearly all retrospective [23].

Not surprisingly—because it has been regarded as a general criticism of the European principle of field stabilization—the study by Bickell et al. [10] led to confusion on the utility of such treatment. For hypotensive patients with penetrating torso injuries, Bickell et al. found that immediate fluid resuscitation in the field and during transport compared with a delayed fluid resuscitation in the hospital setting resulted in higher mortality and increased incidence of postoperative complications. There is evidence that it was not time delay but rather fluid resuscitation itself that worsened the outcome in this group of patients [10], but with the narrow parameters studied, conclusions can only be drawn for a special subgroup of patients (young and otherwise healthy) sustaining a distinct mechanism of trauma (penetrating torso injury).

The issue of volume replacement is just one—and probably not the most important—topic of the scoop-and-run versus stay-and-play discussion. Airway management, cervical spine support, and pain control are important treatment areas. Moreover, if advisable, invasive treatment can be performed at the accident scene, although awareness of time is an essential common denominator in unstable, severely injured patients. Pepe et al. have shown in a busy urban paramedic system that the time factors involved in prehospital management and transport directly to a trauma center did not adversely affect outcome, at least if they did not exceed the first hour after injury. This was true even for the most severely injured patients [24].

Only a small percentage of trauma victims attended by EMS personnel have immediately life-threatening problems. The majority of patients require only meticulous basic life-support techniques, such as neck and back immobilization or splinting of extremity fractures [20]. Even if subsequent emergency department evaluation shows no evidence of spinal fractures in the great majority of cases, the absence of such an abnormality is difficult if not impossible to determine clinically, particularly in the field.

In the ATLS® protocol, ''airway and cervical spine control'' have evolved as entities. The same perspective should also be held in the prehospital setting. In the United States, spinal injuries are estimated to number about 10,000 annually. Half of all spinal injuries occur in the cervical region and may result in quadriplegia [25]. Managing the airway in the presence of potential spinal injury therefore has a high priority and requires skill and awareness of possible hazards [26–28]. In one study, the rescue team did not suspect spinal injury in 14% of trauma patients with clinical evidence of injury to the cervical column [29]. Muckart et al. report two cases of spinal cord injury as a possible result of endotracheal intubation in patients with undiagnosed cervical spine fractures [30].

Field stabilization thus should not be regarded as a mere stay-and-play, but rather be recognized as an essential component of good prehospital care. It should therefore include high-flow oxygen, aggressive airway management (if necessary), ventilation, immobilization, venous access, and (if reasonable) volume replacement ''en route'' [20]. Experienced emergency physicians can provide early anesthesia and tracheal intubation even in previously responsive patients, thereby preventing pain, panic, and potential secondary physiological and psychological trauma during extrication and transport.

Even in the presumed scoop-and-run group, in patients with penetrating injuries the provision of a safe airway in the prehospital setting, preferably by endotracheal intubation, is one intervention that correlates with improved outcome [31]. In a study of 131 patients who suffered cardiopulmonary arrest in the field secondary to trauma, the ''survivors were young, intubated, and penetrated'' [31]. Almost all of those with blunt injuries died. The average response, scene, and transport time in this study was about 21 minutes, however. Pepe suggested that the classic ''golden hour'' for this group of patients should be condensed into a ''platinum half hour,'' which prioritizes aggressive airway and surgical interventions as the chief goals [20]. The difference of opinion on the controversial issue of stay-and-play versus scoop-and-run could thus perhaps be harmonized to a *play-and-run*.

C. Trauma is Not a Generic Disease: Different Trauma Patients in Different Countries

Comparisons of outcome after major trauma between different countries are difficult if not impossible due to different rescue systems, geographical and demographic reasons, political issues (primary transport to regional hospitals or specialized trauma centers), investigators' biases, and different predominant injury patterns. This complex background has hindered the development of a uniform pattern of criteria and definitions. Different systems cannot readily be compared because data are often incompatible. Therefore—similar to the consensus guidelines of the European Resuscitation Council for data following cardiac arrest—recommendations for uniform reporting of data following major trauma—the ''Utstein style''—have been published recently [32].

Whereas in the United States penetrating injuries outweigh blunt trauma, in Europe high-velocity automobile crashes are more common with their accompanying increase in the severity of the injuries. The care for victims of blunt trauma often involves many additional variables, such as vehicle extrication time and the need for meticulous splinting and immobilization. Although variable in presentation, depending on anatomical involvement, patients with penetrating injuries still represent a more homogeneous group with fewer management variables. Also, most of these patients require early operation (laparotomy or thoracotomy), making the readily available resources of a trauma center more appropriate [24], but even victims of blunt trauma often present with hypovolemia due to ongoing hemorrhage with the need of rapid transfer to an adequate definitive treatment facility. The tragic death of the princess of Wales in the automobile crash in Paris in the summer of 1998 reinforced the stay-and-play versus scoop-and-run discussion.

Before outside ''experts'' attempt to assist countries in their emergency system development it is important to understand their existing health care systems, the national health care priorities, their economic development, and the societal structure. There is no ''one size fits all'' emergency system for all countries. Even within a country, each city and hospital may need to be considered separately [33].

D. How to Be Prepared for the Prehospital Environment: Clear Protocols or Clinical Experience?

In 1993, Sampalis et al. presented a prospective observational study evaluating the association of prehospital and in-hospital care with trauma-related mortality [17]. The study was conducted in the Montreal metropolitan area, and—unique for North America—only physicians, if available, were authorized to perform ALS in the prehospital setting. In agreement with Trunkey's position against attempts at on-site stabilization [34], the study failed to show any associated benefit in reducing the odds of dying with respect to the use of on-site ALS for severely injured patients. There was not a standard treatment protocol, however, and every physician individually decided what ALS procedures to perform on the basis of personal attitudes, beliefs, previous experiences, distance from the hospital, and perceived urgency of the situation. As stated above (see Sec. II.A), prehospital care provided by paramedics, at least in North America, is more standardized and consistent compared with that of physicians. Perhaps physicians are better suited for the role of supervising and teaching paramedics than for providing the treatment [19].

On the other hand, physicians have accepted the necessity of standardized procedures and priorities for the in-hospital setting as well as the level of performance as established by the American College of Surgeons subcommittee on trauma through the ATLS® principles. Furthermore, that these principles of treatment should be practiced routinely and implemented effectively has been accepted by physicians in more than 30 countries.

Training and simulation according to clear protocols offers the opportunity to realize problems and hazards and to shorten the time at the accident scene. Sampalis et al. demonstrated a significant increase in scene time associated with the use of ALS, secondary to the lack of a specific protocol [17], but this does not automatically include the delay to definitive in-hospital care for trained teams who are well aware of increased trauma mortality in the presence of excess prehospital time. Spaite et al. demonstrated that extremely short scene times could be attained without foregoing potentially lifesaving ALS interventions in an urban EMS system with strong medical control [35]. ATLS® has professionalized emergency room performance and offers principles for safe transfer procedures. For the prehospital environment, as uncontrolled and dynamic as it may be, clear protocols and an established priority list, if performed in a consistent and straightforward manner, should be lifesaving and time-saving at the same time.

In an Israeli study of the evacuation of injured people from crashes of motor vehicles, professional evacuation by a medical team specially trained in extrication procedures was shown to be more rapid than nonprofessional involvement [36]. On the other hand, ATLS® training per se does not guarantee improvement; even though 80% of the Montreal physicians had passed the course, ALS provided by physicians was not associated with reduced mortality [22]. Specific, predetermined protocols for the on-site management of trauma victims may be the key, including a high awareness of the importance of time, at least for the most critically injured patients.

Following a retrospective study of 1000 deaths from injury in England and Wales [37], the National Health Service Management Executive tried to implement quality-of-care improvement strategies for in-hospital accident and emergency departments. Besides other measures, guidelines were considered fundamental to ensure organizationwide quality. Practice guidelines can facilitate evidence-based care (see Sec. II.E) and thus improve patient outcome. There is a substantial body of literature about guideline development, implementation, and evaluation.

The importance of the views of the potential users of practice guidelines has only recently been acknowledged [38]. The results of a survey investigating the compliance of accident and emergency staff toward practice guidelines showed that the benefits of practice guidelines were appreciated and that evidence-based and ''user-friendly'' guidelines were wanted [39]. On the other hand, it was concluded that unless the guidelines were rigorously developed, clear, and easy to use, they were unlikely to be implemented in accident and emergency departments in the United Kingdom. This investigation reflects the conflicting attitude of physicians, educated in the traditional medical philosophy of individualized personal decision making, which depends on personal thoughts, beliefs, and experiences.

This attitude is even more likely for prehospital care providers: ''Under the uncontrolled circumstances of the prehospital environment, cookbook protocols are often difficult to follow and sound clinical judgement has become an essential ingredient in the decision-making process'' [19].

In emergency situations, however, physicians should act on certain generally acknowledged guidelines and principles of treatment, even if they otherwise prefer to make their own independent decisions. Primary and secondary survey algorithms can be adequate and time-saving approaches for trauma victims, and persistent training in communication skills, special prehospital techniques, and awareness of time consumption may improve long-term performance. Following a study evaluating preventable deaths occurring in patients with major trauma, Sampalis et al. emphasized the necessity of clear prehospital care protocols, prompt transport, and specific on-site care algorithms [40].

In a small percentage of emergency situations, however, the given case itself or the surrounding conditions will not comply with existing protocols, and the rescue team's experience, reactivity, creativity, and intelligence will be challenged. Here flexibility and time management are the keys.

E. Do We Need Scientific Proof?

A new paradigm for medical practice is emerging. ''Evidence-based medicine'' de-emphasizes intuition, unsystematic clinical experience, and pathophysiologic rationale as sufficient grounds for clinical decision making and instead stresses the examination of evidence from clinical research [41]. In the field of emergency medicine, this evidence from clinical research contributes to probably less than 50% of all emergency procedures performed on a daily basis [42]. Therefore, ''evidence-based emergency medicine'' [43], involving skills of problem defining, searching, evaluating, and applying original medical literature, will gradually change our prehospital attitudes, but on the other hand, will also require new skills for the physician. Evidence-based medicine relies mainly on the results of randomized control studies, which are the gold standard in clinical research.

The interpretations of results from previous studies on prehospital care are substantially hampered by a large number of less urgent missions that actually do not utilize ALS and thus blur the effect of an advanced medical service [44]. Prospective randomized ''controlled'' trials are extremely difficult to perform in the prehospital setting, which is per se an "uncontrolled" environment. Differences associated with trauma patients include the following: demographics, mechanism and extent of injuring forces, anatomical location of injury, and time course of treatment following the moment of injury. These in turn are dependent on available communication resources and location (rural or metropolitan site of the incident), bystander availability, quality of basic life support, first responders' and EMS personnel's qualifications and treatment rendered, type of hospital referred to, and time elapsed between trauma, beginning of treatment, transport, emergency room, and definitive in-hospital care. Furthermore, patients are taken to different hospitals, and it is perceived that it may be impossible to control all of the variables or ensure study compliance with regard to key actions that can affect outcome [45].

In order to identify influences of a single variable (e.g., prehospital amount of volume replacement) in this heterogeneous population, large numbers of patients have to be evaluated to guarantee comparability of well-defined subgroups with regard to type and degree of injury, age, lack of coexisting disease, similar physiologic parameters, and time course of prehospital and in-hospital support. Contradicting results from studies using only small numbers of patients have caused confusion [17], or have been biased for obvious reasons by their authors. Because many randomized trials are too small to give definitive answers, bias has simply been moved up the chain. Where previously cases were chosen to make a point, trials are now chosen the same way.

Evidence-based medicine has arisen from the realization that answers to clinical problems are more likely to be valid if there is an effort to track down all the relevant trials, not just the trials reviewers know about or the trials reviewers choose to know about [46].

Ethics play an important role in scientific studies. They are a difficult concept to handle, but contrary to law, ethical considerations are individual. For randomized groups of patients it is not easy to provide comparable treatment, because treatment must meet the needs of the individual patient. With respect to time control, one responsive victim with extreme pain will require some pain relief even with a short delay needed for venous access, medication, and setting of a dislocated fracture, while others with complete adrenergic stimulation are nearly free of pain until arrival in the emergency room, and are therefore delivered more rapidly.

Lack of informed consent by trauma patients, an issue present in most prehospital settings, imposes strict limitations on the design of these studies and requires special and careful evaluation by ethical committees. Many, if not most, diagnostic and therapeutic principles in emergency medicine are not at all evidence-based. The question will arise as to whether or not the performance of randomized controlled trials is ethically justifiable if control groups are included whose treatment leaves out traditional generally recommended and recognized principles [42].

Another major point of concern is the issue of valid endpoints for measuring effectiveness of prehospital treatment. Mortality in a reasonable range of time (e.g., six days following trauma) is a well-accepted endpoint, whereas improvement of physiological status (as resulting from ALS at the scene) [47], does not necessarily prove a direct association between on-site ALS and decreased mortality.

On the other hand, "surrogate endpoints" of meticulous prehospital efforts such as pain relief, performance of safe general anesthesia in previously responsive multiply injured patients, quality of airway management, prevention of secondary neurological damage by careful and professional splinting, and immobilization may not lead to a reduction in mortality.

For a long time, even in a much more homogeneous group of emergency patients as compared with the victims of trauma (e.g., a group of patients suffering from cardiac arrest), prehospital data of resuscitation efforts have not been comparable due to different terminologies and methods of the reporting institutions. As a result, after an intensive discussion and consensus process, the European Resuscitation Council and comparable organizations on other continents have issued guidelines for uniform reporting of data following out-of-hospital and in-hospital cardiac arrest; that is, the Utstein style [48]. Unfortunately, in most systems, cardiac arrest accounts for only 1 to 2% of all EMS responses. The lack of development of even the basic data elements and terminology for the other 98 to 99% of EMS responses clearly reveals the vacuum in our understanding of out-of-hospital care systems [49]. In the United States, Spaite and colleagues published a report in 1995 from the Uniform Prehospital Emergency Medical Services Data Conference that set out the principles of data collection using ''core'' and ''supplemental'' information in an effort to provide useful information for quality improvement and research in prehospital care [12]. For trauma patients, the International Trauma Anesthesia and Critical Care Society (ITACCS) developed similar guidelines—''Recommendations for uniform reporting of data following major trauma, i.e., the Utstein Style''—which will be introduced later in this textbook [32].

On the whole, out-of-hospital research is better established in the United States as compared to European countries. In contrast to the concerns stated above, for some research projects Pepe feels the prehospital environment to be better suited than the hospital setting [45]. Emergency Medical Service programs in the United States, particularly fire department programs, are often paramilitary in nature. In addition, paramedics tend to follow accident scene protocols meticulously because such protocols are their routine work. An important rationale for conducting prehospital research relates to the Hawthorne effect. This principle, borrowed from industrial quality assurance studies, states that by simply implementing a study, one will observe improved outcomes in *both* study and control groups. Dramatic improvements in survival for both study and control groups have been demonstrated in several prehospital studies. Because the researchers are scrutinizing the protocol, related patient care improves [45].

Although much information exists on prehospital trauma care, superior methods with which to answer questions of efficacy and cost-effectiveness have not been developed. The approaches that have been used to develop the current prehospital trauma literature do not permit the development of a consensus on the impact of each system component on patient outcome. In fact, most prehospital trauma research has emphasized the wrong issues, asked the wrong questions, and used the wrong methods [49].

III. DIRECTIONS OF FUTURE DEVELOPMENT

A. The Team Approach: Shared Responsibility Versus Leadership

In 1966, Donabedian suggested a classification of the components of a system (structure, process, and outcome) that provided an outline for such data collection, and formed the basis of quality assurance activities [50]. ''Structure'' represented the environment, equipment, personnel, and administration. ''Process'' represented tasks and methods. ''Outcome'' represented evaluation of what had been done and how well.

In both medicine and all other technical professions, it has been found that the majority of accidents and critical incidents involve failures in team performance [51]. It is thus of equal importance that in addition to the above quality assurance components, interpersonal and team skills be assessed and training provided. Such assessment of the dynamics of interactions among EMS personnel, between patients and rescue team, and between EMS and other prehospital teams (e.g., fire brigade or police) can be achieved through an evaluation of the following:

Individual effectiveness in team activities
Team effectiveness
Critical incidents

Establishment of a quality assurance system for prehospital purposes will be a task for the responsible EMS director.

The team approach should define clear responsibilities, but leadership in the traditional sense will be modified. For the helicopter-based team, for example, the pilot is in charge of all aspects of flight safety and navigation, and should by no means be influenced by decisions other than safety as to whether or not the aeromedical mission should be flown. Pilots must be delegated the sole authority to make such decisions, and some would go so far as to leave them ''blinded'' as to the nature of the request for service or the urgency of the request [20]. On scene, the most experienced medical staff member (i.e., emergency physician or paramedic) will be responsible for evaluation and resuscitation of the patient, although when technical problems are encountered technical team leaders like fire brigade officers may temporarily organize rescue procedures, as is necessary in difficult extrication situations. At the same time, as soon as the engine is switched off and the rapid safety check completed, the pilot may be available for transport of medical equipment to the site of the accident, now following the instructions and needs of the other crew members. Medical technicians are often responsible for procedures such as splinting and immobilization of the injured patient, based on their extensive expertise in this area.

The link for flexible leadership structure is communication. Like technical skills, communication skills have to be practiced, assessed, and evaluated. If possible, a short briefing on the way to the scene of an accident and necessary debriefing after finishing a mission should become implemented parts of all missions.

Working in a true team interferes with basic social and psychological effects that should be recognized. Team members, especially leaders, can be considered in terms of their tasks or goals and their interpersonal or emotional orientation. The ''democratic'' style, showing consideration for others and their problems, is likely to be appropriate when things are going well. The ''autocratic'' style may predominate if difficulties or emergencies occur and the demands of the task override the requirement for interpersonal consideration. Problems arise if an individual is either too demanding and inconsiderate or fails conversely to assert proper leadership because of concerns about upsetting colleagues. It is particularly hard for a relatively junior member of a team to make demands of a senior one, who may even have a conflicting interest. On the other hand, members of a group are likely to recognize the best solution when presented, even though only one of them may have solved the problem. Therefore it is crucial that everyone involved should be able to offer opinions and ideas [52].

The overall goal—usually safety of the operation in all aspects (i.e., the patient and the team)—should be kept in mind. Ideally, an individual's contribution should never be affected by personal feelings. Unfortunately, individuals can let someone they dislike continue on an inappropriate course of action hoping that he or she will get into serious trouble [52]. This is why crew resource management should implement psychodynamic structures as well as technical aspects [53] (see Sec. III.C.).

B. Awareness Culture: Training for Hazards and Pitfalls

''Error in medicine'' is a well-known feature of the hospital environment [54,55]; nonetheless high error rates have not stimulated much concern or efforts at error prevention. One reason may be a lack of awareness of the severity of the problem. Contrary to errors in the oil and gas industry or in aviation, errors in medicine are dispatched and individualized, and usually not reported in the newspapers. Although error rates probably are substantial, serious injuries due to errors are not part of the everyday experience of physicians, nurses, or paramedics, but are perceived as isolated and unusual events (i.e., an ''outlier''). Furthermore, most errors do no harm; either they are intercepted or the patient's defenses prevent injury.

The most important reason health care providers have not developed more effective methods of error prevention is that they have a great deal of difficulty in dealing with human error when it does occur. The reasons are to be found in the culture of medical practice [56]. Socialization in medical school and during residency emphasizes perfection in diagnosis and treatment, and physicians are expected to strive for an error-free practice. By the end of one's medical education, a sense of duty to perform faultlessly is strongly internalized. Unfortunately, all humans, physicians included, err frequently. Systems that rely on error-free performance are doomed to fail. There is, in fact, usually a ''human error'' that is the last cause leading toward a critical incident, but the potential of critical incidents that evolve to true accidents or even catastrophes strongly depends on safety regulations within a team and organizational culture, and thus often lies well beyond the individual's control.

Although few data are available for the prehospital setting, the circumstances for error-free performance are very disadvantageous [14]. The emergency environment provides troublesome conditions, is rather noisy and is usually thermally uncomfortable, with the need to communicate with severely ill or injured people and their upset relatives, and usually at the worst time of the day. In addition, fatigue is important, resulting either from long duty hours or from working at a time (usually at night) inappropriate to the circadian rhythm of the individual. Trauma is a nocturnal phenomenon, and although familiar skills and drills are relatively insensitive, a general reduction in cognitive or mental resources results in poorer judgment, problem solving, and decision making. The catastrophic decisions at Chernobyl and Three Mile Island, and a disproportionately large number of motorway accidents occur between 2 and 6 a.m., the lowest ebb of the human circadian cycle [52]. Emergency-care providers are regularly exposed to stress-burdened conditions, and stress is likely to affect the behavior of all individuals.

Within the aviation community, safety management strategies, including defined standard procedures, checklists, and simulator training and assessment to demonstrate continued competence, are formalized and well accepted worldwide. There is much reason to believe that medical teams with different tasks and procedures but with comparable needs of decision making and functioning under stress-prone, hostile conditions, divergent and simultaneous sensory inputs, time pressure, and group conflicts, would comparably benefit from a system's change. The balance of responsibility between an individual operator and the general management of an organization has to be shifted toward organizational structures, enabling all members to realize critical situations, to be aware of pitfalls and hazards, and to interact adequately regardless of hierarchical barriers. A ''safety culture'' has to implement all mechanisms available to reduce risks for the patient and the team, including the risk of human error on the part of a single team member.

C. Human Factors: How do We Employ Risk Management Strategies in Emergency Procedures?

Human factors is an evolving discipline that dealt originally with the interface between the human and the machine with a focus on improving safety and usability through improved design. An important aspect of human factors research is the use of a systems perspective that considers both the influence of individual and group characteristics and the contribution of organizational and national cultures [50]. Not surprisingly, human factors research was implemented into quality management by industry; namely, gas, oil, and aviation. Errors were expensive in these fields of enterprise. The delay of risk management strategies in medicine is well explained by the fact that medical errors usually are more individualized and therefore less expensive. Today, three primary forces drive health care policy not only in America but in most developed countries: namely, efforts to control costs, to improve access, and to produce and assure delivery of high-quality care. For continuous quality improvement, investments need to be made in organizational structures, but in the long run, comparable with industrial experiences, investment in risk management may be cost-saving.

In medicine, risk management was initially considered only as a means of controlling litigation, but safety culture is not just ''caution'' when dealing with a patient. Safety culture is a special type of an organizational culture in totality, and with a view to the emergency situation, one cannot always be merely cautious when a job has to be done, especially when it must be done fast.

Until recently, adverse outcomes were predicted primarily by patient factors, but inquiries, such as the United Kingdom's study on preventable deaths following trauma [37], indicate that complication rates alone are a poor measure of provider quality. As pointed out by Longnecker for the field of anesthesiology, failure to rescue was a better measure of provider quality than mere complication rates, presumably because it examined the clinical skills required to rescue the patient from underlying disease [57]. Both death rates and failure to rescue were negatively related to the proportion of board-certified anesthesiologists on the anesthesia provider staff. Stated in the positive, the more board-certified anesthesiologists involved in the delivery of anesthesia care, the better the outcomes as measured by survival rates and rescue from complication.

Investment in the quality of care providers is thus a necessary prerequisite of improved outcome. For the emergency community, quality requirements refer to paramedics as well as to emergency physicians. The education and training of both groups should be continued, ignoring the fruitless discussion of which of these groups is superior. A good EMS system operates with good radios, good vehicles, good medical directors, good defibrillators, good paramedics, and good EMTs [19], but this is only halfway up the hill. Even good paramedics and good emergency physicians do not always act error-free. In order to manage risk effectively, we first have to understand the nature and etiology of the adverse events that can be encountered.

There are two kinds of accidents: those that happen to individuals and those that happen to organizations [58]. The most important factor distinguishing individual from organizational accidents is the number, quality, and diversity of the defenses preventing known hazards from causing harm or loss. Individual accidents happen in conditions in which the dangers are close, and the main source of protection resides in the skills, experience, and risk perceptions of the workforce. On the other hand, organizational accidents occur in systems in which the operators are separated from direct hazard by many layers of defenses.

Defenses preventing individual and organizational failure should be implemented in regionalized EMS, with the purpose to view human error more as a consequence than as a cause. Errors are the symptoms that reveal the presence of latent conditions in the system at large. They are important only insofar as they adversely affect the integrity of the defenses. Today, catastrophes in the medical business are usually accompanied by the first question: ''Who did it?'' When there is a bad outcome, somebody must be blamed. This ''heads must roll'' mentality produces defensive behavior but not quality in medicine. Therefore, if we are to succeed in implementing risk management philosophy, the first question should be: ''How can we save the next patient?''

IV. CONCLUSION

Prehospital trauma care is strongly influenced by military experiences, and modern principles of field stabilization, rapid evacuation, and basic and advanced life support techniques have been painfully learned from the long history of wars and conflicts. In prehospital fluid resuscitation, aggressive volume restoration has been questioned in patients with penetrating torso injuries and ongoing hemorrhage.

Two major models of emergency medicine exist today, the Anglo-American and the Franco-German models. Parallel to the paramedic or physician-based system, an ongoing controversy on scoop-and-run versus stay-and-play principles has for a long time prevented clear protocols for prehospital trauma care.

Evidence-based emergency medicine will gradually change our prehospital attitudes, and EMS team performance can be improved by implementing crew resource management strategies. Flexible leadership, awareness culture, and risk management could become part of quality-improvement programs for prehospital emergency care providers.

REFERENCES

1. F Blaisdell. Medical advances during the civil war. Arch Surg 123:1045–1050, 1988.
2. S Neel. Medical Support of the U.S. Army in Vietnam, 1965–70. Washington, DC: U.S. Army, U.S. Government Printing Office, 1973, pp. 70–79.
3. R Rozin, J Klausner. New concepts of forward combat surgery. Injury 19:193–197, 1988.
4. D Perkins, B Condon. Post-Vietnam U.S. conflicts: Grenada, Panama, and the Persian Gulf. In: Grande CM (ed.) Textbook of Trauma Anesthesia and Critical Care. St. Louis: Mosby-Year Book, 1993, pp. 1322–1324.
5. M Jevtic, M Petrivic, D Ignjatovic, N Ilijevski, S Misovic, G Kronja, N Stankovic. Treatment of wounded in the combat zone. J Trauma 40:173–176, 1996.
6. W Canon, J Fraser, E Cowell. The preventive treatment of wound shock. JAMA 70:618–621, 1918.
7. Y Henderson. Acapnia and shock-failure of the circulation. Amer J Physiol 27:152–156, 1910.
8. A Keith. Blood Volume Changes in Wound Shock and Primary Haemorrhage. London: Her Majesty's Stationery, p. 1919.
9. B Riley. Battlefield trauma life support: Its use in the resuscitation department of 32 field hospitals during the Gulf War. Mil Med 161:542–546, 1996.

10. W Bickell, M Wall, P Pepe, R Martin, V Ginger, M Allen, K Mattox. Immediate versus delayed resuscitation for hypotensive patients with penetrating torso injuries. New Eng J Med 331:1105–1109, 1994.
11. A Hirshberg, M Wakk, K Mattox. Planned reoperation for trauma: A two-year experience with 124 consecutive patients. J Trauma 37:365–369, 1994.
12. D Spaite, R Benoit, D Brown, R Cales, D Dawson, C Glass, C Kaufmann, D Pollock, S Ryan, E Yano. Uniform prehospital data elements and definitions: A report from the uniform prehospital emergency medical services data conference. Ann Emer Med 25:525–534, 1995.
13. D Demetriades, L Chan, E Cornwell, T Berne, J Asensio, D Chan, M Eckstein, K Alo. Paramedic vs. private transportation of trauma patients: Effect on outcome. Arch Surg 131:133–138, 1996.
14. W Ummenhofer, U Boenicke, D Scheidegger. Transport trauma. Trauma Care vol. 7, Oct., 1997.
15. J Arnold. International emergency medicine and the recent development of emergency medicine worldwide. Ann Emer Med 33:97–103, 1999.
16. W Baxt, P Moody. The impact of a physician as part of the aeromedical prehospital team in patients with blunt trauma. JAMA 257:3246–3250, 1987.
17. J Sampalis, A Lavoie, J Williams, D Mulder, M Kalina. Impact of on-site care, prehospital time, and level of in-hospital care on survival in severely injured patients. J Trauma 34:252–261, 1993.
18. U Schmidt, M Muggia-Sullam, M Holch, C Kant, C Brummerloh, S Frame, D Rowe, B Enderson, M Nerlich, K Maull, H Tscherne. Primaerversorgung des Polytraumas. Vergleich eines deutschen und amerikanischen Luftrettungssystems. Unfallchirurg 96:287–291, 1993.
19. P Pepe, R Stewart. Role of the physician in the prehospital setting. Ann Emer Med 15:1480–1483, 1986.
20. P Pepe, R Stewart, M Copass. Prehospital management of trauma: A tale of three cities. Ann Emer Med 15:1484–1490, 1986.
21. R Ivatury, M Nallathambi, J Roberge, M Rohmann, W Stahl. Penetrating thoracic injuries: In-field stabilization vs. prompt transport. J Trauma 27:1066–1073, 1987.
22. J Sampalis, A Lavoie, J Williams, D Mulder, M Kalina. Standardized mortality ratio analysis on a sample of severely injured patients from a large Canadian city without regionalized trauma care. J Trauma 33:205–211, 1992.
23. D Spaite, E Criss, T Valenzuela, H Meislin. Prehospital advanced life support for major trauma: Critical need for clinical trials. Ann Emer Med 32:480–489, 1998.
24. P Pepe, C Wyatt, W Bickell, M Bailey, K Mattox. The relationship between total prehospital time and outcome in hypotensive victims of penetrating injuries. Ann Emer Med 16:293–297, 1987.
25. R De Lorenzo, J Olson, M Boska, R Johnston, G Hamilton, J Augustine, R Barton. Optimal positioning for cervical immobilisation. Ann Emer Med 28:301–308, 1996.
26. P Wood. PGP Lawler. Managing the airway in cervical spine injury. Anaesthesia 47:792–797, 1992.
27. A Reber, I Castelli, W Ummenhofer. Management bei zervikalen Wirbelsäulenverletzungen. Notarzt 4:109–111, 1994.
28. T Majernick, R Bieniek, J Houston, H Hughes. Cervical spine movement during orotracheal intubation. Ann Emer Med 15:417–420, 1986.
29. L Lampl, M Helm, M Winter. Zum Problem der präklinisch nicht erkannten Wirbelsäulenverletzung. Notarzt 8:99–103, 1992.
30. D Muckart, S Bhagwanjee, R Van der Merwe. Spinal cord injury as a result of endotracheal intubation in patients with undiagnosed cervical spine fractures. Anesthesiology 87:418–420, 1997.
31. M Copass, M Oreskovich, M Bladergroen, CJ Carrico. Prehospital cardiopulmonary resuscitation of the critically injured patient. Am J Surg 148:20–26, 1984.

32. ITACCS: Recommendations for Uniform Reporting of Data Following Major Trauma—The Utstein Style. Baltimore: ITACCS, 1999.
33. T Kirsch. Emergency medicine around the world. Ann Emer Med 32:237–238, 1998.
34. D Trunkey. Editorial: Is ALS necessary for pre-hospital trauma care? J Trauma 24:86, 1984.
35. D Spaite, D Tse, T Valenzuela, E Criss, H Meislin, M Mahoney, J Ross. The impact of injury severity and prehospital procedures on scene time in victims of major trauma. Ann Emer Med 20:1299–1305, 1991.
36. M Avitzour, I Ronen, L Epstein. Professional evacuation of persons injured in road accidents in Israel is fast but underused. Isr J Med Sci 31:405–411, 1995.
37. I Anderson, M Woodford, F De Dombal, M Irving. Retrospective study of 1000 deaths from injury in England and Wales. BMJ 296:1305–1308, 1988.
38. E Dickinson. Using market principles for healthcare development. Qual Healthcare 4:40–44, 1995.
39. R Hardern, S Hampshaw. What do accident and emergency medical staff think of practice guidelines? Eur J Emer Med 4:68–71, 1997.
40. J Sampalis, S Boukas, A Lavoie, A Nikolis, P Fréchette, R Brown, D Fleiszer, D Mulder. Preventable death evaluation of the appropriateness of the on-site trauma care provided by Urgences-Sané physicians. J Trauma 39:1029–1035, 1995.
41. Evidence-based medicine. JAMA 268:2420–2425, 1992.
42. W Dick. Evidence-based emergency medicine. Anaesthesist 47:957–967, 1998.
43. JF Waeckerle, WH Cordell, P Wyer, HH Osborn. Evidence-based emergency medicine: Integrating research into practice. Ann Emer Med 30:626–628, 1997.
44. J Schou. Major interventions in the field stabilization of trauma patients: What is possible? Eur J Emer Med 3:221–224, 1996.
45. P Pepe. Out-of-hospital research in the urban environment. Prehosp Disas Med 8 (suppl.): S21–24, 1993.
46. N Goodman. Anaesthesia and evidence-based medicine. Anaesthesia 53:353–368, 1998.
47. L Jacobs, A Sinclair, A Beiser, R D'Agostino. Prehospital advanced life support: Benefits in trauma. J Trauma 24:8–13, 1984.
48. R Cummins, D Chamberlain, MF Hazinski, V Nadkarni, W Kloeck, E Kramer, L Becker, C Robertson, R Koster, A Zaritsky, L Bossaert, JP Ornato, V Callanan, M Allen, PA Steen, B Connolly, A Sanders, A Idris, S Cobbe. Recommended guidelines for uniform reporting of data from out of hospital cardiac arrest: The Utstein style. Resuscitation 34:151–183, 1997.
49. D Spaite, E Criss, T Valenzuela, J Guisto. Emergency medical service systems research: Problems of the past, challenges of the future. Ann Emer Med 26:146–152, 1995.
50. A Donabedian. Evaluating the quality of medical care: Part 2. Milbank Q 11:166–206, 1966.
51. R Helmreich, J Davies. Human Factors in the Operating Room: Interpersonal Determinants of Safety, Efficiency, and Morale. London: Balliere Tindall, 1996.
52. R Green. The psychology of human error. Eur J Anaesth 16:148–155, 1999.
53. W Ummenhofer, H Pargger, U Boenicke, D Scheidegger. Extrication and immobilization of the severe trauma victim: How it is done. In: R Goris, O Trentz, eds. The Integrated Approach to Trauma Care: The First 24 Hours. Berlin: Springer Verlag, 1995, pp. 25–39.
54. K Steel, P Gertman, C Crescenzi, J Anderson. Iatrogenic illness on a general medical service at a university hospital. New Eng J Med 304:638–642, 1981.
55. E Schimmel. The hazards of hospitalization. Ann Intern Med 60:100–110, 1964.
56. L Leape. Error in medicine. JAMA 272:1851–1856, 1994.
57. D Longnecker. Navigation in uncharted waters: Is anesthesiology on course for the 21st century? Anesthesiology 86:736–742, 1997.
58. J Reason. Managing the Risks of Organizational Accidents. England, Ashgate: Aldershot, 1997.

2

Prehospital Trauma Care: Demographics

KIM J. GUPTA and JERRY P. NOLAN

Royal United Hospital, Bath, United Kingdom

MICHAEL J. A. PARR

Liverpool Hospital, University of New South Wales, Sydney, Australia

I. INTRODUCTION

Injury may be defined as physical harm or damage to the body resulting from an exchange of mechanical, chemical, thermal, or other environmental energy that exceeds the body's tolerance. The terms injury and trauma are interchangeable. Commonly used major subdivisions of trauma deaths are homicide, suicide, and unintentional. The latter term is preferred to accidental, which implies that injuries occur by chance and cannot be prevented.

Trauma has been a significant cause of death and disability throughout history [1]. One of the earliest attempts at organized prehospital care for trauma in the United Kingdom was made in 1774 when a society was founded to revive drowned people pulled from the river Thames in London. This became the Society for the Recovery of Persons Apparently Drowned, before it changed its name to the Humane Society in 1776. Trying to restore life to a victim of sudden trauma was a new idea and represented a dramatic shift of emphasis in the practice of medicine at the time. In France, Baron D. J. Larrey, who was Napoleon's surgeon in chief, developed the idea of triage and rapid evacuation of casualties. In the same manner as the flying artillery, he created a ''flying ambulance,'' which was a mobile field hospital that followed the advanced guard. Urgent surgery within hours of the injury and before transport back to base hospitals was a revolutionary concept.

Since then trauma has become one of the most serious public health problems facing developed societies today. In this chapter, the scale of the trauma epidemic is defined with a review of trauma data from across the world. Trauma figures are reviewed by cause and intent. The outcome for its victims, the costs it incurs, and the mechanisms for its prevention are explored.

II. SOURCES OF TRAUMA DATA

Many countries have reliable death registration systems and produce mortality statistics that are published annually by the World Health Organization (WHO), a specialized agency of the United Nations with primary responsibility for international health matters and public health [2]. Such medically certified vital-registration data are, however, available for less than 30% of the deaths that occur worldwide each year. Mortality information for the remainder comes from small-scale population data and sample-registration data from selected countries. These have been combined with vital registration data to develop worldwide cause of death estimates such as those presented in the Global Burden of Disease Study [3].

Many individual countries also record and publish their own mortality data. For example, in the United Kingdom the Office of Population Censuses and Surveys (OPCS) publishes annual mortality statistics [4], as do the Centers for Disease Control and Prevention National Center for Health Statistics (CDC/NCHS) in the United States. Many non-government public service organizations also publish data, such as the National Safety Council (NSC) in the United States, which publishes data on the previous year's unintentional injuries in *Accident Facts* [5]. A global subsidiary of the NSC, the International Safety Council produces *International Accident Facts* [6], which provides international comparisons of accident data drawn from several sources. Other groups attempting to collate international comparisons of trauma data include the International Collaborative Effort (ICE) on Injury Statistics [7], sponsored by the CDC/NCHS. Data specific to individual groups or causes of trauma are also available. For example, data concerning motor vehicle accidents are available from the American Automobile Manufacturers Association and the National Highway Traffic Safety Administration (NHTSA) in the United States and the Department of the Environment, Transport and the Regions in the United Kingdom [8]. Much information is now widely available via the World Wide Web. Many of the organizations mentioned above have Websites on the Internet and publish updated data on a regular basis.

International and national comparisons of trauma mortality are more meaningful if there is comparability in the collection, processing, classification, and presentation of data. The WHO aims to provide such a standard in the form of the *Manual of the International Classification of Diseases, Injuries, and Causes of Death*, commonly known as the *International Classification of Diseases*, or ICD. The underlying cause of death is defined as "the disease or injury which initiated the train of morbid events leading directly to death, or the circumstances of the accident or violence which produced the fatal injury" [9].

Since its introduction in 1900, the ICD has been revised ten times to incorporate changes in the medical field. The tenth revision (ICD-10) was published in 1992 [10]. The differences between the ninth (ICD-9) and tenth revisions far exceed those between earlier successive revisions, reflecting a conceptual shift in the structure and content of the classification. It is anticipated that the United States will implement the ICD-10 with 1999 data.

The statistics used for this chapter are mainly derived from the ninth revision, which was instituted in 1979 [9]. For deaths due to injury and poisoning, ICD-9 provides a system of "external cause" codes (E-codes), to which the underlying cause of death is assigned. External causes of injury and poisoning are represented by codes E800 to E999, which permit precise information on the cause of injury to be recorded. The ICD system also includes a basic tabulation of two-digit codes that also cover all causes of death. The WHO tends to use this simpler system for displaying annual international health statistics. Codes E47 to E56 cover causes of trauma.

The ICD system, however, affords only cautious comparability of international statistics. Differences between countries still exist in definitions, recording systems, reporting practices, and interpretation of coding rules. A further problem is that it only presents cause-specific statistics for unintentional injury and not for deaths from suicide, homicide, or where intent is not determined. It therefore does not provide information on *both* cause *and* intent for all injury-related deaths.

One must also consider the demographic, social, geographic, economic, and cultural differences that exist between countries. For example, crude population death rates (usually expressed as death rate per 100,000 population) do not adjust for the age distribution differences that exist between countries. This requires the use of standardized populations, such as the "world standard" population [2].

III. INTERNATIONAL TRAUMA

Approximately 50 million people die in the world each year. It has been estimated that approximately 10% of this global mortality is attributable to trauma; for example, 5.1 million people died from injuries in 1990 [3]. Approximately 0.9 million of these trauma deaths are recorded in the WHO registered statistics.

Trauma is thus among the top five leading causes of death in the world. In the vast majority of the countries submitting data to the WHO, heart disease and malignant neoplasms are the top two causes of death. Trauma ranks usually from third to fifth place, along with cerebrovascular disease and respiratory diseases [6]. Table 1 shows the leading five causes of death in the world according to data from the 1990 Global Burden of Disease Study [3]. The impact of infectious and parasitic diseases is profound when compared to WHO data. This reflects the incidence of this problem in the developing world, from which few certified vital-mortality data are available.

Table 2 shows an international comparison of mortality rates from external causes (i.e., trauma) and other major categories of disease for the countries that submit appropriate mortality data to the WHO. The information is ranked according to the trauma death rate. The range in trauma death rate is wide, with that in the Russian Federation being over

Table 1 Leading Causes of Death Worldwide (1990)

Cause of death	Number (×1000)
Total	50,467
Cardiovascular disease	14,327
Infectious and parasitic disease	9329
Respiratory disease and infections	7316
Malignant neoplasms	6024
Injuries	5085

Source: Ref. 3.

Table 2 Age-Standardized Death Rates (per 100,000 Population) for Selected Causes

Country	Year	External causes (E47–56)	Diseases of the circulatory system (E25–30)	Diseases of the respiratory system (E31–32)	Malignant neoplasms (E08–14)	Total (all causes)
Russian Federation	1995	204.6	501.2	56.5	142.5	1071.4
Latvia	1995	175.2	471.7	36.1	137	978.2
Estonia	1995	169.2	416.6	29.8	140.5	886.7
Lithuania	1995	154	365.1	32.5	140.8	812.7
Kazakhstan	1995	140.8	502.1	106.1	143.5	1074.7
Colombia	1994	120.7	201	49.2	92.7	609.3
Kyrgyztan	1995	111.9	433.7	147.7	86	1032.9
Republic of Moldova	1995	109.3	471.9	73.4	117.4	1092.5
Hungary	1995	78.1	369.9	34.5	191.9	827.1
Venezuela	1994	77.5	248.7	48.1	95.8	665.5
Brazil (selected parts)	1992	75.2	253.1	74.8	97.2	744.4
Tajikistan	1992	71.5	333.9	134.4	72.4	839.3
Romania	1995	71.2	451	65.2	116.2	833.3
Cuba	1995	71.1	221.6	47	108.4	557.3
Mexico	1995	68.7	174.7	67.6	81.2	667.7
Belize	1995	66.5	197.8	65.4	63.9	611
Slovenia	1995	66.1	215.8	39.4	146.9	576.3
Chile	1994	64.5	154.8	62.8	120.3	565
Finland	1995	64.1	211.3	32.2	107.2	495.8
Poland	1995	63.8	323.6	23.3	149	708.7
Costa Rica	1994	56.2	188.3	58.9	113.4	556.2
Trinidad & Tobago	1994	52.7	308.9	51.6	102.5	796.1
France	1994	51.7	107.9	23.2	130.8	423.9

United States	1994	50.5	187.5	41.6	130.8	521.9
Argentina	1993	50.4	267.8	44.2	119	650.5
Mauritius	1995	49.9	346.2	75.1	68.8	787.1
Azerbaijan	1995	48.9	410.2	100.2	77.5	794.9
Portugal	1995	48.5	204	38.5	114.3	568.5
Belgium	1992	46.9	158.6	37.5	142.5	501
Luxembourg	1995	46.4	168.6	28.6	136.8	468.5
Austria	1995	46.1	216.2	18.1	125.1	481.2
Canada	1995	37.3	142.1	32.6	126.1	428.8
Bahamas	1995	36.4	211	56.7	112.9	681
Greece	1995	35	196.7	22.7	109.4	449
Australia	1994	34.6	168.3	32	126.2	440.6
Germany	1995	34.4	202.6	26.5	130.8	493.5
Norway	1994	33.6	174.4	35.9	121.7	451.4
Singapore	1995	33.2	186.6	94.7	130.8	517.7
Spain	1994	32.7	143.8	33.8	120.8	438.5
Barbados	1995	32.6	200.3	38.5	106.3	610.6
Italy	1993	32.6	166	22.1	133.7	450
Ireland	1993	32.4	241.7	69.6	145.1	569.8
Sweden	1995	32.3	172.8	25.5	106.6	408.6
Israel	1995	30	183.7	18.3	114.6	467.9
Former Yugoslav republic of Macedonia	1995	25.7	362.6	32	104.9	698.7
United Kingdom	1995	24.4	192.6	63.7	137.1	495.8
Netherlands	1995	23.9	160.9	35.8	136.7	461.3

Note: Mortality rates are based on a world standard population and ranked in order of mortality rate for external causes.
Source: Ref. 2.

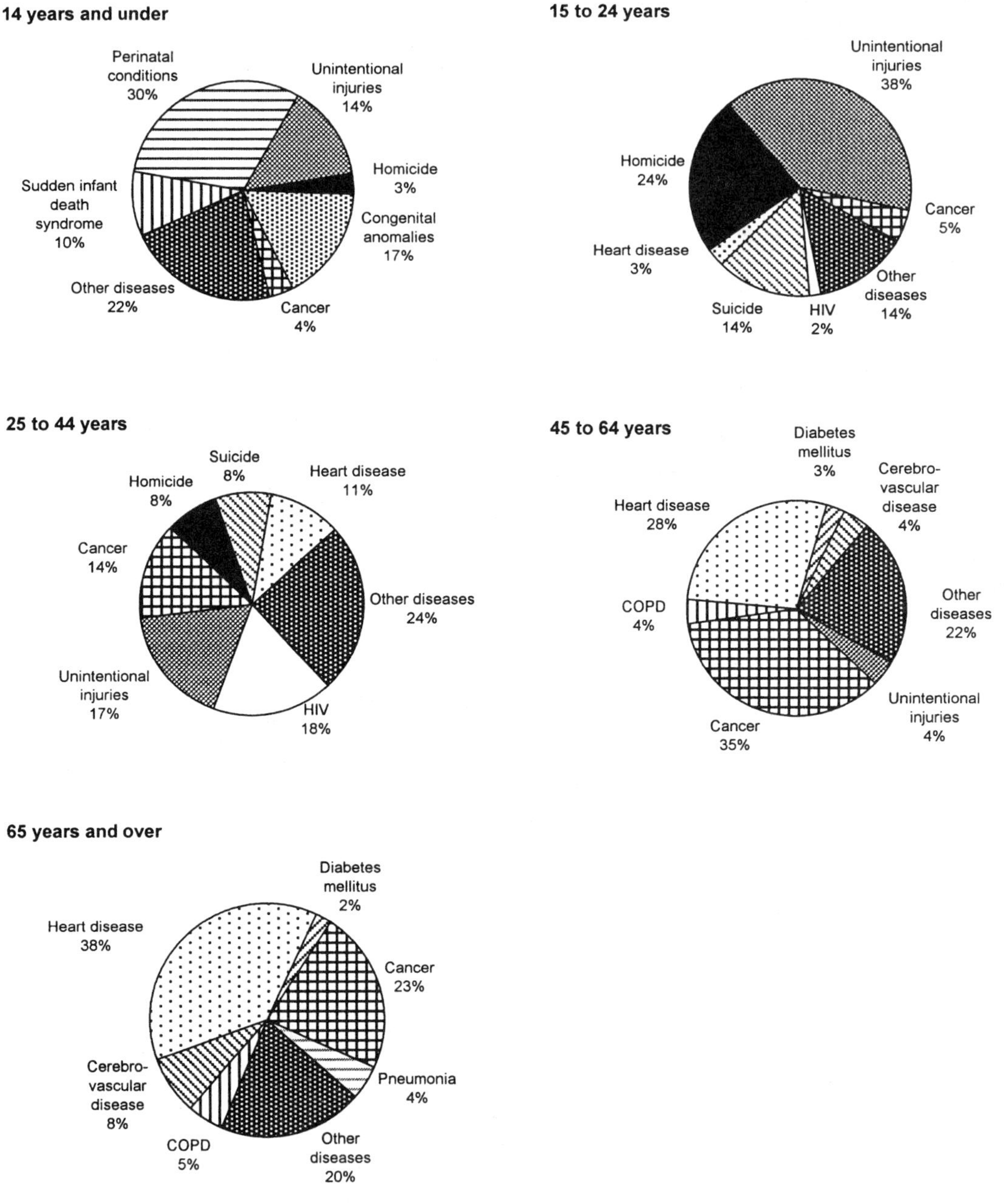

Figure 1 Causes of death by age group (U.S. 1993). (From Ref. 5.)

eight times that in the United Kingdom. The United States is often perceived as having a relatively high level of trauma, but actually falls toward the middle of the list, with a rate of less than one-third that of the top four countries.

The risk of death from injury varies strongly by region, sex, and age. Regional differences can be seen in WHO data from many of the newly independent republics emerging from the former Union of Soviet Socialist Republics (USSR). Many of these countries appear to have extremely high trauma rates. Similarly, global data reveal that in the established market economies injuries from violence caused about 6% of all deaths in 1990, compared with 12 to 13% in sub-Saharan Africa and Latin America and the Caribbean [3]. Worldwide there are about two male deaths from violence for every female death (3.3 million, compared with 1.7 million), and injuries account for about 12.5% of all male deaths, compared with 7.4% of female deaths.

It is well recognized that trauma tends to effect a younger population, and this is clearly demonstrated in the U.S. data in Fig. 1, which shows the principal causes of death in different age groups. Unintentional injuries are the leading cause of death among all persons aged 1 to 38 years in the United States and trauma is responsible for 76% of all deaths in the 15 to 24 age group [5]. This is similar in the United Kingdom, where trauma is the leading cause of death among all persons aged 1 to 34 years [11].

Crude mortality rates give equal weight to all deaths, but time-based measures such as years of life lost (YLL) add significance to premature deaths and the loss of productive life that results, thus while injuries accounted for 10% of global mortality in 1990, they accounted for 15% of YLL [3]. In the United States calculation of the ''years of potential life lost'' before the age of 65 (YPLL-65) emphasizes the significance of deaths among younger people by positively weighting deaths that occur at younger ages. Ranked in this way, unintentional injuries are the most significant cause of death in the United States, accounting for an estimated 2 million YPLL in 1994, with intentional injuries accounting for a further 1.7 million years.

IV. MODES OF TRAUMA

In Table 3 the trauma fatality rates for each nation reporting to the WHO are subdivided into separate categories: all deaths from external causes, motor vehicle accidents (MVA; the major subgroup of accidents), suicide, and homicide. These are age-standardized death rates based on world standard population as defined by the WHO [2]. Table 4 shows the causes of death from trauma (crude death rate) for the 11 countries analyzed in the International Comparative Analysis of Injury Mortality Data produced by the ICE Collaborators [7]. In Table 4 the comparatively high death rate from poisoning and falls in Denmark may be influenced by the use of ICD-10 data by this country.

A. Motor Vehicle Accidents

In 1990, MVAs accounted for the death of one million people globally ranking it the ninth most common cause of death in the world, and representing the largest subgroup of trauma deaths. WHO vital-registration data are available for approximately 210,000 of these. Table 3 shows that Latvia, Venezuela, and Estonia have the highest mortality rates from MVAs, at 27.7, 24, and 22.7 deaths per 100,000 population, respectively. Portugal is fourth, at 21.8 per 100,000 population, although this represents a much higher proportion of total trauma deaths than it does in the first three countries. The range across western

Table 3 Age-Standardized Death Rates (per 100,000 Population) for Selected Causes of Trauma

Country	Year	External causes (E47–56)	Motor vehicle traffic accidents (E471)	Suicide (E54)	Homicide and injury purposely inflicted by others (E55)
Argentina	1993	50.4	10.1	6.2	4
Australia	1994	34.6	10	11.2	1.7
Austria	1995	46.1	12.8	16.6	1
Azerbaijan	1995	48.9	3	0.7	8.7
Bahamas	1995	36.4	5.8	0.6	13.3
Barbados	1995	32.6	7.6	6.3	5.9
Belgium	1992	46.9	14.9	14.1	1.5
Belize	1995	66.5	20.7	8.8	0
Brazil (selected parts)	1992	75.2	20.7	4.6	19.1
Canada	1995	37.3	9.8	11.6	1.5
Chile	1994	64.5	12.1	5.6	2.8
Colombia	1994	120.7	18.6	3.5	73
Costa Rica	1994	56.2	18.2	5.2	5.4
Cuba	1995	71.1	16.7	17.5	6.8
Estonia	1995	169.2	22.7	32.6	19.8
Finland	1995	64.1	6.9	22.6	2.7
Former Yugoslav republic of Macedonia	1995	25.7	—	—	—
France	1994	51.7	12.9	15.8	1.1
Germany	1995	34.4	10.7	11.3	1.1
Greece	1995	35	19.8	2.7	1.1
Hungary	1995	78.1	14.9	24.3	3
Ireland	1993	32.4	10.6	8.7	0.6
Israel	1995	30	10.2	6.1	1.4
Italy	1993	32.6	12.4	5.8	1.5
Kazakhstan	1995	140.8	13.3	28.4	19
Kyrgyzstan	1995	111.9	12.2	16.1	14.3
Latvia	1995	175.2	27.7	33.5	16
Lithuania	1995	154	18.2	38.9	10.2
Luxembourg	1995	46.4	15	12.1	0.6
Mauritius	1995	49.9	17.6	13	1.2
Mexico	1995	68.7	16.2	3.4	17.7
Netherlands	1995	23.9	6.9	7.8	1.1
Norway	1994	33.6	5.9	10.7	0.7
Poland	1995	63.8	16.7	12.4	2.5
Portugal	1995	48.5	21.8	5.9	1.6
Republic of Moldova	1995	109.3	16	16.9	15.6
Romania	1995	71.2	—	10.5	3.7
Russian Federation	1995	204.6	20.4	35.3	26.6
Singapore	1995	33.2	7.6	12	1.5
Slovenia	1995	66.1	17.3	22.4	2.2
Spain	1994	32.7	12.4	6	0.8
Sweden	1995	32.3	4.9	11.8	1
Tajikistan	1992	71.5	10.3	4.9	12.4
Trinidad & Tobago	1994	52.7	10.4	11.8	11.4
United Kingdom	1995	24.4	5.6	6.2	1
United States	1994	50.5	14.9	10.3	9.4
Venezuela	1994	77.5	24	5.6	15.1

Note: Mortality rates are based on a world standard population.
Source: Ref. 2.

Table 4 Average Annual Injury Death Rate (Crude Death Rate per 100,000 Population) by Mechanism

	Motor vehicle traffic	Firearm	Poisoning	Fall	Suffocation	Drowning	Unspecified	All other injuries
Australia	11	2.9	6.8	2.9	4.4	2.2	3.5	6
Canada	10.5	3.9	6.7	5	6.1	2.1	4.9	5.5
Denmark[a]	10.5	2.1	13.4	25.7	7.8	3	0.6	6.8
England and Wales	6.2	0.4	6.4	4.4	3.8	1.1	4.9	3.3
France	14.9	6.3	4.6	7.1	14.1	4.2	18.6	4.9
Israel	10.3	2.8	0.7	2.6	3.1	1.2	8.7	3.5
Netherlands	7.7	0.5	2.4	4.2	4.9	1.6	9.2	2.7
New Zealand	21.3	3.1	5.9	7	5.6	3.7	1.4	7.8
Norway	7.2	4.3	6.1	6.4	5.3	4.7	16.4	7
Scotland	9.8	0.6	7.9	11.8	5	3.2	3.9	7.7
United States	16.2	13.7	6.2	4.3	3.9	1.9	3	7.1

[a]ICD-10 data (all other countries ICD-9).
Source: Ref. 7.

Europe is very large, with Portugal and Greece at one extreme and Sweden and the United Kingdom at the other, with a death rate approximately four times lower. The United States falls twenty-first out of the 47 countries listed in Table 3, with a rate of 14.9 per 100,000 population in 1994.

Such mortality data can be misleading. Many factors affect the mortality rate from MVAs, including the volume of traffic, number of vehicles, population density, distance traveled in vehicles, and definitions of cause of death. A fatality rate together with a ratio of population to vehicles is more meaningful, as is information derived by comparing the figures for deaths on the basis of distance traveled. Table 5 shows information from several developed countries that produce such data [8].

The type of vehicle also has a profound influence on MVA injury statistics. In the United Kingdom, road accidents caused a total of 310,506 casualties (i.e., any person killed or injured in an MVA) in 1995, along with 3621 fatalities [12]. Motorcyclists constituted 12% of the fatalities and 7.5% of the casualties. When analyzed per distance traveled, however, motorcyclists have a casualty rate more than 10 times higher than car drivers (573 compared with 55 casualties per 100 million km) and a fatality rate more than 20 times that of car drivers (10.8 compared with 0.5 deaths per 100 million km). Motorcycles are also associated with a higher mortality in the United States, where the death rate has been calculated to be 14.9 per 100 million km of motorcycle travel, some 17 times higher than for other types of vehicles [5]. It may be that this rate is higher than in the United Kingdom because of the lack of compulsory helmet laws in some states; in 1993 only 25 states plus the District of Columbia had legislation requiring compulsory helmet use for riders of all ages [5].

Motor vehicle accidents also account for a huge number of nonfatal injuries every year. Figures from the National Health Interview Survey in the United States (see Sec. IV.E) show that in 1994 over 3 million people were injured as a result of a moving motor vehicle [5]. Approximately 2,300,000 of these had disabling injuries (defined as one that results in death, some degree of permanent impairment, or renders the injured person unable to perform his or her regular duties or activities for a full day beyond the day of the injury). The implication is that for every person killed in a motor vehicle accident, 73 people are injured, and 52 of these will suffer disabling injuries. In the United States motor vehicles account for a death every 12 minutes and an injury every 14 seconds [5].

B. Falls

Most countries report falls as being among the top three causes of death from unintentional injury [6]. International comparison shows a wide range of death rates between countries; Hungary, Denmark, and Switzerland report crude death rates of over 20 per 100,000 population, and Brazil, Jamaica, Spain, Hong Kong, and Singapore report death rates of less than 3.0 [6]. The rate in the United States was 5.1 per 100,000 population in 1993 [5] and in the United Kingdom was 7.4 in 1991 [6]. These figures are of limited value for international comparison because they take no account of the age distribution within each country. The vast majority of deaths from falls occur in elderly people. In the United States, for example, 13,141 people died from falls in 1993. Of these, 8760 (67%) occurred in those over 75 years. In this age group falls are the commonest cause of death from unintentional injuries, with a death rate of 62 per 100,000 population *over 75 years* of age, some 12 times higher than for the nation as a whole. More meaningful results can be obtained if an international comparison is made for death rates in the elderly population.

Table 5 International Comparison of Road Deaths: Number and Rates for Different Road Users (1996)

Country	Total number of road deaths	Road deaths per 100,000 population	Motor vehicles per 1000 population	Road deaths per 10,000 motor vehicles	Car-user deaths per 100 million car km	Pedestrian deaths per 100,000 population
Australia	1970	10.8	NA	NA	NA	1.9
Austria	1027	12.7	565	2.3	1.3	1.9
Belgium	1356	13.4	516	2.6[c]	1.4	1.5
Canada	3082	10.3	575	1.8	NA	1.5
Czech Republic	1568	15.2	393	3.9	NA	4.3
Denmark	514	9.8	419[b]	2.3[c]	0.8[a]	1.3
Finland	404	7.9	438	1.8	0.6	1.4
France	8514	14.7	496	3	NA	1.8
Germany	8758	10.7	591	1.8	1.1	1.4
Greece	2349[a]	22.5	NA	NA	NA	4.5[a]
Hungary	1370	13.4	269[b]	5[c]	NA	4.2
Irish Republic	453	12.4	367	3.4	0.8	3.1
Italy	6688	12.3	NA	NA	NA	NA
Japan	11,674	9.3	586	1.6	0.7	2.6
Luxembourg	68[a]	16.7	NA	NA	NA	1.7
Netherlands	1180	7.6	436	1.7	0.6	0.7
New Zealand	514	14.1	653[b]	2.2	NA	1.7
Norway	255	5.8	540	1.1	NA	1.1
Portugal	2730	28.9	640[b]	4.5[c]	NA	6.6
Spain	5483	14	498	2.8	NA	2.4
Sweden	537	6.1	497	1.2	0.6	0.8
Switzerland	616	8.7	591	1.6[a]	0.7	1.5
United Kingdom	3740	6.4	456	1.4	0.5	1.8
United States	41,907	15.5	760	2.1	1[a]	2

Note: Total deaths adjusted to represent standardized 30-day deaths. Actual definition in parentheses with adjustment: Italy (7 days) = +8%; France (6 days) = +5.7%; Portugal (1 day) = +30%.

[a] 1995 data.

[b] All motor vehicles other than mopeds per 1000 population.

[c] Road deaths (except moped users) per 10,000 motor vehicles (except mopeds).

NA = Not available.

Source: Ref. 8. Crown copyright is reproduced with the permission of the Controller of Her Majesty's Stationery Office.

An analysis of the data from 1981 to 1991 in the over-75 age group shows that in Hungary, Denmark, France, Italy, Norway, and Switzerland the death rate from falls is over 200 per 100,000. In Japan, Korea, Hong Kong, Iceland, Spain, and Singapore (as well as several developing countries) the equivalent death rate is less than 50.

C. Homicide

International age-standardized homicide rates vary widely, ranging from 26.6 per 100,000 population in the Russian Federation to 0.6 in the Republic of Ireland and Luxembourg (Table 3) [2]. In the period from 1987 to 1988 the United States had the dubious honor of being ''top'' of the international league table made up from WHO information, with a homicide rate of 8.6 per 100,000 population. From 1994 data, the United States now lies fifteenth on this table despite a similar homicide rate of 9.4 per 100,000 standardized population. This appears mainly to be due to the emergence of mortality data from many countries not previously reporting to the WHO, who suffer comparatively high mortality rates secondary to intentional injury.

Approximately 80,000 homicides were reported in WHO-certified data in 1993. Many developing countries, however, do not submit mortality figures to the WHO, but appear to have very high mortality rates from intentional violence. For example, in 1990 40% of the world's male homicides were estimated to have occurred in sub-Saharan Africa, with a further 20% having occurred in Latin America and the Caribbean [3]. The total vital-registration coverage in sub-Saharan Africa is thought to be only about 1%, and that in Latin America and the Caribbean approximately 42% [3].

In 1993 the crude death rate from homicide (E960–969, E55) in the United States was 10.1 per 100,000 population, representing 26,009 cases of intentional killing (of which 356 were due to legal intervention). Homicide therefore accounted for 17.2% of all trauma-related deaths and 1.1% of deaths from all causes in the United States that year. In marked contrast, in England and Wales there were 434 homicides in 1993, accounting for only 2.8% of the 15,728 trauma-related fatalities [4] and less than 0.1% of deaths from all causes.

As with MVAs and falls, homicide rates are influenced significantly by the age of the population being studied. For example, homicides account for 23.7% of all deaths within the 15-to-24-year-old age group in the United States (Fig. 1). It is therefore not surprising that homicide ranks as the fifth leading cause of YPLL in the United States. Homicide rates are influenced by many other factors, such as socioeconomic status and race. The influence of race and ethnicity is profoundly demonstrated by the fact that the lifetime chance of becoming a homicide victim in the United States is approximately 1 in 240 for whites as compared to 1 in 45 for blacks and other ethnic minorities [13].

1. Firearms: Impact on Trauma Rates

The presence of firearms in a society can have a profound influence on homicide and trauma rates, as is demonstrated in the United States, where firearms are a major public health problem. The findings of the International Collaborative Effort on Injury Statistics (Table 4) found that the United States had a higher annual firearm death rate than any of the other industrialized nations studied (20 to 30 times that of the United Kingdom and the Netherlands), and a firearm homicide rate more than eight times higher than the other countries. In 1993 firearms were used in the homicides of 18,253 people (more than 70% of all homicides) in the United States and in the suicides of 18,940 people (60% of all suicides) in the United States. In total, firearms alone killed 39,277 people in the United States in 1993, accounting for 26% of all trauma deaths, rivaling the number killed in MVAs. In 1991, deaths from firearms exceeded those from MVAs in seven states and the District of Columbia [14]. The trend is one of a rapid rise and is almost entirely attributable to the increase in firearm homicides in the 15-to-24-year-old age group [15]. It is estimated that if these trends continue firearms will become the leading cause of trauma deaths in the whole of the United States by the year 2003 [14].

Guns are highly lethal. It has been shown that 60% of gun assaults are fatal, compared to only 4% of knife assaults and <1% of assaults with blunt weapons [16]. Similarly, only 8% of victims survive suicide attempts with a firearm, compared with 33% surviving drowning attempts, 73% surviving poisoning attempts, and 96% surviving knife wounds [17]. It is perhaps not surprising therefore that the presence of a gun in the home increases the risk of homicide by a factor of 2.7 and the risk of successful suicide by a factor of 4.8 [18,19]. The risk of suicide in the 15-to-24-year-old age group increases 10 times if there is a gun in the home, yet 49% of U.S. households have at least one firearm [20].

Firearms also account for a large number of nonfatal injuries. In 1992, it was estimated that the rate of nonfatal firearm-related injuries treated in the emergency rooms of U.S. hospitals was 2.6 times the national rate of fatal firearm-related injuries [21].

D. Suicide

In many European countries, in the Americas, and in Asia, suicide rates have been recorded for extended periods of time. The reported rates vary immensely, and certain areas, such as South India and China, are known to have exceptionally high rates. Why suicide rates in China are so high is unknown, but it accounts for almost one in four deaths of females between the ages of 15 and 44 in that country, a number representing 56% of all female suicides in the world in 1990 [3]. The Global Burden of Disease Study estimated that 786,000 people committed suicide in the world in 1990 (ranking it the twelfth most common cause of death) [3]. Countries reporting mortality statistics to the WHO recorded approximately 190,000 suicides around 1993. The highest suicide rates were in Lithuania (38.9 deaths per 100,000 standardized population), the Russian Federation (35.3 per 100,000 population), and Latvia (33.5 per 100,000 population). The lowest rates recorded in the same year were the Bahamas (0.6), Azerbaijan (0.7), and Greece (2.7) (Table 3).

There is some debate on whether or not national suicide mortality statistics can be assumed to be a reliable source of data on which to base comparative epidemiological studies. Methods and criteria used in identifying suicides vary so much between different countries that they may account for the differences in rates. In 1982 a WHO working group examined all the empirical evidence available on the matter [22]. This review indicated clearly that differences in ascertainment procedures do not explain the differences in suicide rates between populations. Overall, it seems that the effects of underreporting, and the errors encountered in reporting mortality figures generally, appear to be a random effect that permits cautious epidemiological comparisons of rates within countries, between countries, and over time [23].

An assessment of international data shows that men are at considerably higher risk of suicide than women. For most countries the male-to-female ratio is above three. This phenomenon is well known and not restricted to any continent or geographic area [23]. It also holds true across age groups. Suicides account for a high proportion of deaths occurring in the younger population. For example, in the United States suicide accounts for almost 14% of all deaths in the 15-to-24-year-old age group (Fig. 1), with a death rate of 13.5 per 100,000 population of this age [5]. Other countries with high adolescent and young adult suicide rates are Canada (15 per 100,000 in 1990), Finland (25.1 in 1991), and Austria and Switzerland (both with rates of 16.2 in 1991) [23]. In many countries the rate of adolescent suicide has shown a marked increase over the last 35 years. This has been particularly high in Ireland, Norway, and the Netherlands, while countries such as Canada, Colombia, and the United States have shown less dramatic increases. Japan is one of the few countries in which a clear decrease in adolescent suicide can be established [23].

It is difficult to know which specific sociocultural or other relevant aspects explain the similarities and differences between suicide rates in different countries. There are clear correlations between suicide and unemployment rates, divorce, crime rates [24], wars [22], and religious affiliation. Suicide rates in Islamic countries are considerably lower than in Buddhist countries, and rates in Protestant northern Europe and North America are higher than in Roman Catholic southern Europe and Latin America [23]. Psychological risk factors, such as mental illness, alcoholism, and financial problems, also exist.

Two factors related directly to the frequency of suicidal acts are easy access to a killing agent or method and publicity about suicidal acts. Examples of the former have been demonstrated in Western Samoa (with the easy availability of the herbicide paraquat) [25], and also in the United States, with its widespread availability of firearms. Increased publicity about suicide tends to increase suicide rates. This has been demonstrated in relation to television and press coverage in Germany and Austria [26]. These factors are important in the epidemiology of suicide because they have wide implications when considering strategies for its prevention.

E. Nonfatal Injuries

Few countries have an adequate national injury surveillance system that provides reliable estimates of nonfatal injury. In the United States, estimates of the number of disabling injuries are made from the National Health Interview Survey conducted by the U.S. Public Health Service. This is a continuous personal interview of households to obtain information about the health status of household members, including injuries experienced during the two weeks prior to the interview. From this, an estimated 60,452,000 people were injured in 1994 in the United States (23.3 per 100 persons per year) [5]. This survey defines an injury for inclusion if it is medically attended to or if it causes one half-day or more of restricted activity.

The NSC uses injury-to-death ratios to estimate nonfatal disabling injuries. The NSC defines a disabling injury as one that results in death, some degree of permanent impairment, or renders the injured person unable to effectively perform his or her regular duties or activities for a full day beyond the day of injury. The estimated number of patients suffering disabling injuries in 1995 was 19,300,000 in the United States. This is roughly approximate to 400 traumatic injuries and 130 disabling injuries for every death due to trauma.

This number of injured people make huge demands on medical services at substantial expense. According to the National Hospital Ambulatory Medical Care Survey conducted for the National Center for Health Statistics, about 40% of all hospital emergency department visits in the United States are injury-related, as are 8% of all hospital discharges [27]. In 1993 there were approximately 90.3 million visits made to emergency rooms, of which about 36.5 million were injury-related. More than one-third of all injuries resulting in emergency room visits occurred at home, the most common place of injury. The street or highway was the place of injury for about 14% of the total, while work accounted for 12% and school for 4%.

V. COSTS OF TRAUMA CARE

Many factors must be taken into consideration when estimating the financial burden trauma represents to a country's economy. Consideration must be given to costs arising from both fatal and nonfatal injuries in the following categories:

1. Medical expenses, including emergency medical service costs
2. Wage and productivity losses
3. Administrative expenses, which include the administrative costs of private and public insurance plus police and legal costs
4. Damage to property and goods
5. Employer costs, representing the financial value incurred by remaining or newly trained workers

Estimated in this way, the financial impact of trauma is found to be immense. For example, in the United States, the costs arising from unintentional injuries alone were estimated to be $434.8 billion in 1995, rising to $444.1 billion in 1996 [27]. Figure 2 shows the cost components of the figure from 1995. These costs include the differential effects of fatalities, permanent partial disabilities, and temporary disabilities.

In order to put these figures into perspective, the estimated total cost is equivalent to 58 cents of every dollar spent on food in the United States in 1995. If the same costing mechanism is applied to injuries arising from MVAs alone, the resultant costs are estimated to be $170.6 billion [5]. This is the equivalent of purchasing 730 gallons of gasoline for every registered vehicle in the United States.

Such economic costs provide a measure of the economic loss to a community resulting from past injuries. Economic costs, however, should not be used for computing

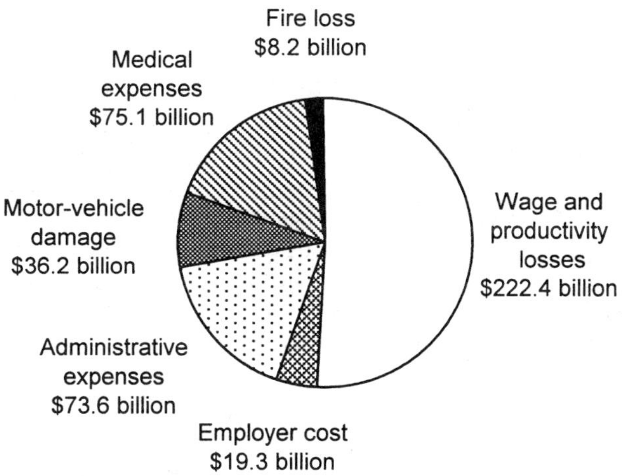

Figure 2 Costs of unintentional injuries by component (U.S., 1995; total $434.8 billion). (From Ref. 5.)

the value of future benefits due to injury-prevention measures, because they do not reflect what society is ''willing to pay'' (an economic concept in its own right) to prevent a fatality or injury. These comprehensive costs should include not only the economic cost components, but also a measure of the value of lost quality of life associated with the deaths and injuries; that is, what society is willing to pay to prevent them. The value of lost quality of life can be estimated through empirical studies of what people actually pay to reduce their health and safety risks, such as through the purchase of air bags or smoke detectors. In the United States, such lost quality of life was estimated to have a value of $775.8 billion in 1995 [5], making the comprehensive cost of unintentional injury in the United States $1,210.6 billion.

VI. OUTCOME AFTER TRAUMA

A. Trimodal Distribution of Death

The trimodal distribution of the timing of death after trauma was based on an analysis of trauma deaths in San Francisco in 1983 [28]. This concept suggested that 50% of trauma deaths occur immediately after the event and are due to overwhelming injury, such as lacerations of the brain, upper spinal cord, heart, or large blood vessels. The second peak accounts for 30% of deaths and occurs up to four hours after injury. These deaths are usually caused by injuries that are considered treatable, and these patients should benefit from a well-organized trauma care system that reduces the time interval between injury and expert definitive treatment. The last peak (20% of deaths) occurs after four hours, but is usually days to weeks after injury. This peak is often the result of sepsis and multiple organ failure (MOF). Appropriate, timely management and aggressive restoration of cellular oxygenation in the resuscitation phase is thought to help reduce this third peak of deaths (see also Chap. 20). Prehospital services and early comprehensive care in the emergency room have been developed with these second two mortality peaks in mind.

Several recent studies have suggested a deviation from the concept of trimodal distribution of deaths. They have implied a bimodal distribution of early and late deaths, where the potential for saving lives by early treatment is much smaller than was previously hoped [29–31] (Fig. 3).

It has been assumed that a considerable proportion of prehospital trauma deaths might be prevented by improved prehospital care. Unfortunately, the number that actually can be prevented is unclear. Hussain and Redmond [32] estimated that death was potentially preventable in at least 39% of those who died from accidental injury before they reached the hospital. Papadopoulos assessed up to 47% of prehospital fatalities as being ''possibly preventable'' [33]. In contrast, there are other studies that emphasize that the majority of deaths occurring prehospital are essentially from unsurvivable injuries and therefore are inevitable [34]. In two large U.K. studies the proportion of deaths that might have been avoided in the prehospital phase was judged to be 1.4% and 3.1% [35,36], and in rural Michigan a maximum preventable death rate of 12.9% among 155 trauma deaths has been estimated, with the majority being in-hospital deaths [37]. A major drawback of most of these studies is that preventable death is a subjective judgment made by expert panels and is not reliably consistent.

The effects of prehospital interventions on longer-term survival are difficult to separate from the effects of in-hospital interventions. An analysis of late trauma deaths, however, suggests that cerebral damage may be a more common cause of death than MOF

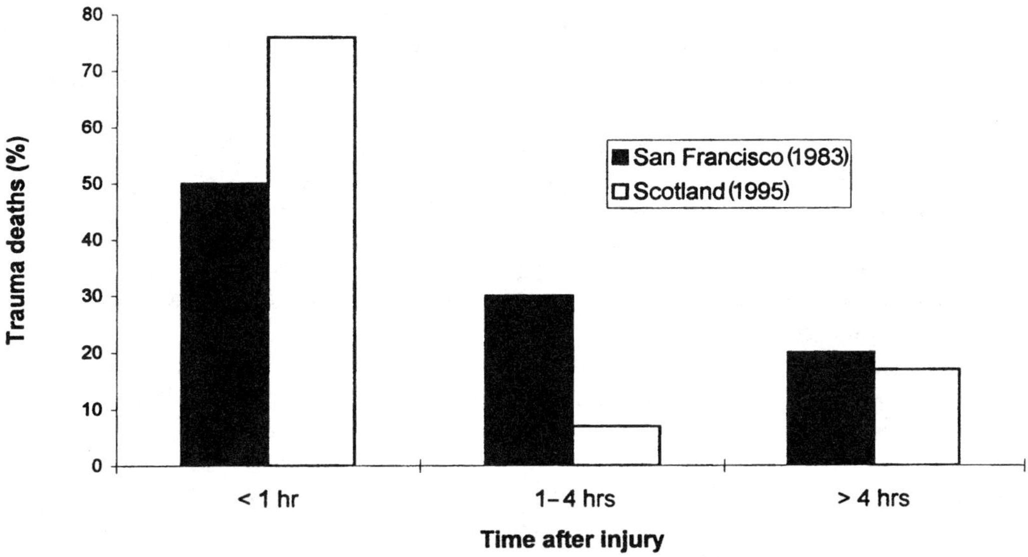

Figure 3 Timing of death after trauma in San Francisco (1983) compared with southeast Scotland (1995). (From Ref. 41).

following multiple nonpenetrating trauma [38]. The contribution of improved prehospital care to this possibly decreased incidence of MOF is unknown. While the debate concerning the benefits of prehospital care proceeds, we should continue to strive to train more bystanders in simple first aid and to reduce the interval between the time of injury and the arrival of emergency services. The philosophy of rapid, systematic, and appropriate management of the trauma victim still remains.

VII. PREVENTION OF TRAUMA

Trauma is responsible for over 5 million deaths in the world each year. In the established market economies it is the most common cause of death in people aged 1 to 38 years. It is also a leading cause of disability and YLL, and a major contributor to health care costs. While much attention has been focused on establishing systems of management that allow faster, more efficient, and higher-quality care for the trauma victim, it is clear that the most effective means of reducing trauma morbidity and mortality lies in prevention.

Internationally there are many epidemiological patterns that raise important questions, such as why suicide rates among women in China are so high, and why women in India are more than twice as likely to die from burns than in any other country. In many countries of the developing world, however, the infrastructure is not adequate to allow the collation of the epidemiological data required to implement meaningful prevention strategies. Much more descriptive epidemiology is urgently needed from the developing world to reveal further patterns and determinants of mortality from injury.

In the developed market economies injuries have until recently been virtually ignored by the public health community. Over the past decade, however, it has become increasingly recognized that many types of trauma are not just chance occurrences, but are in fact quite predictable and therefore preventable. As a result, health care communities, epidemiologists, and economists have collaborated to develop a sophisticated approach to injury control.

Injury can be averted by preventing the event that produces it in the first place (e.g., fire, vehicle crash, fall). If this fails, the next aim is to prevent or minimize the injury that results from the event, by making changes in the person (e.g., preventing osteoporosis, wearing hip padding), the vehicle (e.g., seat belts, energy-absorbing steering wheels), or the environment (e.g., smoke detectors, emergency exits). Finally, if injury occurs, the debilitating effects on the person can be minimized (emergency medical services, public education in resuscitation) [39].

Certain preventive interventions are worth highlighting because of their impact on mortality or their ingenuity. For example, the introduction of three-point seat belts to the United States in 1968 has reduced the risk of severe injury by up to 61% and hospitalization by 33% [40]. The passage of laws enforcing the use of motorcycle helmets reduced the risk of head injury by 34% in California and 22% in Nebraska, and the risk of death by 26% in California and 12% in Texas [39]. Hormone replacement therapy has been associated with a 25% reduction in hip fractures; child-proof pill containers helped reduce the rate of death from salicylate poisoning among children less than 5 years by over half; setting a domestic water heater to 50 degrees centigrade instead of 60 degrees extends the time required for full-thickness burns to occur from two seconds to more than 10 minutes.

Clearly the potential for trauma prevention is enormous and well beyond the scope of this chapter. The introduction of firearm legislation, however, remains an area that requires urgent consideration in order to further reduce trauma mortality in the United States.

VIII. CONCLUSION

Trauma is a major cause of morbidity and mortality worldwide, representing an estimated 10% of global mortality. The associated financial costs to society are enormous.

Meaningful international comparison of trauma epidemiology is extremely difficult. The majority of countries do not have reliable death registration systems, and in those that do, information is readily influenced by reporting practices.

Maximizing survival in trauma victims requires definitive care as soon as possible after injury and a continuing high quality of care to improve long-term survival.

The greatest scope for reducing the number of people dying from trauma lies in its prevention, and resources must be targeted at this as well as at trauma management.

REFERENCES

1. DJ Wilkinson. The history of trauma anesthesia. In: C Grande, ed. Textbook of Trauma Anesthesia and Critical Care. St Louis: Mosby-Year Book, 1993, pp. 199–204.
2. World Health Organization. World Health Statistics Annual, 1996. Geneva: WHO, 1998.
3. C Murray, A Lopez. Mortality by cause for eight regions of the world: Global Burden of Disease Study. Lancet 349:1269–1276, 1997.

4. Office of Population Censuses and Surveys. Mortality statistics, cause: Review of the Registrar General on deaths by cause, sex and age in England and Wales 1993. Series DH2, no. 20, 1995.
5. National Safety Council. Accident Facts. Itasca, IL: National Safety Council, 1996.
6. National Safety Council. International Accident Facts. Itasca, IL: National Safety Council, 1995.
7. LA Fingerhut, CS Cox, M Warner, et al. International Comparative Analysis of Injury Mortality: Findings from the ICE on injury statistics. Advance Data from Vital and Health Statistics, no. 303. Hyattsville, MD: National Center for Health Statistics, 1998.
8. Department of the Environment, Transport and the Regions. Road Accidents Great Britain 1997—The Casualty Report. London: TSO Publications, August 1998.
9. World Health Organization. Manual of the International Statistical Classification of Diseases, Injuries and Causes of Death, ninth revision, vol. 1. Geneva: WHO, 1977, p. 763.
10. World Health Organization. International Statistical Classification of Diseases and Related Health Problems, 10th revision. Geneva: WHO, 1992.
11. Department of Health. On the State of the Public Health, 1995: A report from the Chief Medical Officer. London: Her Majesty's Stationery Office, 1996.
12. Office for National Statistics. Annual Abstract of Statistics, no. 133. London: Stationery Office, 1997.
13. MI Rosenberg, JA Mercy. Homicide: Epidemiologic analysis at the national level. Bull NY Acad Med 62:376–399, 1986.
14. Centers for Disease Control and Prevention. Deaths resulting from firearm and motor-vehicle related injuries—United States, 1968–1991. MMWR 43:37–42, 1994.
15. Centers for Disease Control and Prevention. Trends in rates of homicide: United States, 1985–1994. MMWR 45:460, 1996.
16. J Hedboe, AV Charles, J Neilson, et al. Interpersonal violence: Patterns in a Danish community. Amer J Pub Health 75:651, 1985.
17. DW Webster, CP Chaulk, SP Teret, et al. Reducing firearm injuries. Issues Sci Tech spring 73, 1991.
18. AL Kellermann, FP Rivara, NB Rushforth, et al. Gun ownership as a risk factor for homicide in the home. New Eng J Med 329:1084, 1993.
19. AL Kellermann, FP Rivara, G Somes, et al. Suicide in the home in relation to gun ownership. New Eng J Med 327:467, 1992.
20. PB Fontanarosa. The unrelenting epidemic of violence in America: Truths and consequences. JAMA 273:1792–1793, 1995.
21. J Annest, J Mercy, D Gibson. National estimates of nonfatal firearm-related injuries: Beyond the tip of the iceberg. JAMA 273:1749, 1995.
22. World Health Organization. Changing patterns in suicide behaviour. report of a WHO working group (Athens Sept. 29–Oct. 2, 1981), EURO Reports and Studies no. 74 (E,F,G,R), Copenhagen: WHO, Regional Office for Europe, 1982.
23. RFW Diekstra, W Gulbinat. The epidemiology of suicidal behaviour: A review of three continents. World Health Stat Q 46(1):52–68, 1993.
24. RFW Diekstra. Suicide and parasuicide: A global perspective. In: RFW Diekstra, WH Gulbinat, eds. Preventive Strategies on Suicide. New York: EJ Brill, 1993.
25. JR Bowles. Suicide in Western Samoa: An example of a suicide prevention program in a developing country. In: RFW Diekstra, WH Gulbinat, eds. Preventive Strategies on Suicide. New York: EJ Brill, 1993, pp. 126–156.
26. G Sonneck. Subway suicide in Vienna (1980–1990): A contribution to the imitation effect in suicidal behaviour. In: RFW Diekstra, WH Gulbinat, eds. Preventive Strategies on Suicide. New York: EJ Brill, 1993, pp. 215–223.
27. SR Eachempati, L Reed, J St Louis, R Fischer. The Demographics of Trauma in 1995 revisited: An assessment of the accuracy and utility of trauma predictions. J Trauma 45:208–214, 1998.

28. DD Trunkey. Trauma. Sci Am 249:28–35, 1983.
29. H Meislin, EA Criss, D Judkins, R Berger, C Conroy, B Parks, DW Spaite, TD Valenzuela. Fatal trauma: The modal distribution of time to death is a function of patient demographics and regional resources. J Trauma 43:433–440, 1997.
30. J Wyatt, D Beard, A Gray, et al. The time of death after trauma. BMJ 310:1502, 1995.
31. A Sauaia, FA Moore, EE Moore, et al. Epidemiology of trauma deaths. J Trauma 38:185–193, 1995.
32. LM Hussain, AD Redmond. Are pre-hospital deaths from accidental injury preventable? BMJ 308:1077–1080, 1994.
33. IN Papadopoulos, D Bukis, E Karalas, S Katsaragakis, S Stergiopoulos, G Peros, G Androulakis. Preventable prehospital trauma deaths in a Hellenic urban health region: An audit of prehospital trauma care. J Trauma 41:864–869, 1996.
34. H Meislin, O Conroy, K Conn, B Parks. Fatal injury: Characteristics and prevention of deaths at the scene. J Trauma 46:457–461, 1999.
35. J Nicholl, S Hughes, S Dixon, J Turner, D Yates. The costs and benefits of paramedic skills in pre-hospital trauma care. Health Tech Assess 2:1–72, 1998.
36. D Limb, A McGowan, JE Fairfield, TJ Pigott. Pre-hospital deaths in the Yorkshire Health Region. J Accid Emer Med 13:248–250, 1996.
37. RF Maio, RE Burney, MA Gregor, MG Baranski. A study of preventable trauma mortality in rural Michigan. J Trauma 41:83–90, 1996.
38. E Dereeper, R Ciardelli, JL Vincent. Fatal outcome after polytrauma: Multiple organ failure or cerebral damage? Resuscitation 36:15–18, 1998.
39. FP Rivara, DC Grossman, P Cummings. Injury prevention. parts one and two. New Eng J Med 337:543–548, 613–618, 1997.
40. MC Henry, JE Hollander, JM Alicandro, G Cassara, et al. Prospective countrywide evaluation of the effects of motor vehicle safety device use and injury severity. Ann Emer Med 28:627–634, 1996.

3

Mechanisms of Injury in Trauma

ALLYSAN ARMSTRONG-BROWN and DOREEN YEE

Sunnybrook and Women's College Health Sciences Centre, Toronto, Ontario, Canada

I. INTRODUCTION

In this chapter the authors will discuss how consideration of the mechanism of injury (MOI) can assist in making triage decisions in order to optimize care and to determine the disposition of the trauma patient. The biomechanics of trauma will be reviewed. Examination will also be made of the relationship between various mechanisms of injury and clinical injury patterns in order to improve detection of injuries and anticipation of complications. The history of the traumatic event and the physical observations of the trauma scene by prehospital personnel may provide important information in the prehospital and hospital phases of patient care.

II. HOW MECHANISM OF INJURY AFFECTS TRIAGE DECISIONS

Several MOIs have been repeatedly identified as predicting a high risk of significant injury. Many of these MOIs were identified by retrospective studies of blunt trauma. The American College of Surgeons' Committee on Trauma includes consideration of MOIs in their prehospital triage decision scheme [1] (Fig. 1).

It is notable that this scheme does not mandate the use of trauma team alert purely on the basis of MOI. Several authors have attempted to refine this scheme to suit their particular institutions, to reduce the rates of "overtriage" and "undertriage" that may be associated with the use of MOI as a triage tool.

A. Overtriage and Undertriage

It is well established that severely injured patients benefit from expeditious transfer to a tertiary-care trauma center [2]. It is incumbent on any triage system to accurately and quickly identify those patients requiring this highest level of care. There is no evidence that less severely injured patients (ISS < 16) require or benefit from transfer to a trauma center. A perfect triage system will be 100% sensitive (able to identify all seriously injured patients) and specific (able to identify those with non-life-threatening injuries) and assign patients the appropriate level of care. The overtriage (or false-positive) rate is equal to 1−specificity; the undertriage rate (or false-negative) is equal to 1−sensitivity.

It is generally agreed that it is preferable to err on the side of overtriage (i.e., risk sending those with non-life-threatening injuries to a trauma center) rather than to use triage criteria that incorrectly direct seriously injured patients to nonspecialist centers (undertriage). Clearly, the two are reciprocal; as more liberal triage criteria are used, undertriage decreases but overtriage increases accordingly. This may lead to less efficient use of health care resources by overuse of full trauma team activation. This inefficiency is a necessary side effect of avoiding preventable death from trauma.

The ideal under- and overtriage rates would be 0%, but this is not obtainable in practice. Long et al. [3] quote ''next-to-ideal'' criteria as having 15 to 20% overtriage and no undertriage.

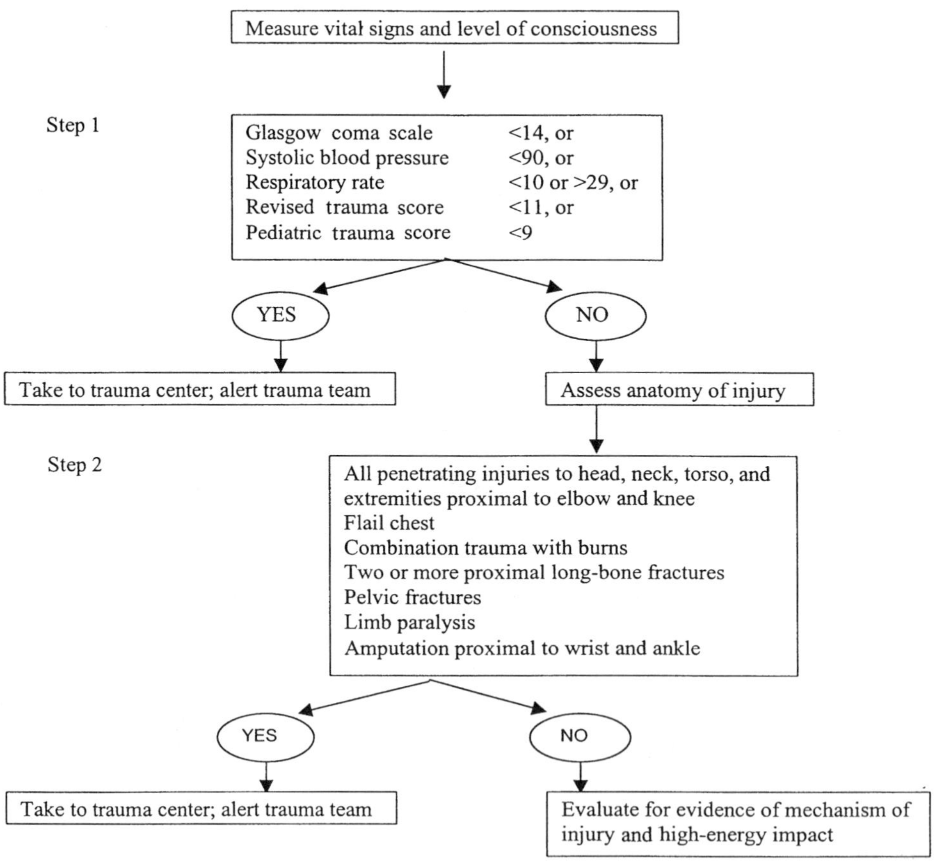

Figure 1 American College of Surgeons' prehospital triage decision scheme. (From Ref. 3a.)

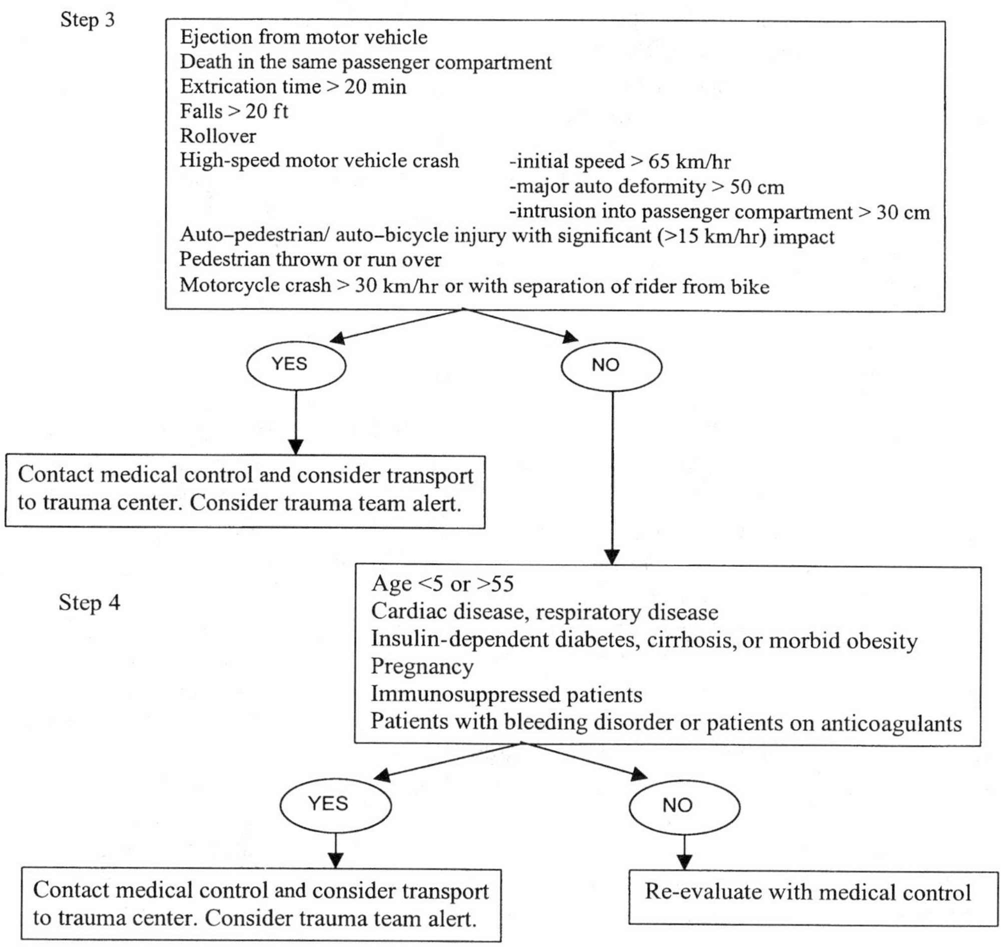

WHEN IN DOUBT TAKE TO A TRAUMA CENTER

Figure 1 *Continued.*

The use of physiologically and anatomically based scores (e.g., trauma score or CRAMS—circulation, respiration, abdomen, motor, speech—score) is discussed elsewhere in this text. The first part of this chapter aims to examine the evidence that certain MOIs can predict the severity of injury and thus the need for transport to a trauma center. Alternatively, MOI criteria may be useful for disposition.

B. Does Mechanism of Injury Criteria Predict Severe Injury?

Analysis of injury mechanism allows those managing the trauma patient from the scene to definitive care to estimate the kinetic energy and forces to which the patient has been exposed, and, by inference, the risk of serious injury. Descriptions of MOI may be inherently flawed, since they are subject to observer error, incomplete availability of information, and poor communication. These may reduce the ability of the tool to differentiate between those at high or low risk of severe injury.

Velocity change (so-called ΔV) shows the strongest correlation with severity of injury [4]. This is not equal to the speed at impact, but takes into account the relative masses of the colliding vehicles, the direction of impact, and the assessment of vehicle damage. Unfortunately for trauma triage assessment, such details are often too time-consuming for measurement by prehospital personnel. Recently developed technologies may make measurement of some of these factors instantly available to trauma personnel (see Sec. III.A.).

Several studies have questioned the ability of MOI criteria to discriminate adequately between patients with minor and severe injuries.

Phillips and Buchman [5] looked at the ability of the American College of Surgeons (ACS) triage criteria to predict admission of a live patient to the ICU or OR (sensitivity, by definition, equal to 100%). This gave a specificity of only 40% (i.e., an overtriage rate of 60%). By modification of predominantly MOI criteria, sensitivity fell to 83%, but specificity rose to 68%. The study by Phillips and Buchman suggested that patients with some anatomical and MOI criteria (e.g., prolonged extrication time or the closing speed of a vehicle alone) can be safely dealt with by a lower level of trauma team response than a full trauma team activation.

In a retrospective review of 347 patients, Simon et al. [6] found that the type of injury mechanism in vehicular trauma was not of itself predictive of the severity of injury. In their urban population, they found that patients exposed to ejection, large deceleration force (>50 km/hr), rollover, significant intrusion, or prolonged extrication were as likely to sustain minor injuries as to be severely injured.

Similarly, Shatney and Sensaki [7] disputed the usefulness of MOI criteria (as described in the ACS protocol) alone. They found that patients with no standard physiological or anatomical indicators of major trauma (i.e., those that had trauma team alerts for MOI alone) had a very low rate of severe injury. Esposito et al. [8] also found that MOI had only an intermediate to low yield when trying to predict major trauma victims.

Conversely, in a prospective study, Bond et al. [9] found that the sensitivity of a physiological triage score (prehospital index; PHI) was improved by the combination of this score with criteria regarding MOI. A PHI alone had a sensitivity of only 41%, and MOI alone had a sensitivity of 73%, but their combination improved sensitivity to 78% with no significant change in specificity (approximately 90%).

In rural California, Karsteadt et al. [10] found that their triage criteria, which included an abbreviated list of MOIs, gave them very low rates of over- and undertriage (0.9 and 6.5%, respectively). Their triage system is run by mobile intensive care nurses or physicians in consultation with emergency medical technicians (EMTs) in the field.

North American triage protocols are generally developed for use by field paramedics. Emerman et al. [11] have suggested that the impressions of EMTs present at the scene may be as accurate as the scoring systems commonly used for predicting the risk of death or the need for urgent operative intervention. Involvement of a trained physician in making the triage call may be useful in minimizing disposition errors [12].

Kaplan et al. [13] found that removing MOI from their triage criteria for a full trauma team alert but retaining a criterion allowing for trauma team activation at the discretion of the attending physician (''any patient/situation deemed appropriate by the responsible attending''), did not significantly alter under- and overtriage rates. Patients who were hemodynamically stable but had a ''significant'' MOI were managed with a lower level of response at the trauma center, with a consequent savings in resource utilization (manpower, emergency department time, and trauma care costs).

Pediatric patients may also differ from adults. Qazi et al. [14] found that at their Level I pediatric trauma center, 74% of trauma team activations were for MOI only. In this population, MOI alone was a poor predictor of serious injury (positive predictive value 2.8% and negative predictive value 90.2%).

C. Conclusions

A confounding factor in the literature is that much of these data are from studies from the United States in the 1970s and early 1980s. Low rates of restraint use from these studies limit their generalizability to other countries and current times, as restraint use often significantly alters injury pattern and severity.

The conflicting results above may be partially explained by differences in study populations and protocols (e.g., rural vs. urban programs, paramedic- vs. physician-controlled triage, retrospective vs. prospective surveys, and regional variations in patterns of restraint use). Most studies had modified the ACS criteria on MOI, and thus were not directly comparable. These factors limit the ability to determine the true utility of MOI as a triage tool.

There is not currently sufficient, reproducible evidence from the literature that some or all of the ACS MOI criteria can safely be deleted from triage protocols. Patients who are physiologically stable at the scene may in fact be severely injured, and in the absence of a more precise triage tool, MOI should still be considered a useful addition to physiological assessment when making decisions about patient disposition.

III. HOW PATTERNS OF INJURY RELATE TO MECHANISM OF INJURY

An essential part of prehospital management of trauma patients is gathering sufficient information on the physical facts of the trauma scene to facilitate management of the patient. Rapidly obtaining a good description of the scene gives important clues as to the pattern and severity of injuries that may have been sustained. For example, in blunt trauma, the factors listed in Table 1 can be extremely informative for both prehospital and hospital personnel. In penetrating trauma, the points listed in Table 2 are relevant.

A. Biomechanics of Injury

It is useful to review some basic physics to allow a better understanding of the process of traumatic injury (Table 3).

In all cases of trauma, there is transfer of energy, in particular to the body's tissues.

1. Biomechanics of Blunt Trauma

A moving vehicle will continue along in motion until an external force acts upon it. The energy of the moving vehicle must be transferred, normally to the braking system, before the vehicle can come to a stop. In a crash situation, this energy is absorbed by deforming the vehicle. The magnitude of energy transferred is dependent on the mass, and particularly the velocity, of the vehicle. The force of the collision is dependent on the mass and deceleration. Injuries are caused by the change in velocity (ΔV). An abrupt deceleration

Table 1 Some Determinants of Likelihood of Severe Injury in Blunt Trauma

Extent and site of deformity of vehicle (internal and external)
Use and types of restraint
Distances involved (particularly for falls and pedestrians struck)
Direction of impact
Surfaces impacted
Body position when found
Injuries to others, particularly if in the same passenger compartment
Seating position in the vehicle
Protective devices (e.g., helmets, leather clothing)
Witnesses' descriptions of the event
Environmental hazards (e.g., toxic chemicals)
Evidence of intoxication

Table 2 Some Determinants of Severity of Injury in Penetrating Trauma

Type of weapon used (e.g., handgun, automatic rifle, switchblade, cleaver)
Caliber of weapon
Type of ammunition used
Distance between victim and weapon

Table 3 Physics Pertaining to the Biomechanics of Injury

A body in motion or a body at rest remains in that state until subjected to an outside force
Energy is never created or destroyed, only transferred
Force = mass × acceleration (or deceleration)
Kinetic energy = (mass × velocity^2)/2

from a high speed (large ΔV) is more likely to cause serious injury than a slow deceleration (small ΔV). A list of injuries associated with a large ΔV is shown in Table 4.

Likewise, an occupant of the vehicle will continue moving at the original speed of the vehicle until the body comes in contact with a stationary object (e.g., lap and shoulder belt, inflated air bag, steering wheel, dashboard, windshield, door panel). An occupant in a collision always tends to move toward the position from which the principal crash force is applied.

2. Emerging Technologies

Sensors located in the air bag are available (though not currently widely installed in vehicles) that act like an active ''black box'' in the event of a crash [15]. These sensors estimate the severity of the crash in order to make an estimation of the probability of major injury to the vehicle's occupants. The measurements (such as ΔV, direction of impact or impacts, rollover, and restraint use) can be transmitted instantly to emergency medical service providers via cellular phones within the vehicle, which transmit the information automatically. The location of the crash is then identified by global positioning system technology. These factors should allow rapid and appropriate deployment of emergency personnel to the scene. These automatic crash notification systems have the potential to significantly reduce

Table 4 Indications of Major Blunt Trauma and of High-Impact ΔV

Two or more long bone fractures
Unstable pelvis
Flail chest
Sternal, scapular, clavicular, upper rib fractures
Falls of 5 meters (15 ft) or more (adult), 4 meters (12 ft) or more (child)
ΔV: 32 km/hr (20 mph) without restraints; 40 km/hr (25 mph) with restraints
Rearward displacement of car by 6 meters (20 ft)
Rearward displacement of front axle
Engine intrusion into passenger compartment
Frame intrusion into passenger compartment: 40 cm (15 in.) on patient side; 50 cm (20 in.) on opposite side
Ejection of passenger
Rollover
Death of another passenger
Pedestrian struck at 32 km/hr (20 mph) or more
"Spiderweb" in windshield
Prolonged extrication

Source: Adapted from Ref. 15a.

response times and thus mortality rates from trauma. Their effects on rates of under- and overtriage remain to be proven.

3. Motor Vehicle Crashes

Frontal Impact

This may be defined as a collision that occurs with an object directly in front of the moving vehicle that abruptly reduces its speed. Included in this category are head-on collisions with another moving vehicle, as well as driving directly into a stationary object. An unrestrained occupant continues to move forward within the vehicle at the original velocity for a few milliseconds after the initial vehicle impact. This motion is quickly ended when contact occurs with the steering column, dashboard, air bag, or windshield. Two patterns of motion have been described in unrestrained drivers, and may occur sequentially (Fig. 2).

1. Down and under motion
   a. Driver slides forward in seat
   b. Knees hit dashboard
2. Up and over motion
   a. Chest strikes steering column
   b. Head hits windshield

Known as the "expressway syndrome" in older literature, the constellation of potential injuries of the lower body arising from the above include fracture dislocations of the ankle, tibia, and knee, as well as fractures of the femur and posterior acetabulum. In the upper body, rib fractures are common; sternal fracture or myocardial injury (contusion, rupture, valvular disruption) may occur. When the head strikes the windshield, cervical spine injuries may occur (by extension, flexion, or axial compression), along with facial

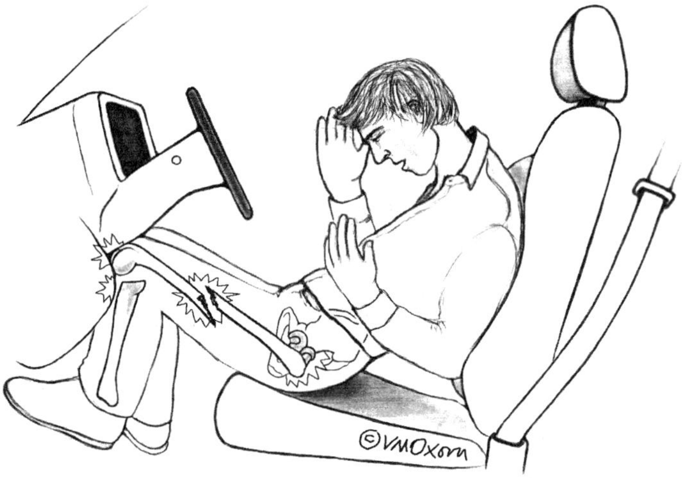

(a)

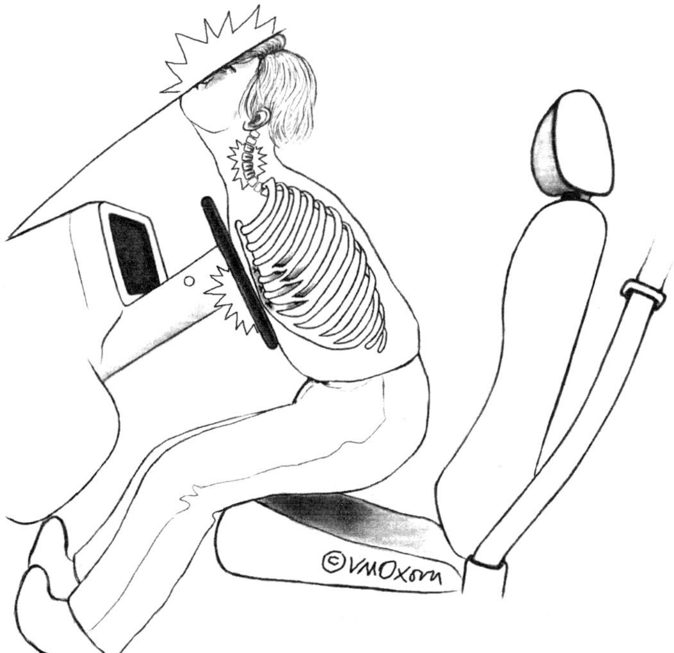

(b)

Figure 2 Potential injuries to the unrestrained driver with a frontal impact. (a) Down and under motion; forces transmitted from the bulkhead may cause fracture or dislocation of the tibia, knee, femur, and acetabulum. (b) Up and over motion; windshield impact causes facial smash and hyperextension cervical injury. Steering wheel may cause rib or sternal fractures, pulmonary contusion, aortic tear, or myocardial injury. (Illustration courtesy of Valerie Oxorn.)

fractures and head injuries. The upper abdomen may also strike the steering wheel, resulting in a possible liver and splenic laceration or "fracture" [16].

Dashboard intrusion, steering wheel deformity, windshield violation, and vehicle irreparability correlate with injury patterns in severely injured patients [17].

The threshold for change in velocity at which an unrestrained driver may incur a serious injury is approximately 40 km/hr; for the unrestrained passenger it is lower (approximately 30 km/hr) [18]. The use of a seatbelt increases the threshold for change in velocity by about 8 km/hr [18].

Lateral Impact

A lateral impact collision occurs when the side of a vehicle is struck perpendicular to its direction of motion. Unrestrained occupants will be first hit by the impacted side of the vehicle, then will be accelerated away from the impact point; the car is "pushed out from under them." The side of the occupant closest to the impact may sustain injury of the ipsilateral clavicle, ribs, pelvis, and abdominal organs (Fig. 3). If the arm is caught between

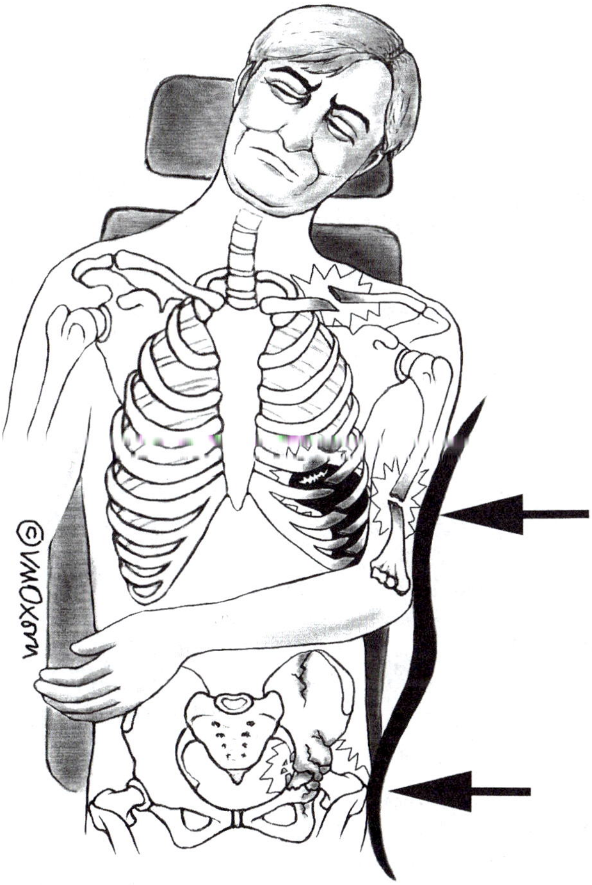

Figure 3 Injuries from a left-lateral impact. Fractures may occur in the clavicle, humerus, ribs, spleen, greater femoral trochanter, and acetabulum. A right-lateral impact may result in liver laceration. (Illustration courtesy of Valerie Oxorn.)

the door and thorax, the humerus may break. The head of the femur may be driven through the acetabulum into the retroperitoneal space, or a fracture of the greater trochanter may occur. Splenic lacerations may occur in the driver, and liver lacerations in the front seat passenger. The head frequently stays "stationary" while the lower body is "pushed out" so that the side of the neck contralateral to the impact may suffer injury involving the ligaments, muscles, and roots of the brachial plexus [19]. The head may flex laterally through a side window to strike the impacting object (e.g., truck grill, pole). Contrecoup injuries may be sustained as the victim is thrown around the interior of the vehicle. Cervical injuries are more common in lateral than frontal or rear impacts, as the cervical spine tolerates lateral flexion less well than extension or flexion. A retrospective review from the Sunnybrook Regional Trauma Unit in Toronto, Canada, also showed that lateral impact collisions were the mechanism of injury in almost half of patients with traumatic aortic rupture [20].

Restraint use appears to have less of a protective effect in lateral versus frontal impact [21], but is still important in limiting lateral movement of the victim around the passenger compartment. A lower change in velocity is required to give the same risk of severe injury in lateral impacts when compared to direct frontal or frontal offset collisions [18]. This is likely due to the limited protection afforded to passengers by the sides of the car frame; lateral supplemental restraint systems such as air bags may be able to modify this.

Traditionally it has been thought that frontal-impact crashes resulted in higher mortality and greater severity of injury [22]. Recent review of the trauma databases from the Maryland Institute for Emergency Medical Services Systems (MIEMSS) showed that drivers in left lateral collisions had higher mortality rates than ones in frontal impacts, despite similar injury severity scores (ISS) [23]. A review from the Sunnybrook Regional Trauma Unit showed that the lateral-impact victims were older, had higher ISS, and more serious thoracic and abdominal injuries than the nonlateral impact group. Mortality rates were similar in both groups, however [24].

Rear Impact

This type of collision occurs when a stationary or slower-moving vehicle is hit from behind by a faster-moving vehicle. Energy transferred to the vehicle that is hit causes acceleration of the vehicle and all the body parts of the occupants (torso, back, and legs) that are in close approximation to the car. The body is pushed out from under the head with the forces transmitted to the neck. If there is an improperly placed or even absent headrest, the occupant's head is initially forcefully hyperextended, followed by a forward flexion, thereby causing tearing and stretching of the ligaments and muscles of the neck (whiplash injury). Cervical spine fractures and spinal cord injuries are uncommon. This initial acceleration is then followed by a deceleration force much like a frontal impact if there is a vehicle in front. Only 8% of collisions causing serious injury are rear-impact ones.

Sideswipe/Rotational Impact

A sideswipe or rotational impact occurs when a vehicle hits something or is hit off-center (obliquely at an angle between frontal and lateral impact). The vehicle experiences a rotational force with the point of impact acting as the center. Occupants are exposed to a centrifugal force that results in combination injury patterns as seen in lateral and frontal, or lateral and rear-impact mechanisms. Lap and shoulder belts have been shown to be very effective in preventing injury from these collisions [25].

Rollover

Rollover collisions produce a complicated spectrum of injuries that range from minimal to severe. In general, the unrestrained occupant will not escape injury as multiple parts of the body strike different parts of the interior of the vehicle. That occupant is also at great risk for ejection. The well-restrained occupant, however (whose deceleration is well coupled with a vehicle), who does not hit any object during the roll, may well escape injury altogether, as the transferred kinetic energy is dissipated over a much longer distance than in frontal- and lateral-impact mechanisms. The degree of roof deformation has been linked to injuries; soft-top vehicles are likely to put occupants at higher risk. Many vehicles now have a central roll bar built in. Other factors that determine severity are the terrain that the vehicle is rolling through and the presence of objects that it may collide with.

Ejection

Occupants who are ejected from the vehicle sustain injuries both during the process of ejection as well as on impact. Ejection may be partial or complete. Partial ejection of a limb from a window may result in a severe crush or total amputation. Total ejection increases the victim's risk of dying sixfold. Almost 8% of ejected victims will suffer a spinal fracture [19].

The Effects of Restraints

Seatbelts. The benefits of correctly applied seatbelts in reducing injury have been repeatedly established [26,27]. It has been estimated that wearing a seat belt offers a 75% reduction in fatal injury and a 30% chance of preventing any injury [22]. Restraints couple the passenger to the frame of the moving vehicle, thus permitting the kinetic energy of the system to be dispersed toward deforming the vehicle for as long as possible [22]. Consequently, this decreases the amount of energy available to be transferred to the passenger (by decreasing the rate of change of the passenger's velocity). As an example, an unrestrained occupant sustains more than ten times the amount of deceleration in one-tenth of the time as a belted occupant in a vehicle that crashes into a cement wall at 55 km/hr (≈35 mph).

There has been a documented decrease in head, facial, thoracic, abdominal, and extremity injuries, particularly since the introduction of the shoulder belt. Seat belts are primarily protective in frontal collisions, which are commonly involved in serious injury.

It is sometimes unclear at the scene of a motor vehicle crash whether or not a restraint has been used. Evidence of restraint use includes stretched and abraded belt webbing from occupant loading, "burns" to seat fabric, abrasions or deformations to the seat back or pillar-mounted belt guides, and deformed motor components of the restraint system, as well as evidence of distinctive marks on the patient's body [21].

Lap–shoulder belts are most effective in preventing death and injury in crashes below 55 km/hr (≈35 mph). The residual deceleration forces are directed to more resilient parts of the body—the pelvis and thorax.

Air Bags. Frontal air bags have been available for over a decade. They appear to protect against serious facial, head, and chest injuries, but only in frontal crashes. The number of severe lower-extremity injuries is unaffected. The air bag serves as an additional restraint to the seatbelt in a frontal collision, with an impact angle within 30 degrees of head-on [28]. Side air bags are becoming more common.

Restraint-Associated Injuries. Despite their proven salutary effects, these protective systems are associated with their own set of injuries (Fig. 4). To function effectively, the lap belt should be worn between the anterior superior iliac spines and the femur. Worn above the iliac spines, the belt could cause compression injuries such as described earlier—mesenteric tear, rupture of hollow viscera, and lacerations of solid organs [29]. Hyperflexion of the torso over the seat belt may cause an anterior compression fracture of the lower lumbar vertebrae (Chance fracture) [30]. Children have an increased incidence of suffering a combination of these injuries [31,32]. It was hypothesized that because of their smaller size and underdeveloped pelvis that the lap belt would ride higher onto a child's abdomen [31].

Even a properly worn shoulder restraint may cause injury in the form of a fractured clavicle or a pneumothorax. If the shoulder belt is worn incorrectly under the axilla, fractured ribs and injuries to the lung, heart, or upper abdominal organs may result [33].

The National Highway Traffic Safety Administration (NHTSA) describes three injury patterns from close-proximity air bag deployment. First are basilar skull fractures, associated with brain stem lacerations and subdural and subarachnoid hemorrhages. Sec-

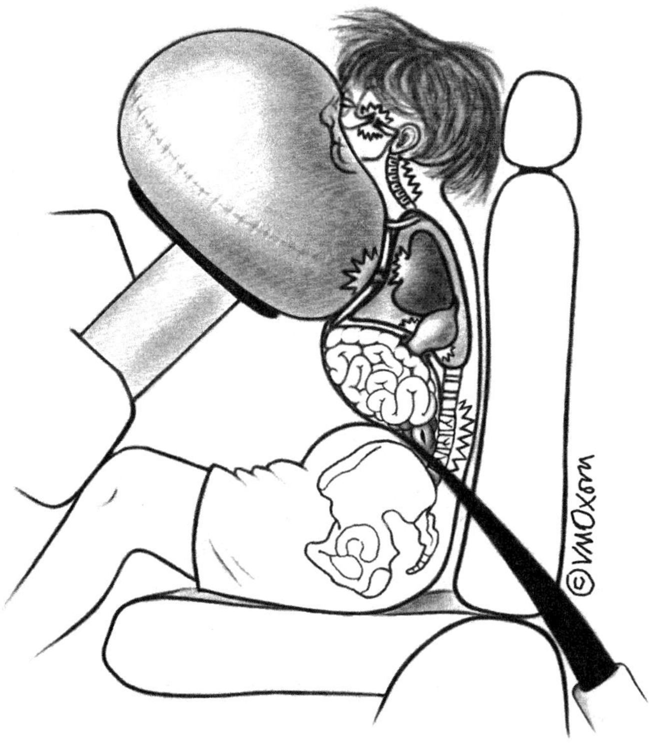

Figure 4 Restraint-associated injuries. Bowel may be ruptured when compressed between an incorrectly placed lap belt and the lumbar spine; hyperflexion of the torso over the lap belt may cause an anterior compression (''wedge'') fracture of the lumbar vertebrae. Airbags have been associated with cervical fracture, facial trauma, and chest injuries, particularly in the unbelted occupant, small adults, and children. (Illustration courtesy of Valerie Oxorn.)

ond are multiple rib fractures, usually bilateral, and often with associated thoracic and abdominal injuries. Third are cardiac and pulmonary injuries without rib fractures [34].

Benefits of air bag deployment are maximal in high-velocity impacts or in unbelted drivers. It has been suggested that in minor to moderate-severity crashes, air bag deployment may sometimes increase the overall likelihood of injury to the *belted* occupant [35]. Ocular, dental, and aural injuries have been described, as have burns to the upper extremity and face.

Recent publicity has been given to reports of deaths caused by air bags in the United States [34]. Because of the low rates of seat belt use in the United States (about 50%), air bags are designed to prevent injury to unrestrained occupants and therefore deploy more rapidly than air bags in other countries. These factors may have contributed to the deaths of 28 children in the front passenger seat and the deaths of 18 drivers (predominantly small women seated close to the steering wheel) up to September 1996. In all but one of the child fatalities, the child was unbelted or improperly restrained, allowing forward travel toward the air bag during precrash braking. It is estimated that up to the end of 1996, 2000 lives were saved by air bags in the United States [34].

The above emphasizes the importance that prehospital personnel should note whether or not restraints were used; *the unrestrained occupant in a crash in which no air bag has been deployed is likely to have been exposed to a much greater energy transfer than a restrained one* (*i.e., using a seat belt or air bag or both*).

4. Motorcycle and Bicycle Crashes

Riders of motorcycles and bicycles are particularly vulnerable in crashes because they do not have the benefit of the steel car frame to absorb the transmitted forces. A massive amount of energy is transferred to the cyclist on impact. The only piece of equipment that is able to redistribute some of the transmitted energy is the helmet, which offers some protection to the brain.

Frontal Impact/Ejection

When part of a motorcycle or bicycle strikes an object and is stopped, the remainder of the bike continues moving, along with the rider. Because the center of gravity (the pivot point) is the axle, the bike will tend to tip forward, causing the rider to go over the handlebars. Any part of the head, chest, or abdomen can be impacted onto the handlebars. Besides the usual blunt abdominal injuries, a traumatic rupture of part of the abdominal wall may occur, causing an acute herniation of abdominal contents. If the rider's feet remain in the footrests, the body may be restrained at the midshaft of the femurs, which will break as they strike the handlebars.

Lateral Impact/Ejection

Open or closed fractures of the extremities may occur on the impacted side. Injuries are similar to those that occur in a lateral impact to a car, only the energy transferred is much greater. Secondary injury occurs when the rider lands.

''Laying Down the Bike''

This is a strategy developed by bikers to uncouple themselves from the speed of the bike and slow themselves down from an impending impact. The bike is turned sideways (90°), then dropped, along with the inside leg, to the ground. Significant soft tissue injuries and road burn may occur in the down limb. This may be decreased to some extent by wearing leather garments and other protective equipment.

Helmets

Helmets have been shown to decrease the incidence of severe head injury in numerous studies. Head injury occurs in more than 30% of all bicycle-related injuries, and is the cause of death in 85% of fatalities. Helmets have been found to decrease fatal head injury by 30 to 50% [36]. They are designed to reduce direct force to the head and disperse it over the entire foam padding of the helmet. There is no evidence that the use of helmets leads to an increased incidence of cervical spine injuries.

5. Pedestrian Injury

This is primarily an urban problem, with more than 80% of such injuries occurring in residential areas. Almost 90% of automobiles that hit pedestrians are going less than 50 km/hr (≈30 mph). Most pedestrians are struck by the front of the vehicle, usually in an offset manner (e.g., by the passenger-side bumper). Most of the victims are children, senior citizens (women), or intoxicated adults (men) [37]. The majority of patients sustain some extremity injury, though the pattern of injury depends on the heights of the victim and the vehicle involved. Chest and abdominal injuries occur in children struck by cars and in adults struck by light vans, while most adults hit by cars have pelvic or lower extremity injuries.

Children tend to be knocked down by the bumper and run over. An adult's higher center of gravity means that he is more likely to be knocked up in the air and run under by the vehicle, especially if the vehicle is traveling at high speed.

The following describes the triad of adult pedestrian impact [22] (Fig. 5):

1. Bumper impact: The initial contact occurs when the bumper hits the pedestrian. Patient versus bumper height determines the nature of the injury. Tibia-fibula fractures, knee dislocations, and pelvic injuries are the most common. Femoral

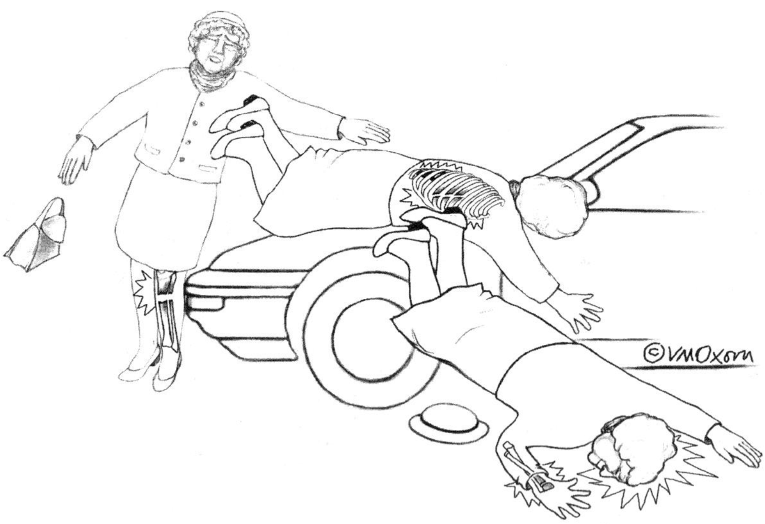

Figure 5 Patterns of pedestrian injury in an adult. Bumper impact causes lower limb or pelvic fractures. Hood and windshield impacts cause truncal injuries (chest and/or abdomen). Ground impact leads to head and facial injuries, and cervical spine and upper extremity fractures. (Illustration courtesy of Valerie Oxorn.)

fractures may be associated with impacts with taller vehicles (e.g., sports utility vehicles, vans, and minivans).

2. Hood and windshield impact: Following the initial impact, the patient is thrown onto the hood and may hit the windshield. Truncal injuries such as broken ribs or a ruptured spleen may result. Alternatively, the patient may be thrown into the air and land some distance away. Other organ compression injuries may also occur.
3. Ground impact: The final phase occurs when the victim slides off the hood and strikes the ground. At this point, he or she may suffer a head injury or upper extremity fractures. Injuries in two of the three areas of the body (e.g., head and lower extremity) should alert the physician to look for truncal injury as well.

6. Falls

Falls are the most common cause of nonfatal injury and the second leading cause of neurologic injury (brain and spinal cord) [38]. They can be categorized as a form of blunt trauma in which injury is caused by an abrupt change in velocity (ΔV). The characteristics of the contact surface and ΔV determine the severity of these injuries. The extent of the deceleration injury depends on

1. The rate of change of velocity, related to the distance of the fall
2. The size of the body surface area over which the kinetic energy is dissipated
3. The viscoelastic properties of the body tissues (i.e., how much ''give'' the body tissues have: bone vs. visceral organs)
4. The characteristics of the contact surface (how ''flexible'' or giving the surface is—trampoline vs. grass vs. concrete ground)

The position of the person upon landing determines the mechanism of energy transfer and frequently predicts the pattern of injuries sustained. A person who lands on his or her feet has the full force transmitted up the axial skeleton, resulting in calcaneal, tibial, femoral neck, and spinal fractures. Some intra-abdominal organs may be avulsed off the mesentery or peritoneal attachments. If the person lands on his or her back, however, the same amount of energy is transferred over a larger surface area, causing less significant damage. Landing on his or her head with the neck slightly flexed would result in a severe closed head injury and a cervical spine fracture, since most of the energy would be transferred to the skull and to the point where the neck is flexed.

Survival has been linked to falls from various heights. The LD_{50} (lethal dose—height at which 50% of the population will be killed) is estimated to be four stories or 48 feet, and the LD_{90} is estimated to be seven stories [39].

B. Penetrating Trauma

1. Stab Wounds

Most stab wounds can be defined as a crushing force caused by a sharp instrument that disrupts tissues. The degree of tissue damage depends on the shape, sharpness, size or length, and degree of penetration of the instrument. A description of the length and thickness should be obtained if it is no longer in the patient. With duller instruments, a degree of blunt trauma or crush injury is also present. The severity of the wounds depends on the location of the wound, the underlying structures, and the direction of the blade. Thoracic or abdominal wounds, and greater than four stab wounds have been correlated to serious injury. Most fatalities arise from chest wounds.

2. Gunshot Wounds

The availability of firearms to the public in many countries has unfortunately resulted in gunshot wound victims ending up in trauma units increasingly frequently. Where it is available, it is important to note the type of weapon used, the type of bullet, and the distance from weapon to victim. Police officers and witnesses may be useful in providing this information.

Some basic knowledge of ballistics and firearms is helpful in the assessment, triage, and management of these patients.

Ballistics

As in blunt trauma, the physical principles governing energy and its transfer are the same. Determinants of the degree of tissue damage from a bullet include the *amount* of energy transferred to the tissues from the bullet, the *time* it takes for the transfer to occur, and the surface *area* over which this energy transfer is distributed.

The energy that the bullet imparts upon the victim is defined by the same basic formula:

$$\text{Kinetic energy} = 1/2\ (\text{mass} \times \text{velocity}^2)$$

As is evident from this formula, the velocity of the missile is the most important factor in determining its wounding potential. Doubling the velocity results in a quadrupling of the kinetic energy, while doubling the mass of the missile only doubles the energy. The average distance between the victim and assailant in civilian shootings is about 7 meters, or 21 ft [40], therefore the impact velocity of the bullet on the victim is similar to the velocity of the missile as it leaves the muzzle of the firearm. Muzzle velocities may be classified into low ($<$1100 ft/sec, $\approx$335 meters/sec), medium (1100–2000 ft/sec, $\approx$335–600 meters/sec), and high ($>$2000 ft/sec, $>\approx$600/meters sec).

The caliber of a gun refers to the *internal diameter* of the gun barrel and may be measured in millimeters (9-mm Luger) or fractions of an inch (.357 Magnum). Larger barrels accommodate larger and heavier bullets. Magnum bullets contain more gunpowder, thereby increasing the muzzle velocity.

A variety of bullets are also in use in conjunction with the different kinds of firearms. Plain lead bullets come in different shapes and sizes and are used in low-velocity guns. Missiles shot from higher-velocity arms require a hard copper or copper alloy jacket because plain lead bullets are partially stripped before they leave the muzzle. A full-metal jacket bullet is one where the lead is entirely encased in copper. Partial-metal-jacketed bullets that have the lead tip exposed are known as soft points.

A shotgun shell is usually a cylindrical piece of plastic tubing filled with lead or steel pellets where the caliber is measured in ''gauges.'' Smaller gauges mean a larger size barrel. A larger caliber holds smaller and more numerous pellets. The denotation of the type of shot often gives a clue to the size of the pellets, as well as informs one what the weapon was designed to hunt. For example, birdshot pellets are smaller than buckshot pellets. A ''slug'' or a ''sabot'' is a large single piece of metal almost like a giant bullet. It is designed to be fired from a shotgun, and can produce a large, gaping wound at short range.

Firearms

The majority of firearms in civilian use can be classified under one of the following:

1. Handguns
2. Rifles
3. Shotguns

The first two classes of firearms are available in manual, semiautomatic, and automatic models. Manual weapons require cocking the hammer before each firing and are usually revolvers or target-shooting weapons. Semiautomatics house bullets in a magazine inserted into the handle of the weapon and will fire each time the trigger is pulled. These weapons can be handguns or rifles. Automatic weapons will continuously fire as long as the trigger is depressed.

Handguns are usually low- or medium-muzzle-velocity weapons (700–1500 ft/sec, $\approx$200–450 meters/sec). An example of this is the .357 Magnum. Rifles are high-velocity weapons ($>$2000 ft/sec, $\gtrsim$600 meters/sec). The notorious AK-47 is a Russian-designed rifle that has automatic and semiautomatic modes. Shotguns have a medium-muzzle velocity (1200 ft/sec, $\approx$365 meters/sec) and cause a massive amount of tissue destruction at close range ($<$9 ft, $\approx$3 meters). After firing, the pellets disperse in a conical formation from the muzzle. The nature of the spherical pellets, however, results in a quick loss of velocity in the air and even more after tissue impact. At moderate range (9–21 ft, $\approx$3–6.5 meters), the pellets cause multiple small superficial wounds; at greater distances ($>$21 ft, $\gtrsim$6.5 meters), minimal wounding occurs.

Wound Ballistics

As a missile travels through the body, it forms permanent and temporary cavities. The permanent cavity is about the same diameter as the bullet. Above the critical velocity of 2000 ft/sec ($\approx$600 meters/sec), missiles cause much greater tissue destruction because they create a temporary cavity in the tissue that is a result of the compressed tissues transmitting shock waves that may extend up to distances 30 times the diameter of the bullet [22]. Tissue damage from a high-velocity bullet may thus occur at some distance from the bullet path.

Other characteristics of the bullet trajectory also affect *how* the energy is dissipated to the tissues. Bullets with partial jackets are designed to flatten or ''mushroom'' on impact. This increases the area of skin contact, causing a more rapid deceleration and subsequently a greater transfer of energy over a shorter period of time, resulting in greater tissue damage. Other modifying factors are related to various motions of the bullet that are nonlinear or off its axis of translation. One example is *yaw*, the deviation of the bullet motion from its longitudinal direction of flight. The presence of yaw leads to *tumbling*, which again increases the area of contact with tissues, and increases the amount of energy transferred over a shorter time. Fragmentation of the missile works by the same principle.

The final determinant of the extent of tissue damage are the viscoelastic characteristics of the penetrated tissues themselves. Temporary cavitation in muscle, a relatively elastic tissue, has less permanent effect than in solid organs, such as the brain, liver, or kidneys. In these organs, the cavitation may become a permanent defect [36].

Missile energy may traverse an intact diaphragm, therefore thoracic injuries may be found with abdominal penetration and vice versa.

Entrance and Exit Wounds

Every victim of a shooting must be examined completely to determine the number of shots suffered. In addition to this, an attempt should be made to determine the path of each bullet from either the entrance to exit or the entrance to wherever the bullet may still be lodged in the tissues. Failure to do this results in missed injuries that are potentially life-threatening. It should not be assumed that the bullet trajectory was linear; missiles follow the path of least resistance and may internally ricochet off bony structures or even tissue planes. With the current weapons in use for civilian crimes, entrance wounds may be identified with a 1- to 2-mm circumferential area that is blackened by a burn caused by a spinning bullet entering tissue. Bullets fired at very close range may inject some gas into the surrounding subcutaneous tissues, producing some crepitus. Powder burns may also occur at the edges of the wound. Exit wounds are usually larger and may be ragged or stellate in appearance as a result of the tearing and splitting of the tissues [22].

C. Explosion Injuries

Explosions occur when the rate of energy production exceeds its rate of dissipation. A small volume of material is rapidly transformed into the gaseous state, resulting in a sudden release of energy and heat. If there are no barriers, the gas products will assume a spherical shape where the pressure in the center of the sphere is much higher than the atmospheric pressure. This expanding sphere of high pressure (as high as several atmospheres) transfers energy, as it causes mass movements of air in an oscillating fashion, but decreases quickly as it moves away from the source. This phase is followed by a negative pressure phase that lasts longer, also causes massive air movements, and is potentially as damaging as the initial blast. Blast waves may be reflected by buildings and other objects.

The nature and extent of the explosion, the distance of the victim from the blast, and evidence of secondary projectiles should be noted. Blast injuries may have characteristics of both blunt and penetrating trauma.

Injuries from explosions are classified into the following three kinds:

1. *Primary*: These injuries arise from the direct effect of the high pressure waves and are most harmful to gas- and water-containing organs [39]. Most vulnerable is the middle ear; the tympanic membrane may rupture if the pressure is above 2 atmospheres. It is unlikely that a serious blast occurred if the tympanic membrane is intact.

   Lung tissue may develop edema, hemorrhage, bullae, contusion, or rupture, and cause a pneumothorax (''blast lung''). Respiratory insufficiency may be delayed until more than 12 hr after the explosion. Air emboli may result from ruptured alveoli or pulmonary vessels and the formation of alveolar-pulmonary fistulae. Air emboli traveling to the coronary or cerebral circulations may be rapidly fatal.

   Other organs at risk include the bowel, which may rupture, and the eye, which may sustain intraocular hemorrhage and retinal detachment. Traumatic amputations of limbs are seen in severe blast injury or in those that are killed.
2. *Secondary*: Injury results from either blunt or penetrating trauma caused by objects rendered ''mobile'' by the original blast.
3. *Tertiary*: Injury occurs when the victim becomes mobile (in part or in whole) as a result of the explosion. Injuries suffered may be similar to those from an ejection or a fall.

Burns may occur as a result of ignition of combustibles in the area or by flash burns produced by the explosion.

D. Thermal Injuries

1. Burns

The assessment and management of the burned patient are addressed in Chapter 29 of this book. Both burn and cold injuries may be associated with trauma.

The history of the injury is essential in assessing the risk of concomitant traumatic injury in the burned patient. Injuries may be sustained when the victim is escaping the fire (e.g., by falls). If there has been an explosion, primary, secondary, and tertiary injuries may have been incurred, as discussed above. Burns may occur from ignited fuels at the scene of motor vehicle, aviation, and other accidents. Inhalational injuries and poisonings from carbon monoxide, cyanide gas, and toxic chemical spills may occur. It should be noted whether or not the patient was trapped in an enclosed space; this greatly increases the risk of inhalational injuries to the lower airway, asphyxiation, and carbon monoxide poisoning. Descriptions of the scene and the involvement of government organizations (where available) to identify toxic substances may improve the index of suspicion for serious traumatic and associated injuries.

2. Cold Injuries

Hypothermia worsens the prognosis in trauma patients. It is important to note the time of injury (and thus the length of exposure), ambient temperature, type of protective clothing, presence of moisture, and evidence of intoxication when assessing the trauma victim.

IV. SUMMARY

In the field, immediate, lifesaving management takes precedence over considerations of mechanism of injury. A careful but rapid gathering of the history of the event by personnel on the scene is extremely important. The physical forces involved in the trauma determine the amount of kinetic energy to which the trauma patient has been exposed. The mechanism of injury can provide clues in the identification of injuries. Important issues to consider may include the speed and direction of impact(s), extent of vehicle deformity and intrusion into the passenger compartment, use of restraints, height of fall or distance thrown, type of weapon, and distance from the assailant. Consideration of the mechanism probably reduces undertriage and therefore morbidity and mortality from trauma. Overtriage rates may be increased, especially in pediatric trauma.

REFERENCES

1. American College of Surgeons Committee on Trauma. Resources for Optimal Care of the Injured Patient: 1993. Chicago: American College of Surgeons, 1993.
2. JS Sampalis, R Denis, P Fréchette, R Brown, D Fleiszer, D Mulder. Direct transport to tertiary trauma centers versus transfer from lower level facilities: Impact on mortality and morbidity among patients with major trauma. J Trauma 43:288–296, 1997.
3. WB Long, BL Bachulis, GD Hynes. Accuracy and relationship of mechanisms of injury, trauma scores, and injury severity scores in identifying major trauma. Am J Surg 151:581–584, 1986.

3a. American College of Surgeons. Resources for Optimal Care of the Injured Patient: 1999. Chicago: American College of Surgeons, 1999.
4. IS Jones, SJ Shaibani. A comparison of injury severity distributions and their application to standards for occupant protection. Proceedings of the 1982 IRCOBI Conference, Cologne, Germany, Sept. 1982, pp. 1–16.
5. JA Phillips, TG Buchman. Optimizing prehospital triage criteria for trauma team alerts. J Trauma 34:127–132, 1993.
6. BJ Simon, P Legere, T Emhoff, VM Fiallo, J Garb. Vehicular trauma triage by mechanism: Avoidance of the unproductive evaluation. J Trauma 37:645–649, 1994.
7. CH Shatney, K Sensaki. Trauma team activation for ''mechanism of injury'' blunt trauma victims: Time for a change? J Trauma 37:275–282, 1994.
8. TJ Esposito, PJ Offner, GJ Jurkovich, J Griffith, RV Maier. Do prehospital trauma center criteria identify major trauma victims? Arch Surg 130:171–176, 1995.
9. RJ Bond, JB Kortbeek, RM Preshaw. Field trauma triage: Combining mechanism of injury with the prehospital index for an improved trauma triage tool. J Trauma 43:283–287, 1997.
10. LL Karsteadt, CL Larsen, PD Farmer. Analysis of a rural trauma program using the TRISS methodology: A three-year prospective study. J Trauma 36:395–400, 1994.
11. CL Emerman, B Shade, J Kubincanek. A comparison of EMT judgement and prehospital trauma triage instruments. J Trauma 31:1369–1375, 1991.
12. HR Champion, WJ Sacco, PS Gainer, SM Patow. The effect of medical direction on trauma triage. J Trauma 28:235–239, 1988.
13. LJ Kaplan, TA Santora, CA Blank-Reid, SZ Trooskin. Improved emergency department efficiency with a three-tier trauma triage system. Injury 28:449–453, 1997.
14. K Qazi, MS Wright, C Kippes. Stable pediatric blunt trauma patients: Is trauma team activation always necessary? J Trauma 45:562–564, 1998.
15. HR Champion, B Cushing. Emerging technology for vehicular safety and emergency response to roadway crashes. Surg Clin N Amer 79:1229–1240, 1999.
15a. JK Stene, CM Grande. Trauma Anesthesia. Baltimore: Williams and Wilkins, 1991, p. 51.
16. BR Boulanger, BA McLellan. Blunt abdominal trauma. Emerg Med Clin North Am 14:151–171, 1996.
17. MA Fox, TC Fabian, MA Croce, EC Mangiante, JP Carson, KA Kudsk. Anatomy of the accident scene: A prospective study of injury and mortality. Am Surg 57:394, 1991.
18. IS Jones, HR Champion. Trauma triage: Vehicle damage as an estimate of injury severity. J Trauma 29:646–653, 1989.
19. NE McSwain Jr. Mechanisms of injury in blunt trauma. In: NE McSwain Jr, MD Kerstein, eds. Evaluation and Management of Blunt Trauma. East Norwalk, CT: Appleton-Century-Crofts, pp. 129–166, 1987.
20. D Katyal, BA McLellan, FD Brenneman, BR Boulanger, PW Sharkey, JP Waddell. Lateral impact motor vehicle collisions: Significant cause of blunt traumatic rupture of the thoracic aorta. J Trauma 42:769–772, 1997.
21. JH Siegel, S Mason-Gonzalez, P Dischinger, B Cushing, K Read, R Robinson, J Smialek, B Heatfield, W Hill, F Bents, J Jackson, D Livingston, CC Clark. Safety belt restraints and compartment intrusions in frontal and lateral motor vehicle crashes: Mechanisms of injury, complications, and acute care costs. J Trauma 34:736–759, 1993.
22. American College of Surgeons, Committee on Trauma. Appendix 2: Biomechanics of Injury, In: Advanced Trauma Life Support Student Manual, 5th ed. Chicago: American College of Surgeons, 1997.
23. PC Dischinger, BM Cushing, TJ Kerns. Injury patterns associated with direction of impact: Drivers admitted to trauma centers. J Trauma 35:454–459, 1993.
24. BA McLellan, SB Rizoli, FD Brenneman, BR Boulanger, PW Sharkey, JP Szalai. Injury pattern and severity in lateral motor vehicle collisions: A Canadian experience. J Trauma 41: 708–713, 1996.

25. M Mackay. Kinematics of vehicle crashes. Adv Trauma 2:21–42, 1987.
26. BJ Campbell. Safety belt injury reduction related to crash severity and front seated position. J Trauma 27:733–739, 1987.
27. R Rutledge, A Lalor, D Oller, A Hansen, M Thomasen, W Meredith, MB Foil, C Baker. The cost of not wearing seat belts: A comparison of outcome in 3396 patients. Ann Surg 217: 122–127, 1993.
28. EH Kuner, W Schlickewei, D Oltmanns. Injury reduction by the airbag in accidents. Injury 27:185–188, 1996.
29. TB Sato. Effects of seat belts and injuries resulting from improper use. J Trauma 27:754–758, 1987.
30. WP Ritchie Jr, RA Ersek, WL Bunch, RL Simmons. Combined visceral and vertebral injuries from lap type seat belts. Surg Gyn Ob 131:431–439, 1970.
31. PF Agran, DE Dunkle, DG Winn. Injuries to a sample of seatbelted children evaluated and treated in a hospital emergency room. J Trauma 27:58–64, 1987.
32. AB Reid, RM Letts, GB Black. Pediatric Chance fractures: Association with intraabdominal injuries and seatbelt use. J Trauma 30:384–391, 1990.
33. T Saldeen. Fatal injuries caused by underarm use of shoulder belts. J Trauma 27:740–746, 1987.
34. R Martinez. Improving air bags. Ann Emerg Med 28:709–710, 1996.
35. DJ Dalmotas, A German, BE Hendrick, RM Hurley. Airbag deployments: The Canadian experience. J Trauma 38:476–481, 1995.
36. DV Feliciano. Patterns of injury. In: DV Feliciano, EE Moore, and KL Mattox, eds. Trauma, 3rd ed. Stamford, CT: Appleton and Lange, 1996, pp. 85–103.
37. JA Vestrup, JDS Reid. A profile of urban adult pedestrian trauma. J Trauma 29:741–745, 1989.
38. GS Rozycki, KI Maull. Injuries sustained by falls. Arch Emerg Med 8:245–252, 1991.
39. CM Grande, JK Stene. Mechanisms of injury: Etiologies of trauma. In: CM Grande, JK Stene, eds. Trauma Anesthesia. Baltimore: Williams and Wilkins, 1991, pp. 37–63.
40. T Lesse. Gunfighting tactics. Surv Guide 6:28, 1984.

4

The Role of the Physician in Prehospital Trauma Care

FREDDY K. LIPPERT

Rigshospitalet, Copenhagen University Hospital, Copenhagen, Denmark

ELDAR SØREIDE

University of Bergen and Rogaland Central Hospital, Stavanger, Norway; and Norwegian Air Ambulance Ltd., Høvik, Norway

I. INTRODUCTION

The organization of prehospital trauma care and the role of the physician in emergency medical services (EMS) systems differ from country to country [1,2]. These variations may be related to available medical resources, legal aspects, educational level of physicians and nonmedical personnel, geographic circumstances, and last but not least, tradition, interest, and commitment. In some systems, medical interventions that are the responsibility of physicians within the hospital are performed by nonphysicians outside the hospital.

In Europe, physicians, especially anesthesiologists, are often part of the prehospital trauma care system [1]. In the United States, however, physicians rarely participate in the initial response team but play a role as medical directors of prehospital EMS systems [3]. This chapter focuses on the role and potential of the physician in prehospital trauma care.

II. CHARACTERISTICS OF PREHOSPITAL TRAUMA CARE FOR THE PHYSICIAN

The principles of initial assessment and management of the injured patient outside the hospital do not differ from those in the emergency department [4,5]. Prehospital trauma care management requires additional skills and experience, however. The doctor must be able to cooperate with other prehospital personnel, such as paramedics, police officers, and firefighters. It is important to be aware of all the safety issues involved with prehospital work in an uncontrolled and often dangerous setting. The physician must be able to improvise, to take medical responsibility alone, and to manage patients, even with limited resources. Time pressure; the urgent need for priority decisions based on limited information; difficult access to the patient; limited space, backup options, and equipment, and limitations imposed by light and weather characterize prehospital work. A substantial difference is the existence of limited backup options, not only of resources and manpower but also of the type of equipment available. Physicians need only know the basic principle of extrication, but more importantly, must know and respect the roles and capabilities of other professionals at the scene [6,7].

III. THE GOALS OF PREHOSPITAL TRAUMA CARE

The primary goal of prehospital trauma care is to bring the patient to the hospital as fast as possible as well as to secure the vital functions without causing further harm to the patient [1,2]. Further, the goal is to provide optimal use of resources by appropriate triage and transport and by activation of those that are necessary and sufficient [4,5].

Only a few guidelines and recommendations have been published for prehospital trauma care [5,8]. The debate over whether to ''scoop and run'' or ''stay and play'' continues [1,2]. The recommendations of the American College of Surgeons state [5] that ''the treatment of the severely injured patient in the prehospital arena should consist of assessment, extrication, initiation of resuscitation, and rapid transportation to the closest appropriate facility.'' These principles apply to all prehospital care providers, and whether use of prehospital emergency physicians improves survival rates is still debated. Improving the survival rate seems to be related to both rapid response and an advanced level of prehospital medical care, combined with rapid transport to the appropriate level of definitive care (a trauma care facility) [9–11].

IV. THE POTENTIAL OF PHYSICIANS IN PREHOSPITAL TRAUMA CARE

Physicians might be involved in prehospital trauma care at different levels: as prehospital care providers at the scene, as on-scene supervisors, or as medical directors [3,7–9,12,13]. The primary roles of the physicians *at* the scene are as follows:

To assess the scene together with other prehospital personnel. Safety first!
To identify and treat immediate life-threatening conditions.
To identify priorities in patient care and transportation (triage).
To prevent secondary injuries (primarily avoiding hypoxia and hypotension).
To ensure safe and fast transport.
To effect correct triage to the appropriate facility.

To be able to fulfill these roles, the physician must be well trained in advanced airway management, establishment of intravascular lines, and administration of different drugs and dosages for emergency medical cases before starting in the prehospital environment. A few essential points concerning the physician's potential as a prehospital care provider will be addressed below.

A. Assessment, Diagnosis, and Medical Triage

It is important to treat life-threatening injuries as early as possible and avoid prehospital delays in treatment and transport [1,2,4,5]. Proper triage is a hallmark of a good trauma system. Triage is dependent on established criteria for mechanisms of injury and signs of anatomic injuries and physiologic deterioration [4,5]. It is well known and accepted that substantial ''overtriage'' is necessary to avoid loss due to ''undertriage.'' Although it is tempting to think that an initial assessment made by a physician should lead to a more correct assessment and triage for the trauma patient, this is not necessarily so. Linn et al. [14] found a significant underdiagnosing of injuries in their study of flight physicians. Regel et al. [8] also found that prehospital emergency physicians frequently misdiagnose and do not perform the indicated emergency interventions. Experience and rapid individual feedback from the receiving hospital probably constitute the best way to improve this situation.

What can be done and what should be done depends on the experience, skills, and judgment of the physician, based on the available medical resources. If diagnoses and individual judgment are necessary, it is important that the physician who is directly involved at the scene or is providing medical advice from a medical control center has some ''street experience'' [9,12,13,15]. Based on this advice, the findings of Rinnert et al. [3] are alarming. They found that only 40% of the medical directors of U.S. flight nurse- and paramedic-staffed helicopter EMS systems had any practical flight experience or training themselves and that only 7% worked full time as medical director.

B. Airway Management, Drugs, and Dosages

Airway obstruction is a major contributing factor in deaths resulting from trauma [16,17]. Early endotracheal intubation and controlled ventilation have a high priority in the initial management of the severely injured patient [18–22]. To secure a definitive airway in severely injured patients is definitely a challenge even to experienced prehospital care providers. In some EMS systems, doctors provide airway management both inside and outside the hospital, while in other systems prehospital care is the responsibility of flight nurses and paramedics. Irrespective of the background of the care provider, a high success rate in advanced airway management (rapid and smooth endotracheal intubation) depends on the use of neuromuscular blocking agents (NMBAs) and some form of sedation to facilitate the intubation and secure the tube in place without the patient being awake, in pain, or paralyzed. The use of NMBAs has been restricted in the out-of-hospital setting because of fear of complications in the hands of inexperienced providers [23]. In some countries, the use of NMBAs is even restricted to anesthesia-trained personnel. There will always be a balance between the potential complications of not intubating or attempting endotracheal intubation without paralysis and the risk of further harm to the patient when these drugs are used by inexperienced personnel [12,23,24].

Prehospital airway management (endotracheal intubation versus mask ventilation in children) was the subject of a recent large controlled study by Gausche and colleagues [21]. The investigators failed to show any improvement in survival or neurologic outcome in severely injured and critically ill children in an advanced paramedic system with the use of endotracheal intubation. The number of interventions per provider was limited, however, and the success rate was poor (57%). Furthermore, the interventions were accompanied by high complication rates, including esophageal intubation and unrecognized dislodgement, even though the patients were those most likely to be intubated successfully (mostly in cardiopulmonary arrest). In a recent review [25] of the topic, Falk and Sayre pointed out that not only intubation success but also the location of the tube when the patient reached the hospital is important. Numbers of unrecognized misplaced endotracheal tubes in adults (esophagus, oropharynx)—as high as 25%—have been reported from paramedic-run systems. This lack of experience and avoiding NMBAs is probably reflected by a high incidence of cricothyroidotomy among trauma patients in prehospital settings in the United States [26,27].

Such data differ from those from the physician-based French EMS system, in which 99% of 691 consecutive prehospital intubations were performed successfully in the field by experienced physicians [22]. The French EMS system has achieved similar success rates in children [28]. This difference probably demonstrates both the importance of experience and maintenance of skills, as well as the importance of being able and allowed to use NMBAs to facilitate endotracheal intubation. Whether or not a physician-based system, all other factors being equal, works better in terms prehospital airway management has never been shown in a controlled trial, and probably never will.

C. Definitive Care

The term *definitive care* is often used exclusively to describe surgical intervention for severely injured patients. The majority of patients suffering from blunt trauma and burn patients do not need immediate surgical intervention, however, but are in need of critical care as provided in the intensive care unit. Victims of head injury constitute a large group of patients for whom definitive care can be initiated and provided at the scene to prevent secondary injury [20,27]. This approach demands proper assessment, diagnosis, and competence to decide to treat in the prehospital arena, which can be better achieved in a physician-based system instead of a protocol-driven EMS system [13,29]. Finally, from a legal point of view, the presence of a physician should make it easier to suspend or withhold treatment in case of futile resuscitation.

D. Mass Casualty and Disaster Management

Management of major incidents and disasters is an important part of prehospital trauma care. It is often necessary to use medical teams in the field. Appropriate decisions concerning triage, transportation, and communication are essential elements in both the effectiveness of the response system and the provision of an appropriate level of care to all victims. Most plans for disaster management include the use of a medical team. We think that to be able to function in this situation, prior prehospital experience is necessary, including participation in disaster exercises. Hospital physicians with no street experience tend to arrive inappropriately clothed and with unrealistic expectations. Personnel who are accustomed to working in the prehospital arena should lead the medical rescue work in mass-casualty situations [30].

E. Research

Most of the research on prehospital trauma care has been initiated by hospital-based physicians working in non-physician-based prehospital EMS systems. Many studies have found that advanced life support and an increase in on-scene time seem to correlate with a delay of time to definitive care and thereby increase mortality and morbidity [31]. Others investigators have found that the relationship between advanced life support, prolonged scene times, and survival is not all that easy to understand [32]. Spaite et al. [32] pointed out that such component-based research models (prehospital phase only) in trauma have led authors to ask the wrong questions and use the wrong methods. Instead Spaite et al. suggest that the whole ''chain of survival'' from the incident scene throughout the hospital stay should be studied together to get a better picture of what is important. The keywords are *overall time use* and *quality of care*. Further, in such studies it is important to differentiate between blunt and penetrating trauma and urban versus rural areas, as the approach to prehospital trauma care must be different [1,2,7]. To allow future research to answer the important questions, we feel it is important that physicians with actual street experience lead the way and present outcome results from their own systems [1,6–9,13,22,27].

V. QUALIFICATIONS NEEDED BY PHYSICIANS

Qualifications and training requirement for physicians involved in prehospital care are often not formally stated. The optimal qualifications include extensive medical experience, formal in- and prehospital training, and the right personal attributes. The ideal qualifications require an experienced and senior physician, but in the real world junior physicians are taking part in prehospital trauma care. As Goethe stated, nothing is more scary than ignorance in action. This certainly would apply to junior doctors who have no formal or practical competence in the prehospital work they have been left to do, but do have the approval to do whatever they feel is necessary. Some minimum training requirements are thus needed.

Formal medical training should include knowledge and skills in the management of life-threatening injuries and conditions. Prerequisites are in-hospital experience in life-saving procedures, including advanced airway management, attaining intravascular access, and skill with various procedures from the emergency department, operating room, or the intensive care unit (e.g., chest drainage). Formal prehospital education and maintenance of prehospital skills are especially important for physicians. This includes safety issues, knowledge of extrication [6], radio communication, and logistics of the casualty scene, including mass casualty management and disaster management. Personal attributes include not only medical skills and knowledge but also the ability to cooperate with other EMS personnel, police officers, and fire brigades. In addition, the ability to improvise and adapt to unusual conditions is very important. No specialty encompasses all of these qualifications, but anesthesiologists, emergency physicians, and trauma surgeons have the proper medical background and serve as prehospital emergency physicians [1,6,7,9,13,22]. For any specialty it is necessary to gain additional education and prehospital experience and to maintain and develop practical skills during continuing practice. The best combination for any physician involved in prehospital trauma care is a mixture of hospital and prehospital work to keep up all the skills needed.

VI. THE FUTURE

Concentrating resources and expertise to care for the severely injured patient has resulted in improved outcome and other benefits for the patients [11]. The role of the physician in the prehospital part of the trauma chain of survival varies from system to system and probably will continue to do so in the future in regard to medical care as well as to the legal, financial, and historical aspects. Still, if prehospital trauma care is to be improved, evolved, and expanded, strong physician commitment is needed and clinical guidelines must be developed. We believe that standardization of qualifications also should be addressed, either in local or national contexts. Challenges in organization of prehospital care are present worldwide for emergency medical systems, and different solutions might be adapted; one of them is a physician-based system.

VII. SUMMARY POINTS

Physicians are directly involved in prehospital trauma care to different degrees in different emergency medical systems.

In some systems, among them many European ones, physicians act as prehospital care providers.

To what extent physician-based systems provide better trauma care is still a matter of debate.

Besides extensive in-hospital experience in practical management of life-threatening injuries, the qualifications of physicians taking part in prehospital trauma care should include formal education, personal fitness, and on-scene experience.

REFERENCES

1. P Carli. Prehospital intervention for trauma: Helpful or harmful? The European point of view. Curr Opin Crit Care 4:407–411, 1998.
2. PE Pepe. Prehospital intervention for trauma: Helpful or harmful? The American point of view. Curr Opin Crit Care 4:412–416, 1998.
3. KJ Rinnert, IJ Blumen, SG Gabram, M Zanker. A descriptive analysis of air medical directors in the United States. Air Med J 18:6–11, 1999.
4. American College of Surgeons, Committee on Trauma. Advanced Trauma Life Support. Chicago: American College of Surgeons, 1997.
5. American College of Surgeons, Committee on Trauma. Resources for Optimal Care of the Injured Patient: 1999. Chicago: American College of Surgeons, 1999.
6. A Ersson, M Lundberg, C-O Wramby, H Svensson. Extrication of entrapped victims from motor vehicle accidents: The crew concept. Eur J Emerg Med 6:341–347, 1999.
7. E Soreide, C Deakin, D Baker. Prehospital trauma management for the anesthesiologist. Anesth Clin North Am 17:33–43, 1999.
8. G Regel, A Seekamp, T Pohlemann, U Schmidt, H Bauer, H Tscherne. Does the accident patient need to be protected from the emergency doctor? Unfallchirurg 101:160–175, 1998.
9. G Regel, P Lobenhoffer, M Grotz, HC Pape, U Lehmann, H Tscherne. Treatment results of patients with multiple trauma: An analysis of 3406 cases treated between 1972 and 1991 at a German level 1 trauma center. J Trauma 38:70–78, 1995.
10. G Sanson, S Di Bartolomeo, G Nardi, P Albanese, A Diani, L Raffin, C Filippetto, A Cattarsossi, F Scian, L Rizzi. Road traffic accidents with vehicular entrapment: Incidence of major injuries and need for advance life support. Eur J Emerg Med 6:285–291, 1999.
11. Skamania Symposium. Trauma systems, evidence, research, action. J Trauma 47(suppl. no. 3), 1999.
12. D Leibovici, B Fredman, ON Gofrit, J Shemer, A Blumenfeld, SC Shapira. Prehospital cricothyroidotomy by physicians. Am J Emerg Med 15:91–93, 1997.
13. U Schmidt, M Stalp, T Gerich, M Blauth, KI Maull, H Tscherne. Chest tube decompression of blunt chest injuries by physicians in the field: Effectiveness and complications. J Trauma 44:98–101, 1998.
14. S Linn, N Knoller, CG Giligan, U Dreifus. The sky is the limit: Errors in prehospital diagnosis by flight physicians. Am J Emerg Med 15:316–320, 1997.

15. PJ Shirley, AA Klein. Sydney Aeromedical Retrieval Service. Prehosp Immed Care 8:233–227, 1999.
16. LM Hussain, AD Redmond. Are pre-hospital deaths from accidental injury preventable? BMJ 308:1077–1180, 1994.
17. IN Papadopoulos, D Bukis, E Karalas, S Katsaragakis, G Peros, G Androulakis. Preventable pre-hospital deaths in a Helenic urban health region—An audit of pre-hospital care. J Trauma 41:864–869, 1996.
18. RM Chesnut, FM Lawrence, MR Klauber, BA Blunt, N Baldwin, HM Eisenberg, JA Jane, A Marmarou, MA Foulkes. The role of secondary brain injury in determining outcome from severe head injury. J Trauma 34:216–222, 1993.
19. RJ Winchell, DB Hoyt. Endotracheal intubation in the field improves survival in patients with severe head injury. Arch Surg 132:592–597, 1997.
20. Brain Trauma Foundation, American Association of Neurological Surgeons, Joint Section on Neurotrauma and Critical Care. Guidelines for the management of severe head injury. 13: 641–734, 1996.
21. M Gausche, RJ Lewis, SJ Stratton, BE Haynes, CS Gunter, SM Goodrich, PD Poore, MD McCollough, DP Henderson, FD Pratt, JS Seidel. Effect of out-of-hospital pediatric endotracheal intubation on survival and neurological outcome. JAMA 283:783–790, 2000.
22. F Adnet, NJ Jouriles, P Le Toumelin, B Hennequin, C Taillandier, F Rayeh, J Couvreur, B Nougière, P Nadiras, A Ladka, M Fleury. Survey of out-of-hospital emergency intubations in the French prehospital medical system: A multicenter study. Ann Emerg Med 32:454–460, 1998.
23. SA Pace, FP Fuller. Out-of-hospital succinylcholine-assisted endotracheal intubation by paramedics. Ann Emerg Med 35:568–572, 2000.
24. JS Bradley, GL Billows, ML Olinger, SP Boha, WH Cordell, DR Nelson. Prehospital oral endotracheal intubation by rural basic emergency medical technicians. Ann Emerg Med 32: 26–32, 1998.
25. JL Falk, MR Sayre. Confirmation of airway placement. Prehosp Emer Care 3:273–278, 1999.
26. LE Jacobson, GA Gomez, RJ Sobieray, GH Rodman, KO Solotkin, ME Misinski. Surgical cricothyroidotomy in trauma patients: Analysis of its use by paramedic in the field. J Trauma 41:15–20, 1996.
27. RF Sing, ME Rotondo, DH Zonies, CW Schwab, DR Kaubder, SE Ross, CCM Brathwaite. Rapid sequence induction for intubation by an aeromedical transport team: A critical analysis. Am J Emerg Med 16:598–602, 1998.
28. GA Orliaguet, PG Meyer, S Blanot, M Jarreau, B Charron, C Buisson, PA Carli. Predictive factors of outcome in severely traumatized children. Anesth Analg 87:537–542, 1998.
29. S Zalstein, PA Cameron. Helicopter emergency medical services: Their role in integrated trauma care. Austr NZ J Surg 67:593–598, 1997.
30. J de Boer, M Dubouloz. Handbook of Disaster Medicine. International Society of Disaster Medicine, 2000.
31. S Feero, JR Hedges, E Simmons, L Irwin. Does out-of-hospital EMS time affect trauma survival? Am J Emerg Med 13:133–135, 1995.
32. DW Spaite, EA Criss, TD Valenzula, HW Meislin. Prehospital advanced life support for major trauma: Critical need for clinical trials. Ann Emerg Med 32:480–489, 1998.

5

The Role of the Transport Nurse in Prehospital Trauma Care

CHARLENE MANCUSO and WILLIAM F. FALLON, Jr.

MetroHealth Medical Center, Cleveland, Ohio

I. THE DEVELOPMENT OF FLIGHT NURSING AS A SPECIALTY

A. Historical Perspective

The role of the nurse in prehospital air and ground transport has evolved principally in the United States. The role of nursing in the transport of patients began much like the role of nursing in general in time of war. Florence Nightingale introduced sanitary science through nursing care in military hospitals from 1854 to 1855. She reduced the death rate in the British Army from 42% to 2%. Miss Nightingale founded the first training school for nurses at St Thomas's Hospital in 1860 and brought professionalism to the art of nursing.

The transport of ill and injured patients first occurred in 1870 during the Prussian siege of Paris, when 160 soldiers were flown by hot air balloon over enemy lines [1]. In 1918 the U.S. Army had an air ambulance in Louisiana and Texas [2].

In 1930 eight nurses served as nurse stewardesses on transcontinental flights. In 1933 Laurette Schimmoler, a licensed pilot, worked with a group of interested nurses to form the Emergency Flight Corps, a group dedicated to the research and development of nurses in aviation to achieve better patient care and improve air ambulance safety [2].

Having recognized the importance of flight nursing, the military began the first training program for flight nursing in conjunction with the 349th Air Evacuation School at Bowman Field, in Louisville, Kentucky in 1943. The initial training course was four weeks long and covered air evacuation, aeromedical physiology, survival tactics, mental hygiene, and field training [3]. Both the army and navy instituted flight-training programs for nurses.

During World War II 1.5 million patients were transported accompanied by in-flight medical attendants. Seventeen flight nurses died in the line of duty, 16 were missing in action, and Brigadier General Grant declared that the success of air evacuation in World War II was due to flight nurses [4]. Since 1942 the Air Force has trained over 10,500 flight nurses (T. Moore, personal communication, August 1985).

The Korean and Vietnam conflicts introduced another aspect of aeromedical transport, the helicopter. Prior to this time, most patient transport was done by airplane. In the mid-1960s Europe instituted the first civilian use of helicopters for patient transport. In 1972 the United States began its first civilian flight program at St. Anthony's hospital in Denver, Colorado, in which registered nurses with critical care experience provided medical care during transport. In 1976 Herman Hospital, in Houston, Texas, introduced the second flight program, which utilized a physician/nurse medical team. In 1980 a national flight organization was created, the American Society of Hospital-Based Emergency Air Medical Services (ASHBEAMS), known today as the Association of Air Medical Services (AAMS). In 1981 the National Flight Nurses Association (NFNA) was created. Today this organization has evolved to include both air and ground nursing professionals and is called the Air and Surface Transport Association (ASTNA) [5]. Because critical care transports are being completed in both air- and ground-based environments, the organization can provide guidance to the transport nurse in either venue. These organizations created minimum standards for the medical transport crew configuration that mandated that at least one member of the medical crew be a specially trained professional registered nurse who had extensive experience and expertise in caring for critically ill and injured patients [6].

II. THE ROLE OF THE NURSE AS A CORE MEMBER OF A MEDICAL TEAM

While in Europe the physician is considered the core member of the transport team, in the United States the registered nurse is the core team member of any critical care transport program. Depending on the geographic area and the mission profile of the program, additional crew members may include a physician, another nurse, a paramedic, or a respiratory therapist. The development of regional referral centers has expanded the transport patient population to include specialty transports, including the neonate, the pediatric patient, the burn patient, and the cardiovascular emergency, including the intra-aortic balloon pump (IABP) patient. Transport nurses are trained to care for critically ill and injured patients of all ages in a variety of settings; for example, a helicopter, a plane, the back of an ambulance, the scene of a crash, the emergency department, or the intensive care unit. Transport nurses practice in advanced, autonomous, independent roles, performing duties and skills consistent with critical care and emergency medicine in medical transport [7]. Their primary education, training, and licensure is therefore of utmost importance.

III. TEAM COMPOSITION

A. The Nurse/Paramedic Team

Internationally, the physician/physician [8] physician/nurse crew [9], or physician/paramedic predominate. In the United States more than half the air medical programs have a medical crew comprising a nurse and paramedic. This trend has been found to be the most cost-effective crew configuration [9]. While nurses and paramedics receive the same flight readiness training and can usually perform the same technical skills, such as intubation, c-spine stabilization, and needle decompression, the nurse brings to the team the emergency/critical care experience from the hospital setting, which makes the nurse accountable for more complex assessment and intervention skills. Managing titrating IV drips, managing pain, and coordinating overall patient care is based on the clinical picture assessed both before and during the actual transfer. The nurse usually assumes the leadership role during interhospital transports because of the clinical critical care expertise that is necessary. The paramedic may take the lead role during prehospital transports because of the required expertise in the field management of patients. The team collaborates by phone or radio with a doctor when available to assure appropriate medical judgments are made. The nurse/paramedic team utilizes protocol developed in conjunction with the transport program's medical director.

B. The Nurse/Physician Team

Based on an air medical survey conducted in the United States in 1994, less than 7% of the air medical programs utilize a nurse/physician medical crew configuration. Substantially fewer physicians in the U.S. environment are part of ground transport teams. Forty-three percent of the physicians flying are in a residency program. Flight physician expertise can range from the level of an interm in training to the expertise of a board certified specialist [10]. As a crew member the physician may be the final medical authority. This is not always the case, however. Collaboration between the nurse and the physician is essential because the nurse is the consistent team member and the physician may be coordinating patient care on interfacility transports or at a prehospital scene. Many programs with physicians as part of the medical crew find it is less important to having standing protocols in place. The literature demonstrates that the physicians' most important contribution to the medical team is the ability to both evaluate patients and make a decision to treat immediately, rather than actually carrying out the treatment, which is usually done by the critical care transport nurse [11].

C. The Nurse/Nurse Team

In most programs using this crew configuration the mission profile of the program includes predominantly interhospital transfers that need the intensive care background of the nurse to maintain the appropriate level of care for patients being transferred from an ICU to a specialty center or tertiary care center ICU, such as a level 3 NICU or a heart transplant center. The nurse/nurse team works through established medical protocols designed for the specific patient population being served. Other team configurations may include the addition of a respiratory therapist, a perfusionist, or a neonatal nurse, depending on the mission profile of the program and the patient population being served.

IV. PREPARATION FOR THE ROLE OF FLIGHT NURSE

The role and responsibilities of the transport nurse include clinical practice, patient advocacy, management, administration, consultation, research, and education. The practice of transport nursing is currently regulated by the governmental or state boards of nursing in accordance with their nursing practice acts, and any government regulations pertaining to prehospital care. The transport nurse also practices in accordance with both ASTNA standards and policies and procedures instituted by medical direction and the program's transport nurses. In a study compiled in 1995 it was shown that one-third of the nurses had baccalaureate degrees (BSN) and had 10 to 15 years nursing experience in critical care and/or emergency nursing [7]. Most U.S. programs hire nurses with at least 2 years of intensive care unit or emergency department experience with certifications in advanced cardiac life support (ACLS), basic trauma life support (BTLS), or prehospital life support (PHTLS), pediatric life support (PALS), and certified emergency nursing (CEN).

There are currently three curriculums that outline the recommended education and skills needed to practice transport nursing. These are the *Flight Nurse Advanced Trauma* course from NFNA [12] the *Air Medical Crew National Curriculum* from the U.S. Department of Transportation [13], and the *National Standard Guidelines for Prehospital Nursing* from the Emergency Nurses Association (ENA) [14]. In 1994 a certified flight registered nurse examination (CFRN) was developed to provide a mechanism of verifying a body of knowledge related to the practice of flight nursing [7].

Because of the variability of patients being cared for, the additional training and skills needed for transport nursing include knowledge of prehospital care such as extrication, disaster scene triage, and scene safety. In most U.S. programs the transport nurse is also certified as an emergency medical technician (EMT). Clinical skills must be learned and maintained that allow the transport nurse to perform such procedures as intubation, cricothyroidotomy, intraosseous insertion, cutdown, central line placement, thoracentesis, chest tube insertion, birthing procedures, and escharotomy. Ventilatory management, IABP management, pain management, medication administration, and complex assessment skills are also necessary skills to master and maintain competency in when functioning as a transport nurse in any setting.

The transport nurse must constantly question, analyze, and evaluate the entire transport process so that organized, efficient, and quality care is provided to the patient. Learning the necessary skills is done through hands-on experience in a hospital laboratory setting or in a monitored patient care setting. Many programs require skills such as intubation, chest tube insertion, and IABP to be performed a certain number of times to remain "competent." The need to keep the transport nurse competent becomes part of the programmatic strategic planning with continuing lectures and hands-on practice sessions that review and update skills in settings such as animal labs, the OR, or simulated situation. Structured lectures with hands-on practice sessions should be routinely scheduled with nurses expected to attend in order to maintain their ability to transport patients of various types.

V. MAINTAINING COMPETENCY IN THE FLIGHT NURSE ROLE

One format used to maintain competency is periodic chart review with the nurse's peers and medical director. An interactive group session is most beneficial, but a review by the medical director and the chief flight nurse is minimally required to assure consistency and competency in the care provided by the medical team. Transports that are high risk or have problem-prone care or those requiring difficult procedural intervention, transports requiring judgments made that may conflict with protocol, or even just a general posttransport review session allows the nursing team members to discuss strategies for improving patient care or delivering more efficient care during the transfer process. Here the team members can review the entire transport with input from their peers that allows for the identification and resolution of potential problems. Ideas are formulated to change specific transfer components to improve the overall process. The process should have an educational component to it as well as a performance-improvement focus.

Other strategies used to keep nursing skills at an acceptable level are to provide periodic skill labs for ongoing training. Whether one uses in-hospital training such as intubating in the OR, cadaver labs, animal labs, or manikin labs, it is very important to stress the need to routinely practice skills that may not be used on a regular basis during transport but must be maintained for those situations that require such expertise.

VI. THE ROLE OF THE PHYSICIAN RELATED TO THE FLIGHT NURSE

In other countries, such as India, the physician may be part of a physician/physician team or a physician/nurse team, or may even be sent out as a single provider of care in the prehospital environment [8]. In rural eastern Africa the African Medical Research Foundation (AMREF) Flying Doctor Service, founded 42 years ago by two surgeons, provides evacuation care and consultation by three surgeons to rural hospitals [15]. In Greece the medical team consists of physicians trained in an advanced trauma life support (ATLS) course and nurses experienced in the ICU [9].

As stated earlier, in the United States physicians function as team members in some flight programs. In most situations, however, the physician's role is that of the program's medical director. In this capacity the physician is responsible for several aspects of the transport program. According to a survey of U.S. air medical directors conducted in 1995 there were six commonly reported areas of involvement:

1. Protocol development (87.6%)
2. Quality improvement activities (86.3%)
3. Medical crew training (80.4%)
4. Administrative negotiations (79.1%)
5. Online medical control (71.9%)
6. Personnel hiring (59.5%) [16]

The Air Medical Physicians Association (AMPA) is considered a forerunner in the development of an educational tool for physicians with publication of the Air Medical Physician Handbook [17].

VII. THE CONTINUOUS PERFORMANCE IMPROVEMENT PROCESS

For the transport nurse, the performance improvement (PI) process is a combination of the traditional QA (quality assurance) process and a QI/QM (quality improvement quality monitoring) process. Quality Assurance in the traditional sense monitored different indicators retrospectively and compared the indicators to some pre-established threshold of acceptance. Many health care organizations performed QA to satisfy externally mandated requirements by regulatory bodies such as the Joint Commission for Accreditation of Hospital Organizations (JCAHO). This process was generally viewed in a negative light because it was built on the premise that individuals were not meeting standards or they were doing a bad job. In many instances critical incidents were reviewed based on incomplete data.

Quality improvement/quality monitoring took a different approach. This process focuses on determining activities that will please the customer. In the health care arena there are expectations of care and care delivery, and programs need to determine what is needed to make a positive impact on the service being delivered. Quality improvement/quality monitoring is more of a team participatory process. It is based on gathering and displaying facts and statistics that pertain to specific areas being monitored. Then a consistent problem-solving methodology is implemented that yields much more productive, reproducible solutions and behaviors than the traditional QA problem-solving did. Every member of the team must be involved in the QI/QM process for it to be beneficial. Team members must have the ability to make constructive decisions or changes with no bureaucratic interference. This means the transport program leadership must take an active role in initiating and maintaining an ongoing QI/QM process.

Quality improvement/quality monitoring was multifaceted, and included some retrospective review of areas that are consistently important to customer satisfaction, such as a review of the team's mission profile and the ongoing continuing education and credentialing. This ensures the program is meeting its own standards. Other general categories of care should be delineated and then a decision made by the QI/QM committee about which ones to monitor and how to monitor and evaluate the different components or processes of care. There should be a written QI/QM plan to use as an organizational tool or template. This assures that whatever component of the QI process is being reviewed, it has a systematic and organized structure to follow. Ongoing multifaceted transport team patient care reviews are another component of QI/QM. In an educational, peer-oriented meeting, cases that display high risk or problem-prone situations should be discussed and methods of care reviewed to determine appropriateness. Also, groups of patients with similar presenting problems whose outcomes are often litigious should be reviewed.

The QI/QM process also incorporated the appropriateness utilizing the transport service. There are several organizations that propose utilization criteria [18]. Each program must develop a method to evaluate the appropriateness of the medical transports undertaken, however. Some criteria to be considered are included in Table 1. These components of utilization review should be done both retrospectively and concurrently.

PI emphasizes a continuous multidisciplinary effort to measure, evaluate, and improve both the process of care and the outcome. A major objective of PI is to reduce any inappropriate variation in care [19].

PI is an ongoing cycle of monitoring, assessment, modification, and reevaluation. There must be reliable data collection methods that can obtain valid and objective information so that opportunities for improvement can be observed through the data collection obtained. There must be

1. Clear authority and accountability for the PI program through leadership
2. Clear organizational structure

Table 1 Examples of Utilization Criteria for Review

Did the patient's condition warrant a transfer?	Y	N
Did the level of medical care needed during transport mandate the air versus ground mode of transportation?	Y	N
What location, geographic, or logistic element made air transport the most reasonable mode of transport?		
Did the weather play a role in the decision to use air transport?	Y	N
Was the patient transported multiple times for the same condition within 24 hours?	Y	N
Did the cost of air versus ground transport play a role in the decision making?	Y	N

3. Appropriate, objective standards used to determine quality.
4. Clear definition of outcomes developed from the objective standards [19]

Monitoring is done through

1. Data collection-registry data
2. PI forms that can be initiated by anybody
3. Peer review data

Assessment of the data may show the standard is being met consistently, or when analyzed the data may show that variation in care is occurring, prompting some type of change or modification be put into place.

The modification could include the following:

1. Protocol or guideline development
2. Educational sessions held for staff
3. Increase in resources
4. Improvement in communications

The PI process must be dynamic and strive to challenge the way patient care is provided. The goal should be to continually improve the process of providing care and to improve patient outcomes.

VIII. MEDICAL AND LEGAL ASPECTS OF FLIGHT NURSING

The unique practice setting in which flight nurses care for patients brings with it the need to understand what constitutes negligence and malpractice. *Negligence* is a deviation from an accepted standard of performance [20]. *Malpractice* is based on a professional standard of care, as well as the professional statutes of the caregiver [20]. Nurses can be charged with criminal offense if they violate either the state nurse practice act or conduct unsafe nursing practices. Nurses can be charged with a civil offense when a patient feels he has been wrongfully injured by the actions taken by the nurse and/or other members of the medical team. The nurse is usually covered by the hospital or independent program that employs her.

Each transport program should have a risk management program and a vigorous performance improvement program. When made a component of the transport program, these two interrelated activities will greatly reduce the risk of untoward legal actions involving the transport nurse.

There are four elements of negligence that must be present for malpractice to have occurred. (see Table 2). Questions usually arise about duty that relate to the point at which care, responsibility, and accountability are transferred from the referring hospital to members of the transport team and/or the receiving hospital. Breach of duty is difficult to determine in any malpractice case. If the care provided was found to be below the "standard" of care, did that substandard care cause the patient's injury? Referring hospital standards of care may be different from those practiced at the receiving hospital, depending on the expertise of the institutions. There may also be times when the transport team cannot treat the patient according to their standard of care because of referring physician objections. Again, detailed documentation of when the transport team assumed care and what did or did not transpire prior to the team's arrival could help establish when the breach of duty, if any, occurred. Establishment of proximate cause is the cause and effect

Table 2 Four Elements of Negligence as They Relate to Transport of Patients

Element	As it pertains to transport	
Duty	This is the patient/provider contract, as it pertains to transport. It is established when the professional assumes care of patient.	Use clear written programmatic protocols, procedures that clarify when the medical transport team takes over care of patient [21].
Breach of duty	Occurs when the professional providing care does so in a manner inconsistent with what any reasonable practitioner with the same level of skill in same type of setting would have provided.	Transport team must document when care was assumed.
Establishment of proximate cause	Determination of what particular activity or intervention actually caused a worsening of the patient's condition or caused a new injury or insult due to the caregiver's actions.	Document initial assessment, stabilization, interventions, changes during transport, and the patient's response to the transport team's intervention.
Determining actual damages	Assessment of damages to include how the damage amount is calculated. 1. Actual damages: Compensates the patient for those injuries directly associated with the action of the caregiver. 2. Special damages: Assessed if liability is determined. This could include paying for the lost wages of a spouse who had to be absent from work to care for the injured patient. 3. Punitive damages: Assigned if the court believes the act was particularly egregious. These are damages assessed to punish.	

component necessary to prove malpractice. Because most transport teams treat critically ill or injured patients in life-threatening phases of their care, it is very difficult to separate the rapid hemodynamic changes associated with the severity of the illness or injury from those that may be due to specific interventions that are usually done in rapid sequence due to necessity. Timed flowsheets that outline a sequence of care can assist in determining the standard of care that was followed by the transport team in the care of the patient. When several parties are named in a malpractice suit, differing state legislation determines how each defendant will be apportioned liability.

IX. CONSENT AND ABANDONMENT

For the transport nurse, the principles related to patient abandonment are important to understand. Abandonment can occur if the care of a patient is transferred to someone less qualified or if there is a perceived demonstration of disregard for the patient's welfare [22]. With the institution of the Examination and Treatment for Emergency Medical Conditions and Women in Labor Act (EMTALA), also known as Section 9121 of the Federal Consolidation Omnibus Budget Reconciliation Act of 1985 (COBRA) to prevent patient dumping [22] it is imperative that patients are appropriately evaluated and stabilized prior to transfer. There must be documentation that both higher-level care is needed to justify the transfer and the mode of transport has the appropriate level of personnel and equipment to perform the transfer.

Understanding the scope of practice one works within is important for the transport nurse. State nurse practice acts and mandatory licensure are the basic regulatory bodies responsible for nursing practice. The transport nurse should also know and understand Federal Aviation Administration (FAA) regulations as they pertain to functioning in the aviation environment. Also, there are Federal Communication Commission (FCC) regulations that control what types of communications can be used over airwaves, and the flight nurse must master the appropriate methods of communication.

X. SUMMARY

The development of transport nursing has evolved from the early days of hot air balloon transports in France to the more independent practitioner role observed predominantly in the United States. The transport nurse role has developed in the United States as the core member of the transport medical team. In many instances the nurse practices with paramedics and respiratory therapists to form the medical team. In a few U.S. programs and in more European programs the team is made up of the physician/nurse or physician/physician team. Licensure, critical care experience, and ongoing education are pertinent to growth in this role. Performance improvement is essential to the development and maintenance of competent transport teams and must be programmatically supported to succeed. The transport nurse must understand the legalities of practicing in the prehospital environment. Documentation of events, interventions, and patient status is essential.

REFERENCES

1. HL Gibbons, C Fromhagen. Aeromedical transportation and general aviation. Aero Med 42: 773, 1971.
2. RE Skinner. The U.S. flight nurse: An annotated bibliography. Aviat Space Environ Med 52: 707–712, 1981.
3. J Barger. U.S. Army Air Force flight nurses: Training and pioneer flight. Aviat Space Environ Med 51:414–416, 1980.
4. HL Gibbons, C Fromhagen. Aeromedical transportation and general aviation. Aero Med 42: 773, 1971.
5. ASTNA http://www.astna.org.
6. Emergency Nurses Association/National Flight Nurses Association. Staffing of critical care air medical transport services. J Emerg Nurs 12:6A–19A, 1986.
7. GB Bader, M Terhorst, P Heilman, JA DePalam. Characteristics of flight nursing practice. Air Med J 14:214–218, 1995.
8. NPS Chawla, K Caroler. Against all odds: Air medical transport in India. Air Med J 17(4): 146–148, 1998.
9. Gamma Air Medical Website; http://www.flightweb.com/programs/gamma/index.html.
10. G Cody. 1994 air medical program survey. Air Med J 13:9, 1994.
11. KJ Rhee, M Strozeski, RE Burney, JR Mackenzie, K LaGreca-Reibling. Is the flight physician needed for helicopter emergency medical services? Ann Emerg Med 15:2, 174–177, 1986.

12. The Flight Nurse Advanced Trauma Course Handbook. rev. ed. DesPlaines: IA National Flight Nurse Association, 1995.
13. DJ Samuels, HC Block. Air Medical Crew National Standard Curriculum. Pasedena, CA: ASHBEAMS, 1988.
14. Emergency Nurses Association. National Standard Guidelines for Prehospital Nursing Curriculum, I. Chicago: ENA, 1991.
15. AMRE home page: http://www.amref.org/.
16. K Rinnert, I Blumen, S Gabram, M Zanker. A descriptive analysis of air medical directors in the United States. Air Med J 18:6, March 1999.
17. R Walker. Qualification and training of the air medical director. In: Air Medical Physician Handbook. Salt Lake City: Air Medical Physicians Association.
18. AAMS Quality Assurance Committee. AAMS resource document for air medical quality assurance. J Air Med Trans 9:23–26, 1990.
19. Resource for Optimal Care of the Injured Patient. Chicago: American College of Surgeons Committee on Trauma, 1998, pp. 69–78.
20. R Hepp. Standards of Flight Nursing Practice. St. Louis: Mosby, 1993.
21. BJ Youngberg. Medical–legal considerations involved in the transport of critically ill patients. Critical Care Clin 8:501–511, 1992.
22. COBRA Statute; 42 USC 1395dd, Section 1867 of the Social Security Act.

6

The Role of the Paramedic in Prehospital Trauma Care

GREGG S. MARGOLIS

The George Washington University, Washington, D.C.

MARVIN WAYNE

Emergency Medical Services, City of Bellingham and Whatcom County, Bellingham, Washington; University of Washington, Seattle, Washington; and Yale University, New Haven, Connecticut

PAUL BERLIN

Pierce County Fire District 5, Gig Harbor, Washington

Paramedics are often the first trained personnel to care for the victims of traumatic injuries. The training, educational level, experience, and work status of these providers varies greatly from country to country, as well as locality to locality. It is the intent of this brief introduction to provide the reader with an overview of the roles that these initial responders have in the spectrum of care provided to trauma patients.

First, some clarification of terminology is in order. The term *first responder* can be confusing. It is often used as a catchall term for the first trained individual to arrive at the scene of an emergency. In this use of the term, the first responding individual may have a wide variety of training, from simple first aid through physician. In some countries, the term is used to describe a course and/or a certification level, usually designed to provide basic initial care in emergency situations (EMT, paramedic, first responder).

Regardless of the level of certification, licensure, training, or experience, the roles of anyone providing care to trauma patients before they reach the hospital can be summarized as (1) control the scene/triage, (2) correct immediate life threats, (3) identify the patient priority, (4) avoid secondary injury, and (5) provide transport. While each of these roles seems to be obvious and straightforward, the challenges of the out-of-hospital setting can make each an extraordinary clinical challenge.

I. CONTROL THE SCENE/TRIAGE

Situations in which people have been injured are often highly chaotic and dangerous scenes. Many of the hazards persist even after initial patients have been injured. Motor vehicle crashes, hazardous materials incidents, explosions, fire, and acts of violence may not be resolved before help arrives. The very first priority of the prehospital care provider is to assess the scene for hazards and assure that no additional injuries occur. While it takes tremendous personal discipline not to rush into a scene to render care to an injured patient, the initially responding personnel have the primary responsibility to assure that neither they nor others are hurt in the process.

In the case of multiple casualties, the prehospital care provider must make difficult decisions as to which patients stand to gain the most from the allocation of limited resources, therefore guidelines for the triage of all patients should be established in advance. In the case of many victims, the initial responders may provide no care, but rather spend their time triaging patients, securing additional resources, and coordinating additional response.

II. CORRECT IMMEDIATE LIFE THREATS

Some injuries and situations are so time-sensitive that they cannot wait to be treated in the hospital. Typically these problems involve the airway, breathing, and/or bleeding, therefore the roles in patient management revolve around the following three priorities.

A. Maintain a Patent Airway

The first priority of patient management is assuring a patent airway. Although overused and trite, trauma patients continue to die every day from failure to have their airways secured. The trauma patient represents significant challenges in airway management. Patient location or entrapment combined with facial, oral, head, neck, or chest trauma complicate an already difficult task. The options for maintaining the airway, depending on the training and experience of the provider, may include manual positioning, suction, oral/nasal airways, endotracheal intubation, multiple lumen airways, and cricothyrotomy.

B. Assure Adequate Ventilation

The goal of providing a patent airway is to assure that ventilation can occur. It is very common for victims of major trauma to be hypoventilating, either as a direct result of their injuries or secondary to mental status changes. After assuring a patent airway, the role of the prehospital care provider must be to provide adequate ventilation. Depending on training and experience, options include exhaled breath ventilations (with or without a barrier device), bag–valve device, flow-restricted, oxygen-powered ventilation devices, and automatic transport ventilators. The most common method, the bag–valve device, is the most difficult to use properly, especially with one person trying to maintain the airway, assure a mask seal, and squeeze the bag.

C. Bleeding Control

While blood loss is a factor in many trauma situations, major bleeding that can be controlled is relatively uncommon. Internal hemorrhage is much more common and insidious than external hemorrhage. In cases in which external hemorrhage is severe, it obviously must be stopped. This is usually accomplished by a combination of direct and indirect pressure. Tourniquets are rarely needed, but should be used if bleeding in an extremity is life-threatening and cannot be controlled any other way.

In most cases, prehospital care providers must assure a patent airway, adequate ventilation, and major bleeding control at the scene. Even with relative close proximity to a hospital, most patients cannot survive without these immediate lifesaving interventions. Airway management and ventilation are the only clinical reasons for delaying transport.

III. IDENTIFY THE PATIENT PRIORITY

The definitive care of multisystem trauma is surgery. While some procedures (e.g., IVs) are possible in the field, they only increase the window of opportunity until the underlying problem can be corrected. For this reason, a major role of prehospital care providers must be the rapid identification of patients requiring immediate surgical intervention. Identifying priority patients is based on the findings of a rapid trauma assessment. The goal of this assessment must be to recognize and correct immediate life threats and identify patients who have a serious risk of rapid decompensation. This typically includes an altered level of consciousness, respiratory compromise, signs of shock, signs of internal hemorrhage, or fractures of the pelvis or femurs.

IV. AVOID SECONDARY INJURY

Moving traumatized patients provides a risk of secondary tissue damage from fractured bone ends. This can be permanently debilitating, especially when it involves nerve damage. Decisions to immobilize the spine and/or extremities have to take into consideration the mechanism of injury, assessment findings, patient condition, as well as the balancing of time vs. the benefit. As a general rule, an unstable cervical spine is assumed, until proven otherwise. When the patient is stable, extremity fractures should be splinted before movement. In the unstable patient, the risk of patient decompensation usually outweighs the benefit of long-bone immobilization.

V. TRANSPORT

Prehospital care providers serve as the link between the scene of the incident and the hospital by providing transportation to patients in a manner that is most consistant with their needs. In unstable patients, the most expeditious method, either by ground with the aid of ''lights and siren'' or by air (if distances are great), should be used. In less critical cases, the risk to patient, provider, and the public outweigh the time saved, and transportation should be less urgent.

Selection of the proper destination is critical to patient survival. Rapid transportation to a facility that is not capable of immediate surgical intervention will result in a suboptimal outcome. In some cases it is perfectly reasonable to bypass the closest hospital in order to take the patient directly to a facility that is prepared to provide immediate surgical care.

VI. SUMMARY

The role of the prehospital care practitioner is critical to trauma patients. It has been demonstrated that with proper education, experience, equipment, and system design, emergency medical systems can have a dramatic effect on the morbidity and mortality from traumatic injuries. By integrating out-of-hospital and in-hospital care, we can provide a continuum of service that provides the best chance for a positive outcome for all victims of trauma.

7

Working in the Prehospital Environment: Safety Aspects and Teamwork

CRAIG GEIS

Geis-Alvarado & Associates, Inc., Novato, California

PÅL MADSEN

Norwegian Air Ambulance Ltd., Høvik, Norway

I. INTRODUCTION

In the prehospital environment, emergency medicine service (EMS) personnel possibly face more significant challenges than in-hospital care providers do. A major difference is the unpredictability of EMS operations. This unpredictability is often due to the limited information available to the team, a lack of knowledge of the cause and extent of the patient's problem, and the nature of the operational environment. Very often the location of the accident scene is ambiguous at the time of turnout, and the medical team is usually unsure of the resources they may need. This results in the team having to gather the information during the execution of the mission.

Another challenge to the prehospital environment is the introduction of the helicopter emergency medical service (HEMS) concept [1]. The HEMS concept describes a setting in which individuals recruited from very different environments work together with each other and technology to achieve the common goal of quality patient care. While each individual on the team possesses different technical skills, team members must be able to effectively interact with each other to make this possible. Effective team interaction requires the seamless integration of safety and teamwork into every phase of the medical response. When fully integrated into a well-organized EMS system the HEMS concept has proven its ability to improve patient outcomes.

II. TRANSPORT CONSIDERATIONS

A. Ground Transport

Emergency medical service providers routinely violate traffic laws when responding to emergencies. Warning systems such as vehicle markings and lights and sirens are used to reduce collision risk. Even with the use of such warning systems, emergency driving represents a risk eight times greater than regular ambulance driving [2]. Data suggest that intersections pose the greatest hazard and associated risk to the emergency vehicle. In intersection accidents, emergency vehicles are more likely to be struck by another vehicle. Norwegian data suggest that 45% of the injuries and fatalities in emergency vehicles occur in the rear compartment of the ambulance [2]. Passenger restraints can significantly reduce the risk of severe injury [3]. Additionally, ambulance-warning systems are important in alerting others, providing vehicle identification, and projecting size, distance, speed, and direction of travel. These warning systems are critical in obtaining proper reaction from other drivers. Studies indicate that lime-green is probably superior to traditional emergency vehicle colors, and that red flashing lights alone may not be as effective as other color combinations [4]. It has also been demonstrated that the siren is an extremely limited warning device.

The safe operation of emergency vehicles using warning lights and sirens requires that both the public and drivers understand and obey relevant traffic laws. There are indications that this area has the potential for improvement [5].

B. Helicopter Transport

During the 1980s, commercial EMS helicopter activity increased sharply. Unfortunately, so did the accident rate. After a series of fatal EMS helicopter accidents in 1985 and 1986, flight safety became a priority in the United States and Europe. The National Transportation Safety Board (NTSB), in Washington, D.C., undertook a safety study to examine the cause factors relating to accidents in the HEMS industry. Fifty-nine EMS helicopter accidents occurring between 1978 and 1986 were investigated and evaluated [6]. The results revealed that the accident rate for EMS helicopters involved in patient transports was approximately twice the rate experienced by nonscheduled helicopter air taxis, and one and a half times the rate for all turbine-powered helicopters from 1980 to 1985. A striking finding is that the fatal accident rate for EMS helicopters for this period is approximately three and a half times that of nonscheduled helicopter air taxis and all turbine helicopters. The injury rate was slightly less than those of other helicopters, indicating that EMS helicopter accidents tend to be more severe.

A study comparing the U.S. and German EMS helicopter accident rates from 1982 to 1987 revealed very similar rates (4.7 fatal accidents per 100,000 flying hours vs. 4.1) [7]. This occurred despite the different operating profiles in the two countries.

The NTSB findings suggest that the cause of the increased accident rates for the EMS helicopter industry may be related to the fact that these helicopters routinely operate in poor weather and at night, land and take off from unimproved landing areas, and depart on missions with little advance notice. Weather-related accidents are the most common and most serious type of accident experienced by EMS helicopters. Fifteen of the 59 accidents investigated involved reduced visibility and spatial disorientation as a factor. Eleven of the accidents resulted in fatalities. Mechanical failure also caused 15 accidents, but only two resulted in fatalities. Twelve of the accidents involved obstacle strikes.

R. B. Low collected data of accidents and incidents at all registered U.S. HEMS programs during a three-year period from 1986 through 1988 [8]. The most conspicuous finding of this study was the eightfold decrease in accidents experienced by the programs that flew more frequently (more than 28 flights per month). Furthermore, IFR (instrument flight rules) capability and proficiency was a factor associated with increased safety [9].

A study regarding pilot instrument proficiency concluded that instrument-proficient pilots would more safely manage a flight into unplanned instrument meteorological conditions (IMC) than would nonproficient pilots [9]. It is important to note that the instrument-proficient pilots lost control less often (15% vs. 67%), maintained instrument standards more often (77% vs. 40%), and entered IMC at a higher altitude (689 ft vs. 517 ft), compared with the nonproficient pilots. In light of this study, operators may wish to consider requiring an instrument rating for pilots or consider providing basic instrument proficiency training.

Safety recommendations, given by different authors and authorities, address these main topics.

1. Weather conditions. Ceiling, visibility, and flight altitude minimums should be established for each program. The minimums must consider both day and night operations and be terrain- and weather-specific. In all cases the minimums established must be strictly adhered to regardless of the nature of the request.
2. Pilot staffing and workload. Regulatory authorities may specify pilot staffing levels. Generally the staffing level consists of a minimum of three to four pilots per aircraft in any 24-hr program. Duty time guidelines should be established and must be monitored carefully. Relief crews should be provided when necessary.
3. Night operations. If the response location is not well known in advance and the scene is not illuminated, responses at night present an additional challenge to the crew. Consideration should be given to establishing clear guidelines for crews to follow in these situations to ensure safety.
4. Pilot training and experience. An instrument flight rating (IFR) for pilots is encouraged. Such training is helpful during night flying and when unexpected poor weather is encountered. Night flights in marginal weather closely approximate IFR. In these conditions the instrument-rated pilot is better prepared to handle routine as well as emergency situations [9].
5. Emergency medical service helicopter equipment installation and performance standards. Clear standards should be developed for interior design, including but not limited to crashworthiness, oxygen system design, patient location and restraint, and medical system design.
6. Personal protective clothing and equipment. Shoulder harnesses should be installed at all crew stations and passenger seats. Those personnel classified as required crew members should wear protective clothing and equipment to reduce the chance of injury or death in survivable accidents. Clothing and equipment should include protective helmets, flame- and heat-resistant flight suits, and protective footwear.
7. Organization and management. Safety committees for each EMS program should be established, composed of representatives from the hospital EMS program administration, commercial EMS helicopter operator, pilot and medical

personnel, helicopter dispatch, and local public safety/emergency response agencies.

8. Flight crew and medical personnel coordination and communication training. Crew resource management (CRM) training is an important safety consideration. This area will be discussed in detail in the second section of this chapter.

C. Incident Scene Considerations

Emergency medical service helicopters are often asked to land as close as possible to the accident site. While this may be desirable, landing as safely as possible must always be the first consideration. Main rotor blades and the helicopter's tail rotor represent a significant safety hazard. The landing site is not always smooth, and a turning rotor is always a serious hazard. Physical and environmental factors also contribute to the scene hazards. Weather conditions, temperature, humidity, and visibility must all be considered. Hazards at the scene can also result from natural forces, traffic, unsecured wreckage, damaged buildings, construction, fire, smoke, and other kinds of pollution.

Table 1 lists some basic safety considerations that should be addressed in team safety training and briefings.

Another consideration is that prehospital care providers are working under challenging conditions with limited access to the patient, limited diagnostic and treatment resources, limited operational space, and insufficient illumination. In addition to time pressure, different kinds of stressors, such as noise and vibration, add to the burden and may lead to distractions.

Obviously, acknowledgment of the unique demands placed on EMS personnel is an important premise of improving safety. Although safety issues must be on each individual's agenda, the primary responsibility for safe operations lies with management. Selection of personnel, training, standards, procedures, quality assurance system, adequate equipment, and an open and supportive attitude have a great impact on safety. Thorough information collection, premission planning, good communication, information transfer,

Table 1 Team Safety Training and Briefing Considerations

Safety considerations
Prior to landing and takeoff the site should be checked for any items that may be blown in the rotor wash.
Professionals from the ambulance service, fire brigade, and police department should be trained to secure the landing zone.
Distance between the scene and the helicopter should be maintained until the helicopter crew gives a clearance signal.
A helicopter with a turning rotor should never be approached from behind.
If possible, aircraft engines should be shut down immediately after landing in order to decrease the chances of injury.
If engines remain running an attempt should be made to maintain visual contact with the pilot at all times.
Helicopter crew members should always consider the possibility that on-scene personnel may suddenly approach the helicopter and should be prepared.
Protective clothing and equipment should be readily available. Helmets, hearing protection, reflective materials, fire-protective suits, gloves, and boots can all protect personnel.

and cooperative teamwork are all factors that are known to enhance not just efficiency, but safety as well.

III. HUMAN FACTOR AND TEAMWORK CONSIDERATIONS

It has been shown that in settings in which individuals interact with each other, human error is still the major stumbling block to achieving the goal of quality patient care. Human error is and will continue to be a major contributing factor to aircraft accidents and adverse medical incidents.

Aircraft accident investigations show that between 65 to 85% of all accidents are the results of human error. An analysis conducted by the Boeing Commercial Airplane Group of 149 accidents occurring between 1988 and 1997 showed that in 70% of the accidents the flight crew was the primary cause factor of the accident [10]. Additional research conducted in operating room theaters, aircraft cockpits the space shuttle program, and nuclear power plants has similarly concluded that human error, not technical competence, continues to be the primary cause of accidents and incidents. It has been demonstrated that human errors made by individuals in each of these settings fall into the categories of team coordination, communication, and leadership, and decision making [11]. These human error categories have come to be popularly known as CRM issues.

A. Human Error

Preventing mishaps and conducting safe operations assumes that we are able to accurately identify the root causes of the errors that cause accidents and adverse medical incidents. The accurate identification of error depends on the extent to which we understand the factors that lead to errors. For most errors, our understanding of the complex interaction between the cause factors is imperfect and incomplete. The key to predicting and controlling human error lies in our ability to understand root cause. The major components of human error can be identified as either latent or active error [12].

B. Latent Error

Latent errors are generally unintentional acts by management or systems deficiencies within the prehospital system. The effects of latent error may not be readily apparent and may therefore lie dormant for a long period of time. Very often these latent errors only become evident when they combine with other factors to penetrate the safety defenses.

1. Management Error

Management error refers to the underlying causes of errors that set other factors in motion. These errors are generally attributable to decisions made by upper, middle, and line management. In the prehospital system, management error can be attributable not only to hospital management and helicopter company management, but also to the caregiver on the scene and the pilot, who assumes a management role during different phases of the mission.

The type of management error we see in Table 2 generally results from failures in planning, organizing, directing, controlling, and staffing.

Two common examples of latent management error are (1) the failure of management to effectively plan for the integration of a new piece of equipment, and (2) the failure of the pilot in command to properly plan the flight. Latent errors created by management

Table 2 Common Types of Management Errors

Job functions	Failures in
Planning	Defining organizational goals
	Developing strategies for achieving those goals
	Developing a hierarchy to integrate and coordinate activities
Organizing	Determining the structure
	Outlining the tasks
	Determining who will do them
	Determining how tasks are grouped
	Determining who reports to whom
	Determining where decisions are made
Directing	Motivating subordinates
	Directing activities
	Selecting modes of communication
	Resolving conflict
	Directing change
Controlling	Ensuring things are going as they should
	Comparing actual performance against previously set goals and objectives
	Taking action to correct deviations if they exist
	Conducting routine inspections/evaluations
Staffing	Ensuring the presence of sufficient qualified individuals to accomplish the task

Table 3 Common Types of Systems Errors

Systems components	Failures in
Task	Arrangement of tasks
	Demands on people
	Time aspects
	Communications
Material	Supplies
	Equipment
	Maintenance
Environment	Work environment (culture)
	Sociological factors
	Environment (peers, family, organization)
	Physical environment
	Facilities
Training	Types: initial, update, and remedial
	Targets: operating, supervisory, and management
	Consideration: quality, quantity
Person	Mental state
	Physical state
	Emotional state
	Psychological factors
	Motivation

form the preconditions for problems within the operating systems of the organization and the team.

2. Systems Error

Systems error refers to the basic causes or origins of the error. These are generally attributable to defects in the organization's operating systems. These errors can create additional latent errors and affect the other operating systems of the organization. This error, described in Table 3, comes from failures in the system concerning the task, material, environment, training, and person. These systems deficiencies have the potential to affect all individuals within the system. A common example of a systems error is the failure of the organization's training system to provide adequate training to team members in the use of new equipment.

C. Active Error

Active error refers to the immediate cause factors of an accident and is generally attributable to team members and the actions they take. Active error is often a symptom of a larger problem and not the problem itself. The true root cause of the problem is often found in latent error. The most common active errors are listed in Table 4.

Table 4 Common Team or Individual Active Errors

Active errors	
1.	Didn't follow instructions
2.	Blundered ahead without knowing how to do the job
3.	Bypassed or ignored a rule, regulation, or procedure to save time
4.	Failed to use protective equipment
5.	Didn't think ahead to possible consequences
6.	Used the wrong equipment to do the job
7.	Used equipment that needed repair or replacement
8.	Didn't look
9.	Didn't recognize physical limitations
10.	Failed to use safeguards or other protective devices
11.	Didn't listen
12.	Didn't pay attention
13.	Improper inspection/search
14.	Improper attention
15.	Failed to recognize
16.	Improper complex physical action
17.	Misinterpreted
18.	Failed to anticipate
19.	Inadequate planning
20.	Improper decision
21.	Improper physical actions
22.	Inadequate communication
23.	Inadequate improvising
24.	Inadequate problem solving
25.	Misjudgment

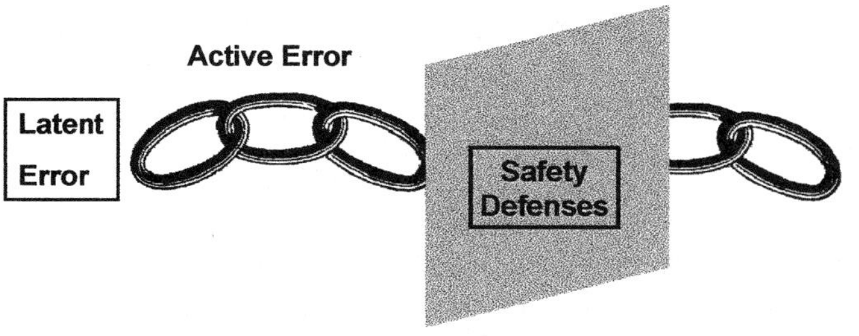

Figure 1 Interaction of latent error, active error, and safety defenses.

An example of active error may be the failure of the individual to follow established procedures. This may be a result or symptom of a lack of standards, impractical standards, overconfidence, an unwillingness to listen to other, more experienced crew members, pressure on the team members to take shortcuts, or simply willful disregard on the part of a team member.

1. Interactions

Latent error forms the preconditions for the team members to commit active errors. When a team member commits an active error, an error chain begins to build. Accident investigations have shown that there is usually a minimum of four, and an average of six, links in an error chain prior to an accident.

When coupled with latent errors the active errors are filtered through the safety defenses set up by the organization, team, or individual. When the defenses work as planned, error is trapped and the error chain is broken (Fig. 1). When the defenses fail, there is a mishap. Minor failures can lead to incidents or adverse consequences.

IV. CRM TRAINING

Crew resource management training has proven to be an effective error-trapping tool for pilots [13], doctors [11], ship captains [14], and other associated team members. A U.S. Coast Guard bridge crew resource management training program [14] begun in 1992 has reduced accidents for boats from 9.5 accidents per 100,000 operating hours to 3.0, and cutter accidents from 5.5 to 1.5.

Very often the individuals associated with these areas of operation have been conditioned to believe that by the nature of their training they are capable of extraordinary feats. The fact is, they are just human and subject to the same human failings that affect everyone else. The ability to use other team members as a resource can help team members compensate for human error.

In the context of the prehospital setting, CRM is broadly defined as the effective use of all available human, informational, and equipment resources toward the goal of providing quality patient care. Crew resource management is an approach to improving organizational, individual, and team performance, which focuses on preventing or managing active and latent error. It works because it facilitates a culture of mutual respect and confidence among the organization and team members. This culture leads to openness, candor, and constructive critique.

Organizations, individuals, and teams can be trained to recognize potential mistakes in judgment and to compensate for them to prevent mishaps. Crew resource management has been demonstrated to increase organizational, individual, and team effectiveness in routine as well as emergency situations. It is a tool to ensure better coordination among the members of the flight crew, ground medical team, and other professionals.

Commercial aviation has achieved an impressive safety record that continues to improve. This record is a direct result of training programs in CRM, which begin with the premise that individual team members are technically proficient. Aircraft and medical accident and incident statistics show that many problems encountered by team members have little to do with the technical aspects of the job task; rather than addressing technical skills, CRM training focuses on the effective use of resources to make optimal decisions.

A. CRM Considerations

As previously stated, a critical factor in the successful integration of the HEMS concept is the consideration of the safety aspects and teamwork of the prehospital team. In developing an effective prehospital system, management must give careful consideration to its decision to implement a CRM training program. This is accomplished by carefully identifying the target audience, selecting appropriate training strategies, determining the course content, evaluating the effectiveness of the training, and addressing specific considerations for the HEMS team.

The decision on what kind of training to provide crew members is management's decision. Crew resource management training has become an industry standard, and in the United States and Europe aviation authorities have mandated the training [13,14]. Even if the training is not mandatory, management should consider the benefits of the training and support its implementation. It has been shown that management support, not only for the training, but also for the team acting in accordance with the learned CRM principles, is instrumental in its success.

Since CRM training is a comprehensive system for improving team performance, training should be directed toward all operational personnel in the prehospital system. As a minimum, this should include the flight crew, medical personnel, communication specialists, and first responders. If resources permit, consideration should be given to expanding the training to management, maintenance personnel, and air traffic controllers.

B. CRM Training Considerations

Selecting an appropriate training strategy is critical to the success of the program. Training success requires a strategy that ensures the active participation of all individuals, concentrates on team member's attitudes and behaviors, and is able to be integrated into all forms of current training. Crew resource management practices must be thoroughly incorporated into operations manuals and standard operating procedures in order to provide team members with clear standards.

While the actual content of effective training programs may vary slightly, effective implementation strategies all have common components. The components include initial awareness training, recurrent practice and feedback, and continuing reinforcement and checking [13].

Initial awareness training is designed to provide the participants with the knowledge of those human factor skills that have been demonstrated to most influence crew performance. The recommended length for this training is three days. The training strategy in this phase should cover a variety of instructional techniques, including lectures, discussion groups, case studies, role playing, and audiovisual presentations. Since classroom instruction does not fundamentally alter attitudes over the long term, this phase of training is only the first step and must be followed approximately 12 to 18 months later by recurrent practice and feedback.

Prior to the recurrent practice and feedback phase, the participants will have had ample opportunity to practice the previously learned skills. Recurrent training is designed to reinforce the initial awareness training, and focuses on the review and amplification of the concepts already learned. The training strategy used in this phase of training can include practice, role playing, and feedback exercises. It is especially beneficial for team members to practice their skills in an operational setting and receive feedback on their performance. This can be done effectively in the classroom, in a work setting, or in a simulator. The recommended length for this training is 1 day, and should be conducted at least every 2 years. To ensure long-term change, continuing reinforcement and checking should follow this training.

Since individual attitudes and norms develop over an individual's lifetime, it is unrealistic to expect a one-time training exposure to the CRM concepts to reverse habits. To develop new habit patterns, continued reinforcement and checking is critical. Crew resources management should be integrated into every stage of each individual's training and further stressed in daily operations. If this is done, continuing reinforcement and checking can facilitate the development of new attitudes and organizational culture [16,17]. During the continued reinforcement and checking phase, it is important to focus reinforcement on the entire team. Segmentation of team members is not appropriate for this phase of training. It is especially beneficial for team members to practice their skills in an operational setting and receive feedback on their performance. This phase should be done in the work setting and not the classroom. The most effective strategy is to set up a system that requires both self- and team critique. Team members can accomplish this after every mission and in work groups on a periodic basis. Self-critique and peer reviews are a critical item in the process.

C. CRM Training Content

Definitive guidance on the topics that have been identified as critical components of effective CRM training can vary, depending on the source. The authors have attempted to include those subject areas that are most common to all successful training programs. This was accomplished by reviewing industry recommendations [18–20,15] and summarizing them in Table 5.

D. CRM Evaluation

Observing specific behaviors can serve as an indicator of how effectively CRM skills are being practiced [21]. The evaluation of CRM skills is part of the continuing reinforcement and checking phase. The key to effective evaluation of the behaviors starts with clear and measurable standards. Standards for evaluating CRM behaviors vary, but must focus on the behaviors associated with the recommended CRM content listed in Table 5. Specific guidelines for evaluation have been published by the Federal Aviation Administration [19].

E. Beyond Basic CRM Training

Crew resource management must be viewed as an ongoing, dynamic development process; it is not a single training event designed for the sake of meeting a requirement. Once

Table 5 General Industry Recommendations for CRM Course Content

Content	Initial training	Recurrent training	Reinforcement and checking
Human error	In-depth	Overview	Observe decision-making process
Types of errors			
Human limitations			
Information processing			
Error chains			
Error trapping			
Decision making			
Communication processes	In-depth	Overview	Observe behaviors
Inquiry			
Advocacy			
Assertion			
Listening			
Conflict resolution			
Crew self-critique			
Briefings and debriefings			
Team building and maintenance	In-depth	Overview	Observe behaviors
Leadership			
Followership			
Concern for the task			
Interpersonal relationships			
Synergy/teamwork			
Group climate			
Duties and responsibilities			
Situational awareness	In-depth	Overview	Observe behaviors
Workload management			
Preparation			
Planning			
Vigilance			
Workload distribution			
Distraction avoidance			
Individual factors	In-depth	Overview	Observe behaviors
Physiological factors			
Psychological factors			
Stress and performance			
Stress management			
Fatigue			
Automation	In-depth	Not required	Observe behaviors
System and human limitations			
Policies for use			
Specific types: advantages and disadvantages			

implemented, CRM can provide the operator with tailored procedures to meet the demands of the operation. The concept of going beyond the basic training of CRM is becoming known as advanced crew resource management (ACRM), which is the operator's way of addressing specific CRM issues and critical team coordination skills. It involves the identification of critical phases of an operation and proceduralization of the skills so that

Table 6 Safety Considerations for Specific Phases of Flight

Phase of flight	Team considerations
Premission/before takeoff	Information collection
	Mission planning
	Crew briefing
	Checklist procedures to include planning for the use of automation
Enroute to pickup	Communications with first responders and communication center
	Routes of flight
	Weather
	Terrain
	Contingency planning
Landing	Communications with ground
	Site description: include wires, trees, buildings, general lay of terrain (slope, flat, soft, plowed, crops, hard surface), minimum area required, factors affecting visibility, vehicle and personnel locations
	Site markings: day/night
	Site evaluation: high/low reconnaissance
	Monitoring responsibilities of other crew members
	Monitoring responsibilities of ground personnel: flight path, clear landing zone
	Performance planning: power management, time to transition from descent to climb
	Forced landing areas
	Noise abatement considerations
	Final obstruction clearance
Ground operations	Control of ground personnel and vehicles
	Clearance around helicopter
	Planned ground time
	Patient transfer
Takeoff	Takeoff briefing
	Aborted takeoff or procedures: snow, dust, wires, vehicles on the landing zone, other
	Monitoring responsibilities of other crew members
	Monitoring responsibilities of ground personnel: flight path, clear landing zone
Enroute to hospital	Communications with hospital and communication center
	Routes of flight
	Weather
	Terrain
	Contingency planning
	Monitoring responsibilities of other crew members
Return to base	Communications with the communication center
	Routes of flight
	Weather
	Terrain
	Contingency planning
	Debriefing/critique of mission and team performance

Table 7 Automation Guidelines for Phases of Flight

Phase of flight	Guidelines
Premission	Briefings include a thorough discussion on applicability, how, and when the crew will use automated systems.
Takeoff/landing	Prior to entering a high-density traffic area, crew takes time to discuss strategies for using the automated systems and plans for backup, should changes occur.
Enroute	Crew does not accept data from automated systems without validation when available.
	Crew plans in advance ways to use automated systems to reduce workload at critical periods of the flight.
	Crew anticipates *early* the need to revert to lower levels of automation to improve situational awareness.
	Crew uses lower levels of automation such as a cross-checking (maps, charts, raw data, etc.) to maintain high levels of situational awareness.
	Crew members do not complicate the use of available automated systems in a manner that causes distractions or confusion among other crew members.
	Crew members demonstrate an in-depth understanding of the capabilities of the automated systems and use this knowledge to help others.
	Crew members update one another routinely after absence or diverted attention without prompting.

they are integrated into policies, procedures, standard operating procedures (SOPs), and/or guidelines.

As an example, Table 6 lists the typical phases of flight for a HEMS mission. Each phase of flight is listed with team safety considerations for the organization, individual, and/or team. In the ACRM phase, the organization could address the permission phase of flight by developing flight crew guidelines for the use of automated equipment. It is important to point out that when an organization develops a procedure, it is not intended to remove the crew from the decision process, but is only intended to provide it with guidelines that have been proven effective. As with any guidelines, the organization needs to tailor them to a specific type of aircraft and to the needs of the organization.

Table 7 describes sample guidelines for the use of automation, which may apply for each phase of flight. The availability of onboard avionics equipment may vary significantly between operators. In general, the guidelines presented apply to the more advanced technology cockpit aircraft that may have an autopilot, a flight director, a flight management system, or a global positioning navigation system.

V. SUMMARY

- The prehospital environment has changed with the introduction of the HEMS concept.
- Changes in the prehospital environment require changes in the system.
- Human error still continues to be the single major cause factor of accidents and adverse medical incidents.
- CRM training can stem the tide of human error mishaps.

Careful selection of CRM training strategies must be accomplished for the training to be effective.

CRM should be proceduralized to ensure attitude and culture change.

VI. CONCLUSION

Crew resource management training has proven to be a valuable method for reducing error and enhancing team performance. It can and should be extended to all forms of training in the prehospital environment. Crew resource management is not a quick fix and cannot be implemented overnight. The benefits in implementing a well-planned and comprehensive system are worth the expenditure of resources. Careful planning on the part of management can foster a new organizational culture and change the attitude of team members. This will result in the team working together toward a common goal to provide the highest level of patient care.

REFERENCES

1. GA Kroesen. Risks and safety standards of flying intensive care units. Acta Anaesthesiol Scand 108 (suppl.):108–109, 1996.
2. P Frøyland Accident Risk in Emergency Driving project number 0–871. Oslo, Norway: Institute of Transport Economics, 1982.
3. PS Auerbach. An analysis of ambulance accidents in Tennessee. JAMA 258:1487–1490, 1987.
4. RA De Lorenzo, MA Eilers. Lights and siren: A review of emergency vehicle warning systems. Ann Emerg Med 20:1331–1335, 1991.
5. JD Whiting, EMT knowledge of ambulance traffic laws. Prehosp Emerg Care 2:136–140, 1998.
6. Safety Study—Commercial Emergency Medical Service Helicopter Operations. report no. NTSB/SS-88/01. Washington, D.C.: National Transportation Safety Board, 1988.
7. Rhee. A comparison of emergency medical helicopter accident rates in the United States and the Federal Republic of Germany. Aviat Space Environ Med Aug.:750–752, 1990.
8. RB Low. Factors associated with the safety of EMS helicopters. Am J Emerg Med 9:103–106, 1991.
9. RC Wuerz, R O'Neal. Role of pilot instrument proficiency in the safety of helicopter emergency medical services. Acad Emerg Med 4:972–975, Oct. 1997.
10. Statistical summary of commercial jet airplane accidents. In: Airplane Safety Engineering Worldwide Operations 1959–1997. Seattle: Boeing Commercial Aviation Group. 1998, pp. 1–23.
11. RL Helmreich, EL Weiner, BG Kanki. The future of CRM training in the cockpit and elsewhere. In: E Weiner, B Kanki, RL Helmreich, eds. Cockpit Resource Management. San Diego, CA: Academic, 1993, pp. 479–502.
12. J Rasmussen, OM Pedersen. Human factors in probabilistic risk analysis and risk management. In: Operational Safety of Nuclear Power Plants, vol. 1. Vienna: International Atomic Energy Agency, 1984.
13. Federal Aviation Administration. In: Crew Resource Management Training. advisory circular no. 120–510. Washington, DC: U.S. Department of Transportation, 1998.
14. MJ Alvarado, CE Geis. Team Coordination Training. U.S. Coast Guard pamphlets nos. A64502, A64503, A64601, A64602, A64701, A64801, A64901. International Safety Institute, August 1998.
15. Joint Aviation Administration. JAA Administrative & Guidance Material, Section Four: Oper-

ations, Part Three: Temporary Guidance Leaflets (JAR-OPS 1, subpart N), leaflet no. 5: Crew Resource Management—Flight Crew, 1998.

16. TR Chidester, RL Helmreich, CE Geis. Selection for optimal crew performance: Identifying performance-relevant clusters of professional pilots. 4th International Symposium on Aviation Psychology, Columbus, OH, April 26–30, 1987.
17. CE Geis. Changing attitudes through training: A formal evaluation of training effectiveness. 4th International Symposium on Aviation Psychology, Columbus, OH, April 26–30, 1987.
18. Civil Aviation Authority. Crew Resource Management. aeronautical information circular 117/1998. Hounslow, Middlesex: Aeronautical Information Service, 1998.
19. Federal Aviation Administration. Special Federal Aviation Regulation no. 58—Advanced Qualification Program (draft material only). Chap. 9. Crew Resource Management. Washington, DC: U.S. Department of Transportation, 1998.
20. Human Factors Group of the Royal Aeronautic Society. Quality crew resource management. a paper by the Human Factors Group of the Royal Aeronautical Society, 1996.
21. CE Geis, MJ Alvarado. Crew Resource Management Evaluation Skills Handbook. Napa: International Safety Institute, 1994.

8

Disasters and Mass Casualty Situations

CHRISTOPHER M. GRANDE

International Trauma Anesthesia and Critical Care Society (ITACCS), Baltimore, Maryland; Harvard Medical School and Brigham and Women's Hospital, Boston, Massachusetts; West Virginia University School of Medicine, Morgantown, West Virginia; and SUNY Buffalo School of Medicine, Buffalo, New York

JAN DE BOER

Free University of Amsterdam, Amsterdam, The Netherlands

J. D. POLK

MetroHealth Medical Center, Cleveland, Ohio

MARKUS D. W. LIPP

Johannes Gutenberg University of Mainz, Mainz, Germany

I. INTRODUCTION TO DISASTERS AND MASS CASUALTY SITUATIONS

A disaster is an event that overwhelms the ability of a community, state, or country to meet the medical needs of its victims. During the past 20 years, disasters have affected the lives of more than 800 million people and have been the cause of more than 3 million deaths worldwide [1,2].

Three types of unpredictable events will cause mass casualties and thus demand an organized medical response:

1. *Cataclysmic events*, both natural (e.g., earthquake, tsunami, tornado) and man-made (e.g., nuclear reactor meltdown, chemical spill)
2. *War*, either full-scale or more insidious, such as a civil dispute within a nation (guerilla warfare or low-intensity conflicts)

3. *Terrorist actions*, often connected with either of the two situations listed above (e.g., the release of a chemical or bacteriologic toxin or the bombing of an airliner)

A. Cataclysmic Events

Incidents such as earthquakes and chemical spills tend to surprise the communities involved, although their occurrence can be reasonably predicted by evaluating the environment and performing a ''risk assessment'' or ''threat analysis.'' (See Sec. III.) For example, a community located near an earthquake fault is at an increased risk of experiencing a disaster, which will not only result in a mass casualty situation but also severely compromise the ability of the local emergency medical services (EMS)/medical system to respond and function as it would under normal conditions. In a true disaster, any EMS/medical response will be forced to depend on assistance from outside the general area, assuming that exogenous rescue teams will be able to access the disaster locale.

Cataclysmic events can be anticipated based on a risk assessment, and direct relationships can be drawn between the risk and the disaster situation that can result. Some typical examples are as follows:

Airport → air crash → mass casualties with many survivors suffering brain injury, smoke inhalation, and conventional trauma.

Chemical weapons development in laboratory → accidental release of agent(s) → mass casualty situation with victims ultimately suffering compromise of airway patency or respiratory, circulatory, and neurologic system failure. (See below.)

Sports stadium → bleacher collapse → mass casualty situation with multiple fractures, head and spine injuries, as well as crush syndrome.

The resulting situation will be horrific in any of these cases, and the response with which they will be met depends on an accurate and complete appreciation of the risks, followed by realistic development and availability of both local (immediate) and external (delayed) assistance. (Disaster response planning, including simulations and drills, is covered more completely in a separate section.)

B. War

Caring for battlefield casualties differs from any other form of medicine. Infrastructure may be severely damaged or destroyed, and health care providers may be in danger themselves, if not under direct attack. Overwhelming numbers of casualties may present continuously for days or weeks. Treatment of casualties may have to be delayed or treatment facilities may need to be relocated in response to tactical situations. Medical personnel may be called away from patient care in order to defend the facility or unit. Tactical commanders have top priority in supply, communications, and manpower, at times causing severe shortages in all three areas. Information can be scarce, and much of it may be misinformation—the ''fog of war'' [3]. Enemy soldiers may be among the casualties the providers are expected to treat, resulting in the problem of preventing attacks from within and the need to ensure that injured enemy soldiers are disarmed of grenades, small arms, and other weapons that could be used against care providers. Additional levels of stress are generated by fear, fatigue, and confusion. Practicing medicine on the battlefield requires more adaptability to changing conditions than in any other setting. Under these conditions, the clinical examination skills that are learned in medical school but are often underused become increasingly important.

Military health care facilities and equipment designed for use in forward locations are generally characterized as follows:

Simple
Easy to maintain
Mobile
Lightweight
Able to function independently of local infrastructure

Well-rounded emergency physicians (including surgeons and anesthesiologists) working under combat/battlefield conditions must be familiar with the equipment and be able to deliver a safe anesthetic with less technological sophistication than in a typical operating room in a civilian environment during peacetime [4]. A modern anesthesia machine provides a wealth of information, but it is not exceedingly portable and its sensitive electronics may not survive battlefield conditions nearly as well as a bag-valve mask and an IV pump.

C. Terrorist Actions

A terrorist attack can occur anytime and anywhere. Terrorist attacks include

The conventional, such as small arms and bombs of varying strength and sophistication, which can cause hundreds of casualties
The unconventional, such as biological, chemical, and nuclear attacks, which may produce many thousands of casualties

Terrorists rarely give advance warning of their attacks; therefore, facilities, systems, and providers caring for the casualties are likely to be unprepared for the event. If the number of injured people is minimal, the medical system can often treat them without invoking a contingency plan. When the number of casualties overwhelms the available treatment capacity, a mass casualty situation has been created. Under mass casualty conditions, adequate contingency plans, well considered in advance, are essential to minimize loss of life and limb. These plans must comply with the wartime mass casualty principles discussed below. Additionally, in the event of an unconventional attack, a system must be in place to protect the health care providers and prevent them from becoming additional casualties.

Community disaster plans can be implemented during and after a terrorist attack, provided they are well designed and practiced. Some aspects of a terrorist attack, however, such as the potential for further attacks or acts of sabotage, are not relevant in a natural disaster. Military assistance can be an invaluable asset for the provision of expertise, rescue, security, personal protective gear, decontamination, materiel, additional manpower, and organization of available resources. Contingency plans for a terrorist attack must include methods of activating and coordinating these resources.

In its most fundamental form, terrorism imposes coercion through atrocity; therefore, a terrorist attack achieves maximal psychological impact when it attracts media coverage, reaching a large population. This fact makes terrorist actions much more likely during an event that receives extensive media coverage, such as a visit from a dignitary, a sporting event, or any large gathering of people. These situations require much more precise planning and training in preparation for a more specific threat. It is advisable to obtain expert advice and professional help toward minimizing the increased risk that these events bring to a community.

Emergency care providers may be called upon to treat the victims of a terrorist attack [5,6]. Treating these victims is not unlike treating war victims, although usually on a smaller and less extended scale. The casualties usually outnumber the care providers, mandating efficiency of triage. Because of the mechanisms of wounding, the injuries will be similar in nature and severity. Anesthesiologists in these scenarios must usually work under substandard conditions, with equipment and monitoring not considered ''standard of care,'' and in most situations to provide care for more than one patient at a time. To minimize the morbidity and mortality of casualties, the anesthesiologist (and all other physicians) must be able to adapt to changing conditions and to improvise when necessary.

II. TACTICAL EMERGENCY MEDICAL SERVICES (TEMS)

The specialty of tactical emergency medical services (TEMS) is a recent development in the arena of disaster management. Developed mainly to deal with high-risk warrant service, raids, and other dangerous law enforcement activities, TEMS has its origins in military counterterrorist units and their activities. The history and present applications of TEMS are discussed more fully elsewhere in this volume (see Chap. 37) [7]. A few salient features are covered here.

The TEMS mission and environment involve high-powered firearms, explosives and other pyrotechnic devices, and chemical agents and contaminants, all of which can create serious individual injuries as well as mass casualties. Immediate stabilization of the scene may assume great importance, because evacuation could be protracted, depending on the tactical environment.

Three main components of TEMS that could involve emergency physicians concern personnel issues; that is, the selection, training, and deployment of medical specialists. In the United States, the majority of these functions are undertaken by nonphysician extenders. In Europe, the opposite situation exists, as summarized by the following complementary cross-training:

TACMED (tactical/medical)—Tactical law enforcement/military personnel receive supplemental medical training to enable them to provide emergency care to the wounded.

MEDTAC (medical/tactical)—Persons with primarily medical backgrounds receive supplemental training in the tactical components of these activities.

Regardless of which approach is adopted (TACMED or MEDTAC), it is essential for medical and tactical personnel to have extensive training and participate in drills together, for them to be familiar with each other's role and equipment, and to have integrated the ''hospital component'' of the TEMS system into the comprehensive response [8].

Typified by the efforts of the U.S. Secret Service to protect the president of the United States, *VIP/executive protection* is the medical component of dignitary protection efforts. A complex system has evolved over the years, primarily to prevent bodily harm to the protectee but secondarily to deal with injuries if they occur. The same considerations apply in the selection and training of personnel in regard to MEDTAC skills, as well as interface with the prehospital/EMS system and designated hospitals, which must be arranged in advance [5–9].

III. MATHEMATICAL MODELING OF MEDICAL DISASTER MANAGEMENT

Every city, town, district, and region has an infrastructure that may be used to anticipate injury incidents and disasters on any scale. This anticipatory process, the mathematical modeling of medical disaster management [10], offers the advantage of allowing disaster preparedness to be addressed in a focused and effective manner. This will serve to markedly reduce mortality, morbidity, and disability figures as well as costs.

An incident resulting in one or more casualties, N, with varying severity of injuries, S, will be met by medical assistance of a specific capacity, C. Medical assistance comprises aid available at the site, transportation of the victim(s), and aid available in the hospital. In this *medical assistance chain* (MAC), both structured and unstructured aid is provided by all kinds of personnel, trained or otherwise, with specific materials, available or otherwise, according to specific techniques, acquired or otherwise. In an organized context, relevant services such as ambulances and hospitals are available. These services within the MAC have a certain capacity, C, that is sufficient for normal, everyday occurrences. If the number of victims, N, with a specific average severity of injuries, S, exceeds the existing capacity, C, however, a discrepancy arises between the injured and their treatment. In this case, either additional services must be called in from outside or local services must be intensified—in other words, a disaster.

A. Medical Severity Index

A turning point can be reached quickly, depending on the number of casualties, N, and the more serious the injuries, S, are in nature. Conversely, the greater the capacity, C, of the medical assistance services, the later the turning point is reached. In short, it is directly proportional to N and S and inversely proportional to, C. This is illustrated by the following simple formula for the calculation of the medical severity index (MSI) [11]:

$$\text{MSI} = (\text{N} \times \text{S})/\text{C}$$

An MSI $\gg$ 1 is indicative of a disaster.

In addition to distinguishing accidents from disasters, the index reflects in medical terms the serious nature of the former and particulars of the latter. For example, an MSI of 0.4 means a sizeable incident, whereas an MSI of 4.2 indicates a substantial disaster. The MSI is important not only for reviewing the momentary situation in a disaster or in evaluating it afterward but also for application in the preparatory phase (i.e., medical disaster preparedness). Each city, town, or ambulance region can use the MSI to calculate its own particular turning point, and on the basis of the number of casualties involved, determine when an incident has turned into a disaster. From a policy point of view, the MSI serves as an excellent tool in the preparatory phase. Methods for determining N, S, and C are presented in the following sections.

B. Estimating the Number of Casualties in a Disaster (N): Rutherford's Rule

In the 1980s, William Rutherford, a Belfast surgeon, formulated a rule for estimating the number of casualties in a disaster [12]. It implies that the number of casualties in a man-made disaster is often initially *over*stated, probably as a result of stress and other emotional factors. Conversely, the number of casualties involved in a natural disaster is initially *under*stated because only a small percentage of the casualties can be seen by eyewitnesses (e.g., in an earthquake). Disasters involving a known number of people (e.g., plane crashes and ferry sinkings) are exceptions to this rule.

With Rutherford's rule in mind, a table can be created to estimate the number of people in immovable objects or passengers in moving ones (Table 1). This allows extraction of the number of casualties and the number of wounded to be hospitalized (if the S factor [see below] is known). Each city or region can prepare such tables, which can be kept in the dashboard of every fire engine and ambulance; displayed in the telephone exchanges of fire, police, and ambulance services; kept in crisis and management centers; and kept in all regional health authorities.

A single example will illustrate the points made above. In 1992, the crash of a plane into an apartment complex in Bijlmer, outside Amsterdam, produced a whole range of casualty estimates; a figure as high as 1,000 was mentioned. Within half an hour, however, it was known that the aircraft involved was a cargo plane and that 40 apartments had been wrecked. With reference to Table 1, the number of occupants per apartment could be put at 2.1, meaning that the total number of casualties, including the crew of the cargo plane, would be approximately 88, three-quarters of whom would have died immediately as a

Table 1 Determination of the Number of Casualties, N, in a Disaster

			Range
Immovables			
Residential area[a]	Per hectare	Low-rise buildings	20–50
		High-rise buildings	50–200
Business area	Per hectare		0–800
Industrial area	Per hectare		0–200
Leisure area	Per type	Stadium	—[b]
		Discotheque	—
		Camping site	—
Shops	Per type	Department store	—[b]
		Arcade	—
Mobile objects			
Road transport	Per 100 M (length)[c]	Multiple collision	5–50
	Per type[d]	Coach	10–100
Rail transport[e]		Single deck	5–400
		Double deck	10–800
Air transport[f]	Per type	Small	10–30
		Large	150–500
Inland shipping[g]	Per type	Ferry	10–1000
		Cruise ship	200–300

Note: Range depends on date, time, and other local circumstances.

[a] Combination of number of residents per house (1.8–2.8) and number of houses per hectare [30–70].

[b] Awaiting further research.

[c] Per car: length 5 meters and 1.5–3 passengers (see Note).

[d] Articulated local bus or articulated double-decker bus.

[e] Carriages of 3 or 4 wagons (see Note).

[f] Seat occupancy 70%.

[g] Seat occupancy 80%.

Source: Ref. 10.

result of the crash itself and the subsequent fire; thus, the estimate would have been 66 dead and 22 injured, totals very close to the actual figures!

C. The Average Severity of Injuries: The Medical Severity Factor (S)

Estimation of the average severity of injuries is an important factor for the medical management team, since there is a major difference between coping with a large number of seriously injured casualties and treating a large number of people with only slight injuries. Trying to save a leg or an arm can require an operation lasting hours, whereas a cut on the head can be treated in less than 10 minutes. Triage systems (for the classification of casualties on the basis of severity of injury) are based on vital functions, respiration, and blood circulation. Disturbances in these functions can be seen as exponents of the seriousness of underlying injuries (e.g., fractures and hemorrhage).

The triage system (Table 2) is suitable for classifying not only people injured mechanically but also people affected by chemical agents. It is clear that groups T1 and T2 demand more time and necessitate hospitalization, whereas the T3 group can be treated by a general practitioner or nurse. The ratio of casualty groups T1 and T2 to the T3 casualty group, or that between those who require hospitalization and those who do not, is the *medical severity factor*.

$$S = (T1 + T2)/T3$$

A recent study [13] of 416 disasters that occurred during the past 40 years reveals that the S factor (i.e., the number of casualties requiring hospitalization) is, for example, three times higher in cases of fire and acts of terrorism (explosions in closed spaces) than that resulting from traffic crashes (road, rail, land, sea). Again, this factor plays a role in the MSI. (See above.)

D. Capacities (C) in the Medical Assistance Chain

Along the MAC, victims receive medical and nursing assistance between the initial site and the hospital, which can be divided into the following three organizational systems or phases:

1. The site of the incident or disaster
2. The transport of casualties and their distribution among hospitals in the vicinity
3. The hospital

Table 2 Triage: Classification of Casualties Based on Severity of Injuries

T1:	ABC unstable victims due to obstruction of airway (A) or disturbance of breathing (B) or circulation (C). Immediate life support and urgent hospital admission.
T2:	Stable victims to be treated within 4–6 hr; otherwise they will become unstable. First-aid measures and hospital admission.
T3:	ABC stable victims with minor injuries not threatened by instability. Can be treated by general practitioners.
T4:	ABC unstable victims who cannot be treated under the circumstances given.

Source: Ref. 10.

During each phase, personnel work with specific materials, employing specific techniques, with a single aim (i.e., to provide the victim with medical and nursing assistance); therefore, during each phase, personnel, materials, and techniques are providing a certain capacity: the medical rescue capacity (MRC) at the site of the disaster, the medical transport capacity (MTC) during transport to medical facilities, and the hospital treatment capacity (HTC) in the hospital.

The MRC is defined as the number of casualties for whom satisfactory and efficient first aid (basic life support and advanced trauma life support) can be provided per hour. The MTC is the number of casualties per hour that can be transported satisfactorily and efficiently to and distributed among hospitals in the vicinity. The HTC means the number of casualties that can be treated satisfactorily and efficiently in the hospital per hour. The smallest capacity (thus the weakest link) in the chain determines the capacity of the whole. This capacity, C, indicates, among other things, the MSI (see above) and thus the turning point between incident and disaster. The MRC, MTC, and HTC are considered separately in the following sections.

1. Medical Rescue Capacity (MRC)

The MRC is determined by personnel, materials, and techniques employed, or in simpler terms, how many casualties can be ''processed'' per hour by a doctor and a nurse, assisted by one or more first aid staff. We are concerned here with casualties who have been moderately or seriously injured and who therefore require further treatment in the hospital. The ratio of moderately and seriously injured (T1 and T2) can vary from 1:2 to 1:4. An experienced team composed of a doctor/specialist and a nurse, assisted by one or two first aid support staff members, would need approximately 1 hr to perform life- and limb-saving procedures for one T1 and three T2 casualties.

2. Medical Transport Capacity (MTC)

A precise estimate of the number of ambulances needed at the site of a disaster not only avoids their unnecessary withdrawal from normal routine duties and therefore avoids unnecessary financial consequences, but also obviates the confusion resulting from the presence of too many relief personnel and vehicles. A considered answer to the question of transporting casualties is desirable from both a repressive and preparedness point of view.

The number of ambulances, X, required at a disaster is directly proportional to the number of casualties to be hospitalized, N, and the average time of the return journey between the site of the disaster and the surrounding hospital, t, and inversely proportional to the number of casualties to be conveyed per journey and per ambulance, n, and the total fixed length of time, T, during which N have to be moved. Thus

$$X = N \times t/T \times n$$

Since the most serious casualties (T1) have to be stabilized within the ''golden hour'' and the moderately injured casualties (T2) within 4 to 6 hr (the Friedrichian time) in order to be subsequently treated in the hospital, T can be fixed at between 4 and 6 hr. The number of T1 and T2 casualties to be conveyed per ambulance per journey is fixed at one in the Netherlands, although a T3 casualty might also be moved as well. The number of casualties to be hospitalized, N, can be determined by using the method described; however, the problem revolves around the calculation of the average journey time, t. This has recently been resolved, so that the average journey time, t, can be expressed in terms of N and T as follows:

$$t = p\,(\sqrt{N}/\sqrt{T})$$

where p depends on local circumstances (e.g., average speed, average hospital treatment capacity, and number of hospitals per square unit surface area). (In the Netherlands, p equals 0.09.) The number of ambulances required, X, and thus the MTC can be determined.

3. Hospital Treatment Capacity (HTC)

The final phase in the MAC concerns the hospital. In a general hospital (from large [1000 beds] to small [100 beds]), there are doctors, nurses, and paramedics. All such hospitals have the basic specialties, such as surgery and internal medicine. Depending on the nature of the illness or incident, in particular whether the patient has mechanical, chemical, nuclear, or biological injuries, treatment takes up a certain amount of time and resources. The HTC is expressed in terms of the number of patients who can be treated per hour and per 100 beds. For the day-to-day surgery situation, the HTC for patients with mechanical injuries amounts to 0.5 to 1 patient per hour per 100 beds. Within the framework of a practiced disaster relief plan, this number can be increased to 2 to 3 patients per hour per 100 beds. This figure, derived from many exercises for mechanical injuries, is determined primarily by the number of available surgeons, anesthesiologists, and specialist nursing staff and also by the accommodations and medical equipment available.

Table 3 Classification and Assessment of Disasters

Classification	Grade	Score
Effect on infrastructure	Simple	1
(impact site + filter area)	Compound	2
Impact time	<1 hr	0
	1–24 hr	1
	>24 hr	2
Radius of impact site	<1 km	0
	1–10 km	1
	>10 km	2
Number of dead	<100	0
	>100	1
Number of injured (N)	<100	0
	100–1000	1
	>1000	2
Average severity of	<1	0
injuries sustained (S)[a]	1–2	1
	>2	2
Rescue time	<6 hr	0
(rescue + first aid + transportation)	6–24 hr	1
	>24 hr	2
Total	DSS	1–13

[a] $S = (T1 + T2)/T3$.
DSS, disaster severity scale score.
Source: Ref. 10.

Table 4 Determination of Medical Disaster Preparedness

	Prehospital		Transport		Hospital			
Personnel	Doctors	a	Doctors	a	Doctors	a	No personnel available	1
							Personnel being appointed	2
	Nurses	b	Nurses	b	Nurses	b	Personnel available	3
							Personnel available and trained (certified)	4
	Paramedics	c	Paramedics	c	Paramedics	c	Personnel available; regular drills and upgrading	5
Subtotal	(a + b + c)/e		(a + b + c)/e		(a + b + c)/e			
Material	Ventilation	a	Ventilation	a	Ventilation	a	No materials available	2
							Materials being purchased	2
	Circulation	b	Circulation	b	Circulation	b	Materials available	3
							Materials available and tested	4
	Other material	c	Other material	c	Other material	c	Materials available; regular drills and upgrading	5
Subtotal	(a + b + c)/e		(a + b + c)/e		(a + b + c)/e			
Methods	Attack plans	a	Ambulance assistance	a	Disaster procedures	a	No plan available	1
							Plan in preparation	2
	Triage	b	Patient distribution	b	Triage	b	Plan available	3
							Plan available and tested	4
	Treatment protocols	c	Patient monitoring	c	Simplication standardization	c	Plan available; regular drills and upgrading	5
Subtotal	(a + b + c)/e[a]		(a + b + c)/e		(a + b + c)/e			
Total							Grand total	

[a] e number of items, in this case 3.

Source: Ref. 10.

Naturally, the HTC for mechanical injuries is determined by additional factors. In a disaster situation, hospital staff works harder, with the result that the HTC increases. On the other hand, the tiredness factor in such a situation occurs somewhat later, reducing the HTC. Certain kinds of disasters (e.g., explosions and fires in closed space) result in more seriously injured patients and therefore place a greater burden on the HTC.

E. Classification of Disasters

When the variables N, S, and C of the MSI are known, so too is the turning point between incident and disaster. The internationally accepted definition of a disaster is a destructive event that claims so many casualties (N and S) that a discrepancy arises between the numbers of people involved and the capacity to treat them (C) [14].

A disaster severity scale (DDS) score can be calculated by assigning a value to the parameters listed in Table 3. The values are totaled, yielding a score of 1 to 13. This assessment is useful for the analysis and comparison of disasters, facilitating epidemiologic research.

F. Determination of Disaster Preparedness

Another score indicates a community's or region's level of preparedness for disasters. For this calculation, the personnel, materials, and methods available in each phase of the MAC are analyzed (Table 4) and the subgroup is assigned a value from 1 to 5. (One represents total absence and 5 the optimal situation.) The values are totaled and their sum is divided by the number of items, giving a set of subtotals. These subtotals are then added and divided by the number of subtotals, yielding a ''grand total'' that also ranges from 1 to 5 [15,16].

IV. DISASTER RESPONSE PLANNING

The best way to manage disasters is to be prepared for them [1]. In fact, planning can be the most laborious part of disaster management [17]. Disaster simulations and drills should be mandatory for all EMS personnel. The Joint Commission on Accreditation of Healthcare Organizations (JCAHO) requires all hospitals to have a disaster plan and to test this plan twice a year.

Disaster response plans incorporate a variety of simulations and drills [18–20], including the following:

Simulations—can be staged at various levels, with varying degrees of complexity and associated costs

Computer-based models—the most simple and easy to execute; can employ a local area network (LAN) to link participants

''Tabletop'' or ''sand table'' systems of disaster modeling present a miniaturized scale of an area (often using materials from model railroad sets) to demonstrate a threat. In this type of simulation, participants can view the situation in three dimensions, use an interactive format to discuss the response, and play out a variety of scenarios.

''Full-scale'' or ''real-life'' systems involve life-size modeling, including moulaged victims; actual response; and transport units (ambulances, fire trucks, and helicopters). This type of simulation is very expensive to conduct, requires a great deal of advanced coordination to maximize the value, and is logistically intense. Both prehospital and in-hospital components can participate, both of which must function in an effective disaster response.

''Drills'' are mock alarms designed to test the readiness of a system, usually without advance warning. Drills may include various elements of the types of simulations described above.

The International Trauma Anesthesia and Critical Care Society (ITACCS) stages its international chief emergency physician training course on command incident management and mass casualty disasters annually [21]. This 3-day course, emphasizing leadership and management skills, employs all of the types of simulations discussed above, culminating with a full-scale simulation on the last day. Participants are typically senior physicians, including many anesthesiologists, surgeons, and emergency medicine specialists, of the trauma/EMS systems from which they are selected. It is assumed that they are already proficient in trauma patient management.

In a JCAHO-mandated drill of a hospital disaster plan, a scenario is given to the hospital, and the hospital disaster response is initiated. Extra personnel are summoned, equipment and supplies are made available, and moulaged volunteer victims are brought to the emergency department. To minimize the waste of hospital supplies, either the supplies are not opened or out-of-date materials are used for disaster plan exercises.

Most communities hold disaster drills for EMS, fire, and police personnel as well. The drills are either planned or random. Planned drills have proven to be more beneficial in terms of training. The plan should involve every department and hospital employee.

V. PRACTICAL ASPECTS OF THE PREHOSPITAL MEDICAL CARE ENVIRONMENT

In the United States, it is rare for physicians (including emergency medicine physicians) to be actively engaged in field situations. In response to mass casualty/disaster situations and in situations requiring prolonged extrications, however, many trauma centers formulate ''go teams,'' which travel from the hospital to the scene to perform emergency surgery and administer anesthesia. Conversely, in Europe anesthesiologists commonly work in field environments, routinely providing service on EMS helicopters and land ambulances, including mobile intensive-care units [6].

Any disaster response has three phases: activation, implementation, and recovery.

Activation is the initial response and notification, followed by the establishment of an incident command post (ICP). The first responder on the scene reports

- The nature of the incident
- The number and types of injuries
- The potential hazards for victims as well as rescuers
- The extent of damage to the area
- Possible access routes to and away from the scene

This relay of information is paramount and should be done before any direct medical assistance is provided.

Following initial notification, the ICP is established as close to the scene as safety allows, uphill and upwind in the event of a liquid or airborne hazard. The incident commander has overall authority on the scene and responsibility for organizing the scene. Depending on the community, the commander is typically the fire chief or chief of police.

The primary concern is scene safety, which must be maintained by fire and police officials. Protecting the responders is the utmost priority. Rescues from contaminated areas (see below) are not attempted until the chemical has been identified and proper personal protective equipment (PPE) and trained personnel are available.

Another priority is crowd control. To minimize the chance of bystanders becoming victims, they are maintained at a safe distance from the scene by police personnel.

Implementation involves search and rescue (SAR) followed by triage and initial stabilization. Search and rescue is carried out by specially trained personnel who have the expertise and equipment necessary for hazardous situations. Medical personnel not trained in SAR should wait at the CCP to avoid the possibility of becoming victims themselves. Search and rescue operations vary, depending on geographic location. Urban areas with large structures are very different from suburban areas. Rescue of victims trapped in tons of steel and concrete demands heavy equipment and skilled rescuers knowledgeable in large-scale extrication. Suburban and wilderness SAR is an entirely different entity. Knowledge of rope and vertical rescue is needed for mountainous terrain. Rescuers must be adept at conducting large-scale searches over vast areas in short amounts of time. In general, SAR personnel are trained in the type of rescue they will most likely need to perform in their particular community.

After victims are brought to EMS personnel, triage continues and initial stabilization is given. Medical care is limited to airway management, control of hemorrhage, administration of oxygen, and immobilization of victims on backboards as necessary. Victims are then transported to facilities that can provide definitive medical care.

Recovery is a three-step process: (1) the systematic withdrawal of all personnel and equipment from the scene, (2) the return of all parties to normal operations, and (3) debriefing, an analysis of the event in an attempt to improve future responses as well as an opportunity for rescue personnel to discuss any emotional difficulties they are experiencing as a result of the disaster. The psychological impact of disasters on rescue and medical personnel can be devastating, ranging from very mild disturbances to posttraumatic stress disorder (PTSD). Therapists or counselors should be available to members of the rescue team if needed.

A. Triage

Triage (from the French verb *trier*, meaning "to sort"), a crucial part of the implementation phase, deserves further elaboration. The process was developed by the military as a method of sorting large numbers of patients according to the priority with which they should be treated and transported. Victims are triaged at numerous sites [22]: (1) at the scene by rescuers, (2) by EMS personnel at the CCP, (3) during transport, and (4) at the hospital at which definitive care is given. The goal of triage is to accomplish the greatest good for the most casualties under the special circumstances of warfare or mass casualty incidents.

During a time of mass casualties, conventional standards of care might not apply. Some seriously wounded casualties may not receive the same standard of care as if they had presented as a single admission. "Reverse triage" is the exclusion of patients with lethal injuries, allowing available resources to be allocated to those with the greatest chance of survival. A single severely injured patient requiring 12 hr of surgery for a small chance of survival may inappropriately consume resources, resulting in the deaths of many patients with lesser injuries. It is important to understand that triage applies to both treatment and transport of patients to a higher echelon of care. Within the basic structure of these principles, triage must be adapted to the specific situation [23].

There is great debate over who should perform triage. Many have advocated physicians as the obvious choice, but mass casualty triage does not involve the use of highly sophisticated equipment or procedures and in general could be performed by the most basic medical personnel on scene. The clinical abilities and high knowledge base of physicians and nurses as well as senior paramedics are better utilized in a treatment or medical command role. Many EMS agencies in Europe have physicians and nurses as their first responders, however, and do not have paramedics. In this case, utilization of physicians in a triage role may be the only choice.

One method of triage that has come to be the standard at most mass casualty training exercises is the START (simple triage and rapid treatment) method. It does not require the expertise of a physician, nurse, or paramedic and can be performed in rapid succession. In the START method, each patient's level of consciousness, airway, breathing, and capillary refill are evaluated in a rapid fashion and then the patients are divided into the triage categories based on the findings. (See below.) This method allows quick assessment of multiple victims and follows the basic tenets of the ABCDE (airway, breathing, circulation, disability, and exposure) of the trauma primary survey. Patients who have been involved in a hazardous materials incident should be decontaminated as much as possible prior to being brought to the triage or treatment areas.

All casualties can be classified into four logical categories, referred to in the military as minimal, delayed, immediate, and expectant (Table 5). In many EMS systems in the United States, four triage categories (Table 6), paralleling those used in Europe, are used.

Triage tags should be used by EMS services in a mass casualty situation. The tags serve a dual purpose in that they not only specify what category the patient has been triaged into but also serve as a means of patient identification via the tag identification number. The patient category is identified by a color coding system. Patients in the immediate category (priority/level 1) are signified by a red tag. Those in the delayed category (priority/level 2) are represented by a yellow tag. The minimal/minor category (priority/level 3) is assigned a green tag. The last category, for dead or morbid patients (priority/level 4), is assigned a black triage label.

The main drawbacks to triage tags are that they are seldom available to the person who does the initial triage and are easily dislodged from the patient. Some tags do not allow for the patient's condition to be upgraded or downgraded. After a long review pro-

Table 5 Military Classifications of Casualties

Minimal	Minor injuries not requiring prompt medical attention	Treated/transported after immediate and delayed patients
Delayed	Serious injuries requiring treatment, but not immediately life-threatening	Treated/transported after immediate patients
Immediate	Injuries requiring immediate treatment to save life or limb	Treated/transported first
Expectant	Injuries sufficiently severe that survival under the current situation is unlikely	Comfort measures only

Table 6 Triage Categories Used in the United States

Priority 1—immediate. The highest priority is given to severely injured victims who will most likely survive if given initial stabilization and early transport but who will probably die if stabilization procedures are not performed.
Priority 2—delayed. The next highest priority is given to victims who have moderate injuries—who would not likely die if treatment is withheld but who will eventually need definitive care.
Priority 3—minor. Third highest priority is given to patients with minor injuries, the "walking wounded." These victims must wait at the scene until victims of higher priority have been transported.
Priority 4—deceased. The lowest priority is given to victims who are hopelessly wounded or in cardiac arrest at the time of initial evaluation. This decision is difficult for most medical personnel to accept, but the goal of triage must be kept in mind.

cess and after experiences with the use of triage tags during several mass casualty incidents and drills, EMS officials in the state of Maryland [24] have identified desirable characteristics for the tags, as shown in Table 7. In this era of computers and miniaturization, small electronic tags will no doubt become available in the future.

An additional aspect of triage is the immediate performance of any lifesaving treatment that can be performed quickly (e.g., application of a tourniquet, decompression of a tension pneumothorax). This step may result in reclassification of an "immediate" patient to "delayed" status, thus conserving resources for other casualties. Triage is a process that needs to be ongoing and repeated according to changing conditions, the needs of the victims, and the treatment capability available.

B. Positioning

The positioning of patients is almost as important as triage. The treatment area should be large enough to accommodate the number of patients and caregivers. The treatment areas should be located in such a way that the red and yellow triage categories are closest to their respective modes of transport, whether that be by helicopter or ambulance. The area should be safe from exposure to hazardous materials. Factors influencing the location of the treatment area such as wind direction should be taken into account so that smoke or hazardous materials will not affect the patients or caregivers.

Table 7 Desirable Characteristics of Triage Tags

They must be easily understood by the variety of prehospital/hospital personnel who will see the patient.
They must be of a size that can be attached to a patient easily without being destroyed by extrication or movement of the patient.
They must be durable and waterproof.
They must accept writing from pen, pencil, and other writing implements.
They must be constructed so that their parts will not separate inadvertently.
They must be designed to allow collection of information that is absolutely necessary to manage the patient.
They must be familiar to prehospital personnel.

Source: Adapted from Ref. 24.

Traditionally patients have been stacked in a side-by-side line fashion, like dominoes. This technique poses several logistical problems: it disperses the caregivers, makes procedures to be performed on the patient difficult, and usually causes patients to be removed on a first-come, first-served basis rather than moving the most critical patients quickly. Attempting to intubate the third patient in the second row requires some degree of acrobatics.

An alternative means of patient positioning is the casualty orientation for rapid exam (CORE) method. This technique uses the same premise that is used in most emergency departments and intensive care units; that is, by placing patients in a semicircle, multiple patients can be attended or observed at one time by a minimum number of caregivers.

In the CORE method, victims are not placed side by side, but in a semicircle, with their upper torsos oriented toward the center (core) (Fig. 1). In this way, rescuers or treatment personnel can assess one victim's airway and then move to the next victim with relative ease. It also allows the medical officer in charge of the treatment area to rapidly visualize each victim's airway, breathing, and ongoing treatment and thus be better able to plan for equipment and transport needs. There is an added benefit of creating additional space between each victim, which occurs by design, so that caregivers are not stepping on or over other victims in order to provide treatment. The open portion of the semicircle allows the relatively easy movement of equipment into the center of the circle for use by treatment personnel. The equipment is therefore more visible, eliminating chaotic searches for equipment from mutual-aid vehicles unfamiliar to rescuers from different departments. Victims can be removed from the treatment area for transport by loading them from the outside of the semicircle so as not to disrupt the ongoing treatment of other victims.

C. Transport

The transport officer should set up a loading zone or staging area for transport so that patients can be taken from the treatment area and placed directly into a waiting squad or helicopter. The transport officer will keep a written record of the patients and their respective destinations by recording the triage tag number and assigning a hospital based on the severity of injury. Although the ambulances may drop off personnel and equipment to

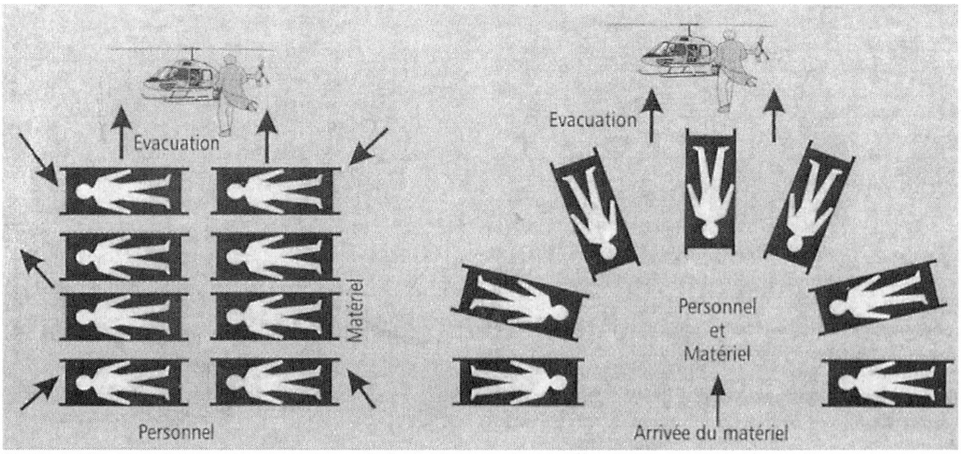

Figure 1 Disposer les blessés: comparaison entre la méthode en ligne et al méthode CORE [disposition of the injured: comparison of the line and CORE methods].

the treatment and triage areas, their vehicles should then be repositioned such that only two ambulances at a time are in the loading zone to minimize chaos and ease traffic patterns. The transport area or loading zone should be in close proximity to the immediate and delayed care areas. Buses and other means of mass transportation should be positioned near the minimal treatment area. Rotor aircraft should be utilized for the immediate care patients when possible. Although most pilots of rotor aircraft prefer to land into the wind, this may not be possible because of hazardous materials or smoke. The landing zone should thus be opposite the wind direction. It is also best to have the ambulance staging area between the patient care areas and the aircraft landing zone. This allows the ambulances to act as a wind break so that the rotor wash does not blow equipment and the triage tags away.

Every effort should be made to transport a patient who has been exposed to hazardous materials by ground ambulance rather than air transport. Fumes from inadequate decontamination could overcome the pilot of an aircraft and cause a mishap. If the cabin is contaminated, the aircraft must be taken out of service for decontamination, and the aircraft will not be able to return to the scene for some time.

D. Public Relations

Representatives of the media will be present at all disasters. Their access to the scene must be limited to protect the privacy of the victims as well as to minimize the possibility of reporters also becoming victims. In regular briefings, an appointed public relations officer should describe the history of the events and generically describe activities related to the response to the incident. A similar officer should be named at the receiving hospital(s). Such designations will improve the flow of information from those in charge at the scene and thus decrease the amount of erroneous information given to the public.

The media can be a valuable resource for announcing possible hazards; the need for evacuation; and even the need for additional fire, medical, rescue, or police personnel. Proper use of the media can also help prevent public hysteria and reactions such as rioting.

VI. HOSPITAL RESPONSE

In a true disaster situation, the decision to implement the hospital disaster response should not be delayed. The hospital could receive large numbers of victims, possibly critically injured, in a very short time. The emergency department should be cleared rapidly, and extra oxygen and crystalloid need to be readily available. Operating room personnel, including anesthesia services, trauma surgeons, and support staff, must be prepared for emergent operations. Extra security will be needed to control family members and the media. A medical triage officer will be needed in the emergency department to set priorities.

VII. NATIONAL DISASTER MEDICAL SYSTEM

In 1984, the National Disaster Medical System (NDMS) was created in the United States to establish a way of caring for large numbers of casualties from military as well as civilian disasters. This was a cooperative effort between the civilian hospital sector of the United States and the Department of Health and Human Services, the Department of Defense, the Federal Emergency Management Agency (FEMA), the Veterans Administration, and state, regional, and local governments.

The NDMS is a two-part system. First is the organization of participating civilian hospitals and health care providers in 74 metropolitan areas. Large numbers of victims can be transported to any of these areas for definitive care. It is equivalent to mutual aid on a national scale. The second part of the NDMS consists of disaster medical assist teams (DMAT)—volunteer health care providers who on request will bring equipment to the scene to support local efforts. During civilian disasters, the NDMS can be employed if the governor of the affected state asks FEMA for assistance and if the request is granted by the president of the United States.

VIII. PREHOSPITAL/RESCUE EQUIPMENT FOR DISASTERS

A wide range of specialized equipment exists for rescue and extrication and is carried by most large-scale, well-supported EMS systems [25]. At times, such equipment is brought to the scene after the initial site survey and may include "jaws of life" (used to pry apart portions of automobiles) and lift bags (filled with air and used to elevate heavy objects).

A full discussion of the types and applications of such equipment is beyond the scope of this chapter, but anesthesiologists who will interact with prehospital care providers and who may be activated in mass casualty/disaster situations should have some familiarity with the terminology and the types of equipment and their use. Equipment having direct applications for the medical component of prehospital emergency services will be discussed here briefly.

A. Basic Life Support

The emergency equipment necessary during disaster conditions varies both in type and in quantity according to the specific situation. Basic equipment that should be always available in the field should include airway equipment (oral and nasal airways, masks, endotracheal tubes, laryngoscopes, and blades), breathing equipment (bag–valve masks, oxygen tanks, tubing, and regulators), and equipment for maintaining circulation (IV fluids, blood, tubing, catheters, tape, drugs). More sophisticated equipment may also be required, contingent upon the level of care to be offered at a specific location [26].

B. Anesthesia/Resuscitation/Advanced Life Support

If anesthesia is to be administered at the incident site, specialized equipment is required [27–29]. Ideally, a state-of-the-art facility would be available and fully functioning; however, the most basic equipment must include apparatus for delivering inhalational, intravenous, and regional anesthetics and for providing oxygenation and ventilatory support. Such equipment can be simple and portable or sophisticated and stationary, as conditions warrant.

Total intravenous anesthesia (TIVA) can be administered with an IV pump, airway/breathing equipment, and monitoring equipment. The equipment is portable, and this technique can be used successfully in a variety of operative procedures. Patients must be monitored closely by properly trained personnel, however.

Regional anesthesia is another option in the field [30,31]. During a disaster, being able to converse with a conscious patient can replace the necessity of extensive monitoring equipment. The equipment and materials needed for performing blocks is simple, portable, and reliable, and most blocks can be placed relatively quickly by trained personnel. When appropriate, subarachnoid and epidural anesthesia, major nerve blocks (e.g., femoral, axillary), and intravenous anesthesia (Bier block) offer the advantage of requiring minimal one-on-one monitoring after the initial placement and establishment of the block. Regional anesthetics that function well can allow anesthesiologists to monitor conscious patients with lesser-trained personnel, thus freeing the anesthesiologists to tend to other patients in the immediate area.

IX. ANESTHETIC MANAGEMENT OF MASS CASUALTY AND DISASTER VICTIMS

Although the actual and specific perioperative and critical care management of trauma patients is beyond the scope of this discussion and covered elsewhere [32], anesthesiologists must be aware that the care of multiple patients is only as good as the care provided for single patients. It therefore follows that an anesthesiologist who might be involved in responding to a mass casualty incident and caring for injury victims must be familiar, hopefully on a routine basis, with the care of severely traumatized patients.

Key areas include heightened awareness of the behavior of hypovolemic patients, specific techniques and strategies for dealing with airway challenges common to trauma patients (e.g., the ''full stomach''), cervical spine precautions, head injuries and cerebral hemodynamics, the prevalence of hypothermia and its implications in trauma, and the impact of pneumothorax and its relationship to hemodynamics as well as to positive-pressure ventilation and anesthetic gases such as nitrous oxide.

If one could choose only one monitoring tool to take to a disaster site, the pulse oximeter might be the device of choice. It is small and low in cost, and can supply the most physiologic data—the state of the arterial blood and tissue oxygenation as well as pulse rate. When there is a decrease in perfusion pressure, the disappearance of the pulse oximeter waveform signals an important clue. The Israeli Defense Force uses the pulse oximeter as its sole monitoring device for critically wounded patients during air evacuation [33].

Similarly, the capnograph may also be used to provide extended information, far more than the level of end tidal CO_2 and respiratory rate, especially for patients who are intubated. Changes in the characteristics of wave form and expired carbon dioxide level may reflect issues of pulmonary dynamics and cardiac output.

X. ANESTHESIA AND ANALGESIA IN PRIMITIVE FIELD CONDITIONS

This section describes various agents and techniques. Their application to specific situations is examined in greater detail elsewhere [34,35].

A. Intravenous Agents

Barbiturates are popular as low-cost induction agents, having especially favorable effects on intracranial pressure. Their use for analgesic purposes and for prolonged infusion is not, however, useful in austere conditions.

Diazepam has positive applications in a variety of field conditions, given via both the intravenous as well as the intramuscular route. Its longer elimination half-life allows it to be administered less frequently, which may be beneficial in mass casualty/disaster situations in which frequent redosing of patients is usually not feasible. Respiratory depression in moderate doses can be avoided and is in fact reversible if desired by using the specific benzodiazepine antagonist, flumazenil.

Midazolam, a newer water-soluble benzodiazepine with good cardiovascular stability, demonstrates variations in dose requirements. Humanitarian and medicolegal concerns related to ''perioperative awareness'' have increased the use of this agent in view of its hemodynamic stability in trauma patients. Its shorter-acting profile, however, may be a relative disadvantage in high-volume trauma scenarios, such as mass casualty/disaster situations, because more frequent dosing might be required. Like midazolam, it is also reversible with flumazenil.

Etomidate is an imidazole induction agent not recommended for prolonged infusion because of adverse affects on steroid synthesis. It is often preferred for anesthetic induction in patients suffering from shock because of its relative cardiostability.

Propofol was introduced in the United Kingdom in 1986 and in the United States from 1988 to 1989. It is suitable as a continuous infusion, either for sedation or as part of a TIVA regimen, and has a short redistribution half-life. Propofol's volume of distribution is similar to that of thiopental and etomidate, but propofol has the highest clearance rate of all induction agents. As with other induction agents, relative cardiovascular depression can be observed in hypovolemic patients, thus warranting caution in patients with serious injury and in patients who may be sensitive to respiratory depression (such as those with head trauma).

B. Inhalation Agents

General characteristics of popular inhalation agents currently in use, as well as their specific applications in trauma, are described elsewhere [32]. Inhalants would be used largely for anesthetic maintenance of patients with traumatic injuries. Because of full-stomach considerations, however, inhalation induction (even with the ''single-breath'' techniques associated with sevoflurane) would largely be avoided, unless other means were unavailable. Desflurane is probably best avoided in trauma patients because of the drug's tendency to induce airway irritability. *Isoflurane* and *sevoflurane* are thus the preferred agents.

C. Analgesic Agents

A wide variety of new nonsteroidal anti-inflammatory agents and nonnarcotic synthetic agents are available. Their mechanisms of actions vary widely, and these drugs can be either additive or synergistic when used in combination with other agents.

The avoidance of central respiratory depression is a primary benefit of these types of analgesics. This characteristic reduces the need for close observation and monitoring and for respiratory support and mechanical ventilation, which are always at a premium in mass casualty/disaster situations.

Parenteral forms are preferred, particularly intravenous, although an intravenous/intramuscular combination regimen can be used to yield immediate onset effects with prolonged duration of action.

D. Mixed Opioid Agonists/Antagonists

Buprenorphine, butorphanol, and *nalbuphine* are attractive for their ceiling on respiratory depression and relative cardiovascular/hemodynamic stability. The potential benefits that apply to nonsteroidal agents (vis-à-vis avoiding the need for close monitoring and respiratory support) are very attractive in the mass casualty/disaster setting; therefore, many military medical services have substituted mixed opioid agonist/antagonist agents for naturally occurring opium derivatives (such as morphine) for field use by medics.

E. Opioids

Fentanyl, one of the first synthetic compounds to become available, is popular among anesthesiologists. Its onset of action and half-life are also attractive when compared with the shorter-acting agents alfentanil and remifentanyl, which would not be appropriate in mass casualty/disaster situations. Sufentanyl, with which profound respiratory depression and chest wall rigidity are experienced, is not warranted for use in these scenarios. European anesthesiologists have made wider use of oxymorphone, propoxyphene, and other synthetic and semisynthetic opioid analgesics that might have applications in these cases.

F. Nonopioid General Analgesics

Ketamine, a phencyclidine derivative, serves as an intravenous anesthetic with analgesic activity. Although a controversial agent and variably popular in various trauma-related settings, ketamine is often regarded as the agent of choice in austere conditions because of its relative portability, extended shelf-life, high relative potency versus dose given, and ability to (relatively) preserve respiratory drive and thus avoid the need for close monitoring and respiratory support [35–39].

Regarded by some anesthesiologists as the ''ideal sole agent'' for unfavorable situations, ketamine can be used in both anesthetic and subanesthetic doses and may be administered intravenously, intramuscularly, or subcutaneously. Various regimens have been described using it as a component of TIVA or in an intramuscular regimen with benzodiazepine for a large group of casualties [36].

Others believe ketamine use to be inadvisable in situations such as military or mass casualty/disaster field situations because of its side effects such as involuntary muscle movements, vivid hallucinations, and hypertension. In addition, its use in patients with head injuries is disputed because of concerns about increasing intracranial pressure.

The inhalation analgesic *nitrous oxide* is generally avoided for in-hospital management of trauma patients. When administered as an analgesic by means of a portable apparatus such as the Entonox device, however (which provides a uniform 50–50 oxygen–nitrogen mixture), the agent has found some use as an analgesic for prehospital and emergency department administration [40]. Nonetheless, the effects of expanding air-filled spaces, as are commonly found in trauma patients (such as a pneumothorax or pneumocephalus), must be kept in mind when considering using this agent.

G. Patient-Controlled Analgesia

Infusion pumps for use as patient-controlled analgesia (PCA) would be at a premium and of limited availability in mass casualty/disaster situations. When applied in a patient-controlled system, however, various regimens can alleviate the need for high nurse : patient ratios and thus help to make queuing for optimal services more tolerable to patients.

XI. ANESTHESIA EQUIPMENT FOR AUSTERE CONDITIONS

It is generally accepted that anesthesia and critical care for trauma victims in out-of-hospital situations can be provided with the same level of sophistication found in hospital operating rooms and intensive care units [27–29]. Thanks to medical device miniaturization, extended battery life, increased durability, and multitasking of equipment, a wide range of capabilities can be condensed within the same package (Fig. 2).

Equipment related to anesthesia and critical care in austere conditions can be divided into those that *provide* a function and those that *monitor* or *measure* a function. Total anesthesia machines, ventilators, and infusion pumps are included in the first category. The second category includes electrocardiogram (ECG) equipment and devices for noninvasive blood pressure (NIBP) measurement; arterial blood gas (ABG) analysis; and blood analysis for electrolytes, hemoglobin, coagulation, and hemoglobin/hematocrit.

There are several options within the first category for providing anesthesia in the field. Anesthesia equipment designed for use under austere conditions should be characterized by portability, durability, serviceability, ease of operation and repair, and low cost. Electrical requirements should be minimal (or even optional), and if possible, fresh gas requirements should also be minimized.

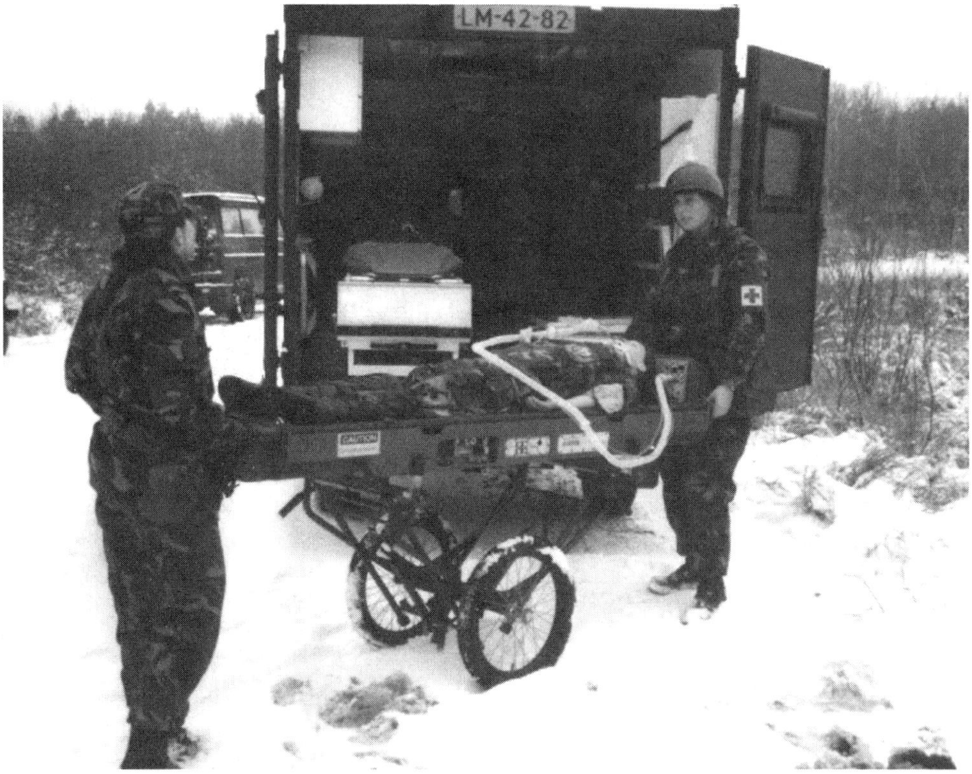

Figure 2 Life Support for Trauma and Transport (LSTAT). An individualized portable intensive care system and surgical platform providing resuscitation and stabilization capability. Features ventilation, suction, oxygen, infusion pump, physiologic monitor, clinical blood analyzer, and defibrillation, complemented by a fully network-capable onboard computer monitoring system and independent power system, packaged on a NATO litter form factor. (Courtesy of Integrated Medical Systems, Inc., Signal Hill, California.)

There are three broad categories of anesthesia delivery systems (which are covered elsewhere in this text): (1) demand flow equipment, (2) plenum or flow equipment, and (3) draw-over equipment. Standard operating room anesthesia equipment utilizes the first type of delivery system. *Closed-circuit techniques* use standard plenum equipment and a circle system, which conserves oxygen supplies and anesthetic agents but which also requires significant amounts of carbon dioxide absorbent. Training and experience are also required. *Draw-over anesthetic systems* allow the administration of a known anesthetic concentration from a calibrated vaporizer using ambient air as the carrier gas. Supplemental oxygen can be added when available, but is not essential for the system's operation. A variety of draw-over systems and modifications exist, used primarily by U. K. Commonwealth members (Britain, Australia, Canada) [41,42] (Fig. 3). This range of devices includes the basic draw-over anesthesia system, as in the Tri-Service Anesthesia (TSA) apparatus, as well as the Portable Anesthesia Complete (PAC) unit (Fig. 4).

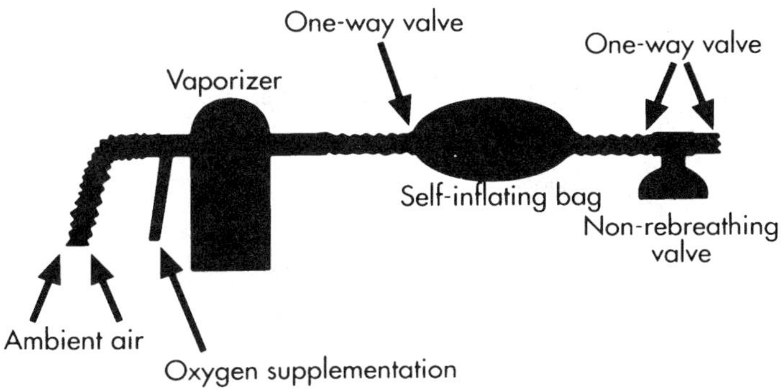

(a)

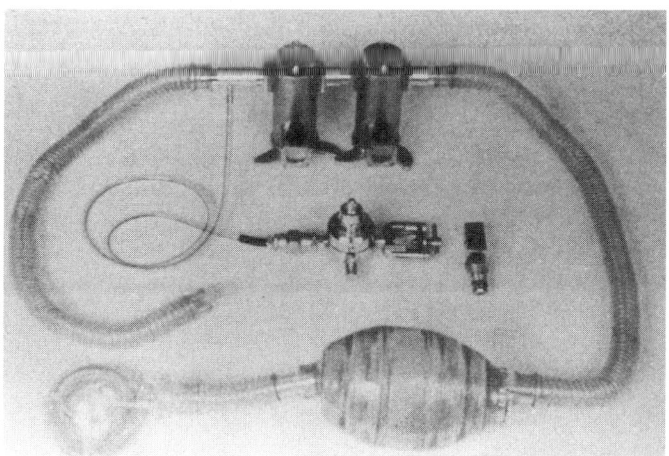

(b)

Figure 3 (a) Components of draw-over anesthesia systems. (b) Tri-Service anesthesia apparatus with Oxford miniature vaporizer unit.

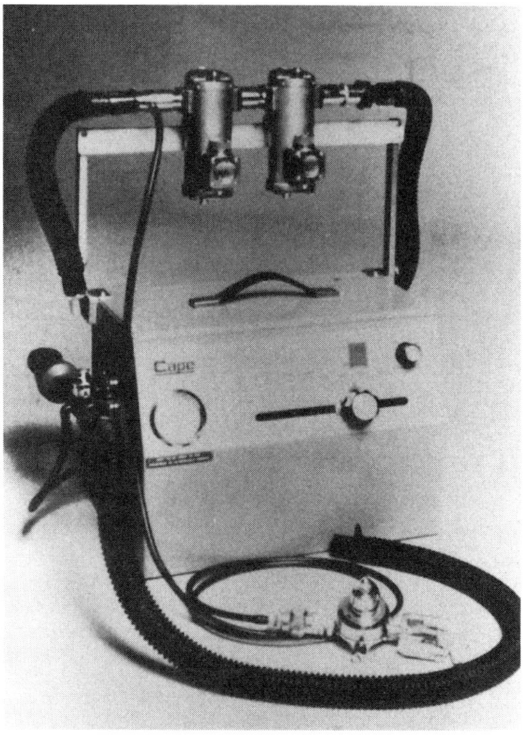

(c)

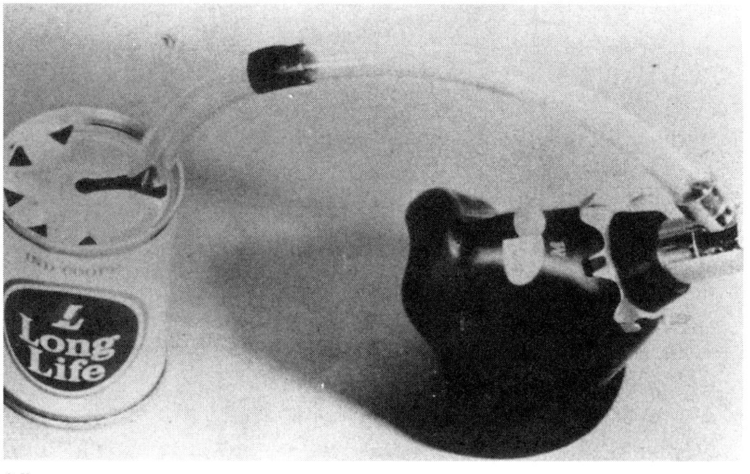

(d)

Figure 3 (c) Mounted on Cape TC50 ventilator. (d) Field expedient system. (From Ref. 42a.)

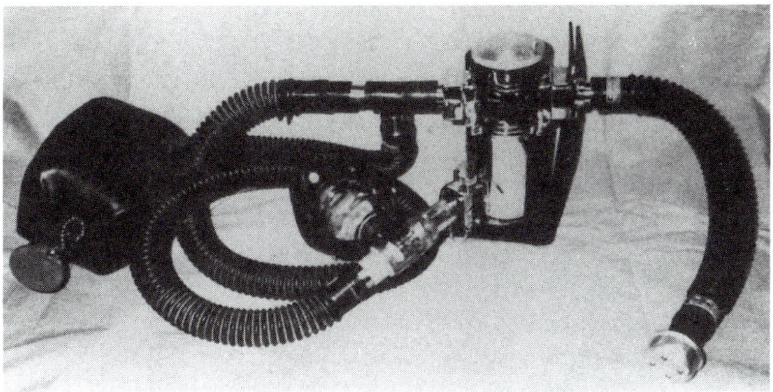

Figure 4 Portable anesthesia complete (PAC) unit vaporizer system. (From Ref. 42a.)

In their standard designs, TSA and/or PAC systems do not incorporate visual signs of the volume of spontaneous respiration. This can be provided, however, by fitting an open-ended reservoir bag to the expiratory port of the one-way valve, or else a scavenging hose for exhaled gases can be fitted to the expiratory port of this valve.

A more conventional but still highly portable (86-lb) anesthetic delivery system is the model 885-A Military Field Anesthesia Machine (Fig. 5) used by U.S. forces. Although it does not meet current American Society of Testing and Materials (ASTM) standards, anesthetics have been administered safely in thousands of cases using this apparatus, which is a continuous-flow, semiclosed circle system similar to the equipment in common use in operating rooms throughout the world.

Suction, a defibrillator, and monitoring equipment must also be available (Table 8; Figs. 6, 7). Monitoring equipment should include pulse oximetry if possible, since this is very portable and provides a great deal of information—pulse, oxygenation status, sufficient arterial blood pressure for the machine to detect, and perfusion of extremities. Additional desirable monitoring equipment includes blood pressure monitors (automatic, manual, and/or invasive), temperature, capnography, gas analysis, electrocardiography, blood gas analysis, and basic laboratory tests. These monitors vary significantly in sophistication and portability, and may not all be available or needed in every situation. Successful anesthesiologists in disaster situations will be able to innovate to use the available equipment, improvise for what is not available, and provide safe anesthetics.

A. Oxygen Supply

Oxygen is perhaps the most essential ''drug'' that may be administered to a trauma patient. In a conventional setting, it is typically supplied by direct pipe to operating rooms. In out-of-hospital situations, oxygen can be carried in a variety of sizes of tanks, which are both heavy and potentially hazardous to transport, particularly in unstable conditions such as those frequently found in mass casualty/disaster situations.

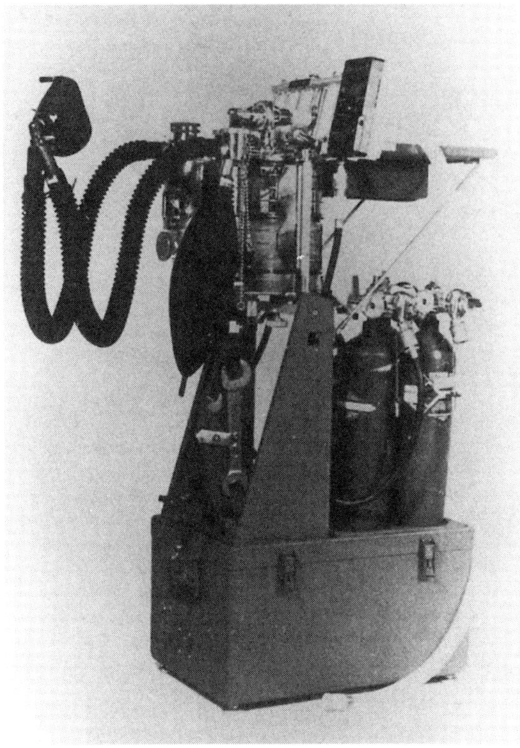

(a)

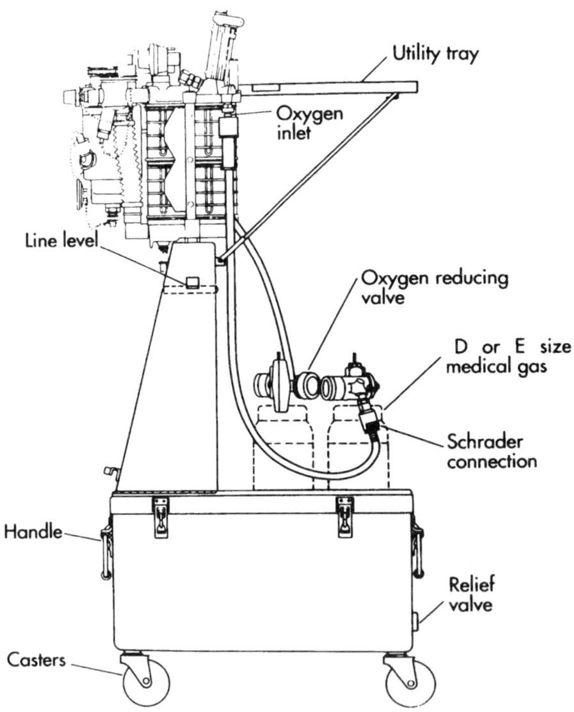

(b)

Figure 5 (a) Model 885-A military field anesthesia machine (Ohmeda BOC). (b) Side view of military field anesthesia machine. Casters provide mobility. Line level on side of support arm. Size E gas cylinder is connected to control head oxygen inlet. (From Ref. 42a.)

Table 8 Equipment for a 100-Person Crew

Mechanical ventilators, allowing the capability of both controlled and assisted ventilation; the maintenance of these should be as simple as possible
Continuous positive airway pressure sets
Warming device to store infusions at body temperature
Several devices allowing both rapid infusion and warming of solutions to be injected
Electrocardiographic machine with defibrillator (automatic or semiautomatic defibrillator, according to local protocols)
Pulse oximeters (possibly with printer)
Adequate stock of rigid cervical collars and splinting devices
Laboratory machine able to perform serum and blood gas analyses
Laboratory machine able to perform antibacterial tests
Portable radiographic equipment (allowing fluoroscopy)
Autoclave
Standard surgical kits (e.g., laparotomy kit, thoracotomy kit, vascular surgery kit)

Source: Ref. 26.

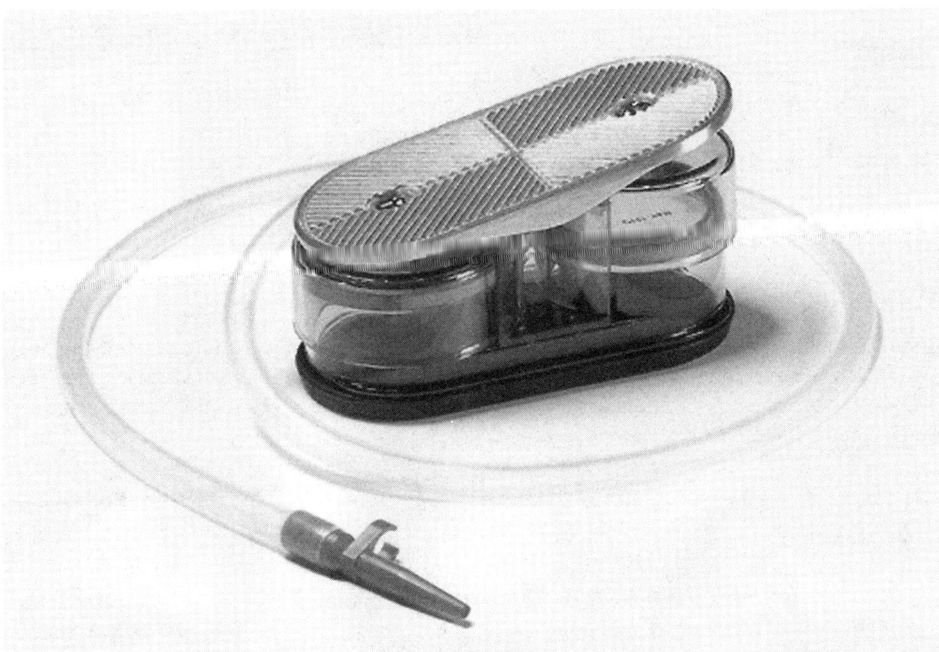

Figure 6 Ambu TwinPump. Manual emergency suction pump, for use in adverse weather conditions, can quickly and effectively aspirate 250 ml of thick fluid in 8 sec. (Courtesy of Ambu International A/S, Brondby, Denmark.)

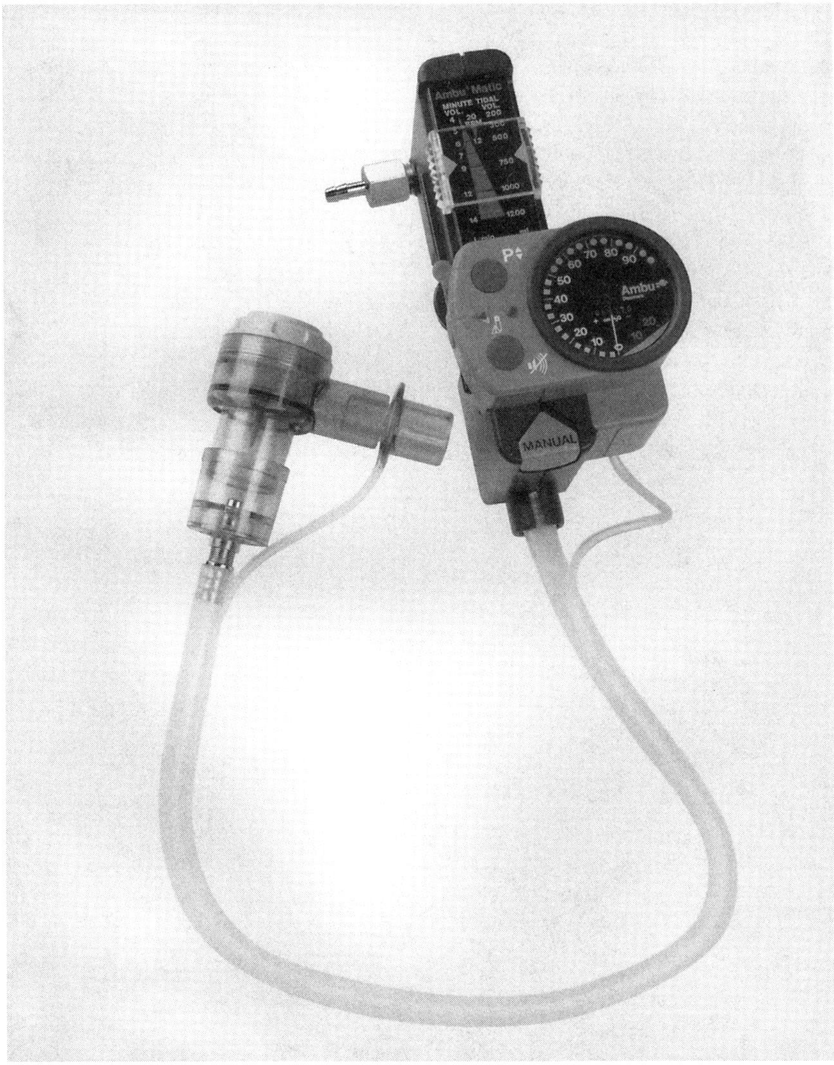

Figure 7 Ambu Matic with ventilation monitor. A compact and lightweight, pneumatically powered ventilator for emergency and transport situations. Ventilation monitor with mechanical and electronic pressure gauge indicating airway pressure (e.g., disconnect, obstruction, leak). (Courtesy of Ambu International A/S, Brondby, Denmark.)

Liquid oxygen is available in containers that weigh approximately 125 lb (56 kilos) and hold approximately 25,000 liters. Using flows of 2 liters/min, such containers can last for up to 8 hr. Liquid oxygen cannot drive a pneumatic ventilator, however, because its operating pressure is too low. Instead, it is useful as a source of oxygen enrichment.

A variety of ''oxygen concentrators'' have been developed and miniaturized as alternatives. These devices are usually more appropriate for mass casualty/disaster settings.

B. Blood Transfusion

Trauma resuscitation often requires blood transfusion or reinfusion. A variety of autotransfusion techniques, many of which are relatively "low-tech" and inexpensive, are gaining increasing popularity. They can be employed in the prehospital setting as well as inside hospital operating rooms or intensive care units as long as sterility is maintained.

Homologous blood transfusion, including screening and testing donors for a variety of diseases, is frequently essential. In some settings physicians must limit the number of units of transfused blood. In austere situations, the severity of injury and the requirement for blood commonly equate survival (or not).

XII. PSYCHOLOGICAL IMPACT OF MASS CASUALTIES

The psychological and emotional repercussions of injury on trauma victims are often considered as part of the holistic care plan. The psychological impact that trauma may have on care providers is often neglected, however [43]. Emergency physicians dealing with trauma patients, whether on an individual basis or in a mass casualty/disaster setting, need to be aware of the psychological and emotional impact of trauma not only upon the patient, but also upon themselves and their colleagues (Table 9).

Steps must be taken to provide supportive care not only to patients but also to relatives and the other people involved. One specific focus unique to anesthesiologists is "perioperative awareness," which must be considered and if possible prevented by the implementation of such strategies as early utilization of benzodiazepines. (The utilization of benzodiazepines per se has not been actually proven to prevent the incidence or diminish the severity of "perioperative awareness," however, nor is there a reliable dose-response curve that can be employed as a guide) [44].

Those involved in horrific situations need to be aware that life-threatening traumatic stress can also be a major event in the life of care providers, potentially resulting in PTSD. A variety of strategies have been developed to deal with and minimize PTSD in care providers, perhaps the most popular of which is the critical incident stress debriefing (CISD) system, based on group discussions and "talking out" emotionally charged issues

Table 9 Sequence of Panic Development

Stage	Description
Preparation	Panic strikes dense concentrations of overwrought people, including many fragile individuals, without any organization or discipline.
Emotional shock	The triggering event, which may be of modest proportion, causes an emotional block.
Reaction	People become agitated and tension explodes in an uncontrolled behavior, the so-called true panic.
Resolution	This stage may be spontaneous or may depend on an energetic outside intervention; resolution gives way to a state of profound prostration.

Source: Ref. 43.

XIII. SUMMARY

In this chapter, the background and overall management of mass casualty and disaster situations have been discussed. Basic appreciation for these instances is important for anesthesiologists, because the surgical management of trauma is frequently a by-product of the circumstances. As opposed to providing excellent care for a single injury victim, in mass casualty and disaster conditions, anesthesiologists must be adept at multitasking. These situations require simultaneous care of several patients, often under adverse and austere conditions. Nevertheless, with advance planning and training, as well as careful selection of program equipment and drugs, the same quality of care available in conventional hospital settings can be achieved.

REFERENCES

1. National Research Council. Confronting Natural Disasters: An international decade for natural disaster reduction. Washington, DC: Academy Press, 1987.
2. Office of US Foreign Disaster Assistance. Disaster History: Significant Data on Major Disasters Worldwide, 1900–Present. Washington, DC: Agency for International Development, 1994.
3. K Von Clauswitz, M Howard, P Paret. On War. New York: Knopf, 1993.
4. R Zajtchuk, CM Grande, eds. Textbook of Military Medicine: Part IV; Anesthesia and Perioperative Care of the Combat Casualty. Falls Church, VA: Office of the Surgeon General of the Army, 1994.
5. D LaCombe, CM Grande. EMS support of executive protection and counter-terrorism operations. In: J DeBoer, M Dubolouz, eds. Handbook of Disaster Medicine. Zeist, the Netherlands: VSP International Science Publishers, 2000, pp. 359–382.
6. R Carmona, CM Grande, D Gonzales. Trauma care support for mass events, counterterrorism, and VIP protection. In: E Soreide, CM Grande, eds. Prehospital Trauma Care. New York: Marcel Dekker, 2001, pp. 719–735.
7. FK Butler Jr, JH Hagmann, eds. Tactical management of urban warfare casualties in special operations. Mil Med 165(4) (suppl):1–48, 2000.
8. RF Lavery, MD Addis, JV Doran, et al. Taking care of the ''good guys'': A trauma center-based model of medical support for tactical law enforcement. J Trauma 48:125–129, 2000.
9. D Carrison, CM Grande. In sickness and in health. Security Management 65–69, March 2000.
10. J de Boer. Order in chaos: Modelling medical management in disasters. Eur J Emerg Med 6: 141–148, 1999.
11. J de Boer, B Brismar, R Eldar, WH Rutherford. The medical severity index of disasters. J Emerg Med 7:269–273, 1989.
12. WH Rutherford, J de Boer. The definition and classification of disasters. Injury 15:10–12, 1983.
13. J de Boer. Tools for evaluating disasters: Preliminary results of some hundreds of disasters. Eur J Emerg Med 4:107–110, 1997.
14. J de Boer. Definition and classification of disasters: Introduction of a disaster severity score. J Emerg Med 8:591–595, 1990.
15. J de Boer. Criteria for the assessment of disaster preparedness. J Emerg Med 7:481–484, 1989.
16. J de Boer. Criteria for the assessment of disaster preparedness—II. Prehospital Disaster Med 12:13–16, 1997.
17. SM Orr, WA Robinson. The Hyatt Regency skywalk collapse: An EMS-based disaster response. Ann Emerg Med 12:601, 1982.

18. CM Grande, PJF Baskett, Y Donchin, et al. Trauma anesthesia for disasters: Anything, anytime, anywhere. Crit Care Clin 7(2):339–361, 1991.
19. E Auf der Heide. The "paper" plan syndrome. In: E Auf der Heide, ed. Disaster Response: Principles of Preparation and Coordination. St. Louis: CV Mosby, 1989, pp. 33–48.
20. CE Smith, E Sinz, CM Grande, eds. New teaching and training methods in trauma care: Present and future role of simulator technology. Am J Anesth 27(4):186–242, May 2000.
21. International Trauma Anesthesia and Critical Care Society. International Chief Emergency Physician Training Course in Command Incident Management in Disaster and Mass Casualty Incidents. Course curriculum and manual. Baltimore: ITACCS, 2000.
22. JS Vayer, RP Ten Eyck, ML Cowan. New concepts in triage. Ann Emerg Med 15:927, 1986.
23. TE Bowen, RF Bellamy, eds. Emergency War Surgery. Washington, DC: U.S. Government Printing Office, 1988.
24. J Donohue. The trouble with triage tags. TraumaCare 10(1):7–11, 2000.
25. M Olds, G Stocks, K Dauphinee. Practical aspects of the prehospital medical care environment. In: CM Grande, ed. Textbook of Trauma Anesthesia and Critical Care. St. Louis: Mosby-Year Book, 1993, pp. 309–318.
26. S Badiali. Extreme environmental conditions; Part 4: Polar conditions. In: CM Grande, ed. Textbook of Trauma Anesthesia and Critical Care. St. Louis: Mosby-Year Book, 1993, pp. 1366–1370.
27. CP Kingsley, C Petty, K Olson. Anesthesia equipment for austere conditions. In CM Grande, ed. Textbook of Trauma Anesthesia and Critical Care. St. Louis: Mosby-Year Book, 1993, pp. 1166–1179.
28. CD Sanders. Anaesthetic equipment in disasters. Br J Clin Equip 2:5–9, 1977.
29. RS Mecca. Anesthesia in field situations. In: FM Burkle, ed. Disaster Medicine: Application for the Immediate Management and Triage of Civilian and Military Disaster Victims. New York: Medical Examination Publishing Co., 1984, pp. 315–322.
30. AR Rosenberg, R Bernstein, CM Grande, eds. Pain Management and Regional Anesthesia for the Trauma Patient. London: W.B. Saunders, 2001.
31. JJ Bonica. Pain control in mass casualties. In: C Manni, SI Magalini, eds. Emergency and Disaster Medicine. Berlin: Springer-Verlag, 1983, pp. 151–166.
32. JK Stene, CM Grande. Anesthesia for trauma. In: RD Miller, ed. Anesthesia, 5th ed. Philadelphia: Churchill-Livingstone, 2000, pp. 2157–2172.
33. Y Donchin, M Wiener, CM Grande, et al. Military medicine: Trauma anesthesia and critical care on the battlefield. Crit Care Clin 6(1):185–202, 1990.
34. A Dow, PJF Baskett. Anaesthesia and analgesia in the field. In: CM Grande, ed. Textbook of Trauma Anesthesia and Critical Care. St. Louis: Mosby-Year Book, 1993, pp. 297–303.
35. J Restall, RJ Knight. Analgesia and anaesthesia in the field. In: PJF Baskett, RM Weller, eds. Medicine for Disasters. Bristol: Wrights, 1988, pp. 87–101.
36. W Dick, WK Hirlinger, HH Mehrkens. Intramuscular ketamine: An alternative pain treatment for use in disasters? In: C Manni, SI Magalini, eds. Emergency and Disaster Medicine. Berlin: Verlag, 1983, pp. 167–172.
37. J Restall, AM Tully, PJ Ward, AG Kidd. Total intravenous anaesthesia for military surgery: A technique using ketamine, midazolam and vecuronium. Anaesthesia 43:46–49, 1988.
38. IW Carson, J Moore, JP Balmer, et al. Laryngeal competence with ketamine and other drugs. Anesthesiology 38:128–133, 1973.
39. IS Grant, WS Nimmo, JA Clements. Lack of effect of ketamine analgesia on gastric emptying in man. Br J Anaesth 53:1321–1322, 1981.
40. PJF Baskett, A Withnell. The use of Entonox in the ambulance service. Br Med J 2:41–43, 1970.
41. RJ Knight, IT Houghton. Field experience with the Tri-Service Anaesthetic Apparatus in Oman and Northern Ireland. Anaesthesia 36:1122–1127, 1981.
42. IT Houghton. The Tri-Service Anaesthetic Apparatus. Anaesthesia 36:1904–1908, 1981.

42a. CM Grande, ed. Textbook of Trauma Anesthesia and Critical Care. St. Louis: Mosby Year Book, 1993.
43. MR Seidel. Psychologic impact of trauma: Implications for the anesthesiologist. In: CM Grande, ed. Textbook of Trauma Anesthesia and Critical Care. St. Louis: Mosby Year Book, 1993, p. 1290.
44. G Lubke, P Sebel. Awareness and different forms of memory in trauma anesthesia. Curr Opin Anaesth 13:161–165, 2000.

9

Research and Uniform Reporting

WOLFGANG F. DICK

University Hospital, Mainz, Germany

I. RESEARCH PROBLEMS

A. Introduction: Lack of Randomized Controlled Trials

In 1991, Jones and Brenneis [1] concluded from an analysis of nine comparative studies that ''In general the studies are limited by heterogeneous levels of service or approach to care. They often study a small specific subset of trauma population and are not randomized.'' Most of the studies contain substandard levels of care with respect to on-scene time and performance of procedures. Spaite et al. [2] came to an almost identical conclusion. ''Current methods for the evaluation of EMS (Emergency Medical Services) systems are fundamentally inadequate for answering important questions because they rely mainly on the traditional medical model.'' Recently Spaite et al. [3] wrote in another article on the subject: ''There is a desperate need for prospective, randomized controlled trials that compare ALS (Advanced Life Support) versus Basic Life Support prehospital care in victims of major trauma.'' Pepe and Eckstein [4] emphasized in an article on prehospital care of the trauma patient that although for the ''use of the PASG (Pneumatic Anti Shock Garments) prospective controlled trials have been recommended,'' ''statistical evidence is still lacking,'' and ''further studies are needed.''

Bissel et al. [5], however, analyzed a variety of primarily American studies on trauma care and outcome [6,7] and found that ''the few large statewide studies that have been completed are in substantial agreement regarding the positive value of ALS-level of care for victims of life-threatening injuries.''

B. What is the Reason for This Predicament?

Basic and advanced care of trauma patients has always been an important aspect of prehospital and immediate in-hospital emergency medicine, demanding a wide spectrum of skills and attracting a plethora of specialties and organizations. Trauma life support continues to be practiced under entirely different conditions and circumstances worldwide. As a result, data on quality of care, outcome, life after survival, and many other criteria differ from publication to publication. This complex background has at least in part hindered the development of a uniform pattern or set of criteria and definitions. Different systems cannot readily be compared because data are often not available or are incompatible, thus precluding the description of a study design for human research projects, reporting on outcome data, or the definition of a responsible emergency medical system.

C. The Utstein Style Concept

The existence of a similarly unacceptable situation was first perceived in CPR (cardiopulmonary resuscitation) research. From 1986 to 1990 the CPR research committee of the European Acadaemy of Anaesthesiology developed recommendations for CPR research in both animals and humans. These recommendations served as the background for the subsequent Utstein style recommendations for reporting data from out-of-hospital and in-hospital resuscitation, from animal research, and from disaster situations [8], as well as for the Utstein style recommendations for uniform reporting of data following major trauma [9].

While ITACCS (International Trauma Anesthesia Critical Care Society) launched this project in 1994, in 1995 Spaite reported on a similar initiative founded on the results of the U.S. Prehospital Emergency Medical Services Data Conference (1992–1994), which provided the basis for an 81-item uniform data set [10].

D. How to Overcome the Crisis in Clinical Research

What can be done to improve the obviously existing inadequate scientific status of emergency medicine research in general and trauma research in particular [11]? The answers to this question can be found in various publications [12–14].

In 1993, the NAEMSP (National Association of EMS Physicians) and the SAEM (Society of Academic Emergency Medicine) published the results of their 1992 winter symposium, Research in Prehospital Care Systems, dealing with basic ethical and pragmatic aspects of prehospital research as well as with data collection and specific criteria for trauma services investigations.

In his book *The Crisis of Clinical Research*, E. H. Ahrens [11] concludes that "in the last 3 decades the focus of clinical investigators has shifted dramatically from integrative to reductionistic research." In contrast to reductionistic research (molecular biology, etc.), "*patient-orientated research (POR)* as part of clinical research is the most time consuming form of clinical research, the most difficult and the slowest." This development may explain why so few current emergency medicine methods, procedures, or drugs are evidence-based; "it is much easier for clinicians to use the narrow research time frame available to them, to move into the laboratory, and to perform reductionistic research rather than invest in POR." Ahrens further elucidates that POR "covers a vast terrain of different objectives, skills, funding, and technical facilities."

It has proven useful to divide this terrain into *basic clinical research and applied clinical research*, as well as into seven study types, with type 2 studies being performed in patients on a prospective controlled basis and investigating the effects of drugs, procedures etc. on the outcome of well described diseases or injuries. Type 7 studies deal with similar topics, but evaluate side effects and cost-effectiveness (Table 1). Research on prehospital trauma care is clearly applied clinical research, although the simulation of individual prehospital scenarios using animal models or even computers can be described as basic clinical research; the interpolation from any simulated model to real life conditions, however, always requires the availability of proven clinical evidence in patients.

Planning and performing research is a time-consuming procedure that needs the careful differentiation between several time points and periods [13,14]. The initial step in a research process consists of a literature search and the review of publications. After the successful conclusion of this first step, a research plan has to be developed and described that considers factors such as ethics, science, statistics, funding, number of patients needing treatment, authorship, publication policy, and conflict of interest problems (especially if research funds are provided by the industry).

Selection of topics: Almost everything in prehospital emergency medicine in general and in trauma care in particular has recently been put into question: for example, the golden hour concept, fluid resuscitation [15–17]–endotracheal intubation [4] [although found useful in cases of airway obstruction and cerebral trauma], blood transfusion as a source of multiple organ failure (MOF) [18], artificial hemoglobins, immobilization, various scoring algorithms (injury severity score [ISS], prehospital severity score [PSS], prehospital index [PHI], Mainz emergency evaluation score [MEES], etc.), the fragmented vs. the integrated approach to trauma care [19,20], paramedic vs. emergency physician approach [4,5], efficacy and effectiveness, and treatment protocols [20].

Objectives/hypotheses: Once a specific topic has been selected, one or more hypotheses (0 hypothesis, nondirectional, uni- or multidirectional) need to be formulated as precisely as possible and related to the topic. The objective of the project has to be described.

Literature search: The literature search should be performed based on at least two computerized sources as well as on hand search because roughly only 50% of references are found using computerized search techniques [14,20]. These publications have to fulfill defined criteria; at this time the use of templates for evidence-based reviews and critical appraisal may be indicated [20].

Methodology [illegible]: The gold standard of a scientific study is the prospective randomized controlled trial (RCT) [14,21]. Other studies should only serve to identify a problem and to provide the background for a prospective trial. Case reports, case control studies, historical reports, observational and retrospective studies, and the like do not meet the gold standard.

A *meta-analysis* may be carried out by statisticians and clinicians if (1) only a few RCTs from different institutions are available, each involving only a limited number of patients, and (2) a large multicenter study is unrealistic to perform. The same strict criteria apply to this type of study as to a controlled single RCT.

Furthermore, it needs to be decided if the study type should be open or single-, double-, or even triple-*blinded*. In the latter case, the patient and investigator as well as the monitor are blinded to the study alternatives.

Consideration should be given to the performance of *placebo-controlled studies* (which are often impossible for ethical reasons) or studies comparing two methods or drugs, one representing the current standard, the other one the study technique. The decision can lead to additional benefits or problems, risks, and even bias.

The selected *measurement criteria* need to be validated with respect to the topic, hypothesis, and objectives. The study population, the number of patients needed to treat in order to save one life, as well as measuring and monitoring criteria (respiratory, cardiovascular, lab tests, radiological material, scores, etc.) need to be characterized before the onset of the study. Care should be taken to avoid any possible bias.

The *size of the study population* needs to be identified before the meticulous planning of the study begins. This presents a particular problem in trauma patients, as the numbers of trauma victims decreases year by year in the industrialized world. (In central Europe only 10% of all emergency patients are trauma patients.) Further questions that need to be answered include, for example, how many patients can be recruited within a given period of time and which age groups are involved.

Trauma studies frequently require a *multicenter approach*, as the required number of patients cannot be collected at a single center within an appropriate period of time (1–2 years). Multicenter studies, on the other hand, presuppose a complex infrastructure; authorship may pose an additional problem in multicenter trials and should be defined at an early stage.

In addition, the suitability of the study site(s) needs to be evaluated (on-scene, mobile life support unit [MLSU], ambulance, helicopter, etc.). It may also be advisable for young researchers to undergo a training program in research methodology for both basic and applied clinical research.

E. Ethics

Before the study design can be finalized it should be checked if the protocol is in accordance with the criteria outlined in the Helsinki Declaration and in the respective national documents as well as in the chapter on ethics in the Utstein document.

Informed consent represents a particular problem in the prehospital arena because in most instances patient consent cannot be obtained and has to be deferred until the victim regains consciousness or a relative is available. The tremendous variation in national regulations needs to be observed.

F. Data Collection

A study nurse or an emergency medical technician (EMT) who is not involved in the treatment modalities should be part of a well-controlled RCT. The most important task is to collect all required data according to the protocol. Tape recording or even video-recording all procedures should be attempted. Throughout the study, prehospital trauma teams should have identical levels of training and comparable skills, unless the objective of the study is to identify staff weaknesses and deficits. This also means that in accordance with the Utstein Style the qualifications and speciality of the emergency physicians (anaesthesiologist, trauma surgeon, internist, etc.) and other trauma team members involved in the study need to be meticulously described.

A *standardized terminology* should be used in order to avoid confusion. It should be based on time points and intervals instead of on downtime and the like.

Primary and secondary *endpoints* need to be defined: return of spontaneous circulation (ROSC) at specific intervals after cardiac arrest, changes in systolic blood pressure in shock patients after fluid resuscitation, and so on.

Secondary endpoints may be outcome in general as well as the duration of ICU (intensive care unit) stay, hospital stay, survival to 6 months, survival to a year, quality of life, morbidity, and disabilities in particular.

The severity of trauma and the extent of treatment (therapeutic intervention scoring system—TISS) serve as a criterion for the comparison of different treatment concepts.

G. Statistics

A statistician needs to be involved as early as possible. If the hypothesis is that meaningful survival can be improved from 10 to 15% using method A instead of method B, it is the task of the statistician to calculate numbers, improve the protocol, and calculate (statistical power, confidence intervals, numbers to treat, odds ratios, p values, etc.). Particularly in emergency medicine research, the numbers necessary to treat in order to save one life may be enormous (up to several thousands, personal communication by L. D. Clayton, 1998).

Randomization may pose both an ethical and a pragmatic problem. For example, in a study comparing prehospital defibrillation by emergency physicians vs. paramedics, only 50% of the involved paramedics were trained in semiautomatic defibrillation to facilitate randomization. If all paramedics had been trained in defibrillation, they would all have had to perform the procedure where indicated for ethical reasons. Randomization can easily be calculated using computers, including even or uneven days, street numbers, addresses, and so on. In a crossover design each patient receives both treatment alternatives (including placebo) in an alternating but specified sequence. Entry as well as exclusion criteria must be carefully described. The ratio of preventable deaths/all deaths is often used for quality management in trauma care.

H. Pilot Trials

A pilot trial should always be planned in order to check whether or not the procedures calculated and the planned protocol can be followed under real-life conditions.

I. Funding

There are principally two sources of funding, by governmental organizations (GOs) and nongovernmental organizations (NGOs). Government funding comprises university funding and financial resources from research institutions. Nongovernmental support includes private funding from companies, donations and awards. In all cases a grant application has to be made that explains to the prospective funder that the described project is in the interest of the donor organization or individual [22]. If private or company research funding is involved, conflicts of interest need to be avoided. Today, researchers working on reductionistic projects compete with clinicians for research money, and GOs often prefer providing money to reductionistic research than to POR.

J. Safety and Data-Monitoring Committee

A data-monitoring and safety committee often has to be involved in a research project, particularly in the case of multicenter and multinational studies. Committee members, consisting of distinguished researchers from neutral institutions, check the data for plausibility, missing information, deviation from protocols, ethical problems, and the like. They decide whether data can be included into the data-processing procedure or not (Table 2).

K. Publication Policy

On completion of a research project it has to be decided when and where to publish the study results. *Impact factors* play an important role in the selection of a particular journal, although the overall impact factor (independent of the scientific specialty and research field) does not necessarily reflect the scientific quality of specific medical research [23]. ''Reductionistic'' research (using, e.g., molecular biological methodology in an experimental laboratory) cannot be compared with POR. It has only recently been concluded by respected international research organizations and journal publishers that a distinction needs to be made between research fields and that specialty and research field-orientated specific impact factors; emergency medicine/trauma research impact factors have to be developed and used. As research money is increasingly provided in relation to the number of publications in high-impact factor journals, this new orientation is of particular importance in obtaining research funds.

If nongovernmental money is involved, the money provider (e.g., a company) may wish to exert influence on the publication policy or even on the conclusions to be drawn from the research results. It should be made clear prior to signing a research contract that the publication policy must be independent of any obvious or hidden influence of the funder (conflict of interest). Finally, it has to be carefully considered when it is justified to transfer research results to clinical and/or prehospital treatment concepts (evidence-based emergency medicine) [24,25].

A final point for consideration should be what is needed to focus on in the future—research people, sources of funding, new procedures, medication, organization, new concepts, and so on.

II. THE ITACCS TRAUMA TERMINOLOGY INITIATIVE

In 1998, ITACCS designed a system similar to the Utstein template for cardiac arrest and resuscitation for ''reporting data following major trauma'' [9]. Such a system has the following features:

A structured reporting system such as an ''Utstein style-based template'' would permit the compilation of comparative statistics and enable groups to challenge any performance statistics that did not take account of all relevant information.

The template would assist studies setting out to improve epidemiological understanding of the problem of trauma. These studies might focus on the factors that determine survival.

The recommendations and template would permit intra- and intersystem evaluation to improve the quality of the program and to identify the relative benefits of different systems and innovative initiatives.

The recommendations and template should apply to both out-of-hospital and in-hospital trauma care.

The present document is structured along the lines of the original Utstein style guidelines publication on prehospital cardiac arrest. It includes a *glossary of terms* used in the prehospital and early hospital phase, definitions, and time points and intervals. The document uses an almost identical scheme (Fig. 1) for illustrating the different time clocks—one for the patient, one for the dispatch center, one for the ambulance, and finally, one for

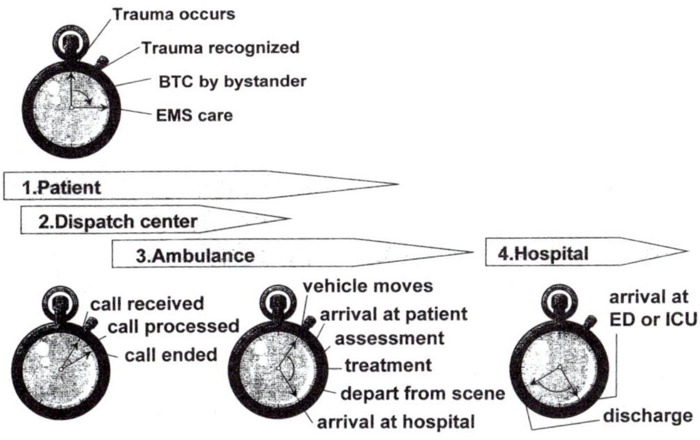

Figure 1 Trauma time clocks. BTG, basic trauma care; EMS, emergency medical services; ED, emergency department; ICU, intensive care unit. (From Ref. 9.)

the hospital. These four clocks and the respective intervals overlap on a number of occasions. The definitions of individual clinical items and outcomes that should be included in reports and recommendations for the description of emergency medical services systems are described together with the input variables, process variables, and outcome variables. These variables may be mandatory (core data = c) or optional (o).

Definitions and terms such as bystander and emergency personnel are defined as in the original Utstein cardiac arrest document and may be referred to in the appropriate publications [7]. The terms corresponding to *BCLS (basic cardiac life support)* and *ACLS (advanced cardiac life support)* in trauma would ideally have been basic trauma life support (BTLS) and advanced trauma life support (ATLS). As, however, ATLS is a trademark held by the American College of Surgeons, the working group decided to use more generic terms; for example, *basic care* and *advanced care*.

In the section on outcome greater attention was paid to details on morbidity and disability. It was not, however, decided on a specific outcome scale but on a variety of scales that investigators may use, including disability and quality of life. The *various parts of the EMS* are described in accordance with the original Utstein documents (i.e., the dispatch system and the first, second, and third tiers). In contrast to the Utstein template used for pre- or in-hospital cardiac arrest, the working group decided not to use a graphic approach but rather a variety of terms and definitions.

Table 1 Seven Categories of Clinical Research

1. Studies of mechanisms in human disease
2. Studies of management of disease
3. In vitro studies on materials of human origin
4. Animal models of human health or disease
5. Field surveys
6. Development of new technologies
7. Assessment of health care delivery

Source: Ref. 11.

Table 2 Composition of a Data Monitoring and Safety Committee for a Multicenter Interdisciplinary Trial

1. Cardiologist (chairman)
2. Intensivist
3. Anesthesiologist
4. Technical adviser
5. Epidemiologist/statistician
6. Ethicist

III. TRAUMA DATA STRUCTURE DEVELOPMENT USING OBJECT-ORIENTATED MODELING

The data to be collected for trauma care is inherently complex. Although the personnel involved in the different stages of trauma care often appear to have different criteria for data collection, there are inherent similarities that allow the development of a single unifying model.

The object-oriented approach used by software engineers may be employed in the development of the model. A flexible data structure is developed not only for recording and analyzing data but also for shaping the way in which trauma care is conceptualized and for designing the language used to describe it. Object-oriented concepts such as ''object inheritance'' can be incorporated to define and refine individual objects within the overall model. In the object-oriented approach, the patient may be regarded as an object with a unique identification number ''traveling'' through time (from the occurrence of the accident) and space (location) with other generic object links such as attendants (personnel involved at different stages), observations (sensors), and interventions (effective).

A. Terms and Definitions in Trauma

The terms used in trauma care have been defined to achieve greater clarity (in documentation and reporting). See Appendix A.

B. Trauma Factors Relating to the Circumstances of the Injury

In general, all trauma is classified as blunt including amputation, crush, laceration, and asphyxia with the exception of stab, spike, or missile injuries, which are classed as penetrating trauma. When more than one injury type is present, the predominant type, i.e., the type primarily responsible for mortality/morbidity will be assessed in hospital at a time considered appropriate. Core data must include information as to whether the trauma is blunt or penetrating. See Appendix B.

1. Severity of Injury

Prehospital Basic Abbreviated Injury Score

The prehospital basic abbreviated injury score attempts to combine anatomical injury with physiological disability. This is core data. More than one score may apply, for example a patient may have a chest injury which is severe but not life-threatening (4.3), plus a head injury which is moderate (1.2), plus a lower limb injury which is severe but not life threatening (8.3).

2. Mechanism of Injury

Core data includes the basic mechanism of injury differentiating between transport, fall, interpersonal, violence, self-inflicted, thermal, asphyxia, etc. Optional data includes details within each of these major groups.

For convenience, explosion, chemical and radiation injuries may be included under thermal injury if that is the major mechanism of injury or they may be included under asphyxia if that is more appropriate.

3. Place of Injury

The place of injury is classed as optional data but may be especially relevant in certain studies. Only the most common places are listed—other places, e.g., on board ship should be specified.

Remote indicates a place not easily accessible by road or more than 100km from EMS base.

C. System Factors

The EMS and Hospital System factors closely mirror those listed in the Utstein guidelines for reporting cardiac arrest. See Appendix C.

–prehospital factors
–interhospital transfer factors
–trauma centre/receiving hospital—factors

1. Patient Factors

These factors have to be recorded under factors relating to the circumstances of injury. There are a number of factors which have been shown to influence trauma patient outcome. These include severity of injury, time to definitive care, the quality of the care provided, and patient factors. Patient factors that influence outcome (morbidity and mortality) are those factors which compromise physiological reserve and include age, gender, and co-morbidity (also referred to as pre-existing disease).

The *patient's age* or best approximation should be recorded in all cases. Age is a predictor of outcome from trauma. Mortality increases between the ages of 45 to 55 years for the same injury severity and is doubled above 75 years. Trauma in the elderly population is also associated with an increased risk of complications, intensive care and prolonged hospital stay.

Gender should be recorded in all cases. The overall death rate from trauma for males is more than twice that of females. This ratio is further increased in intentional trauma and in particular penetrating trauma. The higher rates reflect the greater involvement of males in trauma associated activities, both at work and at leisure. *Height and weight* are core data.

Where appropriate, the *populations* should be defined, for example according to ethnic groups, socioeconomic classification, or *subgroups* (e.g., driver, passenger, cyclist, pedestrian, interpersonal, etc.)

Comorbidity is an important predictor of outcome from trauma but has received little attention until recently. Previous assessments of co-morbidity in trauma patients have used retrospective discharge diagnosis according to the International Classification of Disease (ICD), a limited list of disease states as part of a trauma registry, or a severity of disease classification system. The functional/physiological limitations of the comorbidity have not been clearly defined. An accurate description of all co-morbidity should ideally be included but is likely to be difficult. In the absence of a reliable, simple assessment of co-morbidity the four gradings of comorbidity shown below are proposed which will allow an assessment of the impact of pre-existing disease on physiological reserve.

CO-MORBIDITY GRADINGS

1. Healthy (normal)
2. Systemic illness: non-limiting
3. Systemic illness: limiting normal activity
4. Systemic illness: constant threat to life
5. Intercurrent medication

D. Patient Assessment and Interventions

It is recognized that resuscitation is the priority and that full assessment will not be performed prior to initiation of life saving maneuvers. Consequently, certain assessments and resuscitation may be performed simultaneously. It is also recognized that the physiological status is a dynamic process that is influenced by the interventions. The documentation of the relation of these interventions to the assessments is therefore crucial if the impact of various interventions is to be evaluated. To allow a meaningful interpretation and comparison both anatomical and physiological assessments must be documented. The most commonly used scoring systems in current use are the Prehospital Basic Abbreviated Injury Scale (AIS) from which the Injury Severity Score (ISS) is derived and the Revised Trauma Score (RTS) which is composed of the Glasgow Coma Scale, the systolic blood pressure and the respiratory rate. The ISS and RTS allow TRISS methodology and comparison with the Major Trauma Outcome Study (MTOS). Anatomic assessment by the Abbreviated Injury Scale (AIS 90 is the version most frequently used to allow calculation of Injury Severity Score). See Appendix D.

1. Treatment (Prehospital, Emergency Room, OR, ICU with Time Intervals)

There is a controversy as to whether outcome for trauma patients is influenced by the type of prehospital provider. These uncertainties underline the importance of accurate documentation of treatment and outcome.

Complications/adverse effects/side effects of treatment require documentation for each of the treatment headings. There should be an optional facility to describe details of the complication and its relation to outcome.

E. Outcome Details

Details of outcome are essential to any study. Whilst mortality rates are easier to obtain, every effort should be made to collect information on morbidity, which is defined as *all non-fatal problems* (impairment, disability). See Appendix E.

1. Adverse Factors (Possibly Responsible for Fatal Outcome)

Among others the following factors may be considered as *surrogate measure* of outcome

–time in ICU
–time in hospital
–costs

2. Ethical Issues

Trauma research must be conducted within an ethical framework, which may vary between countries and cultures, although the treatment of the individual patient must always have priority.

In trauma research it is particularly important to depersonalise all data as it is generally easier to connect a specific person to a trauma incident than to a disease process, especially in case reports.

Patient Consent to Trauma Research

All studies should follow the Declaration of Helsinki, and must not be initiated until approved by the appropriate ethics committee. This usually implies that informed consent must be obtained from the patient. This is problematic and presents a unique ethical challenge in trauma research.

Some of the patients will be unconscious, and are thus unable to give their consentor inclusion in many studies. *Surrogate permission*, from family members or legal guardian is found to be unacceptable in some countries and is rarely available in the acute care situation in countries where it is accepted.

Even in conscious patients informed consent is problematic in the acute care setting. Informed consent implies that a competent patient must, to the best of a competent researcher's knowledge, have received and understood all the appropriate information. As the treatment of the patient has first priority, there is frequently insufficient time to ensure quality informed consent in the management of patients with severe trauma.

There are special studies where the act of asking for informed consent causes a bias in itself. This is covered in the *Helsinki Declaration Section* 11.5; thus, if the physician thinks it is essential not to obtain informed consent, the specific reasons for this should be stated in the experimental protocol submission to the independent ethical committee.

3. Documentation/Methodology

Planning for Data Collection

Plans for collecting data on trauma patients should be drawn up prospectively. Full cooperation between prehospital and in-hospital personnel will minimize the possibility of omitting or duplicating relevant data. If the prehospital and in-hospital data can be linked with police or population studies they may provide a means for data verification and validation.

Data Collection

Data collection can be done manually or performed automatically. Some manual techniques are partly automated by using some form of handheld computer with which to record data. In the future, telemetry is likely to become more widely available and will allow continuous automated collection of data from both the prehospital and inhospital areas.

Manual Collection

Real time data collection is the ideal, but requires the continual presence of a dedicated data collector. A single data collection form for both prehospital and inhospital phases may be seen as ideal, but most trauma systems will utilize multiple forms. These need to be linked by a unique identifier. The primary identifier should be a number. This will be supported by secondary identifiers compromising name and time. Links are required between the prehospital, inhospital forms, audit forms, and forms at any secondary hospital to which the patient has been transferred.

Data may be derived from audio and or videotape but this would generally be too labor intensive to use for routine audit. This technique may be a valuable research tool.

Personnel in the control/dispatch center are likely to be able to collect and record some of the relevant prehospital data.

Data Collection Forms

With developing technology, the principle should be to avoid cumbersome forms. Data collection forms should be of ''tick box'' design where possible. The best format is to ask closed questions with yes, no, don't know, and other options. Multiple, color, coded copies will allow the data to be distributed to appropriate personnel. It would seem sensible if the EMS record were also the prehospital audit form.

Data Entry

The entry of data into a database may be performed manually or with optical readers. There should be regular quality checks to ensure data reliability and accuracy, and to eliminate bias. The gold standard for data entry is a validated, primary electronic system.

Electronic Data Collection

Electronic notepads will record the time and location (using GPS) automatically and continually. In addition, they have a manual capability and are likely to include voice recognition software in the future.

Bar code readers are already in common use in hospitals. They may contribute to more efficient and accurate data collection. Data can be downloaded from monitors and a variety of other patient care devices.

Training in Data Collection and Entry

All data collectors and enterers should receive appropriate training. These personnel may be EMS staff, nurses, or doctors. Data validation is important. Intra-rater and inter-rater variation may be minimized with appropriate training.

Common Database

If data collection is standardized, the data may be downloaded to a common database. This could be a national database, such as the Major Trauma Outcome Study (MTOS) or an international database which could be termed the International Trauma Audit (ITA). Appropriate steps should be taken to ensure patient confidentiality; patient and hospital identifiers should be removed before data are downloaded to a common database outside the hospital.

REFERENCES

1. SE Jones, AT Brenneis. Study designs in prehospital trauma advanced life support–basic life support research: A critical review. Ann Emerg Med 20:857–860, 1991.
2. DW Spaite, EA Criss, TD Valenzuela, et al. Emergency medical service systems research: Problems of the past, challenges of the future. Ann Emerg Med 26:146–152, 1995.
3. DW Spaite, EA Criss, TD Valenzuela, HW Meislin. Prehospital advanced life support for major trauma: Critical need for clinical trials. Ann Emerg Med 32:480–489, 1998.
4. PE Pepe, M Eckstein. Reappraising the prehospital care of the patient with major trauma. Emerg Med Clin North Amer 16:1–15, 1998.

5. RA Bissel, DG Eslinger, L Zimmerman. The efficacy of advanced life support: A review of the literature. Prehosp Disas Med 13:69–79, 1998.
6. CG Cayten, JG Murphy, WM Stahl. Basic life support vs. advanced life support for injured patients with an injury severity score of 10 or more. J Trauma 35:460–467, 1993.
7. D Potter, G Goldstein, S Murray. A controlled trial of prehospital advanced life support in trauma. Ann Emerg Med 17:55–61, 1988.
8. W Dick. Uniform reporting in resuscitation. Brit J Anaesth 79:241–252, 1997.
9. W Dick, PFJ Baskett, C Grande, H Delooz, W Kloek, C Lakner, M Lipp, W Mauritz, M Nerlich, J Nickoll, J Nolan, P Oakley, M Parr, A Seekamp, E Soreide, PA Steen, L Camp, B Wolcke, D Yates. Recommendations for uniform reporting of data following major trauma—The Utstein style. Trauma Care 9 (suppl.2):1–13, 1999.
10. D Spaite, R Benoit, D Brown, R Cales, D Dawson, Ch Glass, Ch Kaufmann, D Pollock, S Ran, EM Yano. Uniform prehospital data elements and definitions: A report from the Uniform Prehospital Emergency Medical Services Data Conference. Ann Emerg Med 25:525–534, 1995.
11. EH Ahrens, Jr. The Crisis in Clinical Research. New York: Oxford University Press, 1992.
12. National Association of Emergency Physicians. Research in prehospital care systems. Proceedings of the Winter Assembly of the NAEMSP. Prehosp Disas Med 8 (suppl. 1):S3–S50, 1993.
13. RV Aghababian, WG Barsan, WH Bickell, MH Biros, CG Brown, CB Cairns, ML Callaham, DL Carden, WH Cordell, RC Dart, SC Dronen, HG Garrison, LR Goldfrank, JR Hedges, GD Kelen, AL Kellermann, ML Lewis, RS Lewis, JL Ling, JA Marx, JB McCabe, AB Sanders, DL Schriger, DP Sklar, TD Valenzuela, JF Waeckerle, RL Wears, JD White, RJ Zalenski. Research directions in emergency medicine. Ann Emerg Med 27:339–342, 1996.
14. D Yealy, ed. Research in prehospital care systems. Prehosp Disas Med 1 (suppl. 8):S3–S47, 1993.
15. WH Bickell, MJ Wall, PE Pepe, et al. Immediate versus delayed fluid resuscitation of hypotensive patients with penetrating torso injuries. New Eng J Med 31:1105–1109, 1994.
16. MM Krausz. Controversies in shock research: Hypertonic resuscitation—Pros and cons. Shock 3:69–72, 1995.
17. JR Gill Schierhout. Fluid resuscitation with colloid or crystalloid solutions in critically ill patients: A systematic review of randomised trials. BMJ 316:961–969, 1998.
18. FA Moore, EE Moore, A Sauaia. Blood Transfusion. Arch Surg 132:620–625, 1997.
19. RJA Goris, O Trentz, eds. The Integrated Approach to Trauma Care: The First 24 Hours. Berlin: Springer, 1995.
20. LA Van Camp, HH Delooz. Current trauma scoring systems and their applications. Eur J Emerg Med 5:341–[illegible], 1998.
21. D Yates. Randomized controlled trials and evidence based medicine—What's in a name. Editorial Eur J Emerg Med 4:123–124, 1997.
22. J Cullen. Obtaining funds for clinical medical research. Eur J Emer Med 3:208–209, 1996.
23. SE Gisvold. What is happening to the quality of research—and how can quality be measured? editorial. Acta Anaesthesiol Scand 39:1–2, 1995.
24. A Miles. Evidence-based medicine. Eur J Emerg Med 4:156–164, 1997.
25. DL Sackett, WM Rosenberg, JA Gray. Evidence based medicine: What it is and what it isn't. editorial. BMJ 312:71–72, 1996.

APPENDIX A: Terms and Definitions [9]

Term	*Definition*
Blunt injury	Nonpenetrating, but including crush, laceration, amputation, and asphyxia
Penetrating injury	Bullet, knife, or spike
Long-bone injury	Fracture/dislocation of femur, tibia, humerus, ulna, radius, fibula
Major injury	ISS > 15 Compromising At least one severe life-threatening regional injury OR at least two severe non-life-threatening regional injuries OR at least one severe non-life-threatening plus at least two injuries of moderate severity *NB*: These are based on nine regions of the body. (See Appendix B.)
Mixed/combined trauma	Trauma with more than one mechanism of injury
Multiple trauma/polytrauma	Injury to one body cavity (head, thorax, abdomen) PLUS two long-bone and/or pelvic fractures OR injury to two body cavities
Predominant trauma	Injury to one body part of severity >2 (can include up to one other injury with severity <2)

Terms to be Avoided

"Isolated Trauma"/"Pattern of Injury"/"Single-System Trauma"

Triage

The comparative assessment of the individual patient, i.e., needs and priorities in relation to

1. Vital functions
2. Concomitant injuries
3. Age + co-morbidity
4. Circumstances of the event

APPENDIX B: Factors Relating to the Circumstances of the Injury [9] (c = core data; o = optional data)

1. **Type of injury**

   c Blunt ☐ **c** Penetrating ☐

   o Other Factors:

   Burn ☐ Cold ☐ Asphyxia ☐

   Other (specify) ☐ ____________________

   o Crush ☐ Laceration ☐ Amputation ☐

   Radiation ☐ Multiple ☐ Other (specify) ☐

2. **Severity of injury—The Abbreviated Injury Score**

Anatomic	Physiologic Disability
1. Head	0. None
2. Face	1. Minor
3. Neck	2. Moderate
4. Chest	3. Severe not life-threatening
5. Abdomen	4. Severe life-threatening
6. Spine	5. Critical
7. Upper limb	6. Unsurvivable
8. Lower limb (inc. pelvis)	
9. External	

APPENDIX B: Continued

3. **Mechanism of injury**

c Transport

c Motor vehicle ☐ (Car or truck) Motorcycle ☐ Cycle ☐
Train ☐ Plane ☐ Boat ☐
Other (specify) ______________________

c Occupant or rider ☐ Pedestrian ☐

o Position of occupant in vehicle
Passenger ☐ Front ☐ Rear ☐
Driver/Rider/Pilot ☐
Position in train/plane/boat
(Seat number, specify __________________)

o Type of impact Head on ☐ Rear end ☐
Roll over ☐ Side ☐
Ejection ☐ Entrapment ☐
Other (specify) ___________

o Vehicle deformity
Front ☐ Rear ☐
Side ☐ Roof ☐
Other (specify) ___________

o Restraining devices
Seat belt ☐ Air bags ☐
Helmet ☐
Other (specify) ___________

c Fall

o Height ______ Landing surface ___________

c Interpersonal violence

o Blunt ☐ Stab ☐ Bullet ☐ Spike ☐
Other (specify) ______________________

c Deliberate self harm

o Blunt ☐ Stab ☐ Bullet ☐ Spike ☐

o Fall ☐ Laceration ☐ Substance abuse ☐
Other (specify) ______________________

c Asphyxia

o Physical ☐ Hanging ☐ Strangulation ☐
Explosion ☐ Thermal ☐ Chemical ☐
Radiation ☐ Nr-Drowning ☐ Foreign body ☐
Electrocution ☐ Other ☐

APPENDIX B: Continued

4. **Location of injury**

o Home ☐ Work ☐ Public area ☐
Street (road) ☐ School ☐ Sports ☐
Industrial ☐ Farming ☐
Other (specify) ______________________
Urban ☐ Rural ☐ Remote ☐
Other (specify) ______________________

APPENDIX C: Prehospital Factors [9]

(c = core data; o = optional data)

c Incident: ☐ Date ☐ Time ☐
Discovery ☐ by whom? witnessed ☐ unwitnessed ☐
c Bystander care Yes/No Layperson ☐
Professional (doctor, nurse, technician, others) ☐

c Call for assistance:
c Emergency telephone number(s)
—national/regional/local
—dedicated to EMS ☐ Others ☐
c Dispatcher(s)
—use of protocols Yes/No
—specific trauma training Yes/No
—authority in decision-making
—pre-arrival-instructions given? Yes/No
—call handled or transmitted to ________

c EMS response (data collected for each unit separate)
c Crew
—Technician (BLS [e.g., EMT, lifeguard], ALS [e.g., paramedic])
—Nurse (special trauma training—Yes/No)
—Physician (special trauma training—Yes/No)
—No. of crew members _____

c Vehicle Ground ☐ Air ☐ Sea ☐
Patient transport (Yes/No)

c Type of care Basic care = noninvasive ☐
Advanced care = invasive ☐

o Distance (kilometers) Base → hospital ______________________

APPENDIX C: Continued

c Date/Time Points/Time Intervals

- **c** Incident (incident occurs/recognized/care by bystander/EMS care)
- **c** Call for assistance initiated
- **c** Call for assistance received (pick-up-moment)
- **c** Call processed
- **c** Dispatch achieved
- **c** Vehicle moves
- **c** Vehicle stops
- **c** Arrival at patient
- **c** Scene interval (assessment/treatment)
- **c** Vehicle-departure from scene (vehicle moves)
- **c** Arrival at trauma (or emergency treatment) facility
- **o** Diversion from destination hospital

Interhospital Transfer Factors

c Indications
Usual facilities not available
Special facilities not available
Other (specify) ______________________________

c **Date/Time Points/Time Intervals**
Referral call received (optional)
Transfer accepted
Departing from fixed-monitoring-environment (bed → stretcher)
Initiation of transfer (vehicle moves)
Arrival at fixed-monitoring-environment (stretcher → bed)

c Emergency Yes/No

c EMS Response

c Crew —Technician (BLS [e.g., EMT], ALS [e.g., paramedic])
—Nurse (special trauma training—Yes/No)
—Physician (special trauma training—Yes/No)

c Vehicle Ground ☐ Air ☐ Sea ☐
Referral/retrieval/independent

c Type of care Basic Care = noninvasive
Advanced Care = invasive
Intensive

o Distances (kilometers) Base → hospital
Hospital 1 → Hospital 2

APPENDIX C: Continued

Trauma Center/Receiving Hospital (In-Hospital) Factors

- c **Trauma team**
- c Designated trauma team Yes/No prehospital/inhospital/home
- c Designated trauma protocol Yes/No
- c Advance warning Yes/No
- c Trauma alert: One tier (i.e., whole team responds)
  Trauma alert: Multiple tier (only certain members present at a time)
- o Trauma team members (No.)

		Spec. Trauma Training	Trauma Team Coordinator
Emergency physician	☐o	☐	☐
Trauma Surgeon	☐o	☐	☐
Anesthetist	☐o	☐	☐
Neurosurgeon	☐o	☐	☐
Radiologist	☐o	☐	☐
Other physician	☐	☐	☐
Nurse	☐o	☐	☐
Technician	☐o	☐	☐
Paramedic	☐	☐	☐

- o **Facilities available (24 hr)**

Blood bank	☐
CT	☐
Cardiothoracic surgery	☐
Neurosurgery	☐
Laboratory	☐
Designated audit system	☐

- c **Date/Time Points/Time Intervals**
  - c Arrival at facility ___
  - c Arrival of first (responsible) doctor/MD ___
  - c First X-ray (time of initiation) ___
  - o First ultrasound (time of initiation) ___
  - o First CT (time of initiation) ___
    Specify
  - o Leaving ED ___
  - c Arrival operating room ___
  - o Skin incision ___
  - o Skin closure ___
  - o Arrival postanesthesia care unit ___
  - c Arrival ICU ___
  - c Discharge ICU ___
  - c Discharge hospital ___
  - o Discharge inhospital rehabilitation ___
  - o Return to work ___

APPENDIX D: Patient Assessment and Interventions [9]
(c = core data; o = optional data)

c Anatomic assessment by the Abbreviated Injury Scale (AIS 90 is the version in most common use), which allows calculation of Injury Severity Score

o Data from autopsy (also see Outcome)

c Time intervals to be recorded as a minimum
____Scene
____Emergency department
____Operating room
____Intensive care unit
____Ward

c The first AVAILABLE recording of:
- **c** Glasgow Coma Scale (GCS) score
  GCS (recorded as the eye, ventilation, movement components) (assessed prior to drug administration but note the influence of drugs in further assessment [see below])
- **c** Respiratory function
  Spontaneous/Assisted-Rate (per min)—End tidal CO_2 (**o**)
- **c** Heart rate
  Heart-rate (per min)—ECG (**o**)
- **c** Blood pressure
  Preferably automated (method should be described)
  Reading—ooo/ooo
  Document if a reading cannot be recorded
- **c** Pulse oximetry
  SpO_2 (Document if reading is not obtainable)
- **c** Temperature
  Describe method
- **o** Blood gases
  ABG (pH, PCO_2, PO_2, BD, bicarbonate)
- **o** Electrolytes
- **c** Hemoglobin
  Hb/Hct
- **c** Blood sugar
- **o** Other optional investigations depending on status and mechanism of injury, e.g., lactate, HbCO, drug/alcohol

c Cardiac arrest Yes/No Prehospital ☐ Inhospital ☐
c Respiratory arrest Yes/No Prehospital ☐ Inhospital ☐
o Data from autopsy (also see Outcome)

APPENDIX D: Continued

c **Treatment** (with times recorded [**o**])
Prehospital ☐ _______
ED ☐ _______
OR ☐ _______
ICU ☐ _______
Other ☐ _______

c Oxygen therapy (describe method and concentration)

c Immobilisation
Cervical collar ☐ Vacuum mattress ☐
Spine board ☐ Other ☐

c Airway adjuncts
OPA ☐ NPA ☐ LMA ☐ Combitube ☐
Oral tracheal tube ☐ Nasal tracheal tube ☐
Surgical (needle/cricothyroidotomy/tracheostomy) ☐

c Ventilation
Spontaneous ☐ Manual ☐ Mechanical ☐
Chest decompression (needle) ☐ (tube) ☐

c Hemorrhage control Yes/No

c IV access
Attempts ☐ Success (Yes/No) Number ☐

c IO access
Attempts ☐ Success (Yes/No) Number ☐

c IV fluid
Type_______ Volume infused_______
Infusion time period_____ No. of IV lines
Central access (Yes/No) High flow sets used (Yes/No)

c PASG/MAST ☐

c Surgical intervention should be defined in terms of setting and procedure, e.g., amputation, thoracotomy

c Other interventions
DPL ☐ Pericardiocentesis ☐ Intercostal drain ☐

APPENDIX D: Continued

c Drug information (anaesthesia, neuromuscular blocks, analgesia, sedation, vasopressors; others [specify])

Drug (Name)	Dose	Time (**o**)
________	________	________
________	________	________

etc.

c Time to CT, X-RAY, etc.________

c CPR
Closed chest ☐ Open chest ☐
Minimally invasive open chest ☐

c **Complications/Adverse Effects/Side Effects**
(Document each of the treatment headings on a yes/no basis. There should be an optional facility to describe details of the complication and its relation to outcome.)

c	Oxygen therapy	Yes/No
c	Immobilisation	Yes/No
c	Airway management	Yes/No
c	Ventilation	Yes/No
c	Haemorrhage control	Yes/No
c	IV access	Yes/No
o	IO access	Yes/No
c	IV fluid	Yes/No
c	Surgical intervention	Yes/No
o	Other intervention (specify)	Yes/No
c	Drugs (specify)	Yes/No
c	CPR	Yes/No

APPENDIX E: Outcome Details [9]
(c = core data; o = optional data)

c **Outcome** (quality of life, morbidity, etc.)
—at each stage of care
—hospital
—later (3, 6, 12 months)

Widely used outcome scales
—Glasgow Outcome Scales
—Back to work:
Time
Old job
Reduced capacity
—Other scales (e.g., FIM, SF 36)
—Patient's opinion

APPENDIX E: Continued

c **Mortality** (*NB*: "Trauma death" is defined as death within 30 days of incident.)
- c Time/date of death
- c Location of death
  - Found dead ☐
  - Died at scene ☐
  - Dead on arrival at hospital ☐
  - Died in hospital ☐
  - Died after discharge ☐

c **Confirmation of death**

Time of clinical death	
Time of declaration of death	
Withheld CPR?	Yes/No
Withdrawal of CPR?	Yes/No
Withdrawal of treatment?	Yes/No

c **Cause of death**

Patient factors	
Autopsy?	Yes/No
Details_____	

c **Adverse factors** (possibly responsible for fatal outcome)
(state time of problem)
—Airway problems
—Ventilatory problems
—Circulatory problems
—Other
—Infection/sepsis/MOSF (severity score?)
—Co-morbid conditions
—Age
—Other management

The following factors may be considered as surrogate measures of outcome:
—Time in ICU
—Time in hospital
—Costs

10

Trauma Scoring

LUC VAN CAMP

Ziekenhuis Oost-Limburg, Genk, Belgium

DAVID W. YATES

University of Manchester and Hope Hospital, Salford, United Kingdom

Trauma is the consequence of an external cause of injury that results in tissue damage or destruction produced by intentional or unintentional exposure to thermal, mechanical, electrical, or chemical energy, or by the absence of heat or oxygen. Injury is a threat to health in every country in the world and is currently responsible for 7% of world mortality. In the United States, as in most industrialized societies, trauma is the leading cause of death from childhood to the fourth decade of life. Injuries, fatal and nonfatal, result in an important financial and productivity loss while inflicting a tremendous personal burden on the injured and their families. This universal problem needs a worldwide approach.

The principal goal of this approach, known as "injury control," is to reduce injury mortality, morbidity, and disability. This goal can only be reached through implementation of prevention strategies based on recent injury epidemiology and through continuous assessment and improvement of the quality of trauma care.

The purpose of trauma-scoring mechanisms is threefold. First of all, they are used for triage. Second, they become an essential tool in trauma care management where they have been applied in patient outcome evaluation, quality assessment, and resource allocation. Third, they are fundamental in trauma epidemiology.

This section focuses only on the most universally applied trauma scoring and scaling systems and discusses how they can be applied in injury control.

I. OVERVIEW OF EXISTING TRAUMA-SCORING SYSTEMS

Many trauma scores and scales have been developed during the last 25 years. Table 1 gives a comprehensive summary of these scales.

Table 1 Summary of Existing Trauma-Scoring Systems

Name	Abbreviation	Reference
SIMBOL rating and evaluation system	SIMBOL	1
Trauma index		2
Abbreviated injury scale	AIS	3
		4,5
Comprehensive injury scale	CRIS	6
Prognostic index for severe trauma		7
Glasgow coma scale	GCS	8
Renal index		9
Therapeutic intervention scoring system	TISS	10,11
Injury severity score	ISS	12,13
Respiratory index	RI	14
CHOP index		15
Illness-injury severity index	IISI	16
Triage index		17
Modified injury severity scale	MISS	18,19
Anatomic index	AI	20
Hospital trauma index		21
Acute physiology and chronic health evaluation	APACHE	22
Trauma score	TS	23
Penetrating abdominal trauma index		24
Probability of death score	PODS	25
Circulation respiration abdomen motor speech scale	CRAMS	26
Preliminary method	PRE	27
State transition screen	STS	27
Definitive methodology	DEF	27
Mangled extremity syndrome	MES	28
Acute physiology and chronic health evaluation II	APACHE II	29
Prehospital index		30
Revised trauma score	RTS	31
Acute physiology and chronic health evaluation III	APACHE III	32
Trauma score–injury severity score	TRISS	33
Pediatric trauma score	PTS	34
Outcome predictive score	OPS	35
Riyadh intensive care programme	RIP	36
Organ injury scaling	OIS	37
Anatomic profile	AP	38
A severity characterization of trauma	ASCOT	39
Injury impairment scale	IIS	40
An international classification of disease-9 based injury severity score	ICISS	41
New injury severity score	NISS	42

Trauma-scoring systems were initially introduced as an aid to automotive crash investigation and later in the clinical arena to allow comparisons among patient populations and also for triage purposes. More recently, the value of some of them in quality assessment has been recognized.

II. STATE-OF-THE-ART TRAUMA-SCORING SYSTEMS USED FOR QUALITY ASSESSMENT

A. Physiological Trauma-Scoring Systems

Injury can cause physiological changes in a victim's body. These physiological changes are reflected by changes in both vital signs and the level of consciousness, which are normally assessed as part of the first survey. Trauma-scoring systems, based on the measurement of vital signs and/or the level of consciousness, are physiological trauma-scoring systems.

The best physiological trauma severity scoring systems are based on a limited number of valid parameters that are easy to measure (by doctors, nurses, and paramedics), that have a high intra- and interobserver reliability, and that have a good predictive power (correlate well with mortality).

The state-of-the-art physiological trauma-scoring system currently used is the revised trauma score (RTS), which incorporates the Glasgow coma scale (GCS), systolic blood pressure, and the respiratory rate.

1. The Glasgow Coma Scale (GCS)

The Glasgow Coma Scale was developed in 1974 [8]. It became the most widely used system of defining the level of consciousness of patients with craniocerebral injuries because of its simplicity, its predictive power, and its good interobserver reliability [43]. The GCS defines the level of consciousness according to three parameters: eye opening, best verbal response, and best motor response. These parameters comprise three different subscales, which in turn consist of a hierarchy of responses that are assigned numerical values (Table 2). The score

Table 2 Glasgow Coma Scale (GCS)

	Parameter	Value
Eye opening	Spontaneous	4
	To voice	3
	To pain	2
	None	1
Verbal response	Oriented	5
	Confused	4
	Inappropriate words	3
	Incomprehensible sounds	2
	None	1
Motor response	Obeys commands	6
	Localizes pain	5
	Withdraw (pain)	4
	Flexion (pain)	3
	Extension (pain)	2
	None	1

for each subscale is determined by stimulating the patient and observing the best response. Ranging from 3 to 15, the GCS score is the sum of the scores for eye opening, best verbal response, and best motor response.

As this scale can assess brain function, brain damage, and patient progress in consciousness, it correlates with survival and morbidity and is known as a reliable predictive measure, especially in neurotrauma [43]. The GCS not only helps to predict outcome but also serves as a guide in triage and initial patient management.

2. The Revised Trauma Score

In 1980, Champion et al. [17] developed the triage index, using pattern recognition and mathematical and statistical techniques on nearly 60 biochemical and physiological variables that were known to correlate with mortality following blunt trauma. Weighted values of the five most important variables (eye opening, verbal response, motor response, respiratory expansion, and capillary refill) were taken to create this index. The triage index was the first index that could really predict patient outcome [17].

One year after its development, the triage index was modified by the addition of respiratory rate and systolic blood pressure to create the trauma score (TS) (Table 3) [23]. This score ranges from 1 (worst) to 16 (normal). It correlates better with mortality than did the triage index [44], and was found to be as accurate for penetrating trauma as for blunt trauma [45].

The revised trauma score (RTS) [31] was developed to be simpler than its predecessor (i.e., respiratory expansion and capillary refill were no longer included as variables). Field use of the TS revealed that these variables were difficult to assess at night and that the observation of ''retractive'' respiratory expansion had a very poor intra- and interobserver

Table 3 Trauma Score

Parameter		Value
Respiratory rate (RR; per min)	10–24	4
	25–35	3
	>35	2
	0–10	1
	0	0
Respiratory effort (RE)	Normal	1
	Retractive	0
Systolic blood pressure (SBP; mmHg)	>90	4
	71–90	3
	51–70	2
	1–50	1
	0	0
Capillary refill (CR)	<2 sec	2
	>2 sec	1
	No CR	0
Glasgow coma scale (GCS)	14–15	5
	11–13	4
	8–10	3
	5–7	2
	3–4	1

reliability. Further, there was concern that the TS underestimated the severity of some types of head injuries [31].

Currently, the RTS is the best and most universal physiological trauma severity-scoring system. Use of the RTS-coded values in the field can allow rapid characterization of neurologic, circulatory, and respiratory distress and assessment of the severity of serious head injuries [31]. The predictive value of an RTS with any value below normal (positive test) to fatality, reported by Champion et al. [44] was 96.6%. This is better than the positive predictive values reported for the TS. Several studies have criticized the RTS as a triage tool, however, [46]. This will be discussed later.

The coded RTS values are not just powerful tools for triage and the evaluation of a patient's progress; appropriately weighted and in combination with quantified information about the anatomical injuries, the RTS values also play an important role in outcome evaluation and quality assessment. For this type of application the coded values of GCS, systolic blood pressure, and respiratory rate are weighted (to reflect their ability to predict outcome) and summed to yield the RTS, which takes values from 0 (worst prognosis) to 7.84 (best prognosis) (Table 4).

B. Anatomical Trauma-Scoring Systems

A good anatomical scoring system must be based on a complete description of anatomical injuries (obtained from clinical evaluation), radiology, surgery, and/or autopsy. Postmortem examination is particularly important because it often reveals previously undetected injuries [47,48].

Whereas physiological scores are assigned at first contact and repeated to follow a patient's progress, anatomical scores are usually assigned after complete diagnosis (often at discharge or postmortem). This makes them less useful as triage tools or for the assessment of response to therapy. They are mainly used to classify injured patients and/or to

Table 4 Revised Trauma Score

Parameter		Recording weight	Value
Respiratory rate (RR; per min)	10–29	0.2908	4
	>29		3
	6–9		2
	1–5		1
	0		0
Systolic blood pressure (SBP; mmHg)	>89	0.7326	4
	76–89		3
	50–75		2
	1–49		1
	0		0
Glasgow coma scale (GCS)	13–15	0.9368	4
	9–12		3
	6–8		2
	4–5		1
	3		0

Note: RTS = 0.9368 (GCS value) + 0.7326 (SBP value) + 0.2908 (RR value).

quantify injury severity. A score that can classify and quantify injury according to severity (threat to life) can be used for prediction of outcome.

1. Abbreviated Injury Scale

The abbreviated injury scale (AIS) [5] is an expertise- and consensus-derived, anatomically based system that classifies more than 2000 individual injuries by body region on a six-point ordinal severity (threat to life) scale ranging from AIS 1 (minor) to AIS 6 (currently untreatable). The nine AIS body regions are: (1) head, (2) face, (3) neck, (4) thorax, (5) abdomen, (6) spine, (7) upper extremities, (8) lower extremities, and (9) external.

The AIS is not an interval scale; that is, the increase in injury severity from AIS 1 to 2 is much less than the increase from AIS 3 to 4 or 4 to 5.

Regular revision of the AIS has been necessary, as experience in its use draws attention to deficiencies. Over the last 20 years it has been substantially expanded to include penetrating as well as blunt, automobile-inflicted injuries. The AIS90 is the most recent and currently the most used system for scaling the severity of physiological derangement after injury. The most important limitations of the AIS are that the scale does not assess the combined effects of multiple injuries in one patient, that it is not an interval scale, and that for some (secondary) injuries severity scaling is dynamic and can be affected by the moment of diagnosis (e.g., as the volume of an intracerebral hematoma can change over time, the AIS score assigned will depend on the moment that such a hematoma is documented).

2. Injury Severity Score

The injury severity score (ISS) [12,13] is an ordinal ascending summary severity score ranging from 0 (no injury) to 75 (severely injured) that takes into account the effect of multiple injuries in one patient. Any patient with an AIS 6 injury is assigned an ISS of 75; otherwise the ISS is the sum of squares of the highest AIS code in each of the three most severely injured ISS body regions. The six body regions of injuries used in the ISS are: (1) head and neck, (2) face, (3) thorax, (4) abdomen, (5) extremities, and (6) external. Confusingly, these are not the same as the sections in the AIS book referred to above.

Although this score is purely empirical without any mathematical foundation, it correlates well with survival in multiply-injured subjects [12,49].

Limitations include its reliance on the noninterval AIS, its consideration of injuries with equal AIS scores to be of equal severity regardless of body region, and its exclusion of all but the most serious injury to any body region [13]. These deficiencies have led to a search for a better representation of multiple injuries [49]. The new injury severity score (NISS) [42] is the most popular. It permits the scoring of all injuries in each body area, overcoming the drawback of ISS, which only scores the highest in each area. It has not been universally accepted, however, and the ISS remains the most frequently used summary measure of severity of anatomical injuries.

3. Anatomic Profile

Limitations of the ISS and the growing need for greater precision in quantifying injury so that comparison of groups with similar injuries would be possible prompted the development of a four-valued anatomic profile (AP) [38,50,51].

Clinical knowledge and research findings regarding the primacy of injuries to the head and chest to mortality [52,31] motivated the grouping of injuries into components.

Table 5 Anatomic Profile Based on AIS90

	Trauma description		
Component	Injury and region	AIS 6-digit code	AIS
A	Head (without face)	Starting with 1	3-4-5
	Spinal cord	Starting with 63 or 64	3-4-5
B	Thorax	Starting with 4	3-4-5
	Front of neck	Starting with 3	3-4-5
C	All other injuries	Starting with 2, 5, 7, 8, 9 or starting with 6 and second digit different from 3 or 4	3-4-5
D	All other injuries		1–2

Note: AP component (A, B, C, and D) value calculation: $\sqrt{\Sigma(\text{AIS})^2}$.

In the AP, the A component summarizes all serious (AIS ≥3 and AIS <6) head, brain, and spinal cord injuries, the B component considers serious (AIS ≥3 and AIS <6) injuries to the front of the neck and the thorax, the C component covers all other serious injuries, and the D component is a summary score for all injuries that are not considered serious (AIS <3). Patients with injuries that are not currently considered treatable (AIS 6) are not evaluated by AP; they are defined as a ''set-aside'' group. Whereas ISS only takes into account the most severe injuries in the most severely injured body regions, the AP takes all injuries into account.

The AP component values are calculated as the square root of the sum of squares of the AIS scores for all associated injuries. Weighting the values of additional injuries in this way makes the AP more precise than the ISS in describing anatomical injuries. It has been documented that patients with the same ISS but different AP values have markedly different survival probabilities, while the opposite was not true, revealing that the AP describes combined anatomical injuries more precisely than the ISS does [53].

Originally based on AIS85, some modifications of AP have been necessary as a result of the new AIS90, in which the AIS values of some injuries have changed. Table 5 shows the modified AP based on AIS90 [53].

III. APPLICATIONS OF TRAUMA SEVERITY SCORES

The main goal of acute trauma care is first to reduce mortality and morbidity and second to provide the care that will lead to the injured person's maximal functional recovery; that is, to minimize the effects of the injury. The major challenge to health care providers dealing with a trauma patient is to determine the nature and extent of the patient's injuries rapidly and to provide the proper treatment quickly. Severity scaling can be helpful in triage as well as in assessing the quality and effectiveness of trauma care.

A. Triage

Triage is the classification of patients according to medical needs. As pointed out earlier, only physiological scores are suitable for field-triage purposes because precise determination of anatomical damage is usually not possible at the scene of injury. Triage can be done to determine the level of trauma care to which the patient needs to be transported and to help in the decision to conduct an interhospital transfer, and is done in disaster medicine to identify and prioritize patients who will derive the most benefit from treatment.

The RTS is currently the best and most universal physiological trauma-scoring system used for triage purposes. It should be clear, however, that this scale is not perfect. A Dutch study [46] showed that although the possibility of severe injuries increases with the lowering of the RTS, a substantial proportion of patients who are trauma center candidates according to different definitions have a normal RTS (low sensitivity of the RTS).

B. Quality Assessment

To assess the quality of total clinical trauma care, the most obvious and probably the most important parameter is the survival of the patient. Survival, however, is not only the result of the quality of care delivered, but is first of all a function of the severity of the injuries sustained, the physical condition of the patient before the accident, and the time elapsed between the accident and the start of care deliverance. This means that given the same care, the probability of survival of each patient will be different. As a result, unweighted mortality rates are not useful to assess the quality of care. Based on quantified information about the anatomical and physiological condition of each patient, however, it is possible to calculate the probability of survival of individual patients. Based on these probabilities one can assess the quality of individual trauma care and the performance of trauma care systems.

The two logistic regression models that have been developed for the calculation of the probability of survival in trauma patients are the trauma and injury severity score (TRISS) [33] model and a severity characterization of trauma (ASCOT) [39] model. Anatomical as well as physiological scores are incorporated in both models. The anatomical scores count for the anatomical severity of the injuries sustained. In addition to the quantified anatomical severity, the physiological scores count for the physical condition of the patient (i.e., the physiological score of a patient with a bad physical condition will be worse than that of a patient with a good physical condition who has sustained the same injuries). Physiological scores have the potential to change over time, meaning that the first physiological score obtained is also partially determined by the time elapsed between incident and first (para-) medical assessment (start of care).

1. Trauma and Injury Severity Score (TRISS)

Based on the type of injury (blunt or penetrating), patient age (below or above 55 years old), RTS, AIS, and ISS, it is possible to calculate a patient's probability of survival. This TRISS methodology [33] is the state-of-the-art trauma-outcome evaluation system promoted by the American College of Surgeons Committee on Trauma and applied in the U.S. Major Trauma Outcome Study (MTOS) [54] and by the U.K. Trauma and Research Network [55].

TRISS is based on the following logistic model:

$$Ps = 1/(1 + e^{-b})$$

where

Ps = probability of survival
e = 2.7183 (base of Napierian logarithms)
$b = b_0 + b_1\,(RTS) + b_2\,(ISS) + b_3\,(A)$

RTS = revised trauma score at first medical contact
ISS = injury severity scale based on a complete description of all anatomical injuries
A = age value
patient age $\leq 54 \Rightarrow A = 0$
patient age $\geq 55 \Rightarrow A = 1$

and where the TRISS values for weighted coefficients* [57] depend on the type of injury.

	b_0	b_1	b_2	b_3
Blunt	−0.4843	0.8234	−0.0848	−1.8084
Penetrating	−1.9127	0.9066	−0.0744	−0.9637

Note: Exception for patients <15 years of age one always uses coefficients for blunt injury.

TRISS-based norms can be used as indicators for institutional quality management. This method is known as the preliminary outcome-based evaluation (PRE) [27]. In PRE the RTS (Y axis) and ISS (X axis) are plotted on a graph called the PRE chart. Separate PRE charts are developed for each age and injury-type group. The diagonal line across the chart (Ps50 isobar) marks a Ps of 0.5 for the particular age and injury-type cohort. Patients can be plotted on the PRE chart as death (e.g., dot) or alive (e.g., triangle), and patients with ''unexpected outcomes'' (survivors above or nonsurvivors below the Ps50 isobar) can be visualized. Of course the dots represent probabilities and are therefore not precise forecasts. It follows that many patients falling on the ''wrong'' side of the Ps 50 isobar will in fact be expected to be in that section from a statistical perspective. The use of such charts may be misleading, and clinicians are advised to view them in the context of the clinical situation.

Although PRE can be used to provide the basis for a trauma center's internal peer review, it does not allow comparison of the performance of a hospital against a standard or ''norm.'' The definitive outcome-based evaluation (DEF) [27] was created for this purpose.

In DEF, a Z statistic, which is based on the central limit theorem and the normal approximation to the binomial distribution (without continuity correction), is used to compare the actual number A of survivors in a hospital with the expected number, based on current norms.

$$Z = \frac{\left(A - \sum_{i=1}^{n} Ps_i\right)}{\sqrt{\sum_{i=1}^{n} (Ps_i \cdot [1 - Ps_i])}} = \frac{(A - n\pi)}{\sqrt{n\pi \cdot (1 - \pi)}}$$

where n = size of the sample

* Coefficients are based on Walker–Duncan logistic regression in a norm data set of 13,406 patients treated between 1982 and 1989 in four level-1 trauma centers in the United States and recorded in 1993 using AIS90.

For sample sizes of more than 150 patients, Z values between −1.96 and +1.96 (95% confidence interval) indicate no statistically significant difference ($p < 0.05$) between actual numbers of survivors and the norm. A Z value exceeding 1.96 indicates that a statistically significant greater number of patients survived than was expected by the norm, and a Z value less than −1.96 indicates the opposite. The power of the Z statistic increases with sample size. This means that statistically significant Z values may result from slight but statistically discernible differences between actual and expected number of survivors.

The W statistic provides deeper insight into the clinical significance of statistically significant Z values.

$$W = \frac{\left(A - \sum_{i=1}^{n} Ps_i\right)}{(n/100)} = \frac{(A - n\pi)}{(n/100)}$$

where A and n are defined as in Z.

W is the number of survivors more (positive W value) or less (negative W value) than would be expected from norm predictions per 100 patients. A further refinement is to ''standardize'' the W statistic to take into account the variations in the case mix. This is the Ws statistic [56].

$$Ws = \sum_{j=1}^{6} (W_j \cdot F_j)$$

where F_j = fraction of patients in norm dataset in interval j,

$$\text{and where } Wj = \frac{\left(A_j - \left[\sum_{i=1}^{nj} Ps_i\right]_j\right)}{(n_j/100)}$$

Ws represents the W score that would have been observed if the case mix of injury severities was identical to that of the norm data set.

Zs, the score measuring the significance of Ws, is given by

$$Zs = \frac{\sum_{j=1}^{6} (W_j \cdot F_j)}{\sqrt{\sum_{j=1}^{6} VAR(W_j) \cdot F_j^2}} \quad \text{where } VAR(W_j) = \frac{\left(\sum_{i=1}^{nj} [Ps_i \cdot (1 - Ps_i)]\right)_j}{(n_j/100)^2}$$

or

$$Zs = \frac{W_s}{SE(W_S)} \quad \text{where } SE(W_s) = \sqrt{\sum_{j=1}^{6} VAR(W_j) \cdot F_j^2}$$

Finally, in the U.K. MTOS the TRISS methodology has been further improved by expanding the age breakdown into deciles over the age of 55 (see ASCOT) (http://www.hop.man.ac.uk/uktrauma).

2. A Severity Characterization of Trauma (ASCOT)

The limitations of the anatomical component ISS used in TRISS prompted the development of the AP. As a result, ASCOT [39] was developed as a more statistically reliable predictor of Ps than TRISS. ASCOT combines values of the GCS G, systolic blood pressure S and respiratory rate R as coded by the RTS (Table 4) with AP components (A, B, and C), patient age, and type of injury.

ASCOT is based on the logistic model

$$\text{Ps} = 1/(1 + e^{-k})$$

where

Ps = probability of survival
e = 2.7183 (base of Napierian logarithms)
$k = k_0 + k_1 G + k_2 S + k_3 R + k_4 A + k_5 B + k_6 C + k_7$ Age value
G = value for GCS as coded in RTS at first medical contact
S = value for systolic blood pressure as coded in RTS at first medical contact
R = value for respiratory rate as coded in RTS at first medical contact
A, B, and C are AP components

and where the ASCOT values for weighted coefficients‡ [53,57] depend on the type of injury.

	k_0	k_1	k_2	k_3	k_4	k_5	k_6	k_7
Blunt	−1.1570	0.7705	0.6583	0.2810	−0.3002	−0.1961	−0.2086	−0.6355
Penetrating	−1.1350	1.0626	0.3638	0.3332	−0.3702	−0.2053	−0.3188	−0.8365

In ASCOT patient age is modeled more precisely, using not a binary classification as in TRISS, but a five-point scale that further breaks down the 54 to 85-year age group.

$$\text{Patient age} \leq 54 \Rightarrow \text{Age value} = 0$$
$$\text{Patient age } 55\text{–}64 \Rightarrow \text{Age value} = 1$$
$$\text{Patient age } 65\text{–}74 \Rightarrow \text{Age value} = 2$$
$$\text{Patient age } 75\text{–}84 \Rightarrow \text{Age value} = 3$$
$$\text{Patient age} \geq 85 \Rightarrow \text{Age value} = 4$$

ASCOT's reliance on the AP rather than the ISS to quantify anatomical severity more comprehensively by incorporating all severe injuries and their appropriate weighting not only of the anatomical score but also of the RTS variables according to aetiology (blunt or

‡ Coefficients are based on Walker–Duncan logistic regression in a norm data set of 13,406 patients treated between 1982 and 1989 in four level-1 trauma centers in the United States and recoded in 1993 using AIS90.

Table 6 ASCOT Set-Asides and Their Ps

Maximum AIS	RTS	Type of injury	Ps
6	0	Blunt	0.000
6	0	Penetrating	0.000
6	>0	Blunt	0.229
6	>0	Penetrating	0.222
<6	0	Blunt	0.014
<6	0	Penetrating	0.026
≤2	>0	Blunt	0.998
≤2	>0	Penetrating	0.999

penetrating) of injury, facilitates better severity characterization. The Hosmer–Lemeshow goodness of fit statistics indicate that ASCOT is a more reliable predictor of outcome than TRISS [53].

Patients with very severe (AIS = 6) or very minor (AP components A, B, and C = 0) injury are not evaluated by the ASCOT logistic model. These set-aside patient groups are defined, and their respective probabilities of survival are given in Table 6.

The same Z, W, Ws, and Zs statistics as explained for TRISS can be performed, based on the survival probabilities calculated with ASCOT. Z(s) and W(s) statistics, based on TRISS or ASCOT norms allow performance assessment. One should realize, however, that the regression coefficients used in these models are based on data from hospitals in the United States and may not be universal. The U.K. Trauma Audit & Research Network, for example, uses other coefficients (http://www.hop.man.ac.uk/uktrauma).

3. Disability

All the above scoring systems are based on outcome assessment measured only in terms of death and survival. We know that many young trauma victims survive with significant permanent disabilities, however. Attempts to establish effective scoring systems to measure this burden of disease have been largely unsuccessful, but recently an international effort has been made to resolve the problem. A consensus has not yet been reached, but it is probable that the following scales will be used increasingly in pilot studies:

For outcome prediction based on anatomical injury, the injury impairment scale (IIS) [40]

For outcome measurement, the quality of well-being scale [58,59]; short form 36 (SF36) [60]; short form 12 (SF12) [61]; EuroQol [62,63].

C. Injury Epidemiology

One of the core functions in injury control is the collection and analysis of data about injuries in order to document where, when, and how injuries occur, what the risk factors are, who is affected, and what the severity is. This critical information related to patient outcome is needed to design, implement, and evaluate preventive interventions.

Basic epidemiological trauma data include information on the distribution of the severity, mortality, and morbidity associated with each of the causes of injury. Universal anatomical severity scores are essential for severity description in such databases. Only the use of such systems will allow injury epidemiologists to compare trauma patients, to measure preventive interventions, and to share the findings of different studies. Recently, for this purpose, ITACCS has published recommendations for uniform reporting of data following major trauma [64,65].

REFERENCES

1. RE Williams, JL Schamadan. The SIMBOL rating and evaluating system: A measurement tool for injury persons. Ariz Med 16:886–887, 1969.
2. JR Kirkpatrick, RL Youmans. Trauma index: An aid in evaluation of injury victims. J Trauma 11:711–714, 1971.
3. American Medical Association Committee on Medical Aspects of Automotive Safety (AMA CMAAS). Rating the severity of tissue damage. I. The abbreviated scale. JAMA 215:277–280, 1971.
4. American Association for Automotive Medicine (now Association for the Advancement of Automotive Medicine; AAAM). Abbreviated Injury Scale. rev. ed. Des Plaines, IL: AAAM, 1985.
5. Association for the Advancement of Automotive Medicine (AAAM). Abbreviated Injury Scale. rev. ed. Des Plaines, Il: AAAM, 1990.
6. American Medical Association Committee on Medical Aspects of Automotive Safety (AMA CMAAS). Rating the severity of tissue damage. II. The comprehensive injury scale. JAMA 220:717–720, 1972.
7. RA Cowley, WJ Sacco, W Gill, et al. A prognostic index for severe trauma. J Trauma 14: 1029–1035, 1974.
8. G Teasdale, B Jennett. Assessment of coma and impaired consciousness: A practical scale. Lancet 2:81–83, 1974.
9. HR Champion, WJ Sacco, W Long, et al. Indicators for early haemodialysis in multiple trauma. Lancet 1:1125–1127, 1974.
10. DJ Cullen, J Civetta, BA Briggs, et al. Therapeutic intervention scoring system: A method for quantitative comparison of patient care. Crit Care Med 2:57–60, 1974.
11. AR Keene, D Cullen. Therapeutic intervention scoring system: Update 1983. Crit Care Med 11:1–3, 1983.
12. SP Baker, B O'Neill. The injury severity score: An update. J Trauma 16:822–885, 1976
13. WS Copes, HR Champion, WJ Sacco, et al. The injury severity score revised. J Trauma 28: 69–77, 1988.
14. MA Goldtarb, TH Ciurey, TC McAslan, et al. Tracking respiratory therapy in trauma patients. Amer J Surg 129:255–258, 1975.
15. WJ Sacco, AV Milholland, WP Ashman, et al. Trauma indices. Computer Biol Med 7:9–20, 1977.
16. DL Bever, CH Veenker. An illness severity index for non-physician emergency medical personnel. EMT J 3:45–49, 1979.
17. HR Champion, WJ Sacco, DS Hannan. Assessment of injury severity: The triage index. Crit Care Med 8:201–208, 1980.
18. T Mayer, ME Matlak, DG Johnson, et al. The modified injury severity scale in pediatric multiple trauma patients. J Pediat Surg 5:719–726, 1980.
19. T Mayer, MI Walker, P Clark. Further experience with the modified abbreviated injury severity scale. J Trauma 24:31–34, 1984.
20. HR Champion, WJ Sacco, RL Lepper. An anatomic index of injury severity. J Trauma 20: 197–202, 1980.
21. American College of Surgeons Commitee on Trauma. Field categorization of trauma patients and hospital trauma index. Bull Amer Coll Surg 2:28–33, 1980.

22. WA Knaus, JB Zimmerman, DP Wagner, et al. APACHE—Acute physiology and chronic health evaluation: A physiologically based classification system. Crit Care Med 9:591–597, 1981.
23. HR Champion, WJ Sacco, AJ Carnazzo, et al. Trauma score. Crit Care Med 9:672–676, 1981.
24. EE Moore, EL Dunn, JB Moore, et al. Penetrating abdominal trauma index. J Trauma 21: 399–444, 1981.
25. RL Somers. New ways to use the 1980 Abbreviated Injury Scale—The Probability of Death Score (PODS). Internal report University of Odense Denmark, Odense Laboratory for Public Health and Health Economics, 1982.
26. SP Gormican. CRAMS scale: Field triage of trauma victims. Ann Emerg Med 11:132–135, 1982.
27. HR Champion, WJ Sacco, TK Hunt. Trauma severity scoring to predict mortality. World J Surg 7:4–11, 1983.
28. RT Gregory, RJ Gould, M Peclet, et al. The mangled extremity syndrome (MES): A severity grading system for multisystem injury of the extremity. J Trauma 25:1147–1150, 1985.
29. WA Knaus, EA Draper, DP Wagner, et al. APACHE II: A severity of disease classification system. Crit Care Med 13:818–829, 1985.
30. JJ Koehler, LJ Baer, SA Malafa, et al. Prehospital index: A scoring system for field triage of trauma victims. Ann Emerg Med 15:178–182, 1986.
31. HR Champion, WJ Sacco, WS Copes, et al. A revision of the trauma score. J Trauma 29: 623–629, 1989.
32. W Knaus, D Wagner, JE Zimmerman, et al. APACHE III study design: Analytic plan for evaluation of severity and outcome in intensive care unit patients. Crit Care Med 17:S169–S221, 1989.
33. CR Boyd, MA Tolson, WS Copes. Evaluating trauma care: The TRISS method. J Trauma 27: 370–378, 1987.
34. JJ Tepas, DL Mollitt, JL Talbert, et al. The pediatric trauma score as a predictor of injury severity. J Pediat Surg 22:14–18, 1987.
35. MJ Hershman, WG Cheadle, D Kuftinec, et al. An outcome predictive score for sepsis and death following injury. Injury 19:263–266, 1988.
36. RWS Chang, S Jacobs, E Lee. Predicting outcome among intensive care unit patients using computerised trend analysis of daily APACHE II scores corrected for organ system failure. Intensive Care Med 14:558–566, 1988.
37. EE Moore, SR Schackford, HL Pachter, et al. Organ injury scaling: Spleen, liver, kidney. J Trauma 29:1664–1666, 1989.
38. WS Copes, HR Champion, W Sacco, et al. Progress in characterizing anatomic injury. J Trauma 20:1200–1207, 1990.
39. HR Champion, WS Copes, WJ Sacco, et al. A new characterization of injury severity. J Trauma 30:539–546, 1990.
40. Association for the Advancement of Automotive Medicine (AAAM). Injury Impairment Scale. Des Plaines, IL: AAAM, 1994.
41. T Osler, R Rutledge, J Deis, E Bedrick. ICISS: An international classification of disease-9 based injury severity score. J Trauma 41:380–388, 1996.
42. T Osler, SP Baker, W Long. A modification of the injury severity score that both improves accuracy and simplifies scoring. J Trauma 43:922–926, 1997.
43. B Jennett, G Teasdale, R Braakman, et al. Predicting outcome in individual patients after severe head injury. Lancet May 15. 1(7968):1031–1034, 1976.
44. HR Champion, PS Gainer, E Yackee. A progress report on the trauma score in predicting a fatal outcome. J Trauma 26:927–936, 1986.
45. HR Champion, WJ Sacco. The trauma score as applied to penetrating injury. Ann Emerg Med 13:415–418, 1984.

46. J Roorda, EF van Beek, JWJL Stapert, W ten Wolde. Evaluation performance of the revised trauma score as a triage instrument in the prehospital setting. Injury 27:163–167, 1996.
47. JD Harviel, J Landsman, A Greenberg, et al. The effect of autopsy on injury severity and survival probability calculations. J Trauma 29:766–773, 1989.
48. JC Strothert Jr, GBM Gbaanador, DN Herndon. The role of autopsy in death resulting from trauma. J Trauma 30:1021–1026, 1990.
49. JP Bull. The injury severity score of road traffic casualties in relation to mortality, time of death, hospital treatment time and disability. Accid Anal Prev 7:249–255, 1975.
50. WJ Sacco, JW Jameson, WS Copes, et al. Progress toward a new injury severity characterization: Injury profiles. Computer Bio Med 18:419–429, 1988.
51. WS Copes, WJ Sacco, HR Champion, et al. Progress in characterizing anatomic injury. 33rd Annual Proceedings, Association for the Advancement of Automotive Medicine, Des Plaines, IL, 1989.
52. TA Gennarelli, HR Champion, WJ Sacco, et al. Head injury mortality in trauma centers. J Trauma 29:1193–1202, 1989.
53. HR Champion, WS Copes, WJ Sacco, et al. Improved predictions from severity characterization of trauma (ASCOT) over trauma and injury severity score (TRISS): Results of an independent evaluation. J Trauma 40:42–49, 1996.
54. HR Champion, WS Copes, WJ Sacco, et al. The major trauma outcome study: Establishing national norms for trauma care. J Trauma 30:1356–1365, 1990.
55. F Lecky, M Woodford, D Yates. Trends in trauma care in England and Wales 1989–1997. Lancet 355:1771–1774, 2000.
56. S Hollis, DW Yates, M Woodford, P Foster. Standardized comparison of performance indicators in trauma: A new approach to case-mix variation. J Trauma 38:763–766, 1995.
57. M Lawnick. Personnal communication. Washington, DC 1993.
58. RM Kaplan, JW Bush, CC Berry. Health status: Types of validity and the index of well-being. Health Serv Res 11:478–507, 1976.
59. TL Holbrook. Outcome after major trauma: Discharge and 12 month and 18 month follow up results from the Trauma Recovery Project. J Trauma 49:765–773, 1999.
60. JE Ware Jr, CD Sherbourne. The MOS 36-item short-form health survey (SF-36). I: Conceptual framework and item selection. Med Care 30:473–483, 1992.
61. JE Ware Jr, M Kosinski, SD Keller. A 12 item short form health survey: Construction of scales and preliminary tests of reliability and validity. Med Care 34:220–233, 1996.
62. Euroqol Group. Euroqol—A new facility for the measurement of health-related quality of life. Health Pol 16:199–208, 1990.
63. R Brooks. EuroQol Group. EuroQol: The current state of play. Health Pol 37:53–72, 1996.
64. WF Dick, PJ Baskett, C Grande, H Delooz, W Kloeck, C Lackner, M Lipp, W Mauritz, M Nerlich, J Nicholl, J Nolan, P Oakley, M Parr, A Seekamp, E Soreide, PA Steen, L van Camp, B Wolcke, D Yates. Recommendations for uniform reporting of data following major trauma Ugstein style. An International Trauma Anaesthesia and Critical Care Society (ITACCS) initiative. Eur J Emerg Med 6:369–387, 1999.
65. WF Dick, PJ Baskett, C Grande, H Delooz, W Kloeck, C Lackner, M Lipp, W Mauritz, M Nerlich, J Nicholl, J Nolan, P Oakley, M Parr, A Seekamp, E Soreide, PA Steen, L van Camp, B Wolcke, D Yates. Recommendations for uniform reporting of data following major trauma Ugstein style. An International Trauma Anaesthesia and Critical Care Society (ITACCS) initiative. Br J Anaesth 84:818–819, 2000.

11

Organization, Documentation, and Continuous Quality Improvement

KEN HILLMAN

The University of New South Wales, Sydney, Australia

MICHAEL SUGRUE

The Liverpool Hospital, Sydney, Australia

THOMAS A. SWEENEY

Christiana Care Health Services, Wilmington, Delaware

I. INTRODUCTION

In the last decade we have been made increasingly aware of the importance of ischemia and hypoxia on cellular function. At one end of the spectrum, severe hypovolemia and shock can result in rapid death. Even minor degrees of ischemia, however, can cause measurable cellular damage [1]. Moderate degrees of ischemia can predispose to cytokine release and multiorgan failure (MOF) [2]. Severe cellular ischemia can occur in spite of a normal blood pressure [3]. Goris was one of the first to describe the concept of nonbacterial ''sepsis states'' as a result of mediators such as cytokines, prostinoids, and lysosomes [4]. He proposed that trauma is the ''match'' that lights the ''fuse'' (complement) that activates the ''blasting cap'' (the macrophage) that sets off the ''explosion'' of mediators that lead to multiple organ injury.

Understanding the concept of a spectrum of damage caused by cellular hypoxia and ischemia is crucial for the optimal management of trauma. The world's best trauma surgeon can be waiting in his or her operating room for a patient who is languishing at the scene of an accident or in the emergency department. The cascade of cytokines is irreversibly fired off from the moment injury first occurs, resulting in organ failure if not treated early, despite magnificent and heroic surgery.

Unfortunately acute care hospitals and trauma systems can act as disjointed islands of care [5], often with excellent care practiced within those islands but with little in the way of horizontal interaction between various departments, professions, and functions. The management of trauma cannot optimally operate within the paradigm of separate islands of care. The trauma system is only as strong as its weakest point. For example, hospital care for trauma may be well organized, but if hypoxia and ischemia remain untreated in the prehospital situation, patient outcome will be less than ideal.

Trauma management requires an ''integrated approach'' involving every point of care from the scene of the injury to rehabilitation. The medical profession often finds this challenge frustrating, as its training and education is based on the individual patient–doctor relationship and works within the traditional paradigm of history, examination, provisional diagnosis, investigation, diagnosis, and treatment. Trauma management requires a very different approach. Excellent trauma care is based on a ''systems approach,'' through which every point of care is optimized and every part of the system is integrated. The medical profession comprises only one part of this system. The system also involves interaction with services such as dispatch centers, ambulance and on-scene resuscitation personnel, police, and local and regional governments, as well as many different departments and staffs within a hospital. To be part of that system requires a different set of skills to those traditionally taught at medical school.

There must be a mechanism for measuring the effectiveness of this complex system. Outcome—such as mortality adjusted for age, severity of injury, and pre-existing comorbidities—is often used. The parts of the system for which management might be improved must be identified. The most challenging aspect of trauma care is to involve all parts of the trauma system in translating the results and interpretation of such data into action, whereby the system can be continually adjusted and improved. Among many other names, this process is known as continuous quality improvement (CQI) [6].

II. GENERIC COMPONENTS OF PREHOSPITAL TRAUMA CARE

The establishment of a trauma system has one common goal, at least in the initial phase of management—to maintain an optimal flow of oxygenated blood to cells. Every region and nation will have a different approach in achieving that goal [7–9]. The following are some of the key elements [10] that must be carefully examined by the CQI process. The reader is referred to Chap. 10 and two other articles [11,12] for more details on the uniform use of definitions in the prehospital setting.

A. Scene

The system must adjust to any scene within the environment of the region. Existing data analysis should outline the major etiology and source of trauma. There is a need to define the incidence and location, for example, of blunt road trauma, penetrating injuries as a result of violence, work-related injuries, and sports-related injuries. Local assessment of infrequent natural or major disasters should also be conducted, and the trauma center should be integrated with local disaster planning and management. Planning and resource allocation should be focused on the existing major sources of trauma, however, and any tendency to become obsessed with ''possibilities'' rather than reality should be avoided.

B. Activation of Primary Response

Each area covered by the trauma system must establish an efficient method of activating the primary trauma response. The effectiveness of system activation will depend on factors such as population density, public education, and the sophistication of public and private communication systems in the community. For trauma requiring urgent and professional care, a single emergency telephone number that can also alert other services, such as the police or the fire department, is desirable in order to allow the general public easy activation of the trauma system.

C. Options in Primary Response

Primary response options are determined by such factors as distance from the site of definitive care and traffic density. Motor vehicle and rotary or fixed-wing air response are among the available options. Cost also is a factor in determining primary response. Often, however, local politics and history are the major determinants of the options available. For example, enthusiasm among local helicopter lobby groups may be the most important factor in determining response rather than compelling data, logic, or cost.

D. Skills and Levels of Initial Response

Even more important than the response vehicle is the level of skills and knowledge of the attending personnel. Unfortunately, the choice of personnel also can be largely determined by local politics and history rather than by logic. The skills and knowledge required are related to immediate airway, breathing, circulation support, and patient packaging, in combination with experience in operating in the less than ideal world of the out-of-hospital environment.

The medical profession certainly does not have a monopoly in this area; in fact, its undergraduate training in resuscitation is often inadequate [13]. Doctors not specifically trained in all aspects of out-of-hospital trauma resuscitation certainly should not be utilized just because they are doctors. There is an essential set of knowledge and practical skills that is necessary for initial out-of-hospital resuscitation, related to such areas as airway control, cervical spine immobilization, intubation, ventilation, intravenous cannulation, and rapid fluid transfusion. Occasionally bystanders and authorities such as police and fire personnel can contribute as first responders [14], but usually physicians, nurses, or specifically trained paramedics are employed in the initial out-of-hospital resuscitation [15]. Just as doctors with a wide base of medical knowledge require specific training in out-of-hospital resuscitation, personnel with limited medical knowledge require protocols that are flexible enough to enable them to practically apply the protocols in many different situations. There is little evidence to suggest that one alternative is superior to another [15] as long as the area of skill and knowledge is well defined and taught and the person works a majority of his or her time in that setting in order to maintain those skills.

The discussion about "load and go" versus "stay and play" is biased in one direction even in the manner in which it is expressed. It assumes that every trauma patient is dying of surgically correctable bleeding and must be transported immediately to the operating rooms. There are few sound data in this area, and what do exist may be colored by the perspective of the authors. One cannot argue that surgical bleeding does not need to be controlled. Similarly, one cannot argue that prolonged obstruction of the airway, hypoxia, and ischemia is not harmful and does not require immediate management. If basic maneuvers that address life-threatening problems can occur at the scene or on the way to hospital, then they should not be delayed until the patient arrives in the operating room! Similarly, the distance between the scene and the hospital and the skills of those attending at the scene need to be factored into the equation. Patient outcome depends more on why you need to load and go and who is staying and playing rather than on local bias and politics, which reduce complex issues to catchy phrases.

E. Protocols

Trauma care depends on a systemized approach to injury. Whether the initial response is conducted by a clinician, paramedic, or other personnel, it is important that it be conducted within agreed-upon protocols such as those developed by the advanced trauma life support (ATLS) [16]. The protocols must also guarantee the safety of those working at the scene. A process must exist that allows protocols to be flexible and change according to new evidence-based developments in prehospital trauma care.

F. Triage

Triaging trauma patients is an important part of any trauma system [17]. There may only be one hospital in which all trauma patients, no matter what the level of severity, are managed. There may, however, be two or more hospitals working together within a region. Where possible, it is important that all serious, life-threatening trauma is triaged to one center with a 24-hr response capable of dealing with all aspects of trauma management. Apart from any other consideration, a trauma center requires expensive infrastructure in terms of staff and equipment, and this is difficult to duplicate. The system needs to define seriously injured patients in order for triage to effectively occur. The performance of the triage system depends on the sensitivity and specificity of the triage device as well as the degree of compliance of the staff working with the tool.

The ''overtriage'' rate needs to be low enough to minimize disruption of the system and maintain an adequate compliance rate but high enough to capture all potentially life-threatening injuries. This is usually achieved in terms of physiological criteria, such as respiratory rate, level of consciousness, blood pressure, and pulse rate; the circumstances of the injury, such as a pedestrian being hit by vehicle and penetrating trauma; the nature of the injury, such as a head injury and burns; and the extent of the injuries.

Scoring systems have been developed to improve trauma triage, including the prehospital index (PHI) [18] and the mechanism of injury score (MOI) [19]. Bond et al., from Alberta, Canada, have trialed a mechanism of combining the PHI and MOI in order to improve the accuracy of the tool [20]. They found in a prospective study of over 3,000 trauma patients that the PHI/MOI score was better at identifying those patients with injury severity scores (ISS) of 16 or greater.

Other triage tools include the trauma score [21] and CRAMS [22] which involves an assessment of circulation, respiration, and the abdomen, as well as motor and speech function. Although widely used, these triage tools fail to identify the trauma patient who appears to be initially stable and then seriously deteriorates. It is possible that different trauma systems will require individual triage trauma tools and that not all trauma triage tools will fit individual services.

Key components were identified in conjunction with the Emergency Medical Services (EMS) Systems Act as part of an initiative in the United States [23]. These are outlined in Table 1.

Table 1 Key Components for Emergency Services

Training	Audit and quality assurance
Communications	Disaster
Prehospital transport	Mutual aid
Interfacility transport agency	Protocols
Emergency facilities	Financing
Specialty care units	Dispatch
Public information and education	Medical director

Source: Ref. 14.

III. COORDINATION AND INTEGRATION OF TRAUMA CARE

It has been recognized for many years that a regional plan should be developed that deals with the care of the trauma victim from the scene of the injury to rehabilitation. Regions that have adopted these criteria have experienced a dramatic reduction in preventable death rates [9,24,25]. The suggested steps to achieve effective regionalization of trauma services involve [8] the following:

- Establishment of a basic database
- A comprehensive regional plan
- Identification of barriers to change
- Development of a management structure
- Implementation of a plan

The regional plan and management structure will be outlined here. Other challenges will be discussed later in the chapter.

A. Regional Plan

A plan for regionalizing trauma services must involve all the major stakeholders, including the local government and hospitals, as well as ambulance, police, and fire services. Involvement of everyone concerned leads to genuine ownership and a more effective system. Other local issues include funding, population distribution, and geographical considerations, as well as the nature and incidence of trauma.

B. Management Structure

The management structure will be determined by local conditions, such as the way in which government and private agencies interact. The most important factor in determining the degree of success is probably related to the local enthusiasm of one or two champions of a regional trauma system. The management system needs to address issues of how the various components of the system interact, how the system is coordinated, and how the effectiveness of the system is measured and adjusted according to those data. The way the policies and procedures component of the system interacts with quality evaluation depends on local circumstances.

IV. NATIONAL STANDARDS

While not essential for regional trauma care, it is extremely useful for each country to establish its own national standards. The process of establishing national standards in itself engages the major national stakeholders, such as national medical and nursing organizations, as well as national police, fire, and ambulance authorities with national funding and legislative bodies. National standards set a minimum benchmark with which every regional system must comply. There is also an implication that funding must be available for the infrastructure necessary to meet those standards. Funding can also be linked to performance and outcome measurements. The national standard-setting process is also a useful vehicle for the establishment of evidence-based medicine for all aspects of trauma care. National standards could also provide an accreditation process based on those agreed-upon standards. Each country would obviously work with different sets of groups and organizations in order to achieve national standards.

Despite the attraction of establishing national standards for prehospital care and allocating resources to meet those standards, there are few successful working models [26].

V. IMPLEMENTATION

A. Identification of the Barriers to Change

The greatest barriers to change are related to human behavior. This seems to be a general response to any change. People are suspicious of change, and it needs to be managed appropriately. If we are accustomed to dealing with trauma victims in the same way we deal with, for example, elective surgery, and we have no data to state otherwise, the common response will be ''Why change?'' A major change in the way we manage trauma involves participants becoming part of a team rather than controlling most of the process, as occurs with less complex challenges and more focused challenges, such as when an individual doctor treats a patient electively admitted to hospital. Usually a local champion has to convince his or her colleagues that developing a trauma system will not only improve patient care but the system will not be a threat to their own practices, financially or in terms of losing control.

Economic factors are also important, even for prehospital care. In societies driven by the patient's ability to pay, trauma care may be an unattractive option for hospitals and patient retrieval systems. It could be argued that no matter how the national economy is organized, regionalization and rationalization of existing trauma care, so that it performs in a more efficient fashion, may provide better patient care for the same or lower costs.

B. Implementing a Trauma System

Despite convincing studies suggesting that regionalization of coordinated trauma systems decreases preventable mortality, only a small minority of regions have actually achieved full implementation [8].

Some of the reasons for this failure include a lack of funds, resistance by colleagues to changing from individual clinician to team player, a lack of support by health managers, often due to local financial constraints, a lack of awareness by society, failure of local champions to push the service, and an underestimation of the time and effort required to establish a fully coordinated and integrated system.

The steps required to implement an effective regional trauma service include the following [8]:

Defining the authority to implement a regional trauma plan
Defining a management structure to oversee its implementation
Defining the elements of a comprehensive CQI program
Providing adequate resources to implement the plan
Providing appropriate authority to coordinate and integrate the system

VI. THE CONTINUOUS QUALITY IMPROVEMENT PROGRAM

Quality management is a set of principles derived from operations research, statistics, and theories of human motivation and organization behavior. It has been associated with improved quality, productivity, and profitability in diverse industries around the world. Most acute health services have attempted to introduce the concept of quality management into the health industry, but the gap between the attractive theory and the implementation of these principles is variable.

Continuous quality improvement is a statistically based quality management theory that was originally developed based on attempts to remove variation in the production process. Unacceptable variation (poor quality) is thought to result from failures in the design or execution of the process or system rather than from failure by individuals.

Continuous quality improvement in health care is based on certain principles [6], including the following:

1. Clinical leaders must take the lead in ensuring quality.
2. Infrastructure and investment is needed to ensure quality improvement.
3. Respect for the opinions and role of the deliverer of health care is essential for CQI.
4. The receivers and providers of health care must be aware of each other's needs and intentions.
5. Measuring what is done and using those data to continuously improve the system is essential.
6. The quality of health care delivery must be seen as a reality as well as rhetoric and be seen as equally important as the cost of health care delivery.

Table 2 Prehospital Trauma Care Data

Patient demographics (e.g., age, gender, comorbidities)
Intervals from traumatic event to definitive hospital care, including:
Incident to call interval
Call received to dispatch interval
Dispatch to arrival of first treatment team interval
On-scene (assessment/treatment) interval
Vehicle departs scene/arrival emergency treatment facility interval
Demographics of injury (e.g., cause, time, mechanism of injury, place)
Description of injury (e.g., type, severity)
Management of injury (e.g., oxygen, immobilization, airway adjuncts, ventilation, IV access, and fluids)
Outcome (e.g., mortality)

Table 3 Examples of Quality Indicators for Prehospital Care

Time intervals (e.g., receipt of call to unit dispatch, extrication of entrapped patient)
Dispatch of appropriate personnel
Skills of first responder (e.g., basic or advanced life support)
Impact of clinical interventions on on-scene interval
Appropriateness of cervical spine control
IV cannula established and resuscitation fluid commenced in the presence of signs of hypovolemia
Success rate of intubation attempts
Evaluate prehospital component in potentially preventable deaths

Several models or principles of quality assurance have been well documented and evaluated in prehospital care. Of particular note is the Donabedian concept of structure, outcome, and process [27]. Emergency medical services and prehospital care providers have had traditional strength in the structure and process of care but have often failed to look at outcome [27]. The basis for effective CQI is data. Some of the suggested major headings for prehospital data collection are described in Table 2 [15,28–30].

There is little in the way of level 1 or 2 evidence to support specific prehospital performance indicators, however [31].

A uniform approach to collecting prehospital trauma data based on the Utstein style for prehospial cardiac arrests [12] will hopefully provide the basis for an international comparison of data and the establishment of benchmarking practices [11,12].

Examples of possible quality indicators that could be derived from uniform prehospital data sets are listed in Table 3. For example, in relation to prehospital intubation, Thompson and colleagues suggest a threshold for successful intubation be between 90–95% [32].

Another method of viewing performance is through the ''value equation.'' The value relates to the quality of the process, the quality of the outcome, and the cost.

$$\text{Value} = \frac{\text{Quality of process} + \text{Quality of outcome}}{\text{Cost}}$$

Value can be increased by improving the quality of the process or outcome or by decreasing the cost. A modest increase in cost that significantly improves quality can also add value, however. This prospective can help prioritize performance improvements.

VII. DOCUMENTATION AND DATA COLLECTION

No matter what indicators are chosen, the key to implementing CQI is to measure what we do and then provide those data to health care deliverers at all levels and empower them to change the system in order to improve patient care; otherwise CQI becomes yet another management fad with no credibility.

While some studies have examined the issue of prevention in the prehospital component of the trauma system [14,33,34] there are as yet no internationally agreed-upon standard data sets for prehospital care. Many outcome measurements are used to evaluate overall trauma care, but the measurement of the system usually assumes its beginning point is admission to the hospital.

Some of these outcome measures include TRISS [35], ASCOT [21], the Z score [36], and the standardized mortality rate derived from initial trauma scores and at-hospital discharge mortality status. Scores that measure recovery in the community setting include the SF36, a measure of quality of life [37]; the Glasgow coma scale (GCS) outcome score; and FIMMS [38]. It is difficult to distinguish the prehospital phase of trauma management from the overall quality of trauma management using existing outcome indicator data. The American College of Emergency Medicine emphasizes the differences between monitoring the prehospital component of the trauma system as opposed to the hospital component [28].

While there is no single gold standard outcome measurement for the prehospital component of trauma care, some of the process measurements are listed in Table 3.

Using indicators such as these, a threshold level can be assigned. The data then need to be analyzed in order to determine whether or not that threshold was achieved. The next step (and possibly the most difficult one) is to feed those data back to health care deliverers in such a fashion that they can implement and own the changes to the system, which are necessary to improve it and achieve whatever threshold levels are set.

A. Evidence-Based Medicine and Standardization

The concept of evidence-based medicine (EBM) has recently become popular [39–43]. Organizations such as the Cochrane Collaboration support implementation and utilization of EBM. The theory is that if there is evidence that one way of delivering care is better than all the others we all should be standardizing our practice around that evidence. Evidence-based medicine may play an increasingly important role in trauma management. Examples include the single best way to detect intra-abdominal bleeding [44] or to manage a ruptured spleen [45,46]. The Internet offers new resources from professional organizations such as the Eastern Association for the Surgery of Trauma Website [47].

In the prehospital arena, there are a number of different approaches to prehospital management. Many of these are based upon expert opinion and have not been subject to peer review [48]. One of the problems is that it is often difficult to assemble unequivocal evidence to prove that one way of managing is substantially better than another. Examples include the controversy and uncertainty following whether immediate surgery or resuscitation is preferable after penetrating torso injury [49] and whether colloids or crystalloids are better in the initial management of trauma [50]. Although there was evidence presented in these articles, both contained strong opinions, and debate continues about the methodology and conclusion of these studies. This seems a predictable and indeed healthy intellectual process. Where uncertainty exists there will not be standardization or convincing EBM. Where there is unequivocal and overwhelming evidence, however, standardization should follow.

VIII. THE PUBLIC PROFILE OF TRAUMA

Trauma continues to be the leading cause of death in many Western countries for individuals under 40 years of age, and the cost to society is enormous [51].

Opinion leaders and those involved in trauma systems need to make the public aware of what regional and well-organized trauma systems are and how society may suffer if their region does not enjoy the benefits of a well-organized trauma system. Governments must also be aware of the impact of trauma on society and their own responsibility in funding and supporting regional trauma systems. This can be achieved by many means, such as the use of media and of our professional organizations, as well as understanding how health, funding sources, and decision-making processes engage each other and interact. The increasing use of data to measure the effectiveness of our systems and how they compare to others will also be a powerful agent for change.

IX. SUMMARY/CONCLUSION

Generic components of prehospital care include the scene and the primary response options, activation, and skills, as well as protocols and triage.

Coordination of prehospital trauma care involves integration between government and agencies apart from health, including the police and fire departments.

Implementation of prehospital trauma systems involves standard data collection, analysis of those data, and distribution to all those involved in the delivery and organization of the system.

REFERENCES

1. P Wang, ZF Ba, J Burkhardt, IH Chaudry. Measurement of hepatic blood flow after severe haemorrhage: Lack of restoration despite adequate resuscitation. Am J Physiol 262:G92–G98, 1992.
2. WL Biffl, EE Moore. Splanchnic ischaemia/reperfusion and multiple organ failure. Brit J Anaesth 77:59–70, 1996.
3. BF Rush Jr. The bacterial factor in hemorrhagic shock. Surg Gyn Ob 75:285–292, 1992.
4. R Goris, TP te Boekhorst, JK Nuytinck, JS Gimbrere. Multiple organ failure: Generalized autodestruction inflammation? Arch Surg 120:1109–1115, 1985.
5. KM Hillman. Reducing preventable deaths and containing costs: The expanding role of intensive care medicine. Med J Aust 164:308–309, 1996.
6. DM Berwick. Continuous improvement as an ideal in health care. New Eng J Med 320:53–56, 1989.
7. SA Deane, PL Gaudry, I Pearson, S Misra, RI McNeil, C Read. The hospital trauma team: A model for trauma management. J Trauma 30:806–812, 1990.
8. JG West, MJ Williams, DD Trunkey, CC Wolferth Jr. Trauma systems: Current status—Future challenges. JAMA 259:3597–3600, 1988.
9. SR Shackford, P Hollingworth-Fridlund, GF Cooper, AB Eastman. The effect of regionalization upon the quality of trauma care as assessed by concurrent audit before and after institution of a trauma system: A preliminary report. J Trauma 26:812–820, 1986.
10. Committee on Trauma, American College of Surgeons. Hospital and pre-hospital resources for optimal care of the injured patient. Bull Amer Coll Surg 71:4–12, 1986.
11. RO Cummins, DA Chamberlain, MF Hazinski, V Nadkarni, W Kloeck, E Kramer, I Becker, C Robertson, R Koster, A Zaritsky, L Bossaert, JP Ornato, V Callanan, M Allen, PA Steen, B Connolly, A Sanders, A Idris, S Cobbe. Recommended guidelines for uniform reporting of data from out of hospital cardiac arrest: The Utstein style. Resuscitation 22:1–26, 1991.
12. RO Cummins, DA Chamberlain, MF Hazinski, V Nadkarni, W Kloeck, E Kramer, L Becker, C Robertson, R Koster, A Zaritsky, I Bossaert, JP Ornato, V Callanan, M Allen, P Steen, B Connolly, A Sanders, A Idris, S Cobbe. Recommended guidelines for reviewing, reporting and conducting research on in-hospital resusctiation: The hospital "Utstein style," Resuscitation 34:151–183, 1997.
13. GA Harrison, KM Hillman, GWC Fulde, T Jacques. The need for undergraduate education in critical care. Anaesth Intens Care 27:53–58, 1999.

14. LM Hussain, AD Redmond. Are pre-hospital deaths from accidental injury preventable? BMJ 308:1077–1080, 1994.
15. DW Spaite, EA Criss, TD Valenzuela, HW Meislin. Prehospital advanced life support for major trauma: Critical need for clinical trials. Ann Emerg Med 32:480–489, 1998.
16. Committee of Trauma, American College of Surgeons. Advanced Trauma Life Support Instructor Manual. Chicago: American College of Surgeons, 1993.
17. HR Champion, WJ Sacco, DS Hannan, RL Lepper, ES Atzinger, WS Copes, RH Prall. Assessment of injury severity: The triage index. Crit Care Med 8:201–208, 1980.
18. JJ Koehler, LJ Baer, SA Malafa, MS Meindertsma, NR Navitskas, JE Huizenga. Prehospital index: A scoring system for field triage of trauma victims. Ann Emerg Med 15:178–182, 1986.
19. R Knopp, A Yanagi, G Kallsen, A Geide, I Doehring. Mechanism of injury and anatomic injury as criteria for prehospital trauma triage. Ann Emerg Med 17:895–902, 1988.
20. RJ Bond, JB Kortbeek, RM Preshaw. Field trauma triage: Combining mechanism of injury with the prehospital index for an improved trauma triage tool. J Trauma 43:283–287, 1997.
21. HR Champion, WS Copes, WJ Sacco, MM Lawnick, DS Gann, T Gennarelli, E Mackenzie, S Schwaitzberg. The major outcome trauma study: Establishing national norms for trauma care. J Trauma 30:1356–1365, 1990.
22. SP Gormican. CRAM scale: Field triage of trauma victims. Ann Emerg Med 11:132–135, 1982.
23. WR Roush, OM McDowell. Emergency medical services system. In: WR Roush, ed. Principles of EMS Systems: A comprehensive text for physicians. Dallas: American College of Emergency Physicians, 1989.
24. JG West, RH Cales, AB Gazzaniga. Impact of regionalization: The Orange County experience. Arch Surg 118:740–744, 1983.
25. RH Cales. Trauma mortality in Orange County: The effects of the implementation of a regional trauma system. Ann Emerg Med 13:1–10, 1984.
26. PA Oakley. Setting and living up to national standards for the care of the injured. Injury 25: 595–604, 1994.
27. A Donebedian. The quality of care: How can it be assessed. JAMA 260:1743–1748, 1998.
28. American College of Emergency Physicians. Trauma care systems and quality assurance guidelines. In: Guidelines for Trauma Care Systems. Washington, March 1990.
29. M Callaham. Quantifying the scanty science of prehospital emergency care. Ann Emerg Med 30:785–790, 1997.
30. FD Brenneman, BR Boulanger, BA McLellan, DA Redelmeier. Measuring injury severity: Time for a change? J Trauma 44:580–582, 1998.
31. G Regel, M Stalp, U Lehmann, A Seekamp. Prehospital care, importance of early intervention on outcome. Acta Anaesthesiol Scand 110:71–76, 1997.
32. CB Thompson, K Balasz, J Goltermann, et al. Intubation quality assurance thresholds. Air Med J 14:55–60, 1995.
33. IN Papadopolous, D Bukis, E Karalas, S Katsaragakis, S Stergiopoulos, G Peros, G Androulakis. Preventable prehospital trauma deaths in a Hellenic urban health region: An audit of prehospital trauma care. J Trauma 41:864–869, 1996.
34. FT McDermott, SM Cordner. Major trauma management deficiencies in Victoria and their national implications. Med J Aust 170:248–250, 1999.
35. CR Boyd, MA Tolson, WS Copes. Evaluating trauma care: The TRISS method. Trauma score and the injury severity score J Trauma 27:370–378, 1987.
36. JD Flora Jr. A method for comparing survival of burn patients to a standard survival curve. J Trauma 18:701–705, 1978.
37. RA Lyons, HM Perry, BN Littlepage. Evidence for the validity of the short-form 36 questionnaire (SF-36) in an elderly population. Age Ageing 23:182–184, 1994.
38. KM Hull, N Mann, WM High Jr, J Wright, JS Kreutzer, D Wood. Functional measures after traumatic brain injury: Ceiling effects of FIM, FIM+FAM, DRS, and CIQ. J Head Trauma Rehab 11:27–39, 1996.

39. D Cook. Evidence-based critical care medicine: A potential tool for change. New Hor 6:20–25, 1998.
40. RA Smallwood. Evidence-based medicine. Aust NZ J Surg 68:1–2, 1998.
41. DL Sackett, WMC Rosenberg. On the need for evidence-based medicine. J Pub Health Med 17:330–334, 1995.
42. DL Sackett, WMC Rosenberg, JAM Gray, RB Haynes, WS Richardson. Evidence-based medicine: What it is and what it isn't. BMJ 12:71–72, 1996.
43. TC Fabian. Evidence-based medicine in trauma care: Whither goest thou? J Trauma 47:225–232, 1999.
44. TM Scalea, A Rodriguez, WC Chiu, FD Breenneman, WF Fallon Jr, K Kato, MG McKenney, MI Nerloch, MG Ochsner, H Yoshii. Focused assessment with sonography for trauma (FAST): Results from an International Consensus Conference. J Trauma 46:466–472, 1999.
45. M Liu, CH Lee, FK P'Eng. Prospective comparison of diagnostic peritoneal lavage, computed tomographic scanning and ultrasonography for the diagnosis of blunt abdominal trauma. J Trauma 35:267–270, 1993.
46. YG Goan, MS Huang, JM Lim. Nonoperative management for extensive hepatic and splenic injuries with significant hemoperitoneum in adults. J Trauma 45:360–364, 1998.
47. http://www.east.org.
48. TJ Hodgetts, ed. Towards evidence based pre-hospital care. Prehosp Immed Care 2:2, 1998.
49. WH Bickell, MJ Wall Jr, PE Pepe, RR Martin, VF Ginger, MK Allen, KL Mattox. Immediate versus delayed fluid resuscitation for hypotensive patients with penetrating torso injuries. N Eng J Med 331:1105–1109, 1994.
50. G Schierhout, I Roberts. Fluid resuscitation with colloid or crystalloid solutions in critically ill patients: A systematic review of randomised trials. BMJ 316:961–964, 1998.
51. National Committee of Trauma and Committee of Shock. Accidental Death and Disability. The Neglected Disease of Society. Washington, DC: National Academy of Sciences/National Research Council, 1966.

12

Initial Assessment, Triage, and Basic and Advanced Life Support

JEREMY MAUGER

St. George's Hospital, London, United Kingdom

CHARLES D. DEAKIN

Southampton General Hospital, Southampton, United Kingdom

I. INTRODUCTION

The first hour of trauma care has been described as the ''golden hour'' [1], and many severely injured patients spend almost three-quarters of this hour in the prehospital phase. This golden hour concept has more recently been augmented by the idea of the ''platinum ten minutes'' [2], which is the pivotal time for airway care and prevention of traumatic exsanguination. During these first few minutes the basic essentials of airway (with cervical immobilization), breathing, and circulation with hemorrhage control must be rapidly assessed and optimized. It has been suggested that the main aim of the prehospital process is to ensure that the lungs are working effectively, which will allow the ultimate goal of adequate tissue oxygenation.

The key to initial assessment of a trauma victim in the prehospital setting is *anticipation*, which should be coupled with well-rehearsed *preparation*. A team that has regularly rehearsed together, understands a systematic approach to the trauma patient, is fully equipped, and regularly treats patients with multiple trauma is likely to perform more effectively and deliver a better resuscitated and ''packaged'' patient.

The prehospital provider will usually act as part of a small team. Each member should have clear roles, such as team leader, initial assessor, or application of patient monitoring. This rescue team should take every opportunity to practice its work together in order to review current practice and improve management. Regular debriefs with reviews of procedures, timing, and clinical notes will assist all members of the team to improve performance and devise new approaches or techniques for particular situations. This is particularly effective when combined with photographs and video footage.

II. INITIAL ASSESSMENT

Patient assessment commences during the initial emergency call and before the provider sees the patient. Key information in the call may hold clues from witnesses to indicate mechanisms of injury and therefore develop an idea of suspected injuries. This information may also be invaluable in the early choice of an appropriate receiving hospital. For example, burn units may be contacted by control staff at an early opportunity to confirm bed availability. For cases of exsanguination, it may be possible at this stage to initialize the process of getting blood to the accident scene.

The approach to the patient is not only important from the aspect of safety, but will also give key clues about mechanisms of injury, enabling recognition of injury patterns. Careful observation during the approach to the patient may give key information from the surroundings—''reading the wreckage'' (Fig. 1). It can be predicted, for example, that the driver of a car involved in a frontal impact is likely to have head injuries from the windshield, chest injuries from the steering wheel and seat belt, hand and knee injuries from the dashboard, and possibly pelvic or hip injuries. A side impact is likely to cause injuries on that side of the body; for example, limb and rib fractures and spleen or liver injuries (Fig. 2). A patient found on a railway line may not have been injured by a train but instead by jumping from a bridge above the track. This will have implications for the degree of energy transfer in the impact and therefore the severity and pattern of the injuries.

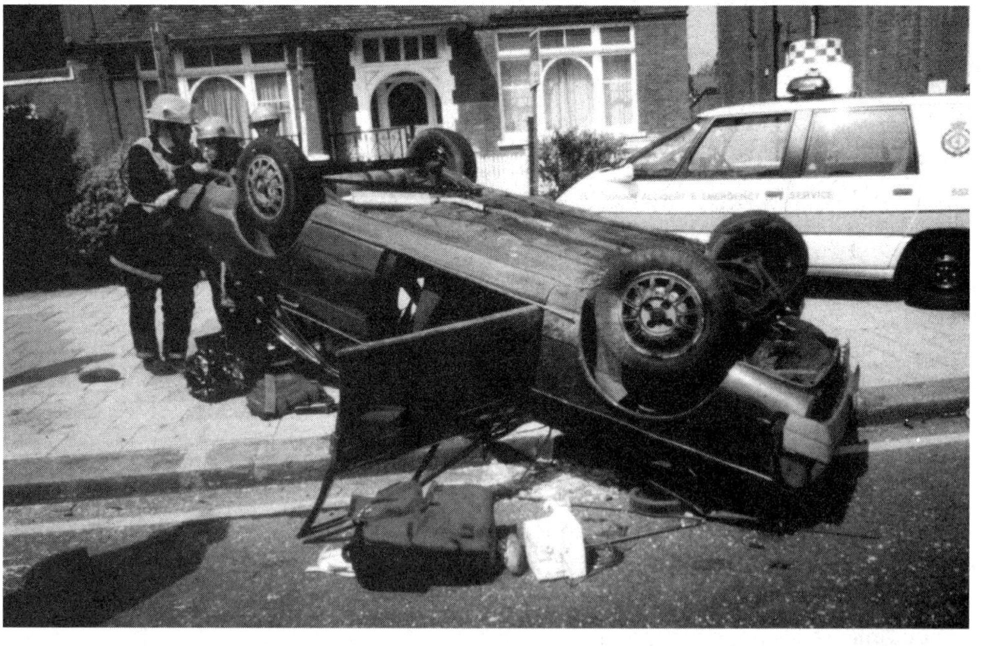

Figure 1 Careful observation of the wreckage and understanding the mechanism of injury can give clues as to the possible injuries.

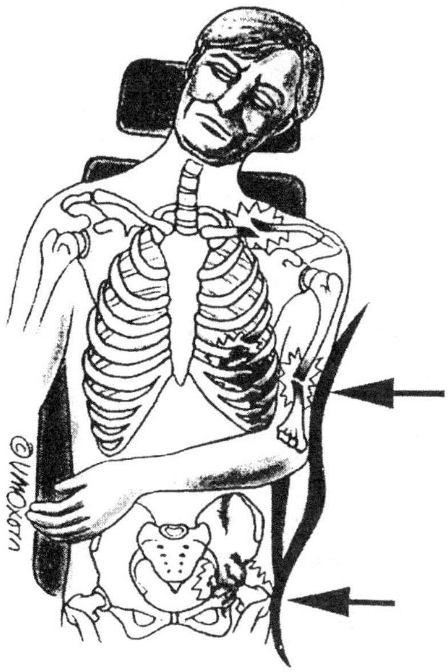

Figure 2 Left lateral impact may cause limb and rib fractures and splenic injury. (From Ref. 2a.)

The other consideration during this stage is the number of casualties affected, as it is very easy to become engrossed in the treatment of a single casualty only to realize that another casualty has been left unnoticed.

The *history* should ideally be taken early at the scene. Whether or not this precedes examination and treatment will depend upon the circumstances. An ambulance crew already on the scene may have obtained the history, so it is essential to liase with them at the earliest opportunity. This may take place during the initial examination. Clues about possible injury may be given from bystanders; the classical missed injury is an unconscious patient with an unrecognized penetrating injury to the back. A useful memory aid for a rapid history is the AMPLE acronym.

*A*llergies
*M*edications
*P*ast medical history
*L*ast ate or drank
*E*vents leading up to the incident.

The *examination* of the patient should commence with the primary survey. This A, B, C, D, E survey looks systematically for life-threatening injuries that should be treated as they are found and before processing to further examination. The entire primary survey should be completed within a very few minutes and will dictate whether the patient needs rapid transport to hospital (load and go) or whether the patient is more stable and can receive initial treatment at the scene (treat then transfer). Some guidelines suggest that this decision should be made within 2 minutes of arriving on the scene. The extent of any further examination will depend upon the situation and is often inappropriate in the prehospital stage of treatment.

The primary survey
*A*irway with c-spine control
*B*reathing
*C*irculation with hemorrhage control
*D*isability
(*E*xposure)

The *positioning* of the patient will dictate the further assessment. This is one of the areas in which prehospital examination differs from in-hospital assessment. Access to the casualty may be very limited. A common mistake is to attempt to move the casualty into the supine position as early as possible, although this may be required in a cardiac arrest situation. The patient may already be lying in a semirecovery position, in which case simple airway maneuvers may allow time not only for further patient assessment but also for the preparation of equipment. In a lateral position the posterior chest may be visualized and auscultated. Examining the patient on his or her side is advantageous because the clothes may be cut up the back to facilitate removal at a later stage, allowing the spine to be assessed for alignment and pain. In addition, further equipment can be prepared; for example, suction in case the patient vomits once moved onto his or her back. Also, drugs prepared for administration and the orthopedic scoop stretcher or extrication board can be placed in an appropriate position ready to roll the patient directly onto the carrying device, thus minimizing patient movement.

A. Airway Management with Cervical Spine Control

1. Assessment

Assessment of the airway is a straightforward procedure that should be complete within only a few seconds. If the patient is able to converse and give a history then this already demonstrates an intact airway. Airway obstruction must be rapidly identified by looking, listening, and feeling. Obvious obstruction from vomit or other fluid should be removed before attempting to open the airway to reduce the risk of aspiration into the lungs. *Sounds* classically associated with partial upper airway obstruction may include *gurgling* if fluid is present in the pharynx, *snoring* from soft tissue obstruction, or *crowing* if there is obstruction at the level of the larynx. Further assessment of the airway should include *palpation* of the larynx to feel for *alignment*, surgical emphysema, or anatomical disruption, which may suggest a laryngeal fracture.

If airway obstruction is found then simple maneuvers should be attempted, such as the *chin lift* or *trauma jaw thrust* (Fig. 3). If this fails, then adjuncts may be required, such as a nasopharyngeal (Fig. 4) or oropharyngeal airway (Fig. 5). Before simple devices were developed, one recommendation a few years ago was to use a safety pin to hold the tongue to the lower lip. Although this now seems bizarre, a similar technique using a suture may be employed when mandibular fractures or soft tissue injury causes the tongue to fall back and obstruct the pharynx if this is not relieved by other techniques. The nasopharyngeal airway has probably been under used in the trauma patient. It has a valuable role to play in the semiconscious patient because the oral airway has a greater chance of causing gagging and coughing, which may aggravate airway obstruction. The nasopharyngeal airway is contraindicated in patients with bleeding disorders and should be inserted

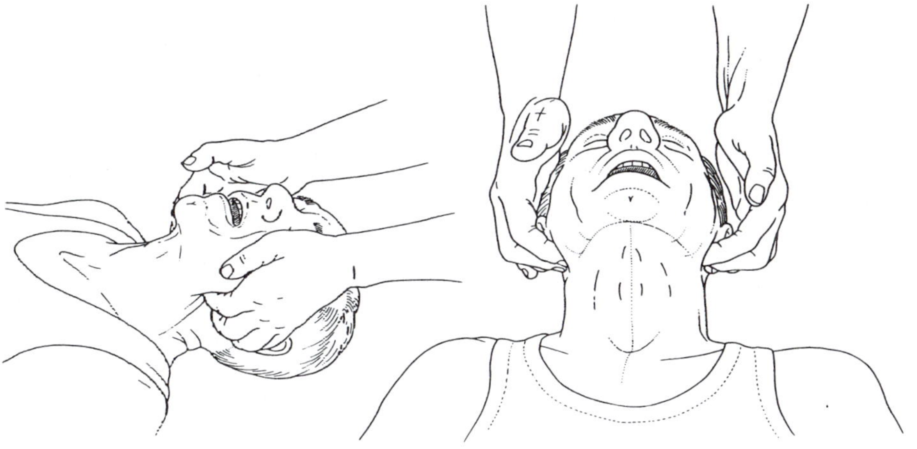

Figure 3 The chin lift or jaw thrust avoids extension of the cervical spine. (From Ref. 2b.)

with caution in patients with potential injuries to the base of the skull because of the small chance of intracranial placement.

Suction is an important tool for clearing airway obstruction by fluids, and should be available early in the assessment process. The correct use of suction is essential, as cosmetic suction around the front of the mouth of a patient with clenched teeth will not clear pharyngeal liquid. The Yankaeur suction tip can be used for clearance at the back of the pharynx but may cause trauma and trigger vomiting or vagal reflexes, particularly in the young. Long, flexible suction catheters can be invaluable in many trauma cases, particularly when a nasopharyngeal airway is already in place.

2. Cervical Spine Precautions

The concern for damage to the cervical spine has been well publicized, so many bystanders are reluctant to perform even the simplest airway maneuvers for fear of litigation. Secondary cervical injury is that which occurs after the initial insult but is caused not only by further movement but also hypoxia. Attention should be paid at all times to consideration of a potential cervical spine injury, but the priority in management is adequate airway care, which may on occasion override absolute immobilization of the neck. If cervical movement is required to open an obstructed airway, then this must be the minimum movement possible to allow airway clearance. The head should be held immobilized by one member of the rescue team with one hand on either side of the head and ideally supported on a hard surface. It should be remembered that the person holding the head will be unable to perform other tasks and therefore should not be the most experienced team member. A semi-rigid cervical collar should be applied, although this does not provide complete immobilization and may worsen intracranial pressure [3] (Fig. 6). Additional support from blocks and tape will also be needed at the earliest opportunity, although they may not provide complete support [4]. A useful technique during resuscitation of the supine trauma patient is to support the head between the knees of a kneeling rescuer, thus freeing the rescuer's hands (Fig. 7). Occasionally a patient in very critical condition may warrant minimal cervical spine protection in the first few moments of a rapid extrication. In this case, immobilization must be applied at the earliest opportunity.

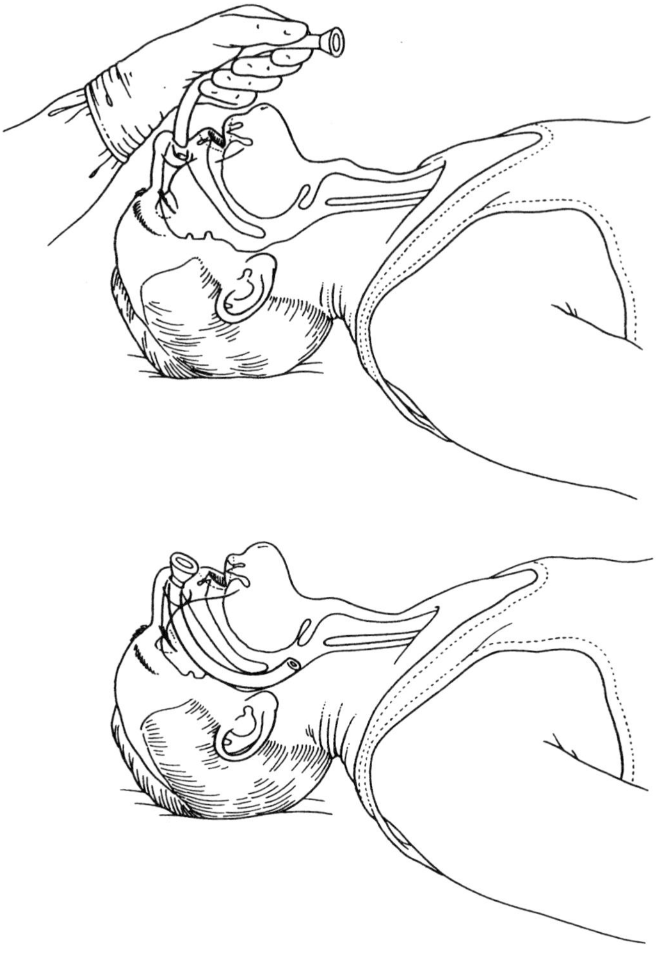

Figure 4 A nasopharyngeal airway may be used when simple airway maneuvers fail. (From Ref. 2b.)

B. Breathing

The chest should be examined for adequacy of respiration. Initially this should be done for up to 10 seconds, as recommended by the International Liaison Committee for Resuscitation (ILCOR) [5]. Respiratory assessment must include an assessment of the rate as well as the *depth* of respiration. The *rate* is often ignored but plays a key role in the revised trauma score. Cyanosis can easily be missed in poor lighting. The ability of a conscious patient to take a deep breath in and out without pain may give an indication of the adequacy of respiration. *Visual inspection* of the chest may reveal penetrating injury, patterns of contusion, or abnormal respiratory movements, such as ''seesaw'' respirations. *Palpation* may reveal surgical emphysema or evidence of rib or sternal fractures, which may indicate severe injury to the underlying organs. The chest is *auscultated*, although this can be very difficult in noisy environments (Fig. 8). *Percussion* can be useful to assist in diagnosis of pneumothorax, flail chest, open pneumothorax, or massive hemothorax. Percussion may be particularly useful when performed simultaneously with auscultation to diagnose pneumothorax [6].

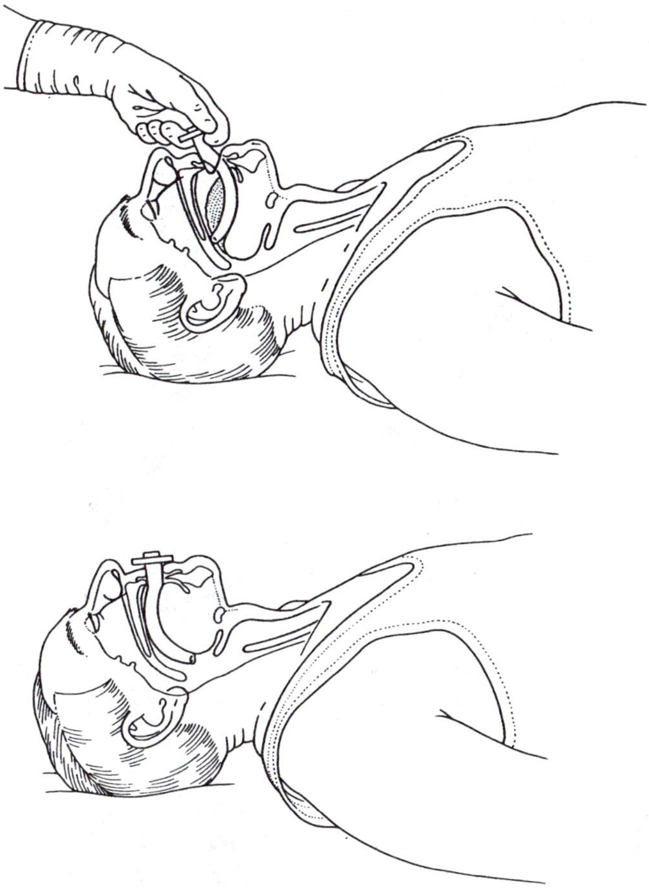

Figure 5 An oropharyngeal (Guedel) airway is also suitable to maintain the airway but requires a greater impaired level of consciousness to be tolerated than is necessary for a nasopharyngeal airway. (From Ref. 2b.)

High-flow oxygen should always be administered via a face mask with a reservoir bag in the spontaneously breathing trauma victim. In order to function effectively, the face mask must provide a good fit around the patient's nose and mouth and have working valves. In addition, the reservoir bag must be inflated rather than cold and collapsed. Oxygen cylinders should be repeatedly checked during an incident to ensure that an adequate supply of oxygen remains available, particularly considering that, for example, a full D-size cylinder containing 340 liters of oxygen will last less than 23 minutes if run continuously at 15 liters per minute.

C. Circulation with Hemorrhage Control

The cardiovascular system can be very difficult to assess in the prehospital phase. Visual assessment of blood loss at the scene is notoriously inaccurate [7] but may give further evidence of the severity of an injury. Intensive care teams struggle to find ways to measure blood flows or end-organ perfusion. It should be remembered that end-organ perfusion is the ultimate aim in any critically ill patient rather than simple pressure measurements,

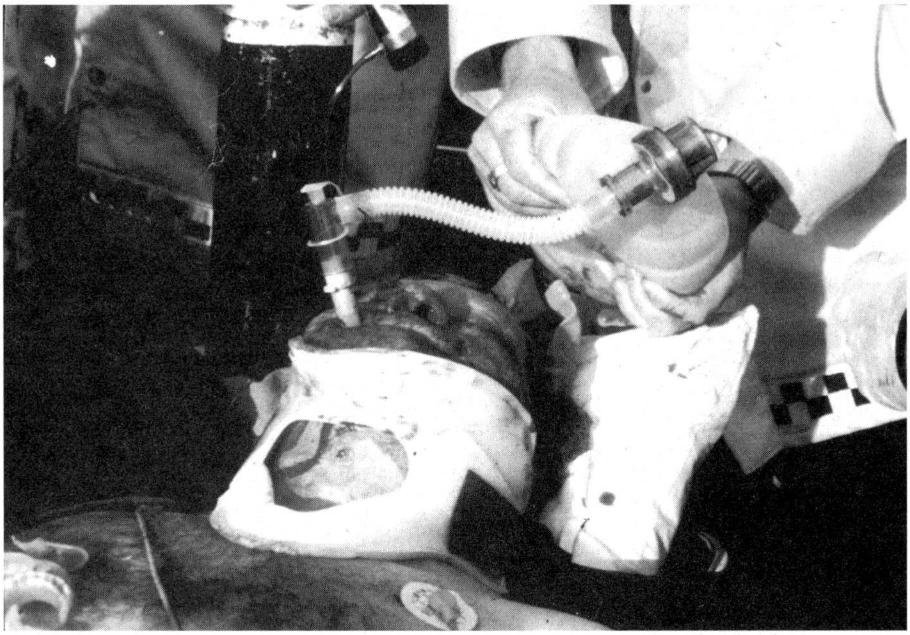

Figure 6 A semirigid cervical collar should be applied, although this does not provide complete immobilization. Additional support from blocks and tape will also be needed.

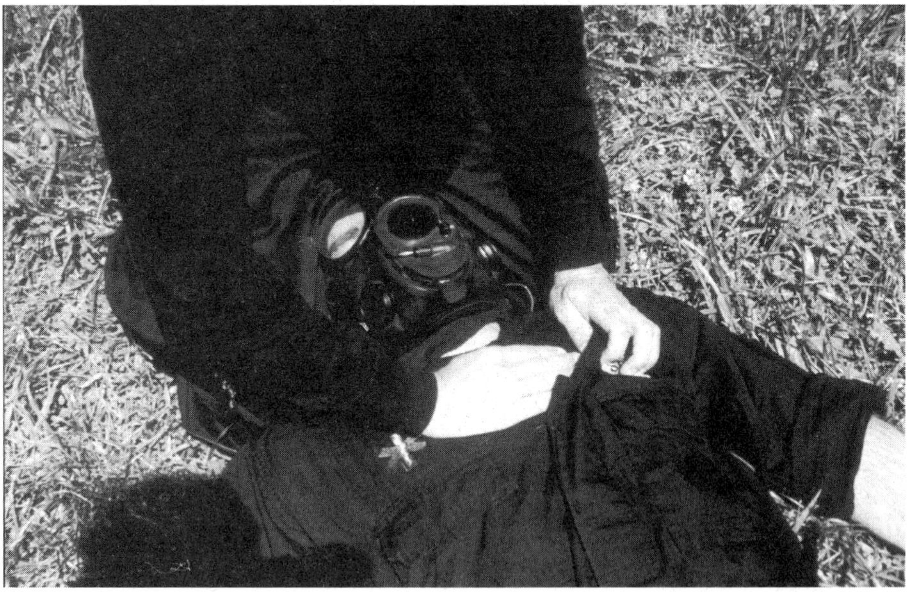

Figure 7 A useful technique during resuscitation of the supine trauma patient is to support the head between the knees of a kneeling rescuer, thus freeing the rescuer's hands.

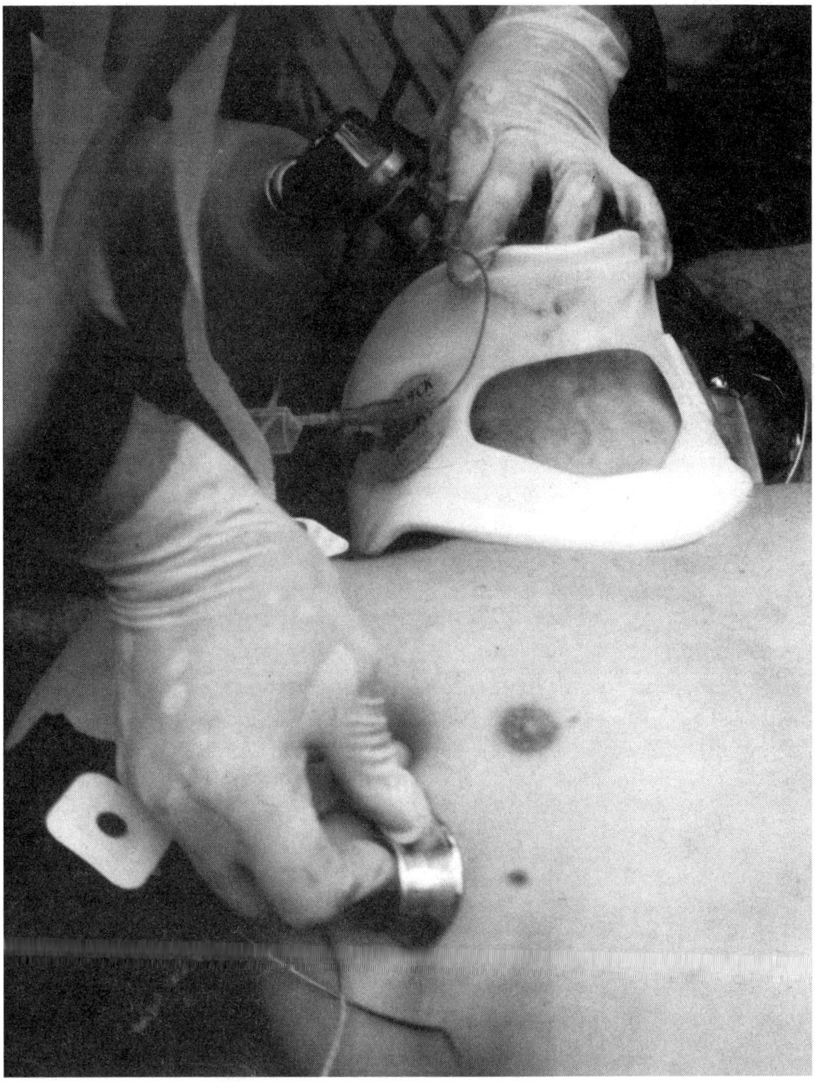

Figure 8 The chest is auscultated, although this can be very difficult in noisy environments.

therefore the whole clinical picture of the cardiovascular system should be considered. An estimation of pulse rate and blood pressure alone will suffice for many patients, but a large group of profoundly hypovolemic patients may have ''normal'' values for these parameters. Inspection of the patient may reveal pallor, lack of sweating, or decreased level of consciousness, any of which may suggest possible hypovolemia.

The *pulse* should be palpated to confirm presence or absence. Absence of pulse should be confirmed only after a pulse check of up to 10 seconds (or longer in the hypothermic patient). *Pulse rate* may be elevated by pain or emotional factors immediately after injury and may not necessarily indicate blood loss. Bradycardia may indicate spinal injury, β-blocking medication and is also occasionally seen in intra-abdominal hemorrhage. A *narrow pulse pressure*, suspected from a thready pulse, may be a better indication of blood loss. The ATLS course teaches that the radial pulse becomes impalpable at a systolic pressure below 80 mmHg, the femoral pulse below 70 mmHg, and the carotid pulse below 60 mmHg. This method has been shown to be very crude and inaccurate and may actually underestimate the degree of hypovolaemia [8]. It is a technique that must be used with caution when estimating systolic blood pressure (Fig. 9).

The *capillary refill test* has been used as an assessment of the cardiovascular system since the early 1980s, particularly in children. The test is performed by gentle manual compression of a nail bed that is held at or just above the level of the heart for approximately 5 seconds. When the compression is released the time taken for the color to reappear is noted and is classically said to be less than 2 seconds, or the time that it takes to say "capillary refill." This test has been shown to be grossly inaccurate in many situations, particularly in cold environments [9]. The basis of the test, however, is that the systemic vascular resistance is increased in hypovolemia. Another useful application, therefore, is to feel for a *temperature gradient* between the core and periphery or along a limb.

Blood pressure measurement has become an integral part of trauma patient assessment. The results of automated devices should be interpreted with caution. The systolic blood pressure is one of the core components of the revised trauma score.

Cardiac tamponade must be considered in the profoundly hypotensive trauma patient. This is classically recognized by *Beck's triad* of distended neck veins, hypotension, and muffled heart sounds. It should be remembered that the hypovolemic patient with coexisting cardiac tamponade may not have distended neck veins.

The emphasis of the cardiovascular assessment is shifting more and more toward the goal of preserving blood volume. Hemorrhage control is therefore a key issue in prehospital care. *Pressure pads* should be applied to stem external bleeding, but also early

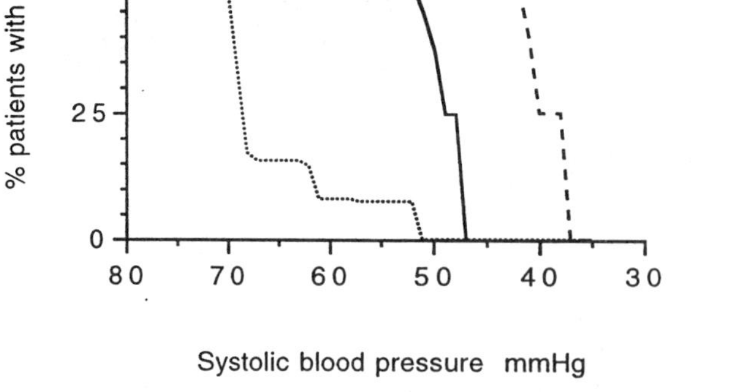

Figure 9 The relationship between palpable pulse and systolic blood pressure. The presence or absence of pulse is an inaccurate guide to systolic blood pressure.

splintage of major pelvic or limb fractures should be considered, and are probably of greater importance than fluid replacement. Traction splints, such as the Sager, Donway, or Hare, are particularly useful for closed femoral fractures, as these will not only provide effective pain relief but also slow blood loss into the thigh. The splint should therefore be applied early. If pelvic injury is suspected from mechanism of injury, examination by rocking the pelvis is seldom useful, since will disrupt clots and cause further hemorrhage. This sort of examination should therefore be avoided. *Limb tourniquets* have been largely condemned, but still have a role to play in life-threatening exsanguination, which is uncontrollable by any other means. Indirect pressure points, such as the brachial or femoral arteries, and limb elevation must also be considered during life-threatening hemorhage.

Military antishock trousers (MAST), also known as pneumatic antishock garments (PASG; Fig. 10), have moved in and out of favor in the prehospital arena [10]. These were initially introduced to improve venous return and splint lower limb fractures. Evidence has suggested that they may increase mortality, possibly by aggravating chest injury, impairing respiratory effort, or disrupting clots. Despite these risks, they may still have a place in the treatment of major lower limb and pelvic crush injury, although if used they should only be removed under strictly controlled conditions.

D. Disability

A brief neurological assessment should be considered as part of the primary survey. A decreased level of consciousness must not be attributed automatically to drugs or alcohol, but hypoxia, hypovolemia, head injury, and hypoglycemia should also be considered. The Glasgow coma scale (GCS) [11] is not only predictive of patient outcome but is also another core element of the revised trauma score [12].

Four years and over		Less than four years	
Response	Score	Response	Score
Eyes			
Open spontaneously	4	Open spontaneously	4
To verbal command	3	React to speech	3
To pain	2	React to pain	2
Unresponsive	1	Unresponsive	1
Best motor response			
Obeys command	6	Spontaneous/obeys commands	6
Localizes pain	5	Localizes pain	5
Flexion to pain	4	Withdraws to pain	4
Flexion abnormal	3	Abnormal flexion (decorticate)	3
Extension	2	Extension (decerebrate)	2
Unresponsive	1	Unresponsive	1
Best verbal response			
Orientated	5	Smiles, follows objects, interacts	5
Disorientated	4	Cries but consolable, inappropriate	4
Inappropriate words	3	Inconsistently consolable, moans	3
Incomprehensible sounds	2	Inconsolable, irritable	2
Unresponsive	1	Unresponsive	1

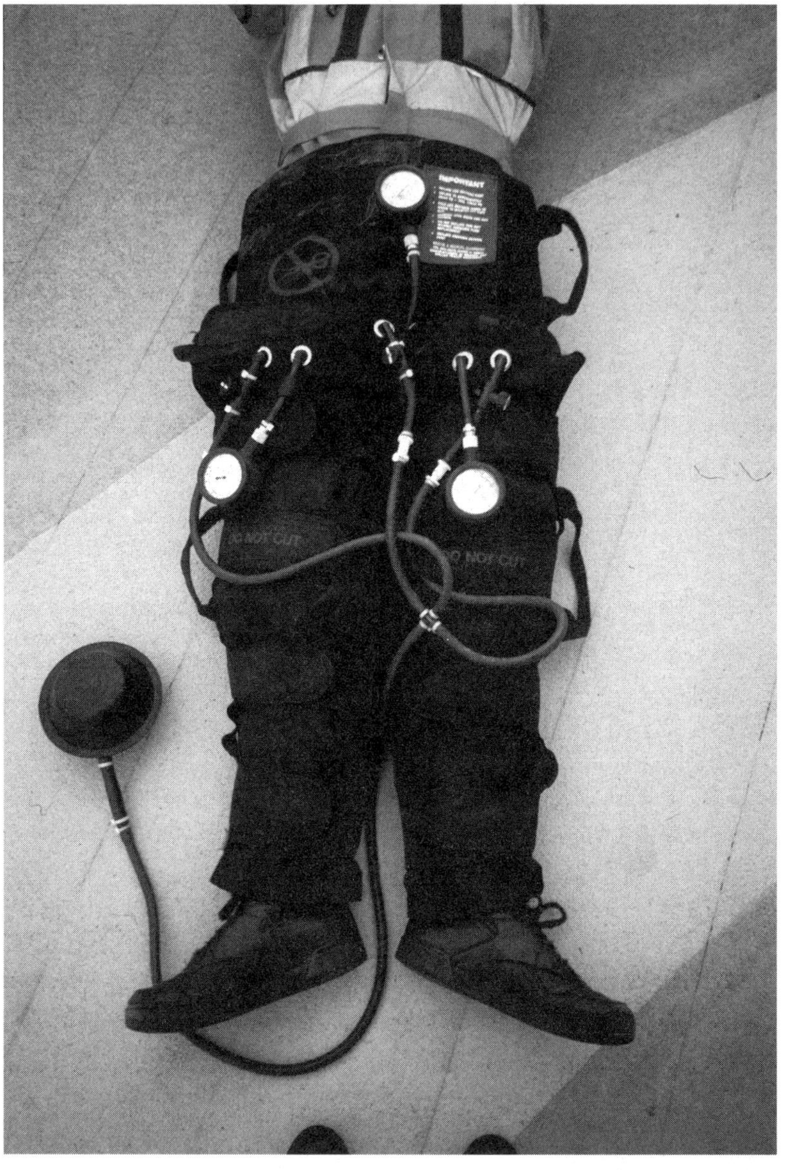

Figure 10 Military antishock trousers (MAST), also known as pneumatic antishock garments (PASG), have moved in and out of favor in the prehospital arena.

A more rapid assessment of conscious level is to consider the AVPU mnemonic.

*A*lert
*V*ocalizing
*P*ain response
*U*nresponsive

In addition to the conscious level, the pupils should be checked for size and equality, and gross motor movements should be confirmed by asking the patient to move his or her fingers or toes.

Rapid neurological examination
AVPU (or GCS)
Pupil size and reaction
Gross motor response (wiggle toes/squeeze fingers)
Gross sensory deficit

E. Exposure

Major injuries should be apparent by the end of the initial assessment, although some will be difficult to discover before a full hospital assessment. In the hospital, the patient will be *fully exposed by removing his or her clothes*, but in the *prehospital* setting a *compromise* will need to be established. A single penetrating wound will usually require little further exposure and full examination would be to the patient's detriment when rapid removal to the hospital becomes the priority. In addition, the removal of clothes may lead to significant cooling and unnecessary public exposure. *Clothes* can be *prepared* to facilitate later *removal* by cutting a slit down the back of a jacket and shirt before the patient is rolled into the supine position. These slits may be made quickly using a seat belt cutter. If similar cuts are made along the back of each trouser leg then clothing can be very rapidly removed with the patient lying on the extrication board or scoop stretcher in the emergency room without further movement.

Hypothermia is common in the trauma patient and should be considered at an early stage. Although mild hypothermia is thought to be beneficial for head injuries, severe hypothermia may lead to coagulopathy, immune dysfunction, cardiac arryhthmias, and acidosis. Trauma patients are at risk because of impaired thermoregulation as well as increased heat loss. Once established, hypothermia can be difficult to correct, particularly in the prehospital phase, and therefore preventative measures must be taken. Warm blankets should be used, and if any intravenous fluids are administered, they should be warmed if possible. Exposure should be minimized and the patient taken early to a prewarmed ambulance.

At some point during the initial assessment it will be necessary to move the patient usually into the supine position. This may need to be done early in the assessment for airway management but can otherwise be delayed. This movement will need to be done with due consideration for the stability of a potential spinal injury. The *logroll* is a seemingly simple procedure but has the potential for catastrophe if not performed correctly. An adequate logroll usually requires four people, so an ambulance crew of two should seek assistance from bystanders, possibly from other emergency services personnel. The sequence of the logroll should be carefully explained, and care should be taken to ensure that all involved understand the procedure. The lead should always be taken by whoever has control of the head and airway, and should ensure that the spine remains in line so that no part of the spine is subject to rotation.

F. Monitoring

Monitoring the trauma victim has become an increasingly integral and sophisticated part of the delivery of prehospital care. Monitoring equipment must be reliable and robust, while at the sometime readily portable with adequate battery life. Most U.K. ambulances are now equipped with three lead *ECG, pulse oximetry*, and *noninvasive blood pressure* monitoring (Fig. 11). The timing of the application of this equipment will depend upon the specific circumstances, but there has to be a considerable degree of common sense

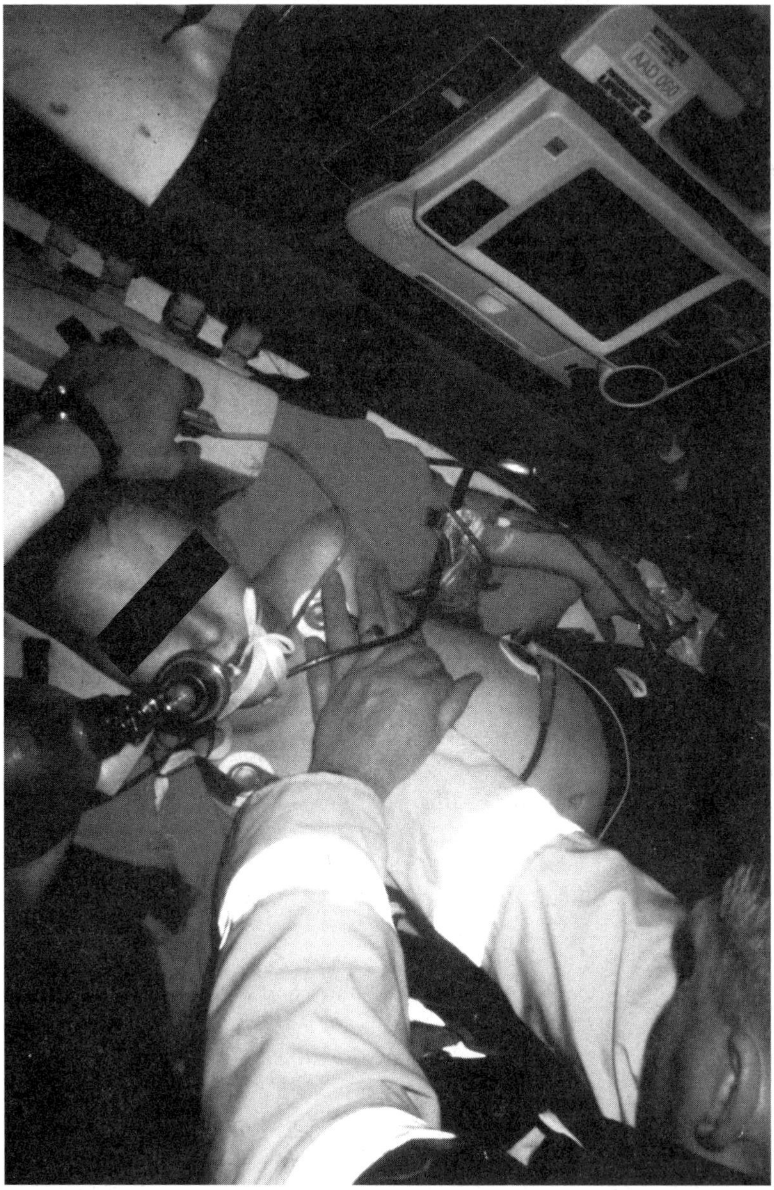

Figure 11 Monitoring the trauma victim has become an increasingly integral and sophisticated part of the delivery of prehospital care.

employed. In the presence of a well-rehearsed team, the monitors can be applied early by a designated team member, particularly in light of the medicolegal aspects of record keeping. Strict guidelines are difficult: while in one extreme early interpretation of VF in the arrested patient will be critical, the accurate measurement of blood pressure in a motorcyclist wearing thick leathers on a cold day should probably be delayed. During a difficult vehicle extrication, monitoring or other unnecessary medical interventions will impede rescue services from access to the vehicle and therefore slow the extrication process.

Harvard Medical School developed minimal monitoring standards for anesthetized patients in the 1980s [13], and this same level of care should now be used for all anesthetized patients outside the operating theater, including the prehospital arena. This equipment should be viewed as an extra tool in the prehospital armory that may enable further interpretation of clinical signs. The limitations should be borne in mind, however, particularly when *potentially erroneous readings* are produced during movement. Pulse oximetry is notoriously difficult in this environment due to movement artefact, interference by bright light, and poor peripheral perfusion due to cold or hypovolaemia. If a low reading is obtained this must be checked against clinical signs before it is assumed that it is artefact.

Anesthesiologists have long considered the single most important monitor to be the *end-tidal CO_2* monitor, and this should ideally be used for all intubated patients, but certainly if anesthetic drugs are employed. The universal application of some form of CO_2 analysis would certainly prevent many of the tragic cases of unrecognized esophageal intubation, and may also lead to early recognition of a significant fall in cardiac output in the ventilated patient.

Following the primary survey, a more detailed top-to-toe examination should be considered. This examination is known as the secondary survey, and it includes a detailed and thorough examination of all injuries. A full clinical examination can take considerable time, however. This more detailed examination is often inappropriate in the prehospital setting for the severely injured patient, when emphasis should be placed on rapid removal from the scene.

III. TRIAGE

Triage has become a key area of prehospital care: getting the right patient to the right facility at the right time. The term triage derives from the French word *trier*, meaning to sort. It was first used medically during the Napoleonic wars as a way of deciding which soldiers to treat so that the greatest number of injured soldiers could be brought back into conflict following treatment.

Triage continues to evolve and is used in the prehospital setting in two main ways.

1. In relation to *sorting multiple casualties* (Fig. 12) and in prioritizing both treatment and order of evacuation to appropriate facilities so that the maximum number of lives are saved.
2. It is used at the scene for *single casualty*, first to prioritize the order of treatment of several injuries and also to decide which hospital facility is most appropriate for that patient.

Triage for the individual casualty is based upon accurate identification of specific injuries together with a good knowledge of the nearest specialist hospital facilities. Many injured casualties can receive optimum treatment at the nearest emergency room, but patients with multiple injuries can be viewed as having a separate disease process that is often better managed at designated trauma centers. This concept has been popular in the United States since the 1970s but has been much slower to evolve in other countries. Some of the studies looking at improvements in mortality and morbidity by dedicated trauma centers have been conflicting, although there is growing evidence that patients with multiple injuries have improved outcome if transferred directly to a trauma center. Patients with major thermal injuries present a complex triage problem and may benefit from direct transfer from the scene to a burn unit. This transfer will depend upon the transport times and level of care available from the transport team as well as the percentage of burn area, anatomical

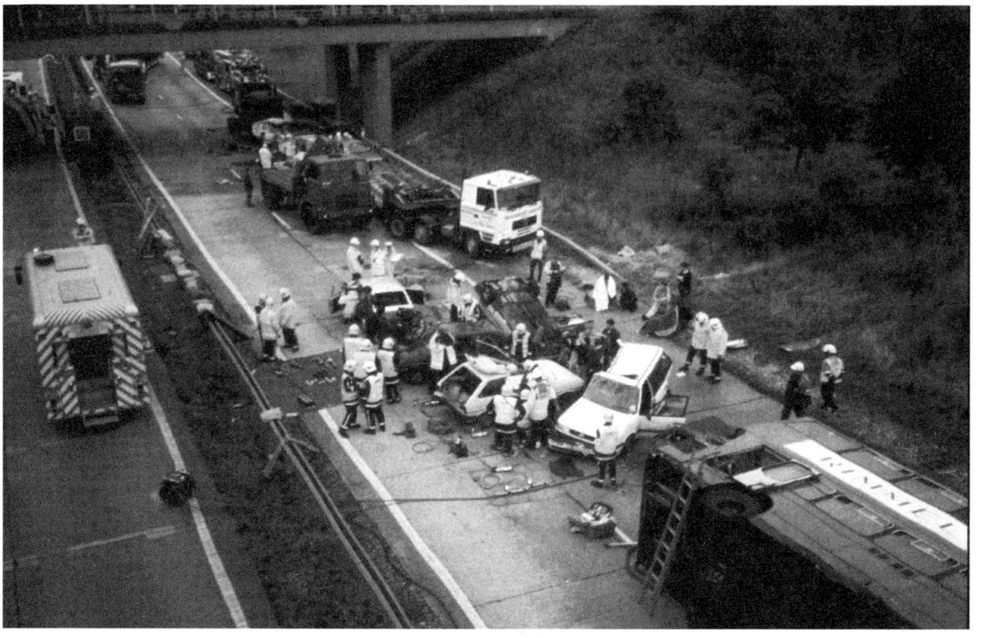

Figure 12 Multiple casualties must be triaged in order to treat life-threatening injuries without delay.

site, and age of the patient. Head injuries, high spinal injuries, cardiothoracic injuries, pelvic injuries, and pediatric patients are all examples of specific situations in which triage to specific facilities can be of potential benefit. If triage of this type is to be performed, then protocols should be arranged in advance, and communication from the scene to a specialist unit is essential.

Triage of multiple casualties is usually into one of four or five groups in order of treatment priority. Many systems have evolved that give the prehospital provider straightforward techniques for mass casualty triage. These systems include the use of decision trees, triage sieves, and triage cards. The provider should be familiar with the local system and ideally rehearse in a simulation role before being faced with a major incident situation. All prehospital providers should be aware of triage categories and criteria. The early phases of a major incident can seem chaotic until cordons and a command structure are established. During this early phase, pocket reference cards can be very useful as an aid to the initial decisions.

IV. BASIC LIFE SUPPORT

One of the key aspects to improved life support is improvement in each link in the *chain of survival*. This concept encompasses not only the hospital phase of resuscitation, but also bystander care with early access to appropriate emergency services and high-quality prehospital medical care. Each link of this chain will require optimal basic life support for improved survival and outcomes. This concept is most often applied to medical cardiac arrest scenarios, but is equally important for optimal trauma care.

The airway in particular is tragically and frequently overlooked in the first few seconds to minutes after major trauma. In one study, evidence of airway obstruction was present postmortem in up to two-thirds of possibly preventable trauma deaths [14]. Lives would be saved by the education of potential bystanders and it would be beneficial to encompass aspects of trauma airway care with cervical spine control in public basic life support courses.

Public first aid courses are a key aspect of improved trauma care, and it has been suggested that first aid questions should become an integral part of all driving tests. Emphasis must be placed on accident prevention before introducing concepts of care. Safe approach to the scene and basic airway management are important concepts that should be focal to any course. The concept of preservation of blood volume is another technique that should be emphasized in first aid courses, including the use of simple pressure, elevation, and splintage.

V. ADVANCED LIFE SUPPORT

Basic techniques in prehospital care cannot be overemphasized, but the application of more advanced techniques should be considered cautiously with attention to the latest evidence base. Two treatment strategies have been suggested. They have become known as *scoop and run* and *treat then transfer*. Clinical evidence now suggests that life-threatening airway and breathing problems must be diagnosed and treated on the scene, whereas circulation is best treated by surgical haemostasis in the hospital. Some patients would therefore benefit from very rapid transfer with minimal on-scene intervention, while others may be fully stabilized at the scene [15]. Further interventions should be applied by experienced providers in order to reduce rather than prolong on-scene times. Clinical judgment must play a major part in determining the optimal point at which transfer should occur, and on-scene interventions must be fully justifiable.

Protocols should be carefully considered and guidelines suggested for specific situations. National cardiac arrest guidelines such as those by the American Heart Association or the U.K. Resuscitation Council and guided by ILCOR are a useful starting point, as the system then becomes a common language for all resuscitation teams both in and out of the hospital. Particular attention should be paid to preventing electromechanical dissociation by recognizing the causes, particularly hypoxia, hypovolemia, tension pneumothorax, and cardiac tamponade.

Physicians who provide prehospital trauma care should have a broad medical background with experience in emergency medicine, anesthesiology, and intensive care, along with surgical skills. Several courses are now available to give newcomers to this arena an idea of the approach, although these courses can also give new insight to experienced practitioners. In the United Kingdom the basic trauma life support (BTLS) course, the prehospital trauma life support (PHTLS) course, the prehospital emergency care (PHEC) course, and the immediate care course all teach a structured approach to the trauma victim, which may lead to an improvement in trauma patient outcome [16]. The advanced trauma life support course was the pioneering trauma course. It started in the United States and has spread around the world. It is aimed at the hospital provider working under very different circumstances to the prehospital provider, who works in hostile environments using different resources. In addition there should be specific training and accreditation in safety procedures, communications, transport medicine, entrapment training, and major incidents.

Advanced airway skills require confidence in oral-tracheal intubation and such emergency airway techniques as surgical cricothyrotomy. Emphasis has been placed on learning to intubate patients in bizarre positions, although with modern rescue techniques and ade-

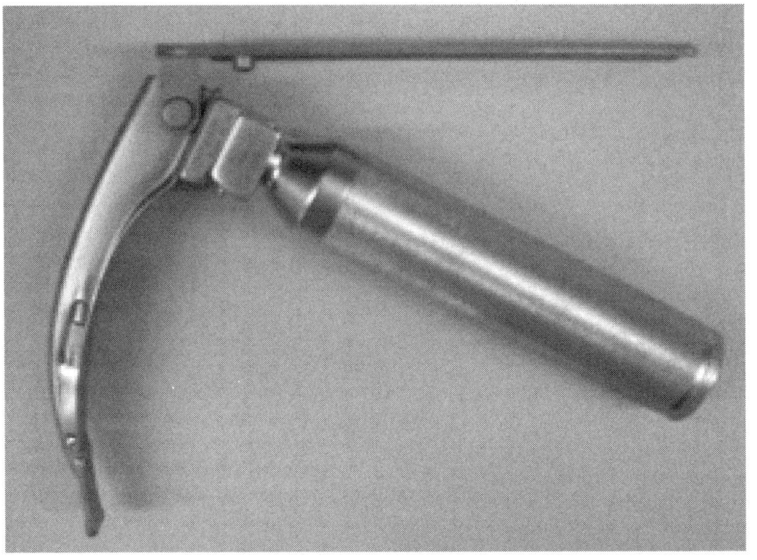

Figure 13 The McCoy laryngoscope improves the view at laryngscopy.

quate basic airway and ventilation skills, it is extremely unusual for patients to require intubation in positions other than supine. Early field intubation of head-injured patients has shown significant outcome benefits [17], but this must then be coupled with optimal ventilation and adequate sedation, if required. Advanced airway skills should ideally be coupled with confident use of intravenous anesthetic agents and paralyzing agents. Many trauma patients present difficult airway problems, therefore difficult intubation procedures should be well rehearsed with readily accessible aids. Some services advocate that trauma patients should be intubated using a McCoy laryngoscope (Fig. 13) and gum elastic bougie (Fig. 14) routinely as the first-line technique, not only to familiarize users with this equipment but also to minimize airway trauma and stress response to intubation [18]. The McCoy laryngoscope has been shown to be useful for patients with potential cervical spine injuries [19]. The laryngeal mask airway (LMA) remains a controversial aid in the trauma victim, due largely to the possibility of gastric aspiration. There is a growing number of case reports indicating the usefulness of the LMA in the prehospital arena, however, particularly when intubation is difficult (Fig. 15).

Poor technique in advanced airway management can be catastrophic if it leads to further trauma, hypoxia, hypotension, and at worst unrecognized oesophageal intubation which leads to death. Every effort must be made to ensure correct endotracheal tube positioning. The provider must also be familiar with all of the potential complications of these techniques and how to correct them. Care should be taken when trying to intubate trapped patients in difficult positions. These situations are usually better managed by allowing rescue services to perform rapid extrication while performing simple airway maneuvers so that better access may be gained to the patient with the ultimate goal of reducing scene times

Surgical cricothyrotomy is a useful prehospital technique in the trauma patient, particularly after failed rapid sequence induction. A 6.0-mm cuffed endotracheal or tracheos-

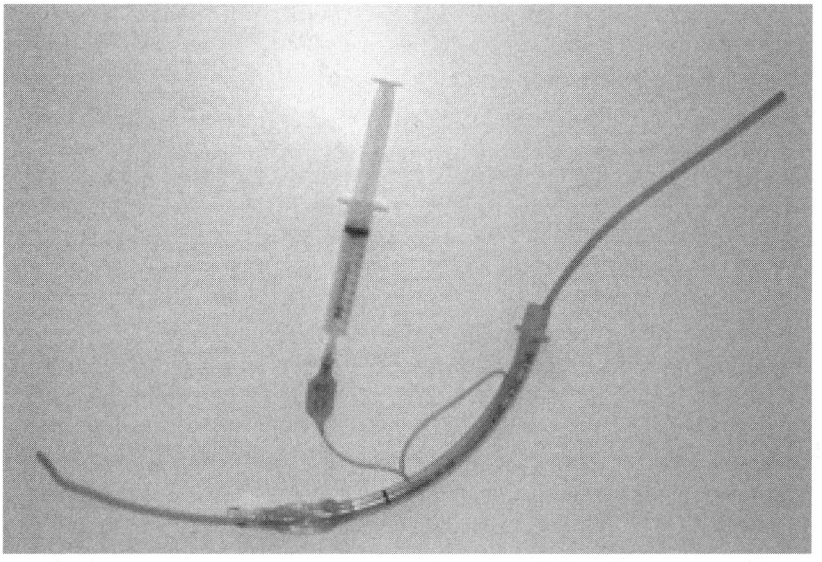

Figure 14 The gum elastic bougie should be used routinely as a first-line technique to minimize the risk of a failed intubation.

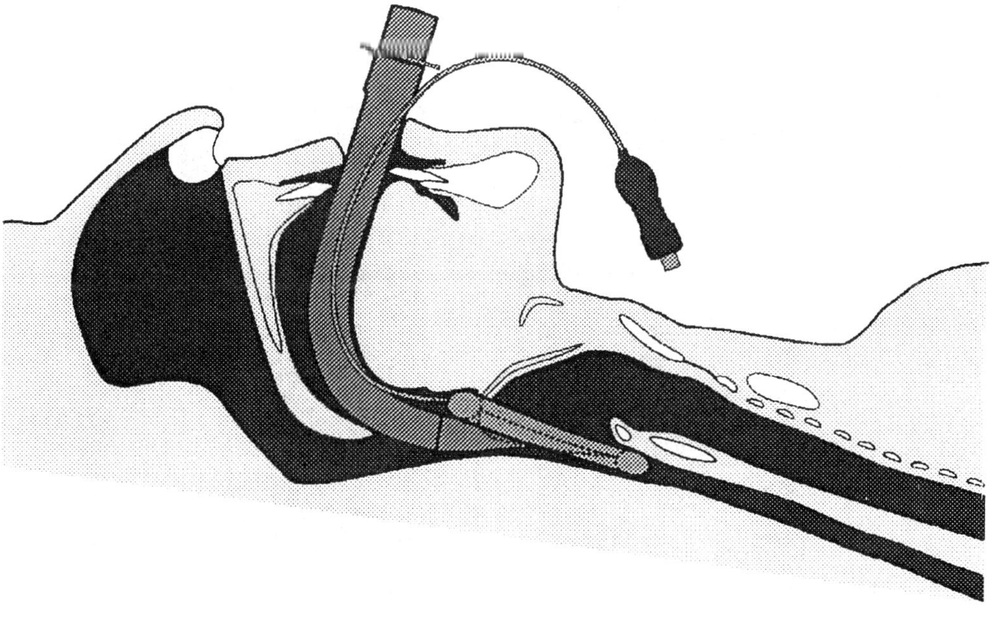

Figure 15 The laryngeal mask airway may be a useful alternative when intubation fails.

tomy tube can be rapidly inserted through a skin incision over the cricothyroid membrane that has been enlarged by blunt dissection down into the trachea. This will enable prolonged ventilation with protection from aspiration until a more definitive airway is established.

Once an optimal airway has been confirmed, *adequate lung ventilation* must be assured. Possible tension pneumothorax should be treated early and aggressively. Needle chest decompression is a useful but limited technique that buys some time before further intervention. The ventilated patient responds well to simple thoracostomy without placement of a chest tube in the prehospital setting [20]. This will allow both a reduction in on-scene time and the ability to ensure that the lung remains expanded during transport by refingering the thoracostomy site in case of further deterioration. Tube thoracostomy can be a useful but time-consuming intervention at the accident site, but should be considered if the patient is breathing spontaneously, if transport time is prolonged, or if there is a massive chest haemorrhage.

Intravenous cannulation was one of the first procedures to be used out of the hospital, and there is now growing evidence that prehospital fluids are detrimental in certain situations, particularly penetrating torso trauma [21]. These studies have given rise to the concept of hypovolaemic resuscitation, and many trauma organizations now advocate an acceptance of lower blood pressure, such as 90 mmHg systolic, in the multiply injured patient during the prehospital phase. This view is often adjusted for patients with head injuries who require optimal cerebral perfusion pressure, such as a systolic pressure of at least 120 mmHg, to maintain oxygenation and prevent secondary brain injury.

Venous access can often be delayed, and may be performed during transport in selected cases to reduce scene times. Specific cases that require early intravenous access include access for drug administration (such as analgesia or anesthesia) and profoundly low blood pressure. In these cases cannulation can be very difficult, but large-bore femoral venous lines in adults and intraosseous needles in children can be lifesaving. Care must be taken with the disposal of sharp objects to prevent hazard to rescue personnel. The type of fluid used in the profoundly hypotensive patient remains a controversial issue, although crystalloids seem to be the more popular choice. Blood brought to the scene can be lifesaving in selected situations, even if massive transfusion is required [22], although the requirement for blood should be considered at an early stage.

The prehospital drug formulary is expanding rapidly, and the provider must be familiar with all emergency drugs and doses. Potent analgesia is a significant benefit that makes initial assessment and patient movement considerably easier.

The momentum created during the prehospital phase by rapid and effective treatment with subsequent packaging will be transmitted to the in-hospital management by setting a train of advanced trauma care into progress.

VI. SUMMARY

A safe approach with consideration of the mechanisms of injury is essential.

A systematic approach to the initial assessment with a well-rehearsed sequence of airway with cervical spine control, breathing, circulation with haemorrhage control, disability, and exposure should be adopted, with particular emphasis on basic airway care.

Careful triage of both a number of casualties and a single casualty to the most appropriate center is a key area of prehospital care.

The initial prehospital assessment of the trauma patient will set the pace for the early treatment of that patient.

REFERENCES

1. DD Trunkey. Trauma. Sci Am 249:28–35, 1983.
2. WC Shoemaker, AB Peitzman, R Bellamy, R Bellomo, SP Bruttig, A Capone, M Dubick, GC Kramer, JE McKenzie, PE Pepe, P Safar, R Schlichtig, JW Severinghaus, SA Tisherman, L Wiklund. Resuscitation from severe hemorrhage. Crit Care Med 24:S12–23, 1996.

2a. Anesthesiology Clinics of North America. Mechanisms of injury. Trauma, March, 1999.

2b. Resuscitation Council (UK). Airway management and ventilation. Advanced Life Support Course Manual, 3d Edition. London: Resuscitation Council.

3. G Davies, C Deakin, A Wilson. The effect of a rigid collar on intracranial pressure. Injury 27:647–649, 1996.
4. I Houghton, P Driscol. Cervical immobilisation—are we achieving it? Prehosp Immed Care 8:17–21, 1999.
5. DA Chamberlain, RO Cummins. Advisory statements of the International Liaison Committee on Resuscitation (ILCOR). Resuscitation 34:99–100, 1997.
6. R Winter, D Smethurst. Percussion—A new way to diagnose a pneumothorax. Brit J Anaesth 83:960–961, 1999.
7. R Birkinshaw, K Zahir, J Ryan. Visual assessment of blood loss at the accident scene. Prehosp Immed Care 2:197–198, 1998.
8. CD Deakin, JL Low. Do Advanced Trauma Life Support guidelines accurately predict systolic blood pressure by palpation of carotid, femoral and radial pulses? An observational study. BMJ 321:673–674, 2000.
9. I Maconochie. Capillary refill time in the field—It's enough to make you blush! Prehosp Immed Care 2:95–96, 1998.
10. PE Randall. Medical antishock trousers (MAST): A review. Injury 17:395–398, 1986.
11. G Ieasdale, B Jennett. Assessment of coma and impaired consciousness: A practical scale. Lancet 2:81–84, 1974.
12. HR Champion, WJ Sacco, WS Copes, DS Gann, TA Gennarelli, ME Flanagan. A revision of the Trauma Score. J Trauma 29:623–629, 1989.
13. JH Eichorn, JB Cooper, DJ Cullen, WR Maler, JH Philip, RG Seeman. Standards for patient monitoring at Harvard Medial School. JAMA 256:1017, 1986.
14. LM Hussain, AD Redmond. Are pre-hospital deaths from accidental injury preventable? BMJ 308:1077–1080, 1994.
15. C Deakin, G Davies. Defining trauma subpopulations for field stabilization. Eur J Emer Med 1:31–33, 1994.
16. J Ali, RU Adam, TJ Gana, H Bedaysie, J Williams. Effect of the prehospital trauma life support program (PHTLS) on prehospital trauma care. J Trauma 42:786–790, 1997.
17. RG Winchell, DB Hoyt. Endotracheal intubation in the field improves survival in patients with severe head injury. Arch Surg 132:592–597, 1997.
18. EP McCoy, RK Mirakhur, BV McCloskey. A comparison of the stress response to laryngoscopy: The Macintosh versus the McCoy blade. Anaesthesia 50:943–946, 1995.
19. SO Laurent, AE de Melo, JM Alexander-Williams. The use of the McCoy laryngoscope in patients with simulated cervical spine injuries. Anaesthesia 51:74–75, 1996.
20. CD Deakin, G Davies, AW Wilson. Simple thoracostomy avoids chest drain insertion in prehospital trauma. J Trauma 89:373–374, 1995.
21. WH Bickell, MJ Wall, PE Pepe, RR Martin, VF Ginger, MK Allen, KL Mattox. Immediate versus delayed fluid resuscitation for hypotensive patients with penetrating torso injuries. New Eng J Med 331:1105–1109, 1994.
22. AA Garner, RA Bartolacc. Massive prehospital transfusion in multiple blunt trauma. Med J Aust 170:23–25, 1999.

13

Advanced Airway Management and Use of Anesthetic Drugs

CHARLES E. SMITH

Case Western Reserve University Medical School and MetroHealth Medical Center, Cleveland, Ohio

RON M. WALLS

Harvard Medical School and Brigham and Women's Hospital, Boston, Massachusetts

DAVID LOCKEY

Frenchay Hospital, Bristol, United Kingdom

HERBERT KUHNIGK

University of Wuerzburg, Wuerzburg, Germany

I. IMPORTANCE OF AIRWAY MANAGEMENT: AN OVERVIEW

Complete compromise of the airway leads rapidly to hypoxia, irreversible brain damage, and death. As a result, management of the compromised airway has the highest treatment priority regardless of the presence of other injuries or medical problems. This is universally accepted practice, and the worldwide expansion of Advanced Trauma Life Support (ATLS) with its ''ABC'' approach to trauma care constantly reinforces this message [1].

While complete airway obstruction is usually easy to detect, partial airway obstruction, particularly when combined with inadequate ventilation, can be much less obvious. The resulting hypoxia commonly encountered at the scene of the accident [2,3] can profoundly influence the outcome of head injuries by creating secondary cerebral injury [4]. In a retrospective case-control study of blunt trauma patients, prehospital tracheal intubation was associated with decreased mortality, especially in patients with severe head injury

[5]. In a retrospective review of injured patients who required intubation within 30 min of admission to the hospital, prehospital intubation had a favorable impact on survival with good neurological outcome [6]. The importance of effective airway management in the prehospital phase of trauma is therefore universally accepted.

What is more controversial is how effective airway management is achieved. Airway obstruction may often be relieved by simple maneuvers such as the jaw thrust or chin lift. The application of supplementary oxygen is also mandatory in trauma patients. Virtually all prehospital emergency medical services (EMS) systems promote this approach. In the event of continued compromise, however, airway protocols around the world vary tremendously [7–9]. Some stop at this point, while others progress to non-drug-assisted tracheal intubation. With increased training, drug-assisted tracheal intubation is possible, and ultimately carrying out a surgical airway is an available option in some systems when all else fails.

If all options are available, prehospital protocol becomes similar to emergency room airway protocol. While this may seem an ideal objective to pursue, there are potential problems, such as the ability of some interventions to make a situation worse. If, for instance, neuromuscular blocking agents are administered but tracheal intubation and ventilation are not possible, death or cerebral hypoxia may result. Good evidence for the benefit of more advanced interventions in the prehospital environment is unfortunately sparse, and a need for clinical trials has been identified for airway and other interventions [10]. Strong medical direction and active continuous quality improvement programs are needed to ensure that prehospital providers learn and practice proper techniques of tracheal intubation, including verification of tube placement with capnography [11].

A number of strategies are available to deal with the challenge to provide advanced airway management training as well as continuing medical education to trauma care providers [12]. Use of simulator technology may help in this regard since the cognitive and psychomotor skills to deal with airway emergencies are difficult to acquire because of a limited number of patients, unplanned admittance, and safety concerns on behalf of the patients [13,14].

The advantages of simulation are as follows: no harm will be done to any patient while training, the same procedure or way of presenting a problem can be trained repeatedly, and the scenarios can be customized to the exact educational level and needs of the trainee [15].

Integrated simulator technology for teaching airway management skills includes a mannequin/manual interactive component, an interactive interface between the mannequin and trainee, computer software for modeling physiologic cause and effect, computer-generated simulations, and teaching modules to expand further upon concepts brought out in earlier stages of the simulation.

Disadvantages of simulation consist mainly of the substantial costs to purchase, house, maintain, and staff the simulator, and the inherent differences between simulated and real emergencies. Also, developing simulations for education and assessment is both costly and time-consuming.

II. INDICATIONS FOR TRACHEAL INTUBATION

The ability to maintain an airway and to exchange gases adequately are the key determinants in the decision to intubate (Fig. 1). Initial evaluation should therefore consist of an assessment of these vital elements.

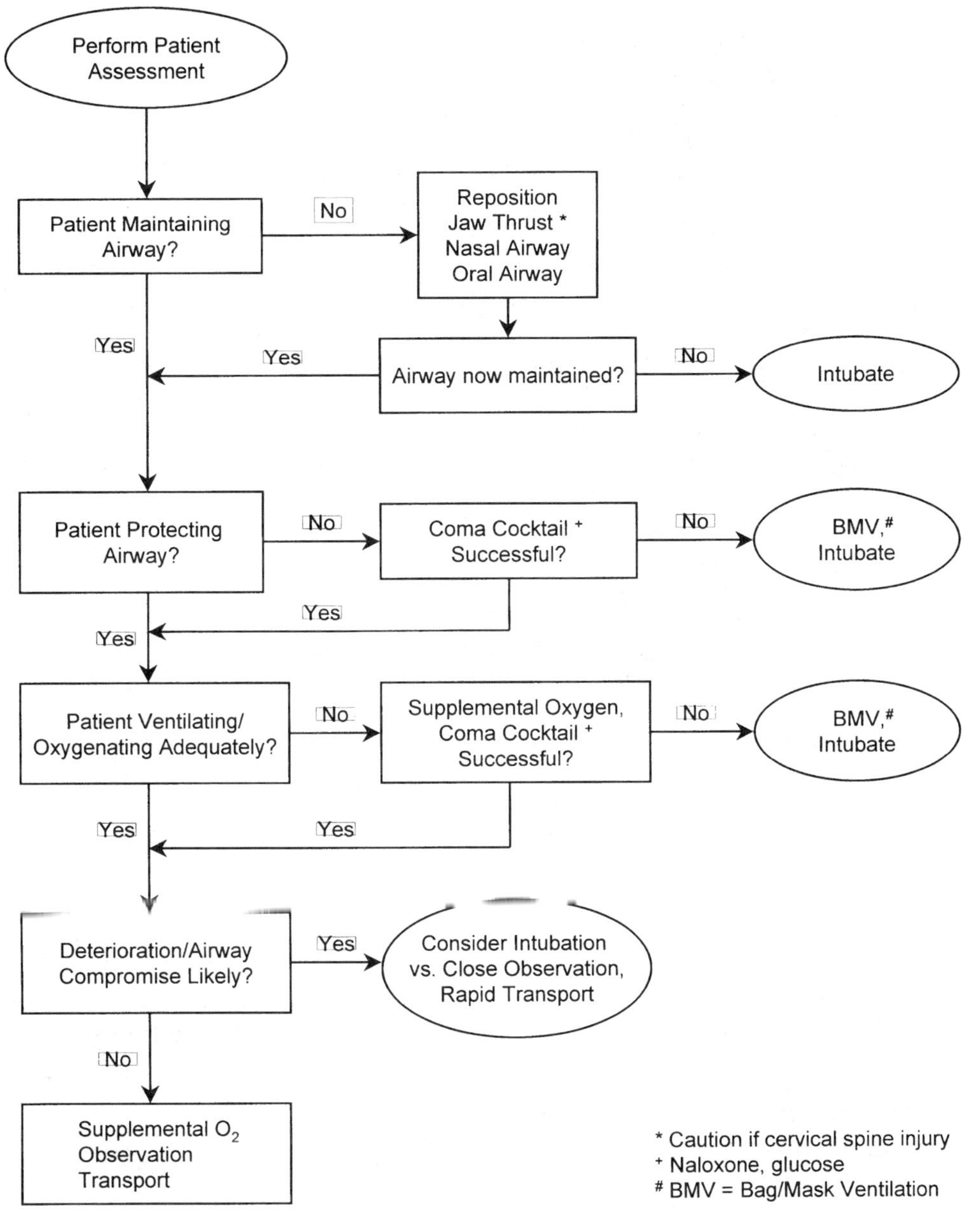

Figure 1 Prehospital airway management decision making regarding tracheal intubation. The algorithm centers on the patient's ability to maintain and protect the airway and the likelihood of airway compromise. (Adapted from Ref. 109.)

1. *Maintenance of the airway.* Airflow in a patent airway is silent. If the airway is not maintained, breathing may be completely obstructed and silent, or more commonly, be partially obstructed with a noisy or ''snoring'' quality. If the airway cannot be maintained, the provider must act immediately. The patient should be positioned maintaining cervical spine precautions if indicated [15,16]. A modified jaw thrust maneuver may be used to establish an upper airway, and oral or nasal airways may also be required. If neither of these techniques work the trachea should be intubated.
2. *Protection of the airway.* In addition to maintaining a patent airway, the lungs must be protected against aspiration. Aspiration of gastric contents can be a very serious complication and carries a high morbidity and mortality rate [17]. The likelihood of aspiration must be weighed against the potential hazards of intervention in the field. In general, if airway protection is poor but airway maintenance and respirations are adequate and there is no active vomiting or other source of aspiration, it may be best to transport the patient promptly to the receiving hospital rather than undertake active airway intervention. If, however, the airway cannot be maintained or if risk of aspiration appears high (e.g., because of recurrent vomiting), then tracheal intubation is indicated.

   An assessment of the ability to protect the airway is difficult. The gag reflex is traditionally used, but up to 20% of the adult population does not have a gag reflex and therefore this sign may be unreliable. In addition, testing the gag reflex may itself stimulate vomiting. A more valuable sign may be observation of the patient's ability to swallow. If the patient is able to sense secretions in the posterior oral pharynx and to swallow these secretions in a coordinated way while lying on his or her back, an adequate level of airway protection is present.
3. *Adequate gas exchange.* Even if the airway is patent and protected, adequate oxygen must be inhaled and adequate carbon dioxide exhaled to preserve vital functions. Of the two, inhalation of adequate oxygen is the most important. Pulse oximetry provides valuable clues to the patient's oxygenation status. In general, pulse oximetry readings above 90% should be considered adequate. All injured patients should receive supplemental oxygen according to ATLS guidelines. Pulse oximetry must, however, be used with caution when assessing

Table 1 Indications for Tracheal Intubation in the Trauma Patient

Airway protection and risk for aspiration
Head trauma and Glasgow coma scale ≤8
Definitive maintenance of airway patency
Mechanical ventilation and respiratory failure
Control over transport conditions
Maintenance of oxygenation or positive end expiratory pressure
Application of advanced cardiac life support and drug administration
Tracheal suctioning
Requirement for general anesthesia/provision of sufficient analgesia and hypnosis

Source: Ref. 112.

respiratory function because supplemental oxygen therapy may permit a normal oxygen saturation in the presence of gross hypoventilation. If oxygen saturation cannot be maintained at 90% despite the use of a nonrebreather-type oxygen mask, then bag-mask assisted ventilation or intubation should be strongly considered.

Certain patients may have adequate oxygenation and ventilation and be maintaining and protecting their airway but may deteriorate before arrival at the receiving center. Examples include expanding hematoma of the upper airway, head injury, shock, chest trauma, or drug overdose with decreasing level of consciousness (Table 1). In such cases, it may be advisable to consider early tracheal intubation.

III. ASSESSMENT OF THE AIRWAY

An orderly approach to airway examination is shown in Figures 2 and 3. Of particular importance is the presence of injuries to the airway itself or injuries to nearby tissue or vascular structures that may distort airway anatomy [18–22]. Patients sustaining severe trauma are frequently confused and obtunded due to head injury, hypoventilation, hypoxia, and shock, and may have an unstable cervical spine [23–27] (Table 2). In addition, trauma patients may present those characteristics that typically predispose to difficulty with mask ventilation, such as facial trauma, facial burns, obesity, and large beards, or to difficult direct laryngoscopy, such as a small mandibular space, limited airway joint mobility, and a small space between the tongue base and epiglottis (Table 3) [22].

Midface fractures permit posterior movement of the hard palate, creating airway obstruction. Basal skull fractures may be associated with central facial fractures and can result in intracranial passage of a nasally placed tube. Mandibular fractures can also result in airway obstruction as well as an inability to open the mouth. Obstruction of the airway due to maxillofacial trauma may be aggravated by soft tissue injury, foreign body (e.g.,

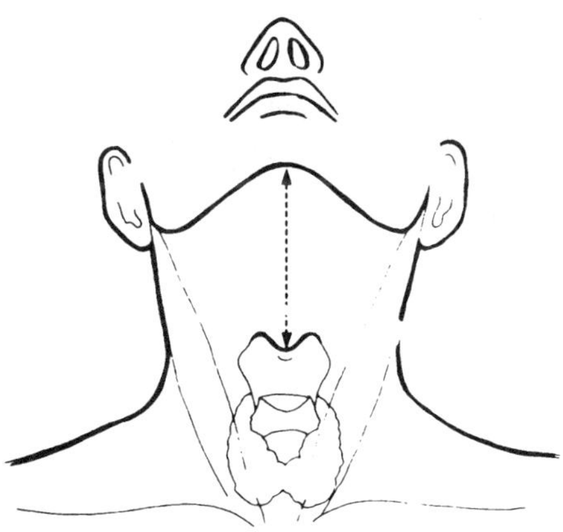

	Yes	No
Nasal Passages Clear		
Submental Angle Narrow		
Submental Swelling		
Submandibular Swelling		
Suprahyoid Notch to Chin Distance <6 cm		
Trachea Deviated		
Neck Swelling		
Neck Scarring		
Antesternal Mass		

Figure 2 Airway examination showing anterior viewing and palpation of the neck. (From Ref. 21.)

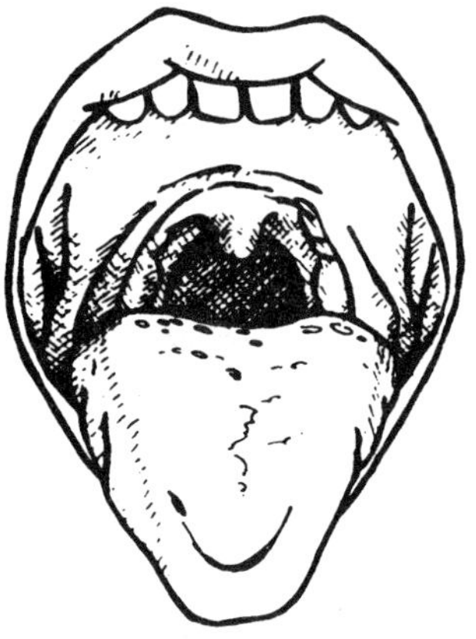

	Yes	No
Mouth Opening Limited		
Width of Mouth Narrow		
Intraoral Cavity Small		
View of Fauces Poor		
Tongue Large		
Cleft Lip/Palate		
Teeth Long		

Figure 3 Airway examination showing view of the mouth, teeth, uvula, tongue, faucial pillars, and interincisor distance. (From Ref. 21.)

avulsed teeth), and upper airway bleeding. Nasal obstruction or injury may be associated with severe epistaxis and prevent nasotracheal intubation. Trauma to the lower airway may vary from laryngeal fracture and tracheobronchial tears to flail chest, severe lung contusion, and hemo- or pneumothoraces.

IV. APPROACH TO TRACHEAL INTUBATION

Once the decision to intubate the trachea is made, an algorithmic approach to the technique of intubation is appropriate. Bag-mask ventilation and supplemental oxygenation should be used before, after, and if necessary during attempts at intubation since failure to oxygenate, not failure to intubate, causes damage to the patient (Fig. 4).

1. *Agonal unresponsive patient.* If the patient is unresponsive and exhibiting only agonal respiratory effort or cardiac activity, then immediate intubation is indicated, and can be accomplished by either the oral or nasal route. If the jaw is clenched, then blind nasotracheal intubation or surgical airway may be preferred. If the jaw is not clenched, then orotracheal intubation without medication

Table 2 Causes of Respiratory Distress in Trauma

Pulmonary aspiration	Shock
Foreign body	Soft tissue obstruction
Airway edema	Airway hemorrhage
Hemothorax/pneumothorax	Neck trauma
Pulmonary contusion	Pulmonary edema
Flail chest	Laryngeal, tracheal or bronchial injury
Spinal cord lesion	Head injury
Poisoning/overdose	Inhalational injury
Cardiac trauma	Pre-existing medical condition

Source: Ref. 23.

Table 3 Assessment for Difficult Direct Laryngoscopy

Reason for difficulty	Objective evaluation
1. Disproportionately increased size of base of tongue relative to pharynx	Mallampati class III; only soft palate visible when patient opens mouth wide and protrudes tongue
2. Decreased mandibular space; larynx relatively anterior to the rest of the upper airway structures	Thyromental distance <6 cm (2.4 in.), measured from the thyroid cartilage (Adam's apple) to the submentum; receding chin
3. Decreased head extension and neck flexion	Head extension <35 degrees; neck flexion <25 degrees; short, thick neck; cervical spine immobilization techniques
4. Decreased mouth opening	Distance between upper and lower incisors <4 cm (1.6 in.); mandibular fractures, especially condylar; rigid neck collar
5. Various conditions and disease states (e.g., rheumatoid arthritis, hypoplastic mandible)	Clinical examination of airway and adjacent structures; prominent maxillary teeth with overbite; long, narrow mouth with high, arched palate

Note: See also Figs. 2 and 3.
Source: Ref. 22.

may be attempted. In either case, bag-mask ventilation should precede the intubation attempt to ensure optimal preoxygenation. If oral intubation without medication is not successful, drug-assisted intubation may be necessary.

2. *Combative/uncooperative patient.* If the patient is combative or uncooperative with intubation attempts, then drug-assisted intubation is required. Blind nasotracheal intubation is relatively contraindicated in a combative or uncooperative patient because of increased risk of complications, particularly nasal and nasopharyngeal trauma with epistaxis. In addition, repeated attempts at nasotracheal intubation can lead to glottic edema and upper airway obstruction. Drug-assisted intubation may take one of the following two forms:
   a. Sedation/hypnosis only (± analgesia or local anesthesia)
   b. Sedation/hypnosis *and* neuromuscular blockade

   These are described in more detail in Secs. VI and VII.
3. *Cooperative passive patient.* If the patient is not combative and uncooperative, then he or she may tolerate intubation directly with minimal amounts of medication together with topicalization of the airway. If the jaw is not clenched then either direct oral intubation without medication or drug-assisted intubation may be used, depending on the patient's response to attempts at laryngoscopy. If attempts at oral intubation are unsuccessful because of excessive patient resistance, the patient should undergo drug-assisted intubation. It should be noted that intubation without judicious use of drugs or without adequate airway anesthesia may result in deleterious patient movements, trauma to the airway, and triggering of airway reflexes (e.g., retching, coughing, vomiting) [28]. In one prospective nonrandomized study of 233 patients requiring emergency intubation, tracheal intubation without paralysis was associated with a greater number and severity of complications, compared with rapid sequence intubation (RSI)

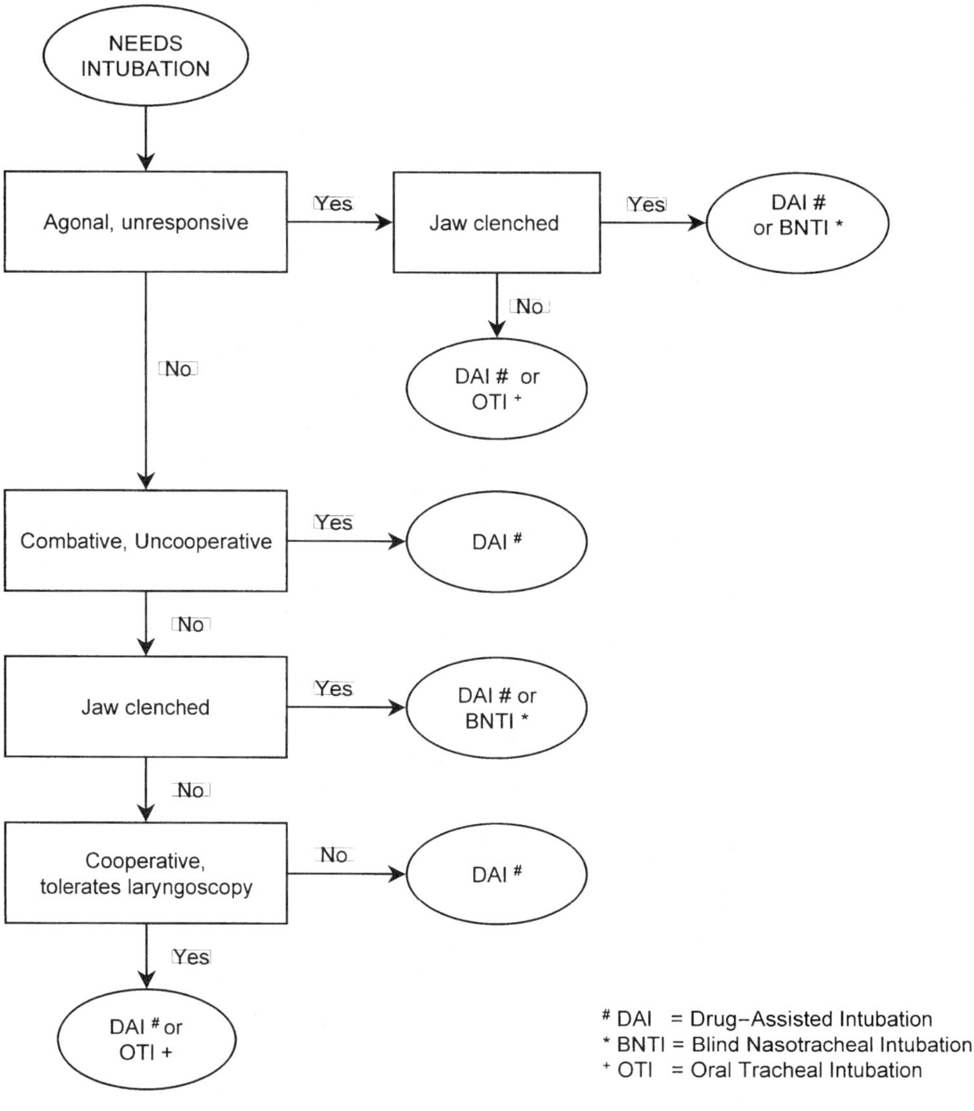

Figure 4 Prehospital approach to the technique of tracheal intubation. Drug-assisted intubation (e.g., sedative-hypnotic and neuromuscular relaxant) is often needed, especially in the combative uncooperative patient or in a patient with clenched jaw.

[29]. Complications in the nonparalyzed group were aspiration (15%), airway trauma (28%), and death (3%). None of these complications were observed in the RSI group [29].

4. *Drug-assisted intubation.* Intubation can be facilitated by using pharmacologic agents such as sedative/hypnotics, analgesics, local anesthetics, neuromuscular relaxants, or some combination of these drugs. Local medical protocols and practice will determine which approach is to be used and in what circumstances.

In general, *neuromuscular blockade-assisted intubation* is easier to perform because the patient is completely paralyzed and offers no resistance to laryngoscopy [30–32]. Airway visualization is superior using neuromuscular blocking agents. The use of *neuromuscular blocking agents*, however, requires the patient to be rendered apneic and completely dependent on successful airway management. Although bag-mask ventilation with an appropriately placed oral airway can often be used to maintain the airway in the event of failed intubation, a good rule of thumb is that a patient should not be paralyzed unless there is considerable confidence on the part of the operator that the intubation will be successful. The approach to drug-assisted intubation without neuromuscular relaxant is simply to administer adequate doses of a sedative or hypnotic drug together with an opioid and topical anesthesia until the patient's airway reflexes are sufficiently obtunded to permit oral laryngoscopy. Great caution must be used, because this level of obtundation generally renders the patient unable to maintain or protect his or her airway adequately, and respirations are often severely compromised.

The use of sedative and analgesic agents carries much of the risk of neuromuscular blocking drugs but without the ultimate benefit of complete paralysis. In addition, some patients, particularly those who are severely ill or compromised, may be rendered completely apneic and unresponsive with relatively small doses of sedative agents. Hypotensive patients may become precipitously worse when a sedative agent is administered. Again, caution and vigilance are indicated.

In all cases before intubation is undertaken, preoxygenation is mandatory. *Preoxygenation* is best accomplished with a nonrebreather mask or with a bag and mask apparatus to administer as close to 100% oxygen as is possible for 3 to 5 min (if there is time) before beginning the intubation attempt. This replaces the nitrogen in the patient's functional residual capacity and allows a much longer period of apnea before oxygen desaturation occurs [33]. Hyperventilation with eight deep breaths of 100% oxygen can also be used to provide maximal preoxygenation [34].

Trauma patients with respiratory distress, pre-existing hypoxia, decreased functional residual capacity, hemoglobin concentration, alveolar ventilation, and cardiac output have a decreased capacity for oxygen loading and will desaturate during apnea more rapidly than healthy patients [33].

V. ENDOTRACHEAL INTUBATION: POSITIONING, ROUTES, TECHNIQUES, AND AIDS

Endotracheal intubation is the gold standard in airway management. It allows for protection against aspiration from blood or vomit, unlimited administration of analgesics and sedative/hypnotics, use of transport ventilators with high oxygen concentrations, use of positive end expiratory pressure, and tracheal suctioning.

Before starting the intubation procedure, equipment and personnel need to be prepared (Table 4). *Backup plans* should be thought out for every possible event during intubation, and all personnel need to be informed about intended procedures in case of a mishap. Alternative airway techniques, such as insertion of a laryngeal mask airway (LMA) or Combitube, or performance of a surgical airway should be available.

Table 4 Equipment for Emergency Tracheal Intubation in Adult Trauma Patients

Masks 3 and 4
Laryngoscope blades 3 and 4
Tracheal tubes size 7.0–8.0 mm
Stylet/gum elastic bougie
10-ml syringe
Adhesive tape to secure the tube
Lubricant
Manual ventilation bag and oxygen source
Stethoscope
IV line with infusion for drugs
Pulse oximeter
End-tidal CO2 detector
ECG monitor

Proper positioning of the patient and the operator can facilitate tracheal intubation. The patient should be in the supine position with the head elevated 10 cm, producing a slight cervical flexion and a small degree of atlanto-occipital extension. This ''sniffing position'' aligns the laryngeal and pharyngeal axes during laryngoscopy. During field conditions, a pillow or a shirt under the head can be used for this purpose.

If the patient is suspected of having a cervical spine injury, head extension cannot be performed and the trachea should be intubated maintaining the neck in a neutral position using in-line immobilization [26]. It should be recognized that in-line immobilization results in a higher incidence of difficuly with glottic visualization using conventional laryngoscopy (22–39% incidence of grade III views) [35–38].

The operator body position during emergency intubation of a supine patient has an effect on the ease of intubation. A left lateral decubitus position is preferable to the kneeling position [39].

Tracheal intubation can be performed via the *oral or nasal route*. Both routes have advantages and disadvantages during field conditions. Ideally, the route chosen should facilitate a fast, easy, and smooth intubation without causing any additional trauma or bleeding. Orotracheal intubation is often preferred for these reasons. Nasotracheal intubation may facilitate taping the tube, but requires more time and can cause nasopharyngeal bleeding, which hinders visualization of the glottis and intubation procedure. Attempts at nasotracheal intubation in patients with basilar skull fractures in the field have not been associated with a higher incidence of complications [40].

The technique of oral intubation can be divided into four steps (Table 5).

1. *Open the mouth.* Sufficient mouth opening is essential for insertion of the laryngoscope. Injuries or pre-existing medical conditions hindering mouth opening such as jaw fractures should be excluded or taken into account before induction of anesthesia or attempting intubation. The rigid cervical collar restricts mouth opening and decreases the likelihood of visualizing the glottis with a MacIntosh laryngoscope [35]. A good option is to remove the collar during intubation and use manual in-line stabilization instead. The mouth should be opened with the fingers on the right hand gently but wide. Care must be taken against having one's fingers bitten in nonanesthetized patients. If a gentle open-

Table 5 Tasks Performed During Emergency Intubation in a Trauma Patient

Physician/paramedic/nurse	Assistant
1. Assess patient with decision to intubate	Prepare IV line, infusion, and monitors
2. Preoxygenate with 100% oxygen and position the head	Prepare intubation equipment
3. Perform laryngoscopy and insert tracheal tube	Give drugs and apply cricoid pressure
4. Confirm correct tube position and secure tube	Ventilate

ing is impossible from jaw rigidity, a deeper level of sedation or neuromuscular blockade is necessary. Caution is required, however, that the limited mouth opening is not a mechanical problem since neuromuscular blockade will not alleviate the problem and can acutely worsen the situation.

2. *Insert laryngoscope.* The laryngoscope blade is inserted into the right side of the mouth without contacting the teeth and moves the tongue to the left side. If the epiglottis is visible, the blade is inserted into the vallecula between the tongue and epiglottis, and the laryngoscope is pulled forward and upward to lift the epiglottis and expose the glottis. A working suction unit is mandatory to remove blood, vomit, or detritus. Visualization of the glottis is facilitated by external laryngeal pressure.
3. *Insert tube.* An adequate size tracheal tube is inserted from the right side of the mouth under direct vision through the glottic opening between the vocal cords. Blind intubation attempts increase the risk of esophageal intubation. In adults, inserting the tip of the tube 2 cm beyond the vocal cords helps to ensure that the tube is above the carina, thus avoiding accidental endobronchial intubation or extubation during movement (Table 6). This usually corresponds to an insertion depth at the upper teeth or gums of 23 cm in males and 21 cm in females.

Table 6 Recommended Endotracheal Tube Size and Insertion Depth for Emergency Intubation

	Internal diameter (mm)	Insertion distance from teeth to midtrachea (cm)
Adult male	8,0	23
Adult female	7,5	21
Child (10 years)	6,5	17
Child (6 years)	5,5	15
Child (2 years)	4,5	13
Newborn	3,0	11

4. *Check placement.* Verification of correct endotracheal tube placement is essential. Sustained presence of end-tidal CO2 (capnograph), auscultation of bilateral breath sounds with absence of air over the epigastrium, adequate chest excursions, and pulse oximetry are used to confirm tube placement. The tube is securely taped, fixing it at the desired length [41].

A. Intubation Aids

Success with any intubation aid or technique relies more on the operator's experience and skill than on the tools themselves [42]. Aids for intubation in the prehospital situation must be simple, robust, and suitable for the skill levels of the operator. Preparation time should be short. Unfortunately, only a few aids fulfill these criteria. Furthermore, equipment and resources in ambulances and in the field are limited. The following two types of aids are often used in the emergency or field situation:

1. Different types and sizes of laryngoscope blades
2. Stylets or tracheal tube introducers

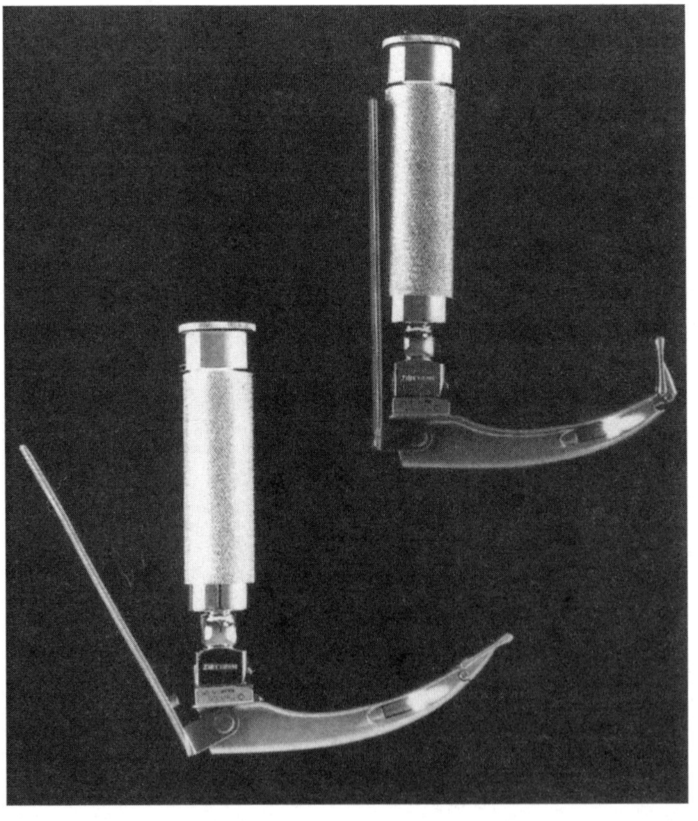

Figure 5 Corazzelli, London, McCoy (CLM) laryngoscope blade. The hinged blade tip is controlled by a lever attached to the blade and uses a standard laryngoscope handle. (From Mercury Medical, with permission.)

B. Laryngoscopes

The laryngoscope introduced by MacIntosh has a curved blade and is the standard in an emergency situation. Straight blades are more often used in children and in cases of limited mouth opening [43]. The choice of blade is an individual decision that depends on experience and familiarity. The correct choice of blade size depends on the age and height of the patient; sizes range from 0 (Miller) and 1 (Macintosh), which are the smallest, up to 4, which is the largest. Sizes 0 to 2 are for children, size 3 is the standard blade for adults, and 4 is an oversized blade for difficult intubations or extremely tall patients. In an adult, the first attempt is usually with a size 3 to explore the larynx. If the larynx is anterior and not visible and the mouth opening is unrestricted, an attempt with a 4 blade may be successful. If the mouth opening is restricted and the larynx is not visualized despite adequate sedation and attempts with two different blades, an alternative technique is necessary.

The McCoy or Corazzelli, London, McCoy (CLM) laryngoscope blade has a hinged blade tip, which is controlled by a lever attached to the blade (Figs. 5 and 6). This new laryngoscopic blade, which attaches to a standard laryngoscope handle, allows the epiglottis to be elevated without requiring excessive lifting force and has been shown to improve the view at laryngoscopy in patients with decreased or absent neck movement (i.e., cervical spine immobilization) [37].

Other specialized laryngoscopes include the Bullard laryngoscope [44–47] and the Wuscope fiberoptic laryngoscope system [48–50]. Both these devices are designed for difficult intubation circumstances, especially in patients with known or suspected cervical injuries [50]. The tubular blade of the WuScope creates more viewing and intubating space

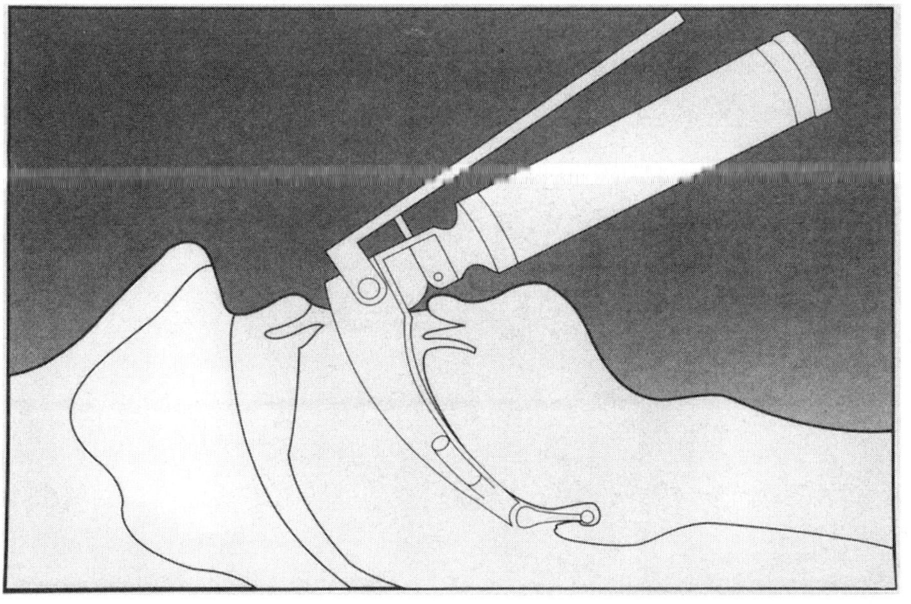

Figure 6 CLM laryngoscope blade. In patients in which visualization of the laryngeal aperture is difficult, the hinged blade permits the epiglottis to be lifted without requiring excessive force. The fulcrum of movement is at a lower point within the pharynx and exposure of the larynx is simplified. (From Mercury Medical, with permission.)

and permits oral intubation in patients with a limited mouth opening without the use of a specialized stylet. At least 20 mm of mouth opening is, however, necessary to insert and manipulate the Wuscope blades. The WuScope also has a separate channel for providing supplemental oxygen, and a portable battery-operated fiberscope is available.

C. Stylets and Gum Elastic Bougie

A *stylet*, which is a rigid implement inserted into the tube, can help to maintain a chosen shape of the tube. Intubation will be easier with a stylet if the glottis cannot be completely visualized or the pharynx is too narrow to insert the tube with its own shape. The preferred shape is described as a hockey stick. With the hockey stick method, the distal 4 to 5 cm of the stylet is bent within the endotracheal tube to form a 45° angle. The hockey stick configuration allows the operator to direct the distal tip of the tube anteriorly. The stylet must be lubricated to allow for easy removal. Another technique is to position 1 to 2 cm of the stylet uncovered outside the distal end of the tube. Depending on the anatomical situation, a more curved shape of the stylet may be preferable. The tip of the stylet is inserted into the larynx and serves as a guide for the tube. Extreme care must be taken when using stylets outside the endotracheal tube in order to avoid airway trauma.

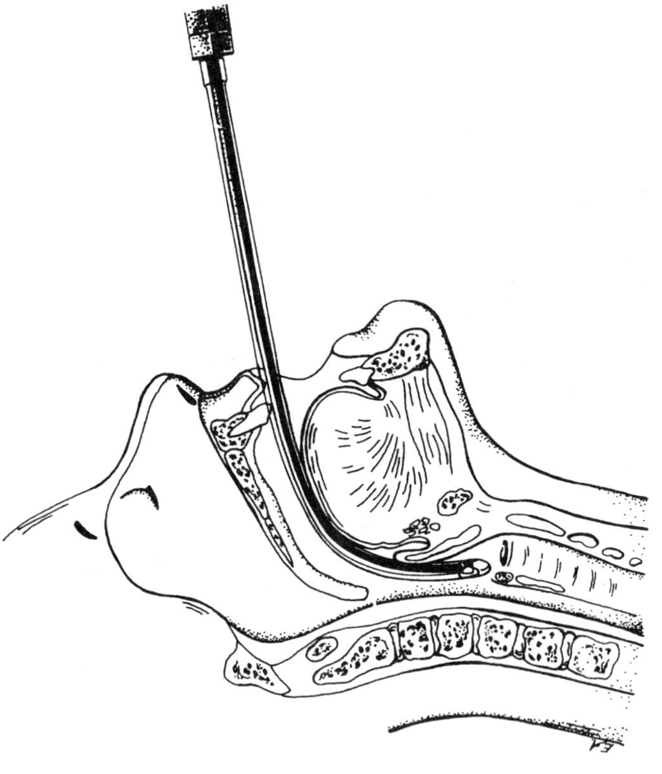

Figure 7 Lighted stylet intubation. The nondominant hand is used to open the mouth and the dominant hand introduces the lighted stylet into the oropharynx from the side and brought into the midline following the midsagittal plane. Anterior mandibular traction is used to pull the base of the tongue and epiglottis forward. (From Ref. 51.)

Lighted stylets may also be useful to facilitate orotracheal intubation (Figs. 7 and 8) [51–53]. Current lightwands have external or internal light sources, and many can accommodate both adult and pediatric tracheal tube sizes [51]. Lighted stylets have been successfully used for orotracheal intubation in patients with cervical spine trauma, micrognathia, jaw immobility, and glossomegaly [54,55]. Problems with using the lighted stylet include the blind nature of technique and a higher failure rate in patients with morbid obesity [55]. Bright sunlight interferes with the ability to visualize the glow of light as the tracheal tube is advanced below the hyoid and between the vocal cords [55].

The *gum elastic bougie* (Figs. 9 and 10) has been used to facilitate tracheal intubation in patients with cervical spine immobilization and in patients with difficult intubation [56,57]. The technique is as follows: direct laryngoscopy is performed and landmarks are identified; the bougie is manipulated under the epiglottis and the tip is directed anteriorly into the trachea until clicks or hold-up is felt. While still maintaining laryngoscopic force, a second operator threads a lubricated endotracheal tube over the bougie and into the

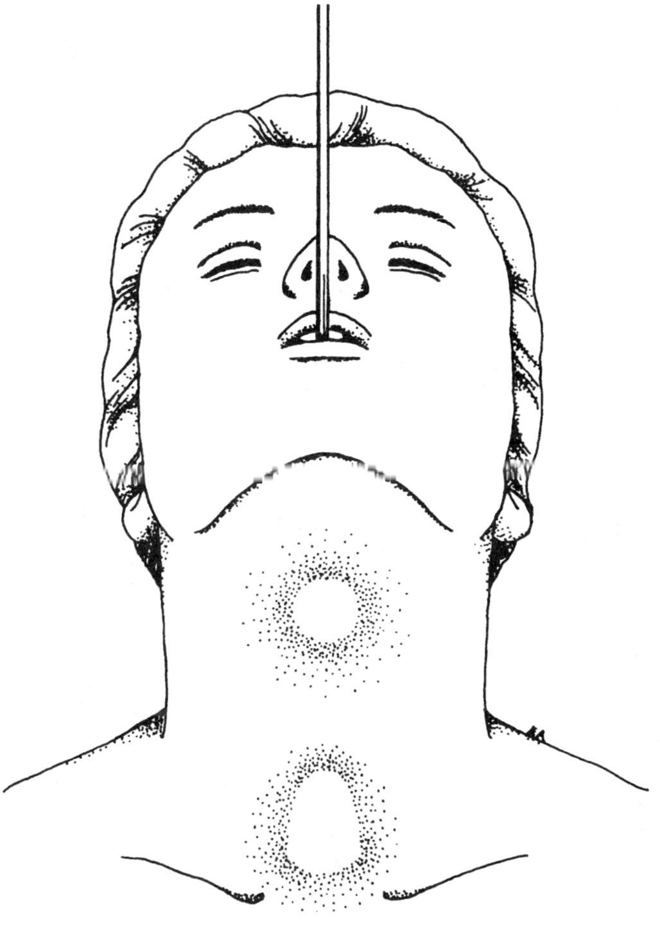

Figure 8 Lighted stylet intubation. The upper glow or well-defined circle of light just above the thyroid cartilage in the midline may change to a cone of light or lower glow as the lighted stylet passes through the glottis toward the suprasternal notch. (From Ref. 51.)

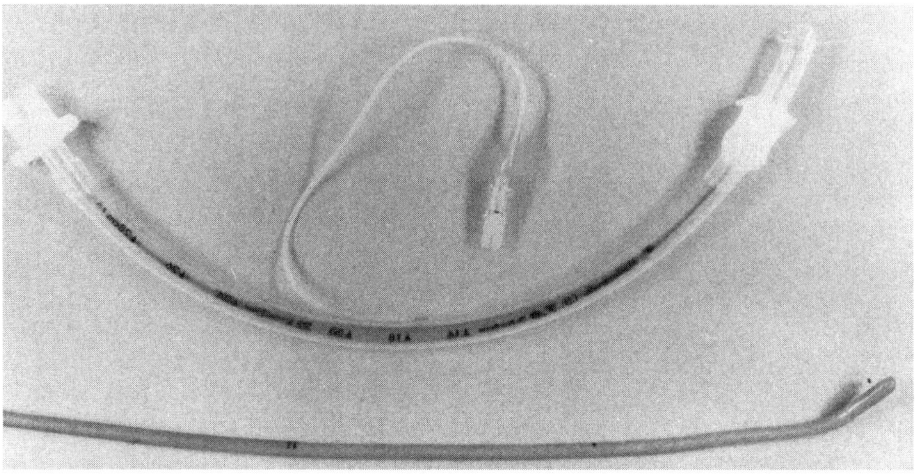

Figure 9 The gum elastic bougie, or Eschmann tracheal tube introducer, consists of a 60-cm-long device composed of a braided polyester base with an outer resin coating. These materials provide both stiffness and flexibility at room temperature. The bougie has an external diameter of 5 mm and can accommodate tracheal tubes with an inner diameter of ≥ 6 mm.

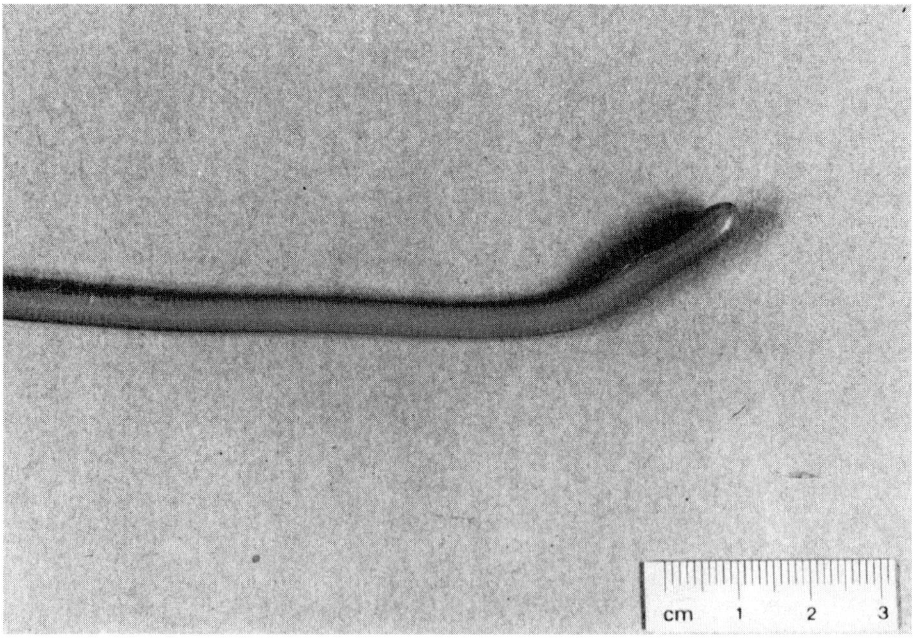

Figure 10 Close-up of the tip of the gum elastic bougie. Note the 35° angle 2.5 cm from the distal end.

airway. If the tracheal tube sticks at the laryngeal inlet, the bougie is rotated 90° counter clockwise.

VI. THE USE OF DRUGS TO FACILITATE TRACHEAL INTUBATION

A. Sedatives

Midazolam is a short-acting potent water-soluble benzodiazepine with sedative, anxiolytic, amnestic, and anticonvulsant properties [58,59] (Table 7). Midazolam is two to four times as potent as diazepam and does not cause local irritation after injection. The onset of action is within 1 to 2 min. Midazolam is metabolized in the liver and excreted by the kidney, with an elimination half-life of 1 to 4 hr. Small incremental doses (1–2 mg IV) are very useful for retrograde and antegrade amnesia and sedation. These doses have minimal if any hemodynamic effects. Midazolam also decreases the likelihood of systemic toxicity produced by lidocaine, which is particularly desirable whenever airway anesthesia is required.

Respiration is depressed by larger doses of midazolam and transient apnea may occur, especially when given in conjunction with opioids or in elderly patients with anemia or chronic obstructive pulmonary disease. Midazolam causes a dose-related decrease in cerebral blood flow and cerebral oxygen consumption. The effects of midazolam are rapidly reversed by the benzodiazepine antagonist, *flumazenil*. The elimination of *flumazenil*

Table 7 Selected Pharmacologic Agents for Sedation During Airway Management

Sedative agent	IV Dose	IM Dose	Maintenance dose	Comments
Midazolam	0.5–1 mg, repeated and titrated to effect	0.07 mg/kg	0.5–1.0 ug/kg/min	Benzodiazepine agent that increases seizure threshold. May cause apnea, which can be reversed with flumazenil
Propofol	0.3–0.6 mg/kg, repeated and titrated to effect	—	10–60 ug/kg/min	Alkylphenol agent with antiemetic properties. May cause apnea, hypotension, and pain on injection.
Ketamine	0.2–0.8 mg/kg, repeated and titrated to effect	2–4 mg/kg	10–20 ug/kg/min	Phencyclidine agent with potent analgesic properties. May cause sympathetic stimulation, vivid dreams, nystagmus, and salivation. These effects may be mitigated by concomitant dosing with benzodiazepines
Droperidol	1.25–5.0 mg, repeated and titrated to effect	2.5–5.0 mg	—	Neurolept agent with antiemetic properties. May cause hypotension, extrapyramidal reactions, and dysphoria.

Source: Ref. 78.

is substantially more rapid than that of midazolam, however, and resedation may occur [60,61].

Droperidol is a butyrophenone that is structurally and pharmacologically related to haloperidol. Butyrophenones such as droperidol act centrally to decrease the neurotransmitter function of dopamine to produce a state of dissociation characterized by reduced motor activity, reduced anxiety, and an indifference to one's surroundings [62]. Droperidol is also a powerful antiemetic. Minute ventilation and the ventilatory response to carbon dioxide are preserved.

The drug is metabolized in the liver with maximal excretion of metabolites within the first 24 hr. Hypotension may occur due to alpha-adrenergic blockade, and the decline in blood pressure may be more pronounced in hypovolemic patients. There is no myocardial depression. Extrapyramidal reactions occur in about 1% of patients, and the drug is contraindicated in patients with Parkinson's disease [62].

B. Opioids

Opioid drugs (Table 8) are useful adjuncts to decrease the pain and coughing associated with direct laryngoscopy and tracheal intubation. The clinical effects of opioid analgesics are exerted via stimulation of the various opioid receptor subtypes at different levels of the neuraxis [63]. Central nervous system effects include sedation and hypnosis, with a reduction in cerebral metabolism, pupillary constriction, and stimulation of the chemoreceptor trigger zone. The cough centers of the medulla are depressed after administration of opioids.

Respiratory effects include a dose-related depression of the ventilatory response to carbon dioxide, an elevated apneic threshold, and a blunted ventilatory response to hypoxemia. Opioids also blunt the stress response to pain, and decrease sympathetic tone, leading to peripheral vasodilation and venodilation. There is no myocardial depression following clinically relevant doses of synthetic opioids such as fentanyl, alfentanil, sufentanil, and remifentanil. Bradycardia may occur due to central vagal nuclei stimulation. Although rarely observed in the prehospital setting, rapid administration of large doses of synthetic opioids can produce skeletal muscle hypertonicity, upper airway closure, and decreased chest wall compliance, leading to difficulty with ventilation [64,65].

Fentanyl is a potent synthetic opioid with minimal hemodynamic or cerebrovascular effects [63]. Onset is within 6 min, with a duration of 45 to 60 min. Fentanyl is rapidly redistributed into a large volume of distribution, which largely determines its duration of action when smaller doses (e.g., 2–5 μg/kg) are given. Elimination is via hepatic transformation and kidney excretion. In a randomized blinded study on sedatives and hemodynamics during RSI in the emergency room, fentanyl, (5μg/kg) provided the most neutral hemodynamic profile during RSI compared with thiopental (5 mg/kg) and midazolam (0.1 mg/kg) [66].

Alfentanil has a smaller volume of distribution and shorter elimination time compared with fentanyl or *sufentanil* [57]. Rapid plasma-effect site equilibration with alfentanil results in a relatively larger peak-effect site concentration. *Remifentanil* is a newer opioid agent. The peak-effect site concentration following remifentanil is approximately 1.5 min, and the drug is rapidly eliminated by plasma esterases.

Many other opioid agonists and partial agonists can be used as adjuncts for airway management in trauma. *Morphine* is a naturally occurring opioid that has been used for analgesia and sedation for centuries. This drug can produce hypotension, however, because

Table 8 Selected Opioid Agents and Lidocaine as Adjuncts to Tracheal Intubation

Agent	Standard dose (mg/kg)	Trauma dose* (mg/kg)	BP	CPP	Comments
Fentanyl	2–6 μg/kg	1–3 μg/kg	Stable	Stable	Minimal hemodynamic or cerebrovascular effects. Useful agent for blunting noxious stimuli (e.g., direct laryngoscopy, tracheal intubation). Half-time of equilibration between the effect site and plasma is relatively slow (5–6 min).
Sufentanil	0.5–1.0 μg/kg	0.1–0.5 μg/kg	Stable	Stable	Similar to fentanyl, but more potent. Faster offset.
Alfentanil	20–80 μg/kg	5–20 μg/kg	Stable	Stable	Similar to fentanyl, but faster onset and offset. Half-time of equilibration between the effect site and the plasma is 1.5 min.
Remifentanil	0.05–1 μg/kg/min	0.05–0.2 μg/kg/min	Stable	Stable	Similar to alfentanil in terms of fast onset. Extremely rapid clearance (3–4 L/min) due to esterase metabolism, which results in rapid and predictable recovery.
Lidocaine	1.5–2.0	1.0–1.5	Stable	Stable or increased	Useful adjuvant agent for blunting airway reflexes. Also blunts BP, ICP, and IOP response to intubation, involuntary muscle movements after etomidate, and injection site pain from propofol and etomidate.

*Dose for hemodynamically compromised patient. Note that trauma by itself does not mandate decreased dosage.
BP = blood pressure, ICP = intracranial pressure, IOP = intraocular pressure, CPP = cerebral perfusion pressure = mean BP − ICP.
Source: Ref. 112.

of histamine release and reduced venous and arterial tone. *Meperidine* is a phenylpiperidine derivative of morphine that has been associated with histamine release, decreased myocardial contractility, and increased heart rate [63].

Partial agonists currently in use include *buprenorphine, pentazocine, butorphanol,* and *nalbuphine*. Nalbuphine (0.3 mg/kg IV) combined with etomidate (0.3 mg/kg) has been used without neuromuscular relaxants to facilitate intubation in the prehospital environment [68]. Buprenorphine has high affinity but low intrinsic activity at the mu receptor, whereas the other agents are antagonists at the mu opioid receptor and agonists at the sigma and kappa opioid receptors [63].

Opioid antagonists such as *naloxone* or *nalmefene* may be used to reverse opioid-induced respiratory depression or to antagonize opioid-induced side effects such as vomiting, pruritus, urinary retention, and biliary spasm [69]. Abrupt reversal of opioid depression may precipitate an acute withdrawal syndrome in persons who are physically dependent on opioids and results in vomiting, tachycardia, sweating, trembling, hypertension, and combative behavior.

In postoperative patients, opioid reversal requires careful titration (e.g., 0.5–1.0 μg/kg), and excessive doses may result in increased plasma catecholamine levels, hypertension, agitation, ventricular tachycardia and fibrillation, and pulmonary edema. The ''naloxone challenge test'' is commonly used in emergency medicine for the diagnosis of suspected opioid tolerance or acute opioid overdosage. The initial IV dose in adults is 0.2 mg, and if no evidence of withdrawal is observed within 30 sec, an additional 0.6 mg can be given. Nalmefene is a new pure opioid antagonist that is structurally similar to naloxone but has a much longer half-life (10.8 hr vs. 1.1 hr). Because the half-life and duration of action of nalmefene is long, renarcotization is less likely following use of this agent. Nalmefene can be administered IV in 0.25 μg/kg incremental doses at 2 to 5 min intervals [69]. Therapeutic plasma concentrations can also be achieved within 5 to 15 min following a 1 mg intramuscular (IM) or subcutaneous (SC) dose.

C. IV Induction Agents

Intravenous induction agents (Tables 9 and 10) are very useful to induce general anesthesia in patients who require RSI.

Table 9 Comparative Pharmacokinetics of IV Induction Agents

Induction agent	Standard dose (mg/kg)	Trauma dose* (mg/kg)	Volume of distribution at steady state (L/kg)	Clearance (ml/min/kg)	Elimination half-life (hr)
Thiopental	3–5	0.5–2	2.5	3.4	11.6
Etomidate	0.2–0.3	0.1–0.2	2.5–4.5	10–20	2–5
Propofol	1.5–2.5	0.5–1	2–10	59.4	4–7
Midazolam	0.1–0.2	0.05–0.1	1–1.5	7.5	1–4
Ketamine	1–2	0.5–1	2.5–3.5	16–18	1–2

*Dose for hemodynamically compromised patient. Note that trauma by itself does not mandate decreased dosage.
Source: Ref. 77.

Table 10 Effects of Induction Agents for General Anesthesia on the Cardiovascular and Central Nervous Systems

Induction agent	Blood pressure	Heart rate	Cardiac contractility	Cerebral blood flow	$CMRO_2$	Intracranial pressure (ICP)
Thiopental	Decrease	Increase	No change or decrease	Decrease	Decrease	Decrease
Etomidate	No change	No change	No change	Decrease	Decrease	Decrease
Propofol	Decrease	No change	Decrease	Decrease	Decrease	Decrease
Midazolam	Slight decrease	No change	No change	Decrease	Decrease	Decrease
Ketamine	Increase	Increase	Increase[a]	Increase	Increase	Increase

[a] Centrally mediated sympathetic response usually overrides direct depressant effects.
Note: $CMRO_2$ = cerebral metabolic oxygen requirements.
Source: Ref. 77.

Thiopental is a rapid onset barbiturate hypnotic with short duration [70]. The rapid onset of effect is due to high lipid solubility and high cerebral perfusion. The maximum effect of a bolus injection is seen within 60 sec. This is followed by a rapid redistribution to other vessel-rich tissues, which accounts for the rapid offset [70]. With higher doses or multiple repeat doses, recovery is delayed because the redistribution mechanism is overwhelmed. Because thiopental may produce hypotension due to myocardial depression and vasodilation, it should be administered in reduced or divided doses to unstable patients. Thiopental decreases cerebral metabolic oxygen consumption, cerebral blood flow, and intracranial pressure (ICP). The rapid onset of thiopental makes this drug useful for treating seizures, although the benzodiazepines provide a more specific anticonvulsant activity.

Propofol is a nonbarbiturate sedative-hypnotic that is formulated in soybean oil, glycerol, and egg phosphatide, similar to parenteral lipid formulations [71]. The onset is rapid, usually within 1 to 2 min. Propofol is metabolized by the liver to glucuronide and sulfate conjugates, which are excreted in the urine. The short duration of this agent is due to its large volume of distribution as well as its high clearance. Patients typically emerge rapidly following anesthesia with propofol and have a low incidence of emesis.

Although propofol has been used in carefully titrated dosages during the acute phase of trauma [72], care must be taken to address cardiovascular and volume status when using this agent because of the risk for hypotension due to myocardial depression and vasodilation. Volume loading can offset some of the cardiovascular effects associated with propofol. In head-injured patients, propofol tends to cause cerebral vasoconstriction and a reduction in cerebral metabolism, cerebral blood flow, and ICP.

Propofol can also be combined with *ketamine* in an effort to minimize the hemodynamic effects of either of these two agents (total intravenous anesthesia, or TIVA). The increased heart rate, blood pressure, and cardiac output associated with ketamine offsets the hypotension and myocardial depression often observed with propofol, resulting in stable hemodynamics [73].

Ketamine is a phencyclidine hypnotic that produces intense analgesia and dissociative anesthesia characterized by electroencephalographic dissociation between the thalamus and limbic system [71]. Ketamine has a rapid onset of action within 60 sec after IV dosages of 1 to 2 mg/kg, and 5 min after IM dosages of 4 to 6 mg/kg. Smaller doses (0.2–0.8 mg/kg IV or 2–4 mg/kg IM) are very useful for sedation and analgesia. Rapid redistribution is responsible for the termination of unconsciousness, whereas the analgesic effects may persist for hours afterwards.

Ketamine produces sympathetic nervous system stimulation with increases in heart rate, blood pressure, cardiac output, and myocardial oxygen demand. In vitro, however, ketamine produces direct myocardial depression. Patients may therefore experience hypotension and decreased cardiac output if catecholamine stores are depleted or if there is exhaustion of sympathetic system compensatory mechanism [74]. Ketamine-induced sympathetic stimulation may be blunted by the coadministration of benzodiazepines and other agents that block the sympathetic outflow.

Ketamine is a potent cerebral vasodilator and leads to an increase in ICP. These cerebral vasodilator effects are particularly undesirable in patients with space-occupying intracranial lesions or in patients with elevated ICP. Ketamine, however, is a noncompetitive NMDA (N-methyl-D-aspartate) receptor antagonist that could theoretically reduce excessive excitotoxic stimuli and brain ischemia following head injury [74–76].

Emergence delirium may occur following ketamine anesthesia, the incidence of which can be decreased by pretreatment with benzodiazepines. Upper airway skeletal muscle tone and reflexes are usually well maintained after ketamine. Salivary and bronchial secretions are increased, although ketamine is a potent bronchodilator in patients with reactive airways disease.

Etomidate is a rapid-onset imidazole hypnotic with short duration. Unlike thiopental and propofol, etomidate has minimal or absent cardiac depressant effects when administered in standard induction dosages. The lack of cardiovascular effects are most likely due to etomidate's lack of effect on the sympathetic nervous system and autonomic reflexes. As with thiopental, etomidate decreases cerebral metabolic oxygen consumption, cerebral blood flow, and ICP. Etomidate is most useful for RSI in both patients with shock or unstable cardiopulmonary status, and patients with head injury [74,77–80].

Problems with etomidate include irritation and phlebitis in the injected vein, myoclonic movements on induction, and a higher incidence of nausea and vomiting after extubation. Involuntary muscle movements (myoclonus) and pain on injection with etomidate can be minimized with lidocaine and small doses of midazolam. Myoclonus is abolished by the simultaneous administration of neuromuscular blocking agents during RSI. Etomidate-induced myoclonus is not associated with epileptiform activity, and appears to be related to disinhibition of subcortical structures that normally suppress extrapyramidal motor activity. These muscle movements can mistakenly be confused with seizures, especially in patients who have sustained head trauma.

Etomidate has been shown to depress adrenal cortical function even after a single dose. Etomidate inhibits adrenal cortisol synthesis by a reversible and concentration-dependent block of 11-beta-hydroxylase and to a lesser extent 17-alpha-hydroxylase [71,81]. This adrenal suppression appears to be related to binding of cytochrome p450 by the free imidazole radical of etomidate, and has been associated with increased morbidity and mortality after prolonged use of etomidate in ICU patients [82]. While the adrenal suppression following single doses of etomidate is of concern, the suppression is apparently short-lived. Nausea and vomiting after etomidate is of little or no consequence when the drug is being given for emergency intubation.

D. Airway Anesthesia

The three main components of airway anesthesia include (1) administration of local anesthetics, (2) a topical vasoconstrictor if the nasal route is chosen, and (3) an antisialagogue.

Because of its potency, rapid onset, moderate duration of action, and versatility, *lidocaine* is the most frequently used local anesthetic. It can be delivered via sprays and atomizers (2%, 4%, and 10%), or 5 ml of 4% lidocaine can be nebulized with oxygen. Lidocaine can also be administered topically as a gargle or 2% jelly or through infiltration to block the superior and recurrent laryngeal nerves. The onset of action is within minutes, and peak blood levels occur at about 15 to 20 min.

Amide local anesthetics such as lidocaine are metabolized by the liver, whereas ester local anesthetics such as tetracaine and procaine are metabolized by plasma cholinesterase and red cell esterase to yield an alcohol and para-aminobenzoic acid. The dose of lidocaine in adults should generally not exceed 5 mg/kg. Most episodes of lidocaine toxicity stem from accidental intravascular injection or from relative overdose. Initial symptoms of lidocaine toxicity are excitatory and include lightheadedness, visual and auditory disturbances, muscular twitching, and convulsion [83]. Eventually central nervous system depression and cardiovascular collapse develop as blood levels increase. Treatment of lidocaine toxicity is supportive and includes airway maintenance and control of seizures with benzodiazepines or barbiturates.

The nasopharynx can also be anesthetized with *cocaine*, which is both a local anesthetic and a vasoconstrictor. Concentrations of 1%, 4%, and 10% have been used. Toxic reactions follow the administration of >3 mg/kg of cocaine, resulting in central nervous system stimulation, convulsions, hypertension, tachycardia, arrhythmias, myocardial ischemia, and cardiac arrest. Because of its toxicity and high potential for abuse, cocaine is rarely used in the trauma population. Dilute *oxymetazoline*, 0.05% or *phenylephrine*, 0.5–1%, are preferred instead of cocaine for vasoconstriction of the nasal mucosa.

Glycopyrrolate is a synthetic anticholinergic agent that is a more potent antisialagogue than *atropine*. Unlike atropine and *scopolamine*, glycopyrrolate possesses a quaternary ammonium structure that prevents it from crossing the blood–brain barrier, thus central nervous system toxicity is unlikely to occur. Glycopyrrolate produces less tachycardia than atropine and less sedation than scopolamine. The dose is 0.2 to 0.4 mg IV, with a duration of 2 to 4 hr. Scopolamine, 0.4 mg IV, is also a potent antisialogogue with sedative, amnestic, and antiemetic properties.

E. Neuromuscular Blocking Agents

1. Depolarizing Agents

Succinylcholine is the most frequently used neuromuscular relaxant in for RSI (Table 11) [84–86]. At the molecular level, succinylcholine mimics the effect of acetylcholine at the neuromuscular junction. Succinylcholine binds to the acetylcholine receptors at the neuromuscular junction, causing conformational change in the receptor. The receptor then remains refractory to acetylcholine, and the sodium channels located in the perijunctional muscle membrane remain frozen in an inactivated state. This ''depolarizing''-type-block persists until succinylcholine diffuses away from the junction and is metabolized by plasma cholinesterase.

Table 11 Selected Neuromuscular Relaxants

Agent	Intubating dose (mg/kg)	Onset time (min)	Time to 25% first twitch recovery (min)	Comments
Succinylcholine	1.0–1.5	1	4–6	Preferred agent for rapid sequence intubation. Several serious side effects may contraindicate its use. (See Tables 12,13).
Rocuronium	0.6–1.2	0.7–1.1	31–67	Intermediate-acting nondepolarizer. Mild vagolysis. No histamine release.
Rapacuronium	1.5–2.5	1–1.5	16	Short-acting nondepolarizer. Rescue reversal possible—shortens recovery time to 8–9.5 min. Mild histamine release.
Vecuronium	0.08–0.1	2.5–3	25–40	Cardiovascular effects unlikely. Higher doses (0.3–0.4 mg/kg) associated with more rapid onset but prolonged duration.
Pancuronium	0.06–0.10	2–3	65–100	Associated with tachycardia and activation of the sympathetic nervous system.

Source: Ref. 112.

Because succinylcholine produces rapid skeletal muscle relaxation within 30 to 60 sec after its administration, it remains the muscle relaxant of choice for RSI, against which all other agents are compared [30]. This is despite several well-described side effects such as hyperkalemia, malignant hyperthermia, arrhythmias, muscle fasciculations, and increased intracranial, intraocular, and intragastric pressures (Table 12) [87].

Table 12 Side Effects of Succinylcholine

Massive hyperkalemia in susceptible patients
Cardiac arrhythmias
Muscle fasciculatione
Myalgias
Rhabdomyolysis
Increased intracranial pressure
Increased intragastric pressure
Increased intraocular pressure
Malignant hyperthermia
Masseter muscle spasm or jaw rigidity
Prolonged apnea, if atypical plasma cholinesterase

Source: Ref. 87.

Succinylcholine acts at the postjunctional neuromuscular membrane to produce the sustained opening of the acetylcholine receptor, which results in leakage of potassium ions from the interior of the cells. In most patients, this results in an increase in serum potassium levels of about 0.5 to 1.0 mEq/L. The literature strongly suggests that succinylcholine be avoided after 24 to 48 hr of injury in patients with burns, massive trauma, crush and degloving injuries, spinal cord injuries, stroke, severe abdominal infections, and tetanus, as well as in patients with neuromuscular disease such as Duchenne's muscular dystrophy, because of the risk of hyperkalemic cardiac arrest (Table 13) [87]. This susceptibility to massive hyperkalemia is most likely a result of the proliferation of extrajunctional nicotinic cholinergic receptors. The administration of small subparalyzing doses of nondepolarizing relaxants prior to succinylcholine prevents fasciculations but does not prevent the development of life-threatening hyperkalemia. Pre-existing hyperkalemia from renal failure or severe acidosis may also predispose to hyperkalemia after succinylcholine [88].

There is evidence that succinylcholine may be safely used in patients with elevated ICP and intraocular pressure (IOP) [89,90]. Although lidocaine is often administered in an attempt to control ICP during RSI, administration of succinylcholine did not result in any change in cerebral perfusion pressure, ICP, electroencephalogram, or middle cerebral blood flow in patients with head trauma and other central nervous system pathologies [89].

It is important to note that both IOP and ICP can be dramatically altered by factors that are not the result of anesthetic drugs and manipulations. For example, crying, coughing, vomiting, rubbing the eye, or squeezing the eyelids closed before induction of anesthesia may increase IOP. Coughing and bucking on the tracheal tube during intubation can increase both IOP and ICP to levels far greater than those observed after succinylcholine.

The short duration of action of succinylcholine results from hydrolysis by plasma cholinesterase. Hydrolysis is so rapid that only a small fraction of the delivered doses actually reaches the neuromuscular junction. In patients with atypical forms of plasma cholinesterase, duration of action of succinylcholine may be increased to 3 hr [91].

Succinylcholine-induced bradyarrhythmias, including asystole, may occur following repeat doses of this agent in any patient, as well as with the initial dose in children and

Table 13 Conditions Associated with Exaggerated Hyperkalemia After Succinylcholine

>24 hr after major burns and multiple trauma
Crush injuries
Metabolic acidosis
Extensive denervation of skeletal muscle
Upper motor neuron injury
Tetanus
Chronic abdominal infection
Subarachnoid hemorrhage
Duchenne's muscular dystrophy
Conditions causing degeneration of central and peripheral nervous systems

Source: Ref. 87.

in conditions of hypoxia or hypercarbia. Pretreatment with atropine prevents these bradyarrythmias in most cases (e.g., atropine, 0.02 mg/kg, given 2–3 min before succinylcholine in children less than 10 years).

Small doses of nondepolarizing neuromuscular relaxants (e.g., d-tubocurare 3 mg) can be give to prevent succinylcholine-induced fasciculations [92]. Pretreatment, however, delays the onset of neuromuscular blockade, decreases the degree of paralysis, and can result in muscle weakness and aspiration [93–96].

2. Nondepolarizing Agents

Nondepolarizing relaxants bind to the acetylcholine recognition sites of the alpha subunits of the acetylcholine receptor at the neuromuscular junction, and competitively inhibit neuromuscular transmission. In contrast to depolarizing relaxants, at the molecular level nondepolarizers do not cause conformational change in the acetylcholine receptor. These receptor channels remain closed, and no current or ions flow. Only rapid-onset nondepolarizing drugs of short to intermediate duration of action are considered appropriate for discussion in this chapter.

Rocuronium is a nondepolarizer alternative for succinylcholine in terms of onset, but has an intermediate clinical duration (37–73 min, range 23–150 min) [97,98]. It has an aminosteroid structure and exerts its effect by binding to the alpha subunits of the postsynaptic cholinergic receptor, which competitively prevents neuromuscular transmission. Like other nondepolarizing relaxants, rocuronium has a small volume of distribution, is highly ionized at physiologic pH, and does not cross the blood–brain barrier. Rapid initial decline in blood levels is caused by redistribution. Elimination is chiefly by hepatic metabolism, followed by renal excretion.

During RSI, it has been found that rocuronium, 0.9–1.2 mg/kg, produced similar onset times and intubating conditions to those of succinylcholine [97]. Time to maximal block after 1.2 mg/kg rocuronium was 55 sec (range 36–84 sec) [97]. Corresponding times were 50 (24–84) sec after succinylcholine, 1 mg/kg [97]. When lower doses of rocuronium are used for RSI (e.g., 0.6 mg/kg), intubation conditions were inferior to those after succinylcholine or after higher doses of rocuronium [99,100].

In anesthetized patients undergoing RSI with thiopental and fentanyl, the incidence of acceptable intubating conditions was similar between rocuronium, 1 mg/kg, and succinylcholine, 1.0 mg/kg, when intubation was done 60 sec after giving the relaxant [100]. The incidence of excellent grade intubating conditions, however, was superior with succinylcholine vs. rocuronium (80 vs. 65%) [100].

The rapid onset time of rocuronium is thought to be due to its lower potency, which allows more molecules of the drug to access the neuromuscular junction during the first few circulation times [30,99]. Unlike succinylcholine, rocuronium does not cause hyperkalemia, malignant hyperthermia, or increased intracranial, intraocular, and intragastric pressures. There is no histamine release [101], although there is a potential for mild vagolysis.

When using rocuronium for RSI after thiopental has been given, it is prudent to flush the drugs through the IV tubing in order to accelerate delivery to the central circulation and in order to avoid precipitation, which can potentially occlude the tubing.

Rapacuronium is a new steroidal low-potency analog of vecuronium. This agent has been associated with the fast onset of tracheal intubating conditions in anesthetized patients [102]. The time to maximal block was 52 sec after a dose of 1.5 mg/kg and duration of action was 16.2 min [103]. Early administration of neostigmine (e.g., rescue reversal) shortened the recovery time to 8.0 to 9.5 min [103]. Early reversal may be beneficial in patients with difficult airway or failed intubation.

Intubating conditions after rapacuronium and succinylcholine were compared in 818 patients in three prospective randomized multicenter trials [104]. Direct laryngoscopy was initiated at 50 sec after giving rapacuronium, 1.5 mg/kg, or succinylcholine, 1.0 mg/kg. Clinically acceptable intubating conditions were somewhat better after succinylcholine than after rapacuronium, occurring in 80–87% of the patients receiving rapacuronium and in 89–97% of the patients receiving succinylcholine [104].

In a prospective randomized clinical trial of 236 anesthetized patients, intubation conditions were excellent or good in 87% of patients after rapacuronium, 1.5 mg/kg, and in 95% of patients after succinylcholine, 1.0 mg/kg [105]. Time to first recovery of the train-of-four response was 8 min (range 2.8–20 min) after this dose of rapacuronium [105].

Adverse events associated with rapacuronium include hypotension (5.2%), tachycardia (3.2%), bradycarida (1.5%), and bronchospasm (3.2%) [104]. These events may in part be related to histamine release [106].

Vecuronium is a monoquaternary steroidal nondepolarizing muscle relaxant. In the usual recommended intubating doses, 0.10 to 0.15 mg/kg, the onset of action is delayed compared with rocuronium and succinylcholine [97]. With the high-dose vecuronium technique, 0.3 to 0.4 mg/kg, onset of neuromuscular blockade is accelerated to 78 to 88 sec (range 60–120 sec), but is associated with a prolonged duration of clinical effect (111–115 min; range 35–208 min) [107].

Vecuronium does have the advantage of being devoid of cardiovascular effects even when large doses are rapidly administered. Vecuronium is metabolized by the liver into three active metabolites, and is excreted in the bile and urine [108].

VII. RAPID SEQUENCE INTUBATION (RSI)

This technique is performed when the patient is at risk of pulmonary aspiration and there is reasonable certainty that intubation will be successful (Tables 14 and 15) [100–112]. Although the success rate for RSI was 99% in over 1200 patients [113] a backup plan for failed intubation is absolutely essential since failure to secure the airway can lead to hypoxia and death. Prior to administering drugs, it is essential to perform a brief neurological evaluation and document the Glasgow coma scale score (Tables 16 and 17).

Sellick's maneuver, also known as "cricoid pressure," is the application of force to displace the cricoid cartilage posteriorly and occlude the esophagus to prevent passive

Table 14 Indications for Rapid Sequence Intubation (RSI) in Trauma

Head trauma with need for definitive airway and mechanical ventilation
Combative patient with compromised airway
At risk for pulmonary aspiration (e.g., full stomach)
Uncontrolled seizure activity requiring airway control
Depressed level of consciousness in trauma patient
Hypoxemia refractory to oxygen therapy

Source: Ref. 12.

Table 15 Technique for Rapid Sequence Intubation (RSI) in Trauma

1. Evaluate the airway. If after evaluation of the airway there is sufficient doubt about the ability to successfully intubate, neuromuscular relaxants should not be administered and consideration should be given to securing the airway in another fashion.
2. Assemble necessary equipment (e.g., laryngoscope, suction, stylet, gum-elastic bougie, equipment for failed intubation) and ensure that a neurological assessment with Glasgow coma scale has been done prior to use of neuromuscular relaxants. (See Tables 16, 17.)
3. Preoxygenate with 100% O_2 or ventilate with bag-mask-valve device and 100% O2.[a]
4. If suspected cervical spine injury, apply manual in-line axial stabilization of the head and neck and remove anterior portion of the rigid cervical spine collar.
5. Give appropriate medications IV, as indicated by the clinical setting and hemodynamic status. Flush IV line with 10 ml of crystalloid solution after each drug to ensure delivery to central circulation and to prevent precipitation within the IV line.
   a. Sedative–hypnotics: etomidate 0.1–0.2 mg/kg, thiopental 0.5–2 mg/kg, or ketamine 0.5–1 mg/kg.
   b. Neuromuscular relaxants: succinylcholine 1.0–1.5 mg/kg, rocuronium 1 mg/kg, rapacuronium 1.5–2.5 mg/kg, or vecuronium 0.3–0.4 mg/kg.
   c. Adjunct medications such as opioids (e.g., fentanyl 1–3 ug/kg) or lidocaine, 1.5 mg/kg are given if needed.
6. Apply cricoid pressure.
7. Intubate the trachea 1 min after the relaxant has been flushed in.
8. Release cricoid pressure only after intratracheal placement confirmed (e.g., visualizing tube passing through cords, sustained presence of end-tidal CO_2), and auscultate the patients' lungs.

[a] Some trauma patients will not tolerate 1 min of apnea without significant oxygen desaturation. For this reason, the lungs can be ventilated with 100% O_2 throughout the RSI procedure using inflation pressures < 20 cm H_2O. Ventilation with cricoid pressure is unlikely to cause gastric distension or increase the risk of regurgitation.
Source: Ref. 12.

regurgitation. This is a key step in RSI and in the ventilation or intubation of any patient who is unresponsive. Cricoid pressure should be applied by an assistant and maintained until the tube is properly placed with the cuff inflated.

Cricoid pressure also prevents gastric insufflation during bag-mask ventilation of the patients' lungs, thus allowing for maximal oxygenation prior to, during, and immediately after intubation [114,115]. Bag-mask ventilation using inflation pressures <20 cm H2O together with cricoid pressure is unlikely to introduce any air into the stomach and is especially important in the trauma setting to prevent oxygen desaturation and hypercarbia [26,27,30,116].

VIII. THE CANNOT-INTUBATE SITUATION

A. Incidence of Difficult or Failed Prehospital Intubation and Management

It is generally assumed that tracheal intubation in trauma patients, and in particular in prehospital trauma patients, is more difficult than in elective surgical patients. Published data from prehospital services around the world support this view. Failed intubation rates are not easily compared because many factors vary among different systems. Factors that may affect the rate of failed intubation are listed in Table 18.

Table 16 The Glasgow Coma Scale (GCS)

	Points	Response
Eye opening (invalid if eyes are swollen shut)		
	4	Spontaneous
	3	To speech
	2	To pain
	1	None
Verbal response: invalid in presence of tracheal intubation		
	5	Oriented
	4	Confused
	3	Inappropriate
	2	Incomprehensible
	1	None
Best motor response		
	6	Follows commands
	5	Localizes
	4	Withdraws
	3	Decorticate
	2	Decerebrate
	1	No movement

Note: The GCS provides a brief, simple, standardized measure of the level of consciousness and motor response. The scores from each category are added together. A GCS ≤ 8 indicates a severe head injury, 9–12 a moderate head injury, and 13–15 a minor head injury.

Table 17 Brief Neurologic Evaluation of the Trauma Patient

1. Glasgow coma scale: level of consciousness and motor response
2. Pupillary equality and response to light
3. Lateralized extremity weakness

Note: The initial assessment provides a baseline for sequential reassessment.

Table 18 Factors Affecting Rate of Failed Intubation

Type of personnel (e.g., paramedic, nurse, doctor)
Level of training of personnel (e.g., for doctors: junior/senior, specialist/generalist)
Patient case mix
Use of neuromuscular relaxants/anesthetic agents
Local protocols e.g., if protocols only allow intubation of the severely injured, failed intubation rates may increase)

In physician-led prehospital services, the rate of failed intubation is remarkably constant. The grade and specialty of physicians varies in different services, but drugs are invariably used to facilitate intubation. Failed intubation rates of 3.8–4.5% in the United States [84,117], 3.3% in Israel [118], 3% in Germany [9], 2.7% in Switzerland [119], 0.9% in France [120], and 2.3% in the United Kingdom [121] have been reported. These rates include some patients for whom laryngoscopy was not attempted, either because the severity of injury indicated the need for an immediate surgical airway, or the position of a trapped patient made laryngoscopy impossible. Removing such patients from the analysis brings the rates of failed intubation following laryngoscopy down to 2.8% for the Israeli series and 0.9% for the U.K. series. All patients in the U.S. study had attempts at intubation. As expected, these rates are considerably higher than commonly quoted in-hospital failed intubation rates for the elective general surgical population (approximately 1 in 2000–3000), and also for the obstetric population (approximately 1 in 300) [42].

In non-physician-led prehospital services, failed intubation rates become much less constant. This may be partly due to the practical skill levels and experience of the personnel involved but is complicated by other factors, such as the fact that drugs are often not used to facilitate intubation. This may considerably reduce success rates. In one recent U.S. study involving 97 prehospital intubations, paramedics had an intubation failure rate of 48% [122]. Drugs were not used. In another small study, U.S. flight nurses had a failed intubation rate of 20% *after* the administration of sedative drugs and succinylcholine [123].

Since the administration of drugs can potentially convert a ''cannot intubate'' situation into a rapidly fatal ''cannot-intubate/cannot-ventilate'' situation (see below), such high failure rates are concerning. It is generally accepted in hospital anesthetic practice that administration of a neuromuscular relaxant is contraindicated in patients for whom intubation is likely to be difficult. It seems appropriate that in most prehospital situations, if neuromuscular relaxants are to be administered, the rescuer should be confident of rapidly achieving a definitive airway by some means afterwards.

A recent paper from Germany demonstrated that in a physician-led service a 97% success rate could be achieved in prehospital tracheal intubation without relaxants [9]. Since large doses of midazolam and fentanyl were administered to facilitate intubation, however, a high risk of prolonged apnea is still present.

Successful management of the failed intubation in the prehospital environment should be as simple as possible and preferably protocol-based. The options available will depend on the skills of the rescuer and the available equipment. The urgency of the situation is essentially determined by whether or not oxygenation can be maintained without a definitive airway. This will be discussed further below.

B. How to Manage the Cannot-Intubate Situation

Management of the cannot-intubate situation in the prehospital trauma patient is fundamentally linked to the issues of oxygenation and ventilation and cannot be considered in isolation (see also secs. V.A, V.B, V.C). Where tracheal intubation cannot be achieved but ventilation (either spontaneous or assisted) is adequate to maintain oxygenation, it is likely that transfer to hospital unintubated is the preferred course of action. There may be occasional exceptions to this, but the principle of not worsening an already serious situation is paramount.

Where ventilation or oxygenation cannot be maintained, a definitive airway must be achieved on the scene rapidly to prevent irreversible cerebral hypoxic damage. The techniques used to achieve this will depend on the skills and equipment available to the rescuer.

Simple techniques such as the adjustment of the head position or the removal or adjustment of the cricoid pressure may be all that is required to allow intubation. Backwards pressure over the laryngeal cartilage or optimal external laryngeal manipulation may help improve the view at laryngoscopy [124]. The *BURP maneuver* may also improve the laryngoscopic view (Fig. 11) [125]. This is accomplished by displacing the larynx in three specific directions: (1) *b*ackwards against the cervical vertebrae; (2) *u*pwards, as far superior as possible; and (3) slightly laterally to the *r*ight.

If available, extra equipment may help. The *McCoy laryngoscope* (Figs. 5 and 6) with a hinged blade tip is easily used by most operators and has been shown to improve the view at laryngoscopy when patients are immobilized in a cervical collar [37].

The *gum elastic bougie* (Figs. 9 and 10) has been recommended where only a small part of the laryngeal aperture can be visualized [56,57]. A *lighted stylet* may be used to direct the tracheal tube into the larynx (Figs. 7 and 8). A variety of special laryngoscopes (e.g., Bullard, Wuscope) are available as well.

Although intubation success rates may be improved by the above measures, they should not unduly delay progress if ventilation is not possible. An alternative to tracheal intubation must be urgently sought.

There are a number of alternatives to tracheal intubation that have been employed in trauma patients. The *LMA* (Figs. 12 and 13) is firmly established in the American

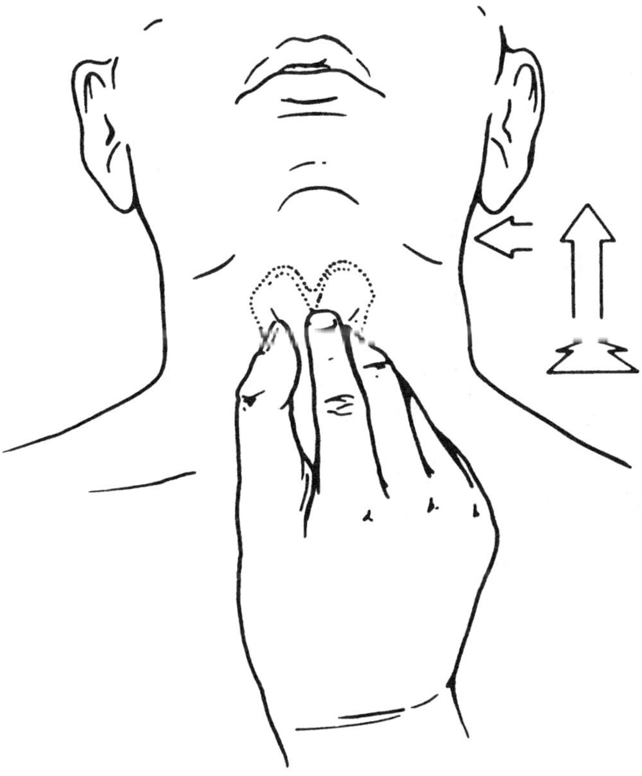

Figure 11 BURP maneuver. The view at laryngoscopy can often be improved by exerting backward, upward, and slightly rightward pressure on the thyroid cartilage. The components of this maneuver can be remembered by the acronym BURP. The arrows indicate the direction of pressure application. (From Ref. 125.)

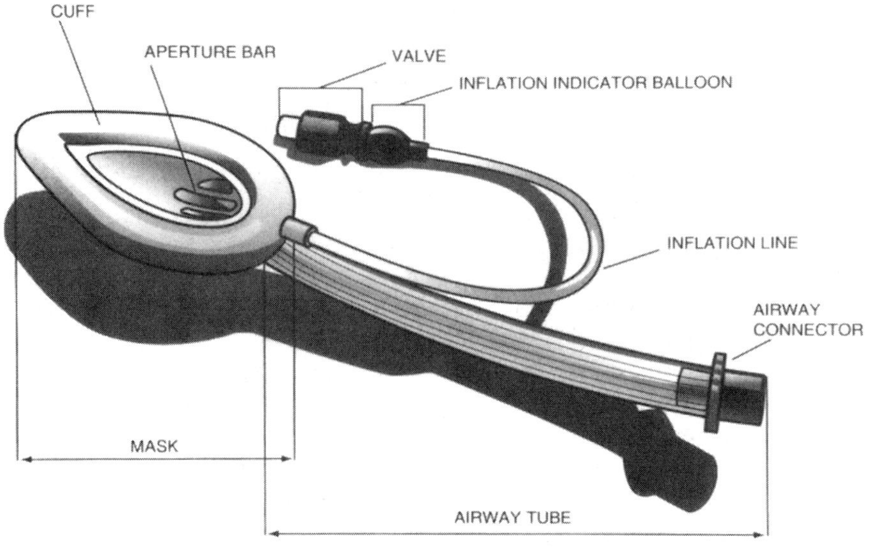

Figure 12 The laryngeal mask airway (LMA) consists of three main components: an airway tube, a mask, and an inflation line. The airway tube has a 15-mm standard male adaptor. The mask is in the form of an elliptical cuff and is designed to conform to the contours of the hypopharynx with the lumen facing the laryngeal aperture. (From LMA North America Inc., with permission.)

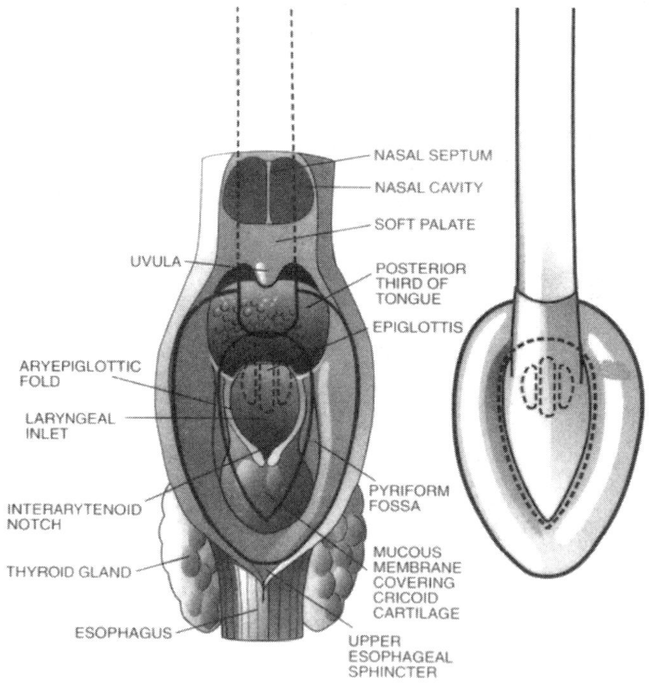

Figure 13 When fully inserted, the distal end of the laryngeal mask airway (LMA) lies with its tip in the inferior recess of the hypopharynx superior to the esophageal sphincter. The sides of the LMA face into the pyriform fossae and the upper body rests against the tongue base. (From LMA North America Inc., with permission.)

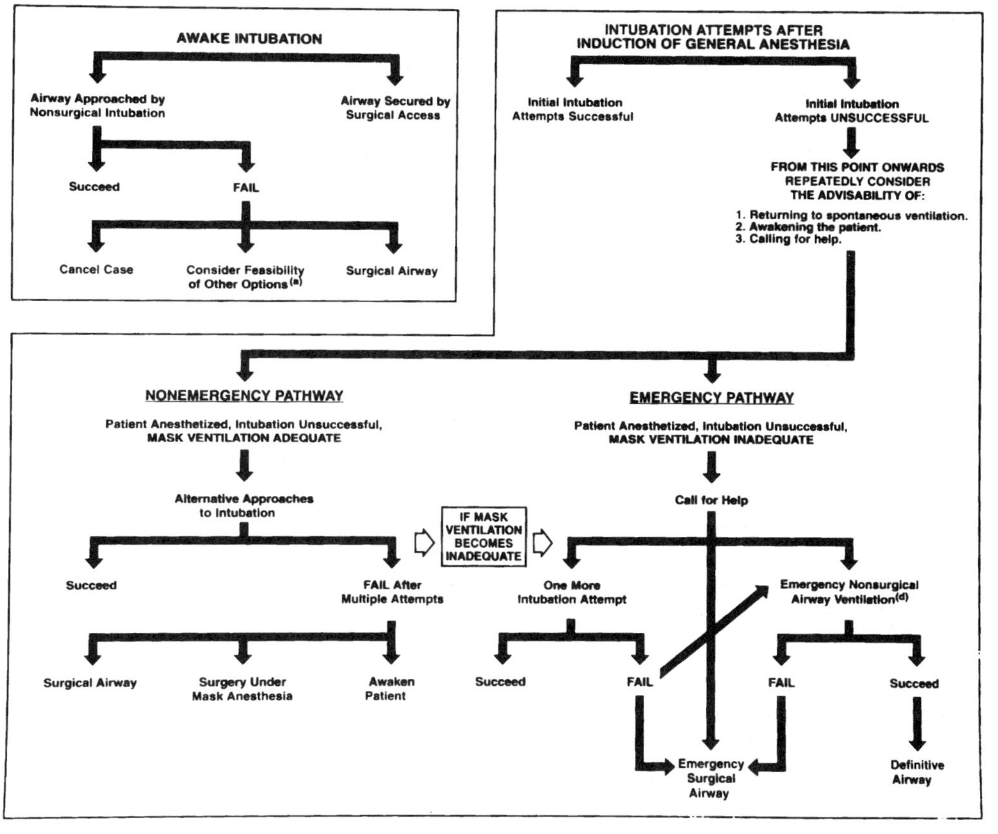

Figure 14 American Society of Anesthesiologists difficult airway algorithm. If intubation and ventilation attempts fail (emergency pathway), the clinician must institute emergency ventilation (laryngeal mask airway, Combitube, transtracheal jet ventilation) or perform a cricothyrotomy. (From Ref. 143a.)

Society of Anesthesiologists difficult airway algorithm [126] (Fig. 14) and in the European Resuscitation Council guidelines [127] as an alternative to intubation. The LMA reliably provides rescue ventilation in cases of failed intubation in both the operating room and in the aeromedical environment [128,129].

It has been shown that paramedics find insertion of the LMA easier than tracheal intubation [130], and an Australian study showed that paramedics have high success rates for LMA insertion in the prehospital environment (Table 19) [131]. Of note, the LMA is available in both adult and pediatric sizes (Table 20).

The *intubating LMA* (iLMA) was designed to have better intubation characteristics than the standard LMA. The cuff portion of the iLMA is identical to the standard LMA, whereas the airway tube has a rigid, silicone-coated stainless steel airway tube (Figs. 15 and 16). The airway tube has a wider diameter and shorter length compared with a standard LMA [132].

The iLMA can be used as an emergency ventilating device or as an aid for ''blind'' or fiberoptic placement of an endotracheal tube of up to 8.0 mm i.d. [133]. Placement of the

Table 19 Laryngeal Mask Airways (LMA)

Mask size	Patient weight (kg)	Internal diameter (mm)	Maximum cuff volume (ml)
1	<5	5.25	4
1 1/2	5–10	6.1	7
2	10–20	7.0	10
2 1/2	20–30	8.4	14
3	30–50	10.0	20
4	50–70	10.0	30
5	>70	11.5	40

Note: LMAs are available in 7 sizes for pediatric and adult use.

iLMA for ventilation may be easier than the standard LMA in patients requiring cervical immobilization [134]. Success rates for blind intubation using the iLMA range from 82–99%. Caution is necessary whenever intubating blindly through an LMA. Blind passage of a tracheal tube through an LMA may convert a partial airway obstruction into a complete one [20]. Laryngopharyngeal injury may occur as well.

Transillumination may enhance the ability to advance the silicone tracheal tube through the iLMA and into the trachea [135]. The mean time to successful intubation after initial placement of the iLMA was 79 sec in 110 patients (range 12–315 sec) [136]. Sixty percent of patients required one adjusting maneuver in order to overcome resistance to passage of the tracheal tube [136].

Because of the more rigid nature of the iLMA, pharyngeal mucosal pressures exceed capillary perfusion pressures [137] and may result in pharyngeal edema [138]. The iLMA is thus unsuitable for use as a routine airway and should be removed after its use as an airway intubator [137].

Table 20 Advantages and Disadvantages of the Laryngeal Mask Airway (LMA)

Advantages	Disadvantages
Easy to insert blindly (direct laryngoscopy not required)	Supraglottic device
Does not require head and neck movement	Risk of aspiration of gastric contents
High skills retention	Requires absent glossopharyngeal reflexes
Multiple sizes: pediatric to adult	Can be dislodged or kinked
No risk of endobronchial or esophageal intubation	Case reports of epiglottic swelling
May protect against aspiration of upper airway material	Leak with positive pressure ventilation, especially if decreased pulmonary compliance
Can be used as a conduit for tracheal intubation	Cannot suction trachea
Less stimulating than tracheal tube	Blind intubation through LMA can cause injury
Disposable LMA available	Rigidity of LMA–Fastrach airway tube can cause pharyngeal edema
Intubating LMA (Fastrach) available	

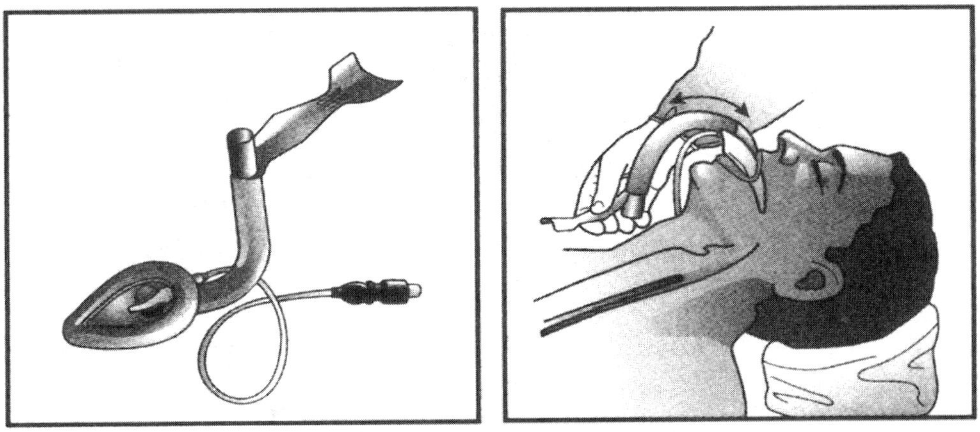

Figure 15 The LMA-Fastrach or intubating laryngeal mask consists of a standard laryngeal mask with epiglottic elevator and a rigid anatomically curved airway. The metal handle facilitates insertion with one hand from various positions without moving the head and neck and without placing the fingers in the mouth. The LMA-Fastrach can be used as a stand-alone airway or as a guide for tracheal intubation. (From LMA North America Inc., with permission.)

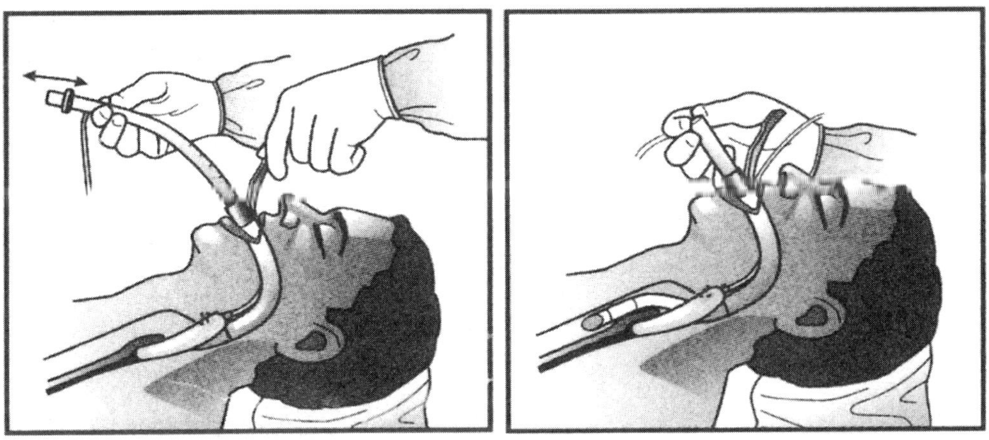

Figure 16 Blind placement of a silicone, wire-reinforced, cuffed tracheal tube through the LMA. Resistance to passage of the tube may be due to a downfolded epiglottis. If this is the case, withdrawing the LMA back outwards (no more than 6 cm) and then reinserting without deflating the cuff can elevate the epiglottis and allow intubation to proceed. Alternatively, a flexible fiberscope can be used. Once successful intubation has occurred, the LMA can be removed. A flexible rod is used to keep the tracheal tube in place while removing the LMA. (From LMA North America Inc., with permission.)

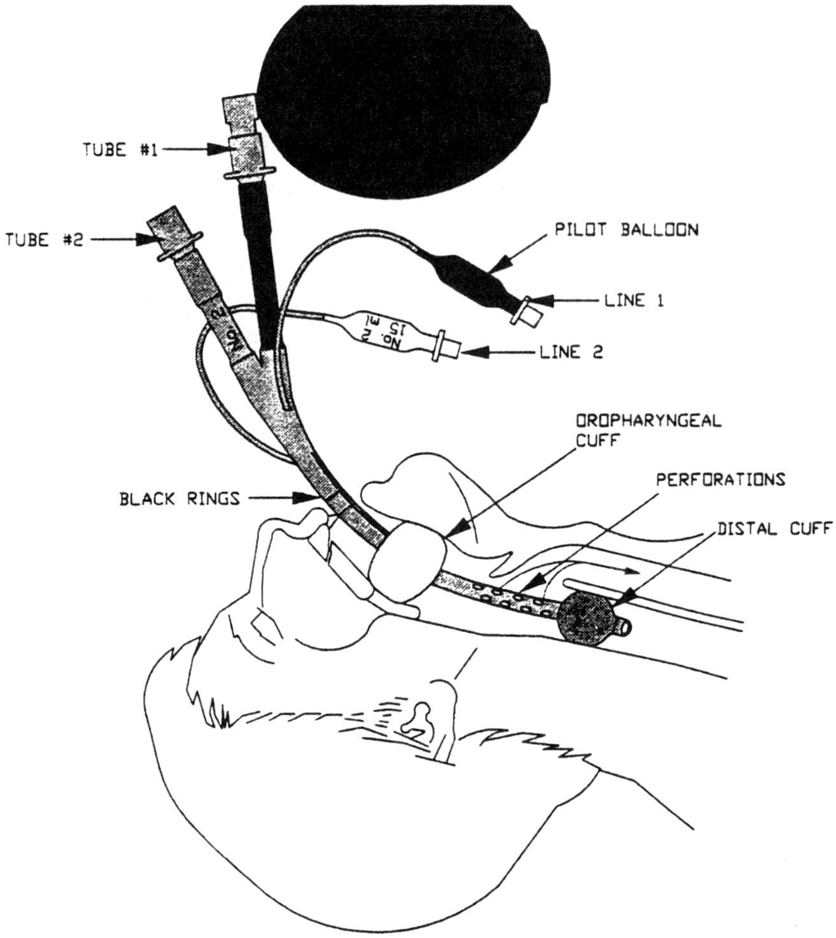

Figure 17 The esophageal tracheal Combitube consists of a double-lumen airway with an outside diameter of 13 mm. After insertion of the Combitube to a point indicated by ring marks on the tube, the oropharyngeal cuff is inflated with 100 ml of air and the distal cuff is inflated with 10–15 ml of air. In the esophageal position, ventilation is via the proximal hypopharyngeal perforations. Note that overinflation of the esophageal balloon (e.g., 40 ml) can lead to esophageal perforation. (From Ref. 123.)

The double lumen *Combitube* (Figs. 17 and 18) has the advantage of blind insertion, and several encouraging studies have been published about its prehospital use [139,140]. Successful insertion and ventilation occurred in 86% of 90 cardiorespiratory arrests [139]. The device has been used effectively in cardiac arrest patients by nurses in intensive care [141]. When used as the airway management technique of first choice by paramedics in the prehospital environment, a success rate of 71% has been reported [142]. More important, in the same study 64% of failed tracheal intubations were successfully managed with the Combitube [142]. In another recent study, in which flight nurses failed to intubate 20% of trauma patients to whom neuromuscular relaxants had been administered, all were successfully managed with the Combitube [123]. In anesthetized paralyzed patients, the

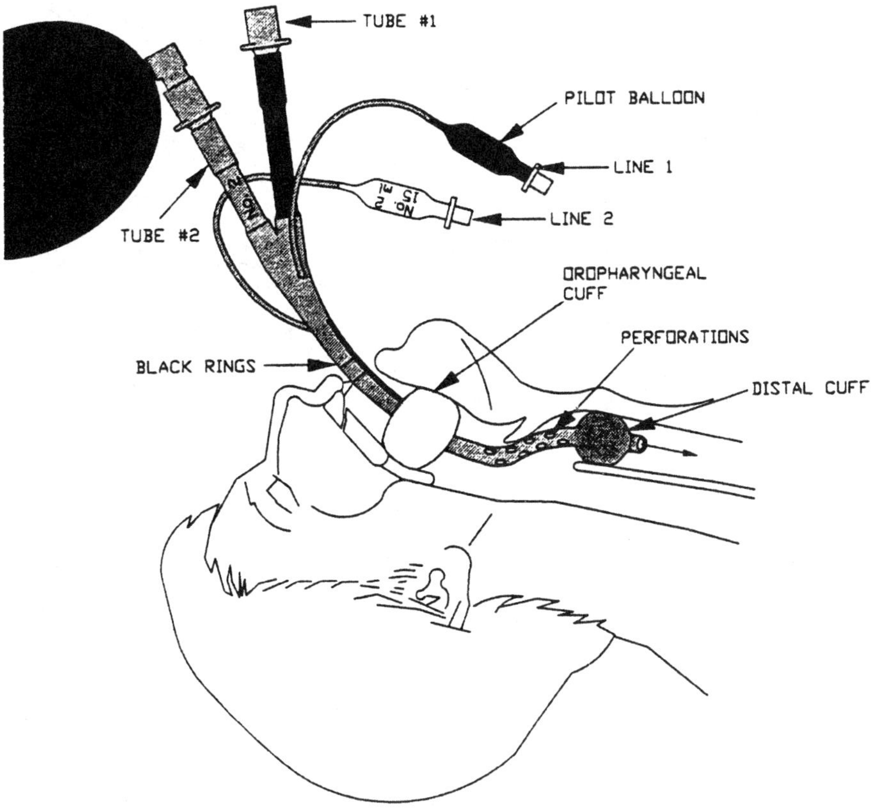

Figure 18 The esophageal tracheal Combitube in the tracheal position. Ventilation is via the distal lumen. (From Ref. 123.)

Combitube was successfully inserted without the aid of a laryngoscope on the first attempt in six of 16 patients (38%) [143]. When a laryngoscope was used, the success rate increased to 94% [143].

Although it was felt by some that the Combitube device might be too complicated to use outside the hospital, these results challenge this view. It may well have a role as an ''airway rescue device'' after failed tracheal intubation, particularly where a rescuer cannot perform a surgical airway. Unfortunately, the Combitube cannot be used in children because it is only manufactured in two sizes: adult (height >5 ft, >1.5 meters) and small adult (height 4–5 ft, 1.2–1.5 meters, Table 21).

Retrograde intubation involves percutaneous puncture of the cricothyroid membrane, threading a guide through the puncture site and out of the mouth, and passing a tracheal tube over the guide and into the trachea [144]. Retrograde intubation allows intubation without head or neck movement and may be effective despite the presence of upper airway trauma, blood, or secretions. Contraindications include a nonpalpable cricothyroid membrane and tracheal stenosis at the puncture site. Relative contraindications consist of goiter, neck abscess, and prominent pyramidal lobe of the thyroid [144].

The last resort in airway management is surgical *cricothyroidotomy* (Fig. 19) [1]. The key to success with this technique is that although it is at the end of most airway

Table 21 Advantages and Disadvantages of the Combitube

Advantages	Disadvantages
Easy to insert blindly	Supraglottic device (esophageal position)
Many protect against aspiration of gastric contents and upper airway material	No pediatric size available; only adult and small adult
Does not require head and neck movement	Requires absent glossopharyngeal reflexes
Allows for tracheal suctioning (tracheal position)	Case reports of esophageal perforation with overinflation of esophageal balloon
Allows for stomach decompression (esophageal position)	Leak with positive pressure ventilation, especially if decreased pulmonary compliance
	May require direct laryngoscopy to facilitate insertion
	Cannot suction trachea (esophageal position)
	Usually needs to be removed prior to tracheal intubation

protocols, where indicated it must be performed early, before hypoxic brain damage occurs. Cricothyrotomy is indicated for emergency airway control in the following settings [145]:

1. Immediate airway required in the blunt trauma patient in whom oral or nasal intubation is not possible
2. Emergency airway required in patients with severe maxillofacial trauma in whom oral or nasal intubation is not possible
3. Immediate airway management in patients for whom other methods fail

A number of studies have been published reporting surgical cricothyroidotomy performed outside the hospital by doctors, nurses, and paramedics. Reports are usually retrospective and involve between 20 and 100 procedures. It is notable that no matter who performs the procedure the success rates are high (between 82% [146] and 100% [117]), perhaps unexpectedly for a procedure that most operators will perform rarely and in difficult circumstances. The proportion of patients having attempted cricothyroidotomy relative to those having intubation is a measure of the failed intubation rate in that system, and by inference, can be a quality assurance indicator.

The lowest rates of surgical airways are seen where doctors administer neuromuscular relaxants [117]. Much higher rates are seen where nurses (18%) [147] or paramedics (15%) [148] attempt to secure the airway (usually without neuromuscular relaxants).

Outcome is not often recorded in these studies, but what is apparent is that patients who have the procedure after cardiac arrest virtually never survive. The other issue is that of training for a rarely performed procedure. It has been estimated that 70% of U.S. paramedics are permitted to perform surgical cricothyroidotomy but that each will on average only do one every 41 years of practice [148]. Where nurses have performed the procedure with excellent success rates [149], it is notable that they have had monthly practical laboratory training.

The single stab through the membrane with a horizontal incision is one that originated (popularly) in ATLS but is not the recommended method [1]. Cricothyrotomy is best performed using a vertical, midline skin incision that is carried down through the anterior cervical fascia, which is located immediately deep to the subcutaneous fat. The

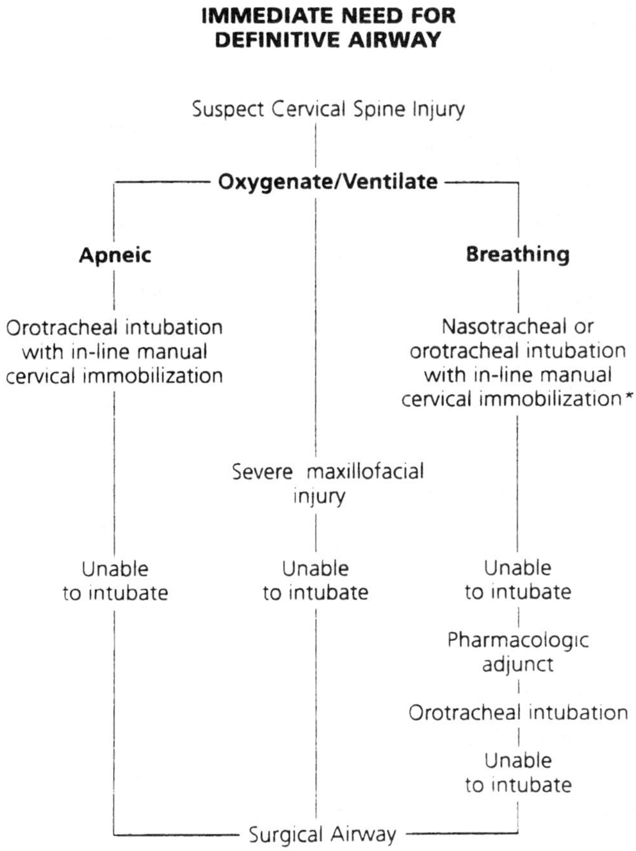

*Proceed according to clinical judgment and skill/experience level.

Figure 19 Airway decision scheme from the Advanced Trauma Life Support Program for Doctors. The algorithm applies to the patient in respiratory distress with a possible cervical spine injury. A surgical airway is generally indicated after failed orotracheal intubation. (From Ref. 1.)

anterior larynx and cricothyroid membrane can then be palpated directly to reconfirm the landmarks. The cricothyroid membrane should be incised transversely (horizontally) through its lower third, because the superior cricothyroid artery and vein traverse the space near its superior extent. After the membrane is opened, the cuffed tracheostomy tube or endotracheal tube can be guided into the airway using a Trousseau dilator and tracheal hook. If the dilator and hook are not available, a large vascular clamp can be used. As with other methods of intubation, confirmation of intratracheal placement with end-tidal CO_2 detection is mandatory [1].

A prepackaged emergency cricothyrotomy catheter set can also be used (Fig. 20). With the Melker set, airway access is achieved utilizing percutaneous entry via the cricothyroid membrane (Seldinger technique) with an 18-G introducer needle and a 0.97-mm stainless steel guide wire with flexible tip. Subsequent dilation of the tract and tracheal entrance permits the introduction of the airway catheter. Thorough familiarity with the cricothyrotomy ''kit'' is recommended before use.

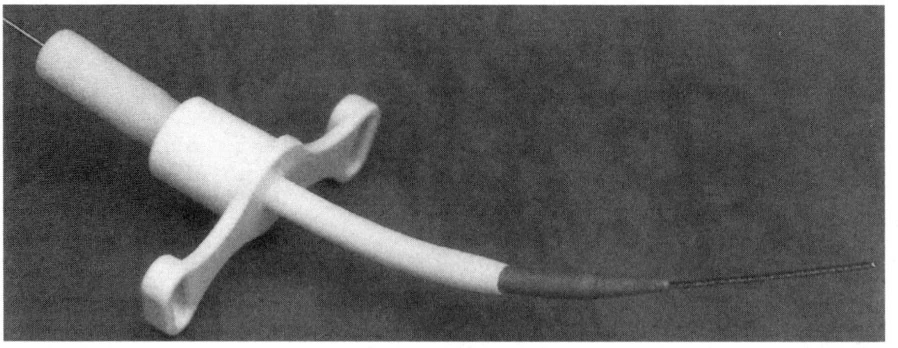

Figure 20 Melker emergency cricothyrotomy catheter set. The airway catheter is positioned over the curved dilator and wire guide. (From Cook Critical Care, Bloomington, IN, 1999, with permission.)

There are few true contraindications to establishing an emergency surgical airway. Relative contraindications to cricothyrotomy include pediatric age group, especially children <10 years old, pre-existing laryngeal pathology, unfamiliarity with the technique, and anatomic barriers such as a large hematoma in the region of the membrane [145].

IX. THE "CANNOT-VENTILATE" SITUATION

Only a few minutes of critical oxygen deprivation are necessary to permanently injure the brain. The often-quoted critical 5 min of apnea in the cardiac arrest patient may in fact be reduced in trauma patients, especially those with head injuries. Hypercarbia secondary to apnea is also an important consideration in victims of head trauma.

An algorithmic approach to the cannot-ventilate situation is shown in Fig. 21. The algorithm presumes that the patient is not ventilating spontaneously on initial assessment. The upper airway should be cleared of any possible foreign body obstruction.

If the patient is conscious on initial assessment but there is both history and evidence of foreign body aspiration and the patient is unable to speak or breathe, then the Heimlich maneuver (subdiaphragmatic abdominal thrusts) should be performed repeatedly until either the foreign body is expelled or the patient loses consciousness. If the patient loses consciousness after unsuccessful attempts at the Heimlich maneuver, direct laryngoscopy should be performed to remove supraglottic foreign bodies, which will then permit bag-mask ventilation and intubation if necessary.

If no foreign body is seen proximal to the vocal cords, the patient should be immediately intubated and the tracheal tube should be pushed all the way down to attempt to move the foreign body into the right (usually) or left mainstem bronchus. The tube is then immediately withdrawn several centimeters to the midtrachea position to permit ventilation of the unobstructed lung [150].

In the absence of an obvious foreign body impaction, the upper airway should be cleared and suctioned, and an oral and nasal airway should be inserted. The patient's head and neck should be repositioned to permit optimal bag-mask ventilation. A tight seal should be obtained with the mask, and if this cannot be done with a one-handed technique, then the most experienced operator should focus on applying the mask to the face and positioning the upper airway using a bilateral jaw thrust technique while an assistant squeezes the bag to provide ventilation.

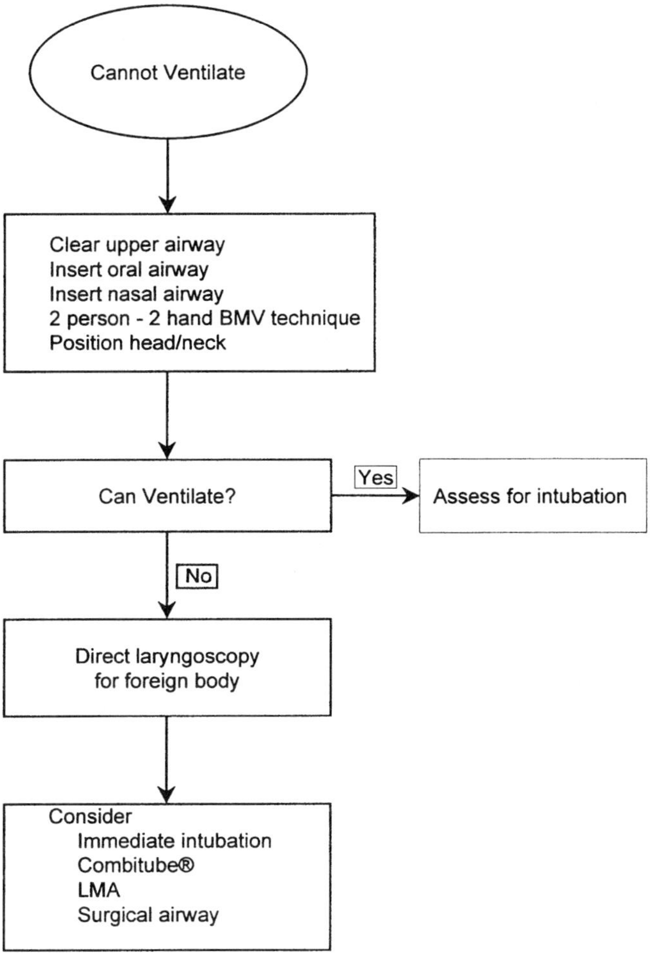

Figure 21 The cannot-ventilate situation is a true emergency. If action is not taken immediately, oxygen saturation will decrease to levels incompatible with neurologic survival. The algorithm assumes that the patient is not ventilating spontaneously. The upper airway should be cleared. Direct laryngoscopy should be performed to remove foreign bodies. If no foreign body is seen proximal to the vocal cords, the trachea should be intubated and the tube pushed all the way down to move the foreign body into a mainstem bronchus. The tube is then withdrawn several centimeters to the midtrachea position to permit ventilation of the unobstructed lung. If intubation is unsuccessful and other methods such as the LMA or Combitube do not establish adequate oxygenation, then local protocols will determine whether cricothyrotomy or needle cricothyrotomy are performed. BMV = bag mask ventilation.

If ventilation is still not successful, additional repositioning should be considered. If the patient cannot be repositioned because of potential cervical spine injury, the risk of this injury must be weighed against the immediate and very real risk of failure of oxygenation. If the risk for cervical spine injury is felt to be low (i.e., low-energy mechanism) then it may be preferable to gently reposition the upper airway, accepting some risk for potential cervical spine injury in order to save the patient's life. This is a judgment call and should be discussed among providers before it is attempted.

Table 22 Causes and Solutions for Ventilation Difficulties in Tracheally Intubated Patients

Cause	Solution/action
Bag malfunction	Replace bag
Endobronchial intubation	Withdraw tube to midtrachea
Endotracheal tube blockage/kink	Suction; if still blocked, replace
Airway obstruction distal to endotracheal tube	Pass endotracheal tube distally into mainstem bronchus, then withdraw to midtrachea and attempt to ventilate again
Tension pneumothorax	Needle thoracostomy/chest drain
Pulmonary resistance (chronic obstructive pulmonary disease, asthma)	Smaller volume, more rapid inspiration, increased expiratory time
Abdominal contents (obesity, term pregnancy)	Reverse Trendelenberg position

If bag and mask ventilation are unsuccessful despite the use of an optimal two-handed technique with the oral and nasal airways in place, then active airway management is required. Active airway management may consist of immediate intubation, placing of a Combitube, placement of an LMA, or other methods according to local protocols. As a blind device to be placed in the esophagus, the Combitube has the advantage of a second lumen to permit ventilation in the unlikely event of tracheal placement. Its predecessor, the older esophageal obturator airway, is a dangerous airway device that has no role in prehospital airway management.

If intubation is unsuccessful and other methods do not establish adequate oxygenation, then local protocols will determine whether cricothyrotomy or needle cricothyrotomy are indicated and possible. Circumstances may arise when the patient cannot be ventilated adequately, even after intubation or placement of a device. In such cases, an orderly assessment should be conducted for correctable causes (Table 22).

X. COMPLICATIONS OF ADVANCED AIRWAY MANAGEMENT

Complications of airway management may be catastrophic (e.g., death; Table 23) or relatively minor (e.g., dental trauma). Reported causes of hypotension after intubation are listed in Table 24. It is reassuring that prehospital maneuvers to secure the airway are usually successful. It falls to those who write local airway protocols and the rescuers themselves to decide on management techniques that are suited to the skill levels of the personnel involved and give good chances of success without an unacceptably high complication rate.

Aspiration of blood or gastric contents into the airway is a major concern in trauma patients and has a significant influence on the way the airway is managed. It is one of the main reasons why a definitive airway (a cuffed tube in the trachea) is the preferred method of securing the airway. The exact incidence and significance of aspiration in various situations is unclear, however. A study in patients who died after cardiopulmonary resuscitation demonstrated pulmonary aspiration in 29%. At postmortem, 49% of the patients had full stomachs [151].

Table 23 Complications of Advanced Airway Management

Hypoxic brain damage and death if airway not secured
Airway compromise by administered drugs (e.g., hypnotics, opioids, neuromuscular relaxants)
Specific complications of administered drugs (e.g., hypotension, arrhythmias, anaphylaxis)
Pulmonary aspiration
Esophageal intubation
Inadvertent extubation/tube displacement
Tracheal cuff rupture
Awareness
Exacerbation of injuries already present (e.g., cervical spine injuries)
Endobronchial intubation and atelectasis
Airway trauma

In trauma patients, several studies have commented on the incidence and significance of aspiration with very different conclusions. Two studies in nonsurvivors of blunt trauma put the incidence of aspiration at 54% [152] and 20% [153]. Another study, which included both survivors and nonsurvivors, documented a rate of 6% [154]. There are two viewpoints on the significance of aspiration. One is that aspiration is a major contributor to preventable trauma deaths [152,155]. The opposing view is that aspiration is of little importance because it occurs only in those patients with non-survivable injuries [153,154]. One point that is clear is that aspiration is usually associated with neurological injury [153–155].

The source of aspiration may also be important. Few papers comment on this. Two small studies suggest that the risk is mainly from blood from the upper airway rather than gastric contents [154,156]. If this is where the major threat of aspiration arises devices such as the LMA could provide protection from aspiration for the majority of trauma patients where a definitive airway cannot be provided.

Table 24 Management of Hypotension After Tracheal Intubation

Cause	Detection	Action
Tension pneumothorax	Increased PIP, difficulty bagging, decreased breath sounds	Needle thoracostomy/chest drain
Decreased venous return	Usually seen in hypovolemic patients or in patients with high PIP and/or PEEP	Fluid bolus, treatment of increased airway resistance (bronchodilators; see also Table 22), decrease tidal volume
Induction agents (e.g., thiopental, propofol)	Usually in hypovolemic patients. Exclude other causes	Fluid bolus, ephedrine, phenylephrine, inotrope, expectant
Cardiogenic shock	Usually in compromised patient. Check ECG. Exclude other causes	Fluid bolus (caution), inotropes

Note: PIP = peak inspiratory pressure; PEEP = positive end expiratory pressure.

XI. SUMMARY OF KEY POINTS

Early and effective airway management can help to prevent secondary complications and improve patient outcome in the prehospital setting.

Endotracheal intubation is the gold standard for airway management. It provides protection of the airway from blood, gastric contents, or swelling, and also ensures a secure airway for general anesthesia and positive pressure ventilation.

Complications resulting from difficulties with airway management include brain injury, myocardial injury, pulmonary aspiration, trauma to the airway, and death.

The presence of shock, respiratory distress, full stomach, airway trauma, cervical spine instability, and head injury all combine to make airway management challenging in trauma.

The administration of drugs to facilitate tracheal intubation is likely to improve failed intubation rates but has potential hazards.

Failed prehospital tracheal intubation has a much higher incidence than in-hospital intubation.

Failure to oxygenate kills, not failure to intubate.

The LMA or Combitube may provide an alternative to tracheal intubation, or rescue the situation after failed intubation.

Surgical cricothyroidotomy should be performed early where indicated.

Adaption of in-hospital procedures for airway management to field conditions continues to evolve.

There is a wide variation in prehospital care systems and prehospital providers.

A worldwide accepted standard for prehospital airway management does not yet exist.

Modified full-scale advanced airway management simulation may provide an excellent means for training prehospital providers.

REFERENCES

1. American College of Surgeons Committee on Trauma. Advanced Trauma Life Support Program for Physicians. Student and instructor manual. Chicago: American College of Surgeons, 1997.
2. N Stocchetti, A Furlan, F Volta. Hypoxemia and arterial hypotension at the accident scene in head injury. J Trauma 40:764–767, 1996.
3. EG Pfenninger, KH Lindner. Arterial blood gases in patients with acute head injury at the accident site and upon hospital admission. Acta Anaesth Scand 35:148–152, 1991.
4. RM Chestnut. Secondary brain insults after head injury: Clinical perspectives. New Hor 3: 366–375, 1995.
5. RJ Winchell, DB Hoyt. Endotracheal intubation in the field improves survival in patients with severe head injury: Trauma Research and Education Foundation of San Diego. Arch Surg 132:592–597, 1997.
6. H Frankel, G Rozycki, H Champion, JD Harviel, R Bass. The use of TRISS methodology to validate prehospital intubation by urban EMS providers. Am J Emerg Med 15:630–632, 1997.
7. T Hatley, OJ Ma, N Weaver, D Strong. Flight paramedic scope of practice: Current level and breadth. J Emer Med 16:731–735, 1998.
8. JS Bradley, GL Billows, ML Olinger, SP Boha, WH Cordell, DR Nelson. Prehospital oral endotracheal intubation by rural basic emergency medical technicans. Ann Emerg Med 32: 26–32, 1998.

9. TG Gerich, U Schmidt, V Hubrich, HP Lobenhoffer, H Tscherne. Prehospital airway management in the acutely injured patient: The role of surgical cricothyrotomy revisited. J Trauma 45:312–314, 1998.
10. DW Spaite, EA Criss, TD Valenzuela, HW Meislin. Pre-hospital advanced life support for major trauma: Critical need for clinical trials. Ann Emerg Med 32:480–489, 1998.
11. JL Falk, MR Sayre. Confirmation of airway placement. Prehosp Emer Care 3:273–278, 1999.
12. B Larmon, DL Schriger, R Snelling, MT Morgan. Results of a 4-hour endotracheal intubation class for EMT-basics. Ann Emerg Med 31:224–227, 1998.
13. A Lippert, FK Lippert, P Foege Jensen, J Nielson. Full-scale simulations in Copenhagen. In: CE Smith, EH Sinz, CM Grande, eds. New Teaching and Training Methods in Trauma Care: Present and Future Role of Simulator Technology. Am J Anesth 27:221–225, 2000.
14. MM Kurrek, JH Devitt, BA McLellan. Full scale realistic simulation in Toronto. In: CE Smith, EH Sinz, CM Grande, eds. New Teaching and Training Methods in Trauma Care: Present and Future Role of Simulator Technology. Am J Anesth 27:226–227, 2000.
15. ET Crosby, A Liu. The adult cervical spine: Implications for airway management. Can J Anaesth 37:77–93, 1990.
16. RH Hastings, JD Marks. Airway management for trauma patients with potential cervial spine injuries. Anesth Analg 73:471–482, 1991.
17. T Kallos, KF Lampe, FK Orkin. Pulmonary aspiration of gastric contents. In: FK Orkin, LH Cooperman, eds. Complications in Anesthesiology. Philadelphia: Lippincott, 1983, pp. 152–164.
18. RS Cicala, KA Kudk, A Butts, et al. Initial evaluation and management of upper airway injuries in trauma patients. J Clin Anesth 3:91–98, 1991.
19. VE Shearer, AH Giesecke. Airway management for patients with penetrating neck trauma: A retrospective study. Anesth Analg 77:1135–1138, 1993.
20. WC Wilson, JL Benumot. Pathophysiology, evaluation, and treatment of the difficult airway. Anesth Clin North Am 16(1):29–75, 1998.
21. JWR McIntyre. The difficult tracheal intubation. Can J Anaesth 34:204–213, 1987.
22. SR Mallampati. Recognition of the difficult airway. In: JL Benumot, ed. Airway Management: Principles and Practice. St Louis: Mosby, 1996, pp. 126–142.
23. JK Stene, CM Grande, CR Barton. Airway management for the trauma patient. In: JK Stene, CM Grande, eds. Trauma Anesthesia. Baltimore: Williams and Wilkins, 1991, pp. 64–99.
24. CE Smith, WF Fallon. Sevoflurane mask anesthesia for urgent tracheostomy in an uncooperative trauma patient with a difficult airway. Can J Anesth [illegible], 2000.
25. RM Walls. Airway management in the blunt trauma patient: How important is the cervical spine? Can J Surg 35:27–30, 1992.
26. JC Criswell, MJ Parr, JP Nolan. Emergency airway management in patients with cervical spine injuries. Anaesthesia 49:900–903, 1997.
27. CM Grande, JK Stene, WN Bernhard. Airwaymanagement: Considerations in the trauma patient. Crit Care Clin 6:37–59, 1990.
28. SC Dronen, KS Merigian, JR Hedges, JW Hoekstra, SW Borron. A comparison of blind nasotracheal and succinylcholine-assisted intubation in the poisoned patient. Ann Emerg Med 16:650–652, 1987.
29. J Li, H Murphy-Lavoie, C Bugas, J Martinez, C Preston. Complications of emergency intubation with and without paralysis. Am J Emerg Med 17:141–144, 1999.
30. CE Smith, JR Peerless. Rational use of neuromuscular blocking agents for emergency airway management in the trauma patient. In: CE Smith, CM Grande, eds. The Use of Neuromuscular Blocking Agents in the Trauma Patient. ITACCS Monograph. New York: McMahon Group, 1996, pp. 3–8.
31. RM Walls. Management of the difficult airway in the trauma patient. Emer Med Clin North Am, 16:45–61, 1998.
32. B Ligier, TG Buchman, MJ Breslow, CS Deutschman. The role of anesthetic induction agents

and neuromuscular blockade in the endotracheal intubation of trauma victims. Surg Gyn Ob 73:477–481, 1991.

33. JL Benumof, R Dagg, R Benumof. Critical hemoglobin desaturation will occur before return to an unparalyzed state after 1 mg/kg intravenous succinylcholine. Anesthesiology 87:979–982, 1997.
34. AS Baraka, SK Taha, MT Aouad, MF El-Khatib, NI Kawkani. Preoxygenation: Comparison of maximal breathing and tidal volume breathing techniques. Anesthesiology 91:612–616, 1999.
35. KJ Heath. The effect on laryngoscopy of different cervical spine immobilisation techniques. Anaesthesia 49:843–845, 1994.
36. RH Hastings, PR Wood. Head extension and laryngeal view during laryngoscopy with cervical spine stabilization maneuvers. Anesthesiology 80:825–831, 1994.
37. DA Gabbott. Laryngoscopy using the McCoy laryngoscope after application of a cervical collar. Anaesthesia 51:812–814, 1996.
38. SC Laurent, AE de Mel, JM Alexander-Williams. The use of the McCoy laryngoscope in patients with simulated cervical spine injuries. Anaesthesia 51:74–75, 1996.
39. F Adnet, RK Cydulka, C Lapandry. Emergency tracheal intubation of patients lying supine on the ground: Influence of operator body position. Can J Anaesth 45:266–269, 1998.
40. KJ Rhee, CB Muntz, PJ Donald, JM Yamada. Does nasotracheal intubation increase complications in patients with skull base fractures? Ann Emerg Med 22:1145–1147, 1993.
41. N Patel, CE Smith, AC Pichak, DE Hancock. Taping methods and tape types for securing oral endotracheal tubes. Can J Anaesth 44:330–336, 1997.
42. ET Crosby, RM Cooper, MJ Douglas, et al. The unanticipated difficult airway with recommendations for management. Can J Anaesth 45:757–776, 1998.
43. DJ Stone, TJ Gal. Airway management. In: RD Miller, ed. Anesthesia, 4th ed. New York: Churchill Livingstone, 1994, pp. 1403–1435.
44. SD Cooper. The evolution of upper-airway retraction: New and old laryngoscopy blades. In: JL Benumof, ed. Airway Management: Principles and Practice. St. Louis: Mosby, 1996, pp. 374–411.
45. PR Saunders, AH Giesecke. Clinical assessment of the adult Bullard laryngoscope. Can J Anaesth 36:S118–S119, 1989.
46. RH Hastings, AC Vigil, R Hanna, et al. Cervical spine movement during laryngoscopy with the Bullard, Macintosh, and Miller laryngoscopes. Anesthesiology 82:859–869, 1995.
47. AD Watts, AW Gelb, DB Bach, DM Pelz. Comparison of the Bullard and Macintosh laryngoscopes for endotracheal intubation of patients with a potential cervical spine injury. Anesthesiology 87:1335–1342, 1997.
48. TL Wu, HC Chou. A new laryngoscope: The combination intubating device. Anesthesiology 81:1085–1087, 1994.
49. CE Smith, TS Sidhu, J Lever, AB Pinchak. The complexity of tracheal intubation using rigid fiberoptic laryngoscopy (Wuscope). Anesth Analg 89:236–239, 1999.
50. CE Smith, AB Pinchak, TS Sidhu, BP Radesic, AC Pinchak, JF Hagen. Evaluation of tracheal intubation difficulty in patients with cervical spine immobilization: Fiberoptic (Wuscope) versus conventional laryngoscopy. Anesthesiology 91:1253–1259, 1999.
51. L Davis, SD Cook-Sather, MS Schreiner. Lighted stylet tracheal intubation: A review. Anesth Analg 90:745–756, 2000.
52. AP Vollmer. Use of a lighted stylet for guided orotracheal intubation in the prehospital setting. Ann Emerg Med 14:324–328, 1985.
53. OR Hung, RD Stewart. Lightwand intubation: I—A new lightwand device. Can J Anaesth 42:820–825, 1995.
54. OR Hung, S Pytka, I Morris, M Murphy, RD Stewart. Lightwand intubation: II—Clinical trial of a new lightwand for tracheal intubation in patients with difficult airways. Can J Anaesth 42:826–830, 1995.

55. HR Paschen. Difficult airway management in trauma—Transillumination devices. Trauma Care 99, Proceedings of the 12th Annual Trauma Anesthesia and Critical Care Symposium, Chicago, May 13–15, 1999.
56. JP Nolan, ME Wilson. Orotracheal intubation in patients with potential cervical spine injuries: An indication for the gum elastic bougie. Anaesthesia 48:630–633, 1993.
57. CE Smith, E Michaels. Tracheal intubation using the gum elastic bougie in an adult patient with epiglottitis: A case report. Amer J Anesthesiol 28:98–100, 2001.
58. SP Nordt, RF Clark. Midazolam: A review of therapeutic uses and toxicity. J Emerg Med 15:357–365, 1997.
59. JK Stene. Midazolam and flumazenil use in trauma patients. In: CE Smith, CM Grande, eds. The use of Midazolam and Flumazenil in Trauma Anesthesia. Baltimore: University of Maryland Medical System, 1999, pp. 2–4.
60. M Lipp, A Thierbach, M Daublander. Perioperative use of midazaolam and flumazenil in trauma. In: CE Smith, CM Grande, eds. The Use of Midazolam and Flumazenil in Trauma Anesthesia. Baltimore: University of Maryland Medical System, 1999, pp. 11–13.
61. J Schou. Midazaolam and flumazenil for prehospital emergency use. In: CE Smith, CM Grande, eds. The Use of Midazolam and Flumazenil in Trauma Anesthesia. Baltimore: University of Maryland Medical System, 1999, pp. 7–9.
62. RK Stoelting. Pharmacology and Physiology in Anesthetic Practice, 2nd ed. Philadelphia: Lippincott, 1991, pp. 368–371.
63. PL Bailey, TH Stanley. Intravenous opioid anesthetics. In: RD Miller, ed. Anesthesia, 4th ed. New York: Churchill Livingstone, 1994, pp. 291–387.
64. JT Abrams, JC Horrow, JA Bennett, et al. Upper airway closure: A primary source of difficult ventilation with sufentanil induction. Anesth Analg 79:913–918, 1993.
65. CE Smith, C Botero, C Holbrook, AC Pinchak, JF Hagen. Rocuronium vs vecuronium during fentanyl induction in patients undergoing coronary artery surgery. J Cardiothor Vasc Anesth 13:567–573, 1999.
66. MLA Sivilotti, J Ducharme. Randomized, double-blind study on sedatives and hemodynamics during rapid-sequence intubation in the emergency department: The SHRED study. Ann Emerg Med 31:313–324, 1998.
67. SL Shafer, JR Varvel. Pharmacokinetics, pharmacodynamics, and rational opioid selection. Anesthesiology 74:53–63, 1991.
68. J Schou. Three techniques for prehospital emergency anaesthesia. JEUR 3:139–145, 1994.
69. American Hospital Formulary Service, Ohmeda Pharmaceutical Products Division. 1995.
70. RJ Fragen, MJ Avram. Barbiturates. In: RD Miller, ed. Anesthesia. 4th ed. New York: Churchill Livingstone, 1994, pp. 229–246.
71. JG Reves, PSA Glass, DA Lubarsky. Nonbarbiturate intravenous anesthetics. In: RD Miller, ed. Anesthesia. 4th ed. New York: Churchill Livingstone, 1994, pp. 247–289.
72. J Nolan. Pharmacology of propofol in the trauma patient. In: CM Grande, CE Smith, eds. Propofol in Trauma Anesthesia: An Evolving Perspective. New York: Intamed, 1996, pp. 8–14.
73. CA Botero, CE Smith, C Holbrook, AM Chavez, NJ Snow, JF Hagen, AC Pinchak. Total intravenous anesthesia with propofol-ketamine during coronary artery surgery. J Cardiothor Vasc Anesth 2000.
74. CP Kingsley. Perioperative management of thoracic trauma. Anesth Clin North Amer 17(1): 183–195, 1999.
75. WE Hoffman, D Pelligrino, C Werner, et al. Ketamine decreases plasma catecholamines and improves outcome from incomplete cerebral ischemia in rats. Anesthesiology 76:755–762, 1992.
76. R Kohrs, ME Durieux. Ketamine: Teaching an old drug new tricks. Anesth Analg 87:1186–1193, 1998.
77. CP Kingsley. Perioperative use of etomidate for trauma patients. In: CE Smith, CM Grande,

eds. Perioperative Use of Etomidate in Trauma. New York: McMahon Group, 1996, pp. 1–7.
78. CM Grande, CE Smith, JK Stene. Trauma anesthesia. In: DE, Longnecker, JH Tinker, GE Morgan, eds. Principles and Practice of Anesthesiology. 2nd ed. St. Louis: Mosby, 1998, pp. 2138–2164.
79. M Lipp, A Thierbach, M Daublander. Use of etomidate in trauma. In: CE Smith, CM Grande, eds. Perioperative Use of Etomidate in Trauma. New York: McMahon Group, 1996, pp. 7–8.
80. F Adnet, B Hennequin, C Lapandry. Induction anesthetique en sequence rapide pour l'intubation tracheale prehospitaliere. Ann Fr Anesth Rean 17:688–698, 1998.
81. RL Wagner, PF White, PB Kan, et al. Inhibition of adrenal steroidogenesis by the anesthetic etomidate. New Eng J Med 310:1415–1421, 1984.
82. IM Ledingham, I Watt. Influence of sedation on mortality in critically ill multiple trauma patients (letter). Lancet 1:1270, 1983.
83. PP Rai, AP Winnie. Immediate reactions to local anesthetics. In: FK Orkin, LH Cooperman, eds. Complications in Anesthesiology. Philadelphia: Lippincott, 1983, pp. 51–74.
84. MA Wayne, E Friedland. Prehospital use of succinylcholine: A 20-year review. Prehosp Emerg Care 3:107–109, 1999.
85. CE Smith. Clinical issues and perspectives: Is succinylcholine obsolete for the intubation of trauma patients? Trauma Care 8(1):17–18, 1998.
86. DR Bevan. Succinylcholine in the emergency department. Trauma Care 8(1):18, 1998.
87. DR Bevan. Complications of muscle relaxants. Semin Anesth 14:63, 1995.
88. DE Schwartz, B Kelly, JE Caldwell, AS Carlisle, NH Cohen. Succinylcholine-induced hyperkalemic arrest in a patient with severe metabolic acidosis and exsanguinating hemorrhage. Anesth Analg 75:291–293, 1992.
89. WD Kovarik, TS Mayberg, AM Lam, et al. Succinylcholine does not change intracranial pressure, cerebral blood flow velocity, or the electroencephalogram in patients with neurologic injury. Anesth Analg 78:469–473, 1994.
90. MM Libonati, JJ Leahy, N Ellison. The use of succinylcholine in open eye surgery. Anesthesiology 62:637–640, 1985.
91. CE Smith, G Lewis, F Donati, DR Bevan. Dose-response relationship for succinylcholine in a patient with genetically determined low plasma cholinesterase activity. Anesthesiology 70:156–158, 1989.
92. AC Pinchak, CE Smith, LS Shepard, L Patterson. Waiting time alters muscle fasciculation response after succinylcholine in adult patients. Can J Anaesth 41:206–212, 1994.
93. DJ Cullen. The effect of pretreatment with nondepolarizing muscle relaxants on the neuromuscular blocking action of succinyclcholine. Anesthesiology 35:572–578, 1971.
94. GD Shorten, BM Braude. Pulmonary aspiration of gastric contents after a priming dose of vecuronium. Paediat Anaesth 7:167–169, 1997.
95. J Musich, LP Walts. Pulmonary aspiration after a priming dose of vecuronium. Anesthesiology 64:517–518, 1986.
96. L Aziz, SM Jahangir, SN Choudhury, K Rahman, Y Ohta, M Hirakawa. The effect of priming with vecuronium and rocuronium on young and elderly patients. Anesth Analg 85:663–666, 1997.
97. T Magorian, KB Flannery, RD Miller. Comparison of rocuronium, succinylcholine, and vecuronium for rapid-sequence induction of anesthesia in adult patients. Anesthesiology 79: 913–918, 1993.
98. N Patel, N Kamath, CE Smith, AC Pichak, JH Hagen. Tracheal intubating conditions and neuromuscular blockade after divided dose mivacurium and single dose rocuronium: A double blinded randomized study in adult patients. Can J Anaesth 44:49–53, 1997.
99. N Patel, C Botero, CE Smith, et al. Tracheal intubating conditions and orbicularis oculi neuromuscular block during modified rapid sequence intubation. Amer J Anesth 25:15–20, 1998.

100. KC McCourt, L Salmela, RK Mirakhur, et al. Comparison of rocuronium and suxamethonium for use during rapid sequence induction of anaesthesia. Anaesthesia 53:867–871, 1998.
101. JH Levy, GK Davis, J Duggan, F Szlam. Determination of the hemodynamics and histamine release of rocuronium (Org 9426) when administered in increased doses under N2)/O2-sufentanil anesthesia. Anesth Analg 78:318–321, 1994.
102. JM Wierda, L Van Den Broek, JH Proost, et al. Time course of action and endotracheal intubating conditions of Org 9487, a new short-acting steroidal muscle relaxant: A comparison with succinylcholine. Anesth Analg 77:579–584, 1993.
103. R Purdy, DR Bevan, F Donati, JL Lichtor. Early reversal of rapacuronium with neostigmine. Anesthesiology 91:51–57, 1999.
104. Rapacuronium package insert. 1999, pp. 1–6. Organon Inc., West Orange, New Jersey.
105. NW Fleming, F Chung, PSA Glass, JB Kitts, H Kirkegaard-Nielson, GA Gronert, V Chan, TJ Gan, N Cicutti, JE Caldwell. Comparison of the intubating conditions provided by rapacuronium (ORG 9487) or succinylcholine in humans during anesthesia with fentanyl and propofol. Anesthesiology 91:1311–1317, 1999.
106. JH Levy, M Pitts, A Thanopoulos, F Szlam, R Bastian, J Kim. The effects of rapacuronium on histamine release and hemodynamics in adult patients undergoing general anesthesia. Anesth Analg 89:290–295, 1999.
107. WC Tullock, P Diana, R Cook, et al. Neuromuscular and cardiovascular effects of high-dose vecuronium. Anesth Analg 70:86–90, 1990.
108. CE Smith, JR Peerless. Use of neuromuscular blocking agents for trauma patients in the intensive care unit. In: CE Smith, CM Grande, eds. Muscle Relaxants in the Trauma Patient. New York: McMahon Group, 1996, pp. 16–21.
109. RM Walls. The decision to intubate. In: RM Walls, et al, eds. Manual of Emergency Airway Management. 3rd ed. Wellesley, MA: Airway Management Education Center, 1999.
110. RM Walls. Rapid sequence intubation in head trauma. Ann Emerg Med 22:1008–1013, 1993.
111. CE Smith. Rapid sequence intubation: Indications and concerns. Clin Pulm Med 2001, in press.
112. CE Smith, CM Grande, MA Wayne, D Gonzalez, MT Murphy, DR Bevan, CR Barton, DM Lacombe. Rapid Sequence Intubation (RSI) in Trauma. Trauma Care 97, 10th Annual Trauma Anesthesia and Critical Care Society Symposium, Baltimore, May 1997.
113. RM Walls, MJ Sagarin, RJ Vissers, JC Sakles, [illegible], ED Barton, RE Wolfe. Confirmation of endotracheal tube placement—Analysis of 1,288 emergency department intubations. Acad Emerg Med 5:482, 1998.
114. BA Sellick. Cricoid pressure to control regurgitation of stomach contents during induction of anaesthesia. Lancet 2:404–406, 1961.
115. EG Lawes, I Campbell, D Mercer. Inflation pressure, gastric insufflation and rapid sequence induction. Brit J Anaesth 59:315–318, 1987.
116. CM Grande, CE Smith, JK Stene. Evaluation of the trauma patient. In: DE Longnecker, JH Tinker, GE Morgan, eds. Principles and Practice of Anesthesiology. 2nd ed. St. Louis: Mosby, 1998, pp. 572–600.
117. RM Miklus, C Elliott, N Snow. Surgical cricothyrotomy in the field: Experience of a helicopter transport team. J Trauma 29:506–508, 1989.
118. D Leibovici, B Fredman, ON Gofrit, J Shemer, A Blumenfeld, SC Shapira. Prehospital cricothyroidotomy by physicians. Am J Emerg Med 15:91–93, 1997.
119. I Fleisch, E Buchser, O Moeschler. Pre-hospital tracheal intubation: A retrospective study of compliance with a set of criteria. Brit J Anaesth 80 (suppl. 1):165, 1998.
120. F Adnet, NJ Jouriles, P Le Toumelin, et al. Survey of out-of-hospital emergency intubations in the French prehospital medical system: A multicenter study. Ann Emerg Med 32:454–460, 1998.

121. London Helicopter Emergency Medical Service, Royal London Hospital. Trauma database. London.
122. SB Karch, T Lewis, S Young, D Hales, CH Ho. Field outcome of trauma patients: Complications, indications and outcomes. Am J Emerg Med 14:617–619, 1996.
123. PA Blostein, AJ Koestner, S Hoak. Failed rapid sequence intubation in trauma patients: Esophageal tracheal Combitube is a useful adjunct. J Trauma 44:534–537, 1998.
124. JL Benumof, SD Cooper. Quantitative improvement in laryngoscopic view by optimal external laryngeal manipulation. J Clin Anesth 8:136–140, 1996.
125. RL Knill. Difficult laryngoscopy made easy with a "BURP." Can J Anaesth 40:279–282, 1993.
126. JL Benumof. The laryngeal mask airway and the American Society of Anesthesiologists difficult airway algorithm. Anesthesiology 84:686–699, 1996.
127. Guidelines for the advanced management of the airway and ventilation during resuscitation: A statement by the airway and ventilation management working group of the European Resuscitation Council. Resuscitation 31:201–230, 1996.
128. JL Parmet, P Colonna-Romano, JC Horrow, et al. The laryngeal mask airway reliably provides rescue ventilation in cases of unanticipated difficult tracheal intubation along with difficult mask ventilation. Anesth Analg 87:661–665, 1998.
129. SE Martin, MG Ochsner, RH Jarman, WE Agudelo, FE Davis. Use of the laryngeal mask airway in air transport when intubation fails. J Trauma 47:352–357, 1999.
130. JH Pennant. Comparison of the endotracheal tube and laryngeal mask in airway management by paramedical personnel. Anesth Analg 74:531–534, 1992.
131. HG Grantham, G Phillips, JE Gilligan. The laryngeal mask in pre-hospital emergency care. Emer Med 1:217–219, 1994.
132. J Nolan. The intubating laryngeal mask airway. Trauma Care 99, Proceedings of the 12th Annual Trauma Anesthesia and Critical Care Symposium, Chicago, May 13–15, 1999.
133. C Schuschnig, B Waltl, W Erlacher, et al. Intubating laryngeal mask and rapid sequence induction in patients with cervical spine injury. Anaesthesia 54:787–797, 1999.
134. T Asai, AU Wagle, M Stacey. Placement of the intubating laryngeal mask is easier than the laryngeal mask during manual in-line neck stabilization. Brit J Anaesth 82:712–714, 1999.
135. V Dimitriou, GS Voyagis. Light-guided tracheal intubation using a prototype illuminated flexible catheter through the intubating laryngeal mask. Eur J Anaesth 16:448–453, 1999.
136. F Agro, J Brimacombe, M Carassiti, et al. The intubating laryngeal mask: Clinical appraisal of ventilation and blind tracheal intubation in 110 patients. Anaesthesia 53:1084–1090, 1998.
137. C Keller, J Brimacombe. Pharyngeal mucosal pressures, airway sealing pressures, and fiberoptic position with the intubating versus the standard laryngeal mask airway. Anesthesiology 90:1001–1006, 1999.
138. K Nakazawa, N Tanaka, S Ishikawa, et al. Using the intubating laryngeal mask airway (LMA-Fastrach™) for blind endotracheal intubation in patients undergoing cervical spine operation. Anesth Analg 89:1319–1321, 1999.
139. CJ Rumball, D MacDonald. The PTL, Combitube, laryngeal mask, and oral airway: A randomized prehospital comparative study of ventilatory device effectiveness and cost-effectiveness in 470 cases of cardiorespiratory arrest. Prehosp Emer Care 1:1–10, 1997.
140. K Tanagawa, A Shigematsu. Choice of airway device for 12,020 cases of nontraumatic cardiac arrest in Japan. Prehosp Emerg Care 2:96–100, 1998.
141. T Straudinger, S Brugger, B Watschinger, M Roggla, C Dielacher, T Lobl, D Fink, R Klauser, M Frass. Emergency intubation with the Combitube: Comparison with the endotracheal airway. Ann Emerg Med 22:1573–1575, 1993.
142. GL Atherton, JC Johnson. Ability of paramedics to use the Combitube in prehospital cardiac arrest. Ann Emerg Med 22:1263–1268, 1993.
143. MJ Bishop, ED Kharasch. Is the Combitube a useful emergency airway device for anesthesiologists? Anesth Analg 86:1141–1142, 1998.

143a. American Society of Anesthesiologists. Practice guidelines for management of the difficult airway. Anesthesiology 78:597–602, 1993.
144. JL Parmet, S Metz, AJ Schwartz. Anesthesiology issues in general surgery: Retrograde endotracheal intubation: An underutilized tool for management of the difficult airway. Contemp Surg 49(5):1–7, 1996.
145. RM Walls. Cricothyrodotomy. Emerg Med Clin North Am 6(4):725–737, 1988.
146. R Oliver, C Rockyvich, SR Petersen. Prehospital cricothyroidotomy in 100 trauma patients. J Trauma 1:159, 1993.
147. W Nugent, KJ Rhee, DH Wisner. Can nurses perform surgical cricothyroidotomy with acceptable success and complication rates? Ann Emerg Med 20:367–370, 1991.
148. JB Fortune, DG Judkins, RPA Scanzaroli, KB McLeod, SB Johnson. Efficacy of prehospital surgical cricothyroidotomy in trauma patients. J Trauma 42:832–838, 1997.
149. MF Boyle, D Hatton, C Sheets. Surgical cricothyroidotomy performed by air ambulance flight nurses: A 5 year experience. J Emerg Med 11:41–45, 1993.
150. AR Thierbach, MDW Lipp. Airway management in trauma patients. Anesth Clin North Amer 17(1):63–81, 1999.
151. EG Lawes, PJ Baskett. Pulmonary aspiration during unsuccessful cardiopulmonary resuscitation. Intens Care Med 13:379–382, 1987.
152. DW Yates. Airway patency in fatal accidents. Brit Med J 2:1249–1251, 1977.
153. A Ottosson. Aspiration and obstructed airways as the cause of death in 158 consecutive traffic fatalities. J Trauma 25:538–540, 1985.
154. BP McNicholl. The golden hour and pre-hospital care. Injury 25:251–254, 1994.
155. LM Hussain, AD Redmond. Are pre-hospital deaths from accidental injury preventable? Brit Med J 308:1077–1080, 1994.
156. D Lockey, T Coats, MJA Parr. Aspiration in severe trauma: A prospective study. Anaesthesia 54:1097–1098, 1999.

14

Oxygenation, Ventilation, and Monitoring

STEPHEN H. THOMAS

Massachusetts General Hospital and Harvard Medical School, Boston, Massachusetts

SUZANNE K. WEDEL

Boston Medical Center/Boston University School of Medicine and Boston MedFlight, Boston, Massachusetts

MARVIN WAYNE

Emergency Medicine Services, City of Bellingham and Whatcom County, Bellingham, Washington; University of Washington, Seattle, Washington; and Yale University, New Haven, Connecticut

I. INTRODUCTION

The second item in the ABCs of resuscitation—breathing—encompasses both oxygenation and ventilation. After the airway is secured, the prehospital care provider must ensure that patients are adequately oxygenated and appropriately ventilated. While not as inherently exciting as achieving a difficult intubation in the field, the securing and ongoing monitoring of oxygenation and ventilation comprise the vital ''follow-through'' to initial airway management. Given the limitations inherent to the use of traditional auscultation in their practice environment, prehospital care providers have learned to employ other means of assessing respiratory performance. Some of these surrogate measures (see Table 1) are low-tech yet effective: observation of patient color, endotracheal tube fogging, or chest rise and resistance associated with bag-valve-mask ventilation. Other measures employed to follow patients' oxygenation and ventilation are even more effective, if somewhat more technical. This chapter will address the prehospital monitoring of oxygenation and ventilation, with emphasis on pulse oximetry and carbon dioxide monitoring, and will also discuss prehospital mechanical ventilation.

Table 1 Nontechnical Means of Respiratory Assessment in the Prehospital Setting

Auscultation (often not feasible)
Observation of patient color
Endotracheal tube fogging
Chest rise with ventilation
Chest resistance with manual ventilation

II. OXYGENATION AND PULSE OXIMETRY

For this chapter's purposes, *ensuring oxygenation* can be operationally defined as optimizing delivery of O_2 to the lungs, from where oxygenated blood flows to the pulmonary and systemic circulations, and ultimately to tissues. The importance of ensuring adequate oxygenation is reflected by the oxygen-critical nature of many injury patterns (e.g., head injury, hypotensive shock) encountered by prehospital care providers.

While there can be no doubt about the importance of assessing clinical correlates of oxygenation, such as patient color or neurologic status, the standard indicator of oxygenation is the blood gas, which reports the partial pressure of oxygen (pO_2) in arterial blood. In the prehospital setting, however, the primary means used to assess and report oxygenation is the percentage of hemoglobin saturated with oxygen—the S_aO_2—as measured by a pulse oximeter.

A. The Pulse Oximeter Device

The pulse oximeter unit consists of a probe, an analytic unit, and a visual display. The probe contains two light sources and two light sensors. It sends two slightly different wavelengths of light through a small area of tissue containing a pulsatile capillary bed. Oxyhemoglobin and deoxyhemoglobin differentially absorb the two wavelengths; it is this absorption information that is used by the analytic unit to calculate the ratio of oxyhemoglobin to reduced hemoglobin, and thus enable the display of the percentage oxygen saturation of available hemoglobin (S_aO_2).

The most common pulse oximeter probe device is one that is placed on the finger. Other probe devices can be placed to assess the vascular beds of the ear, nose, toe, or other sites, depending on the clinical situation.

B. The Use of Pulse Oximetry

As denoted by the classic hemoglobin oxygen dissociation curve (Fig. 1), there is a nonlinear relationship between the oxygen saturation and the total amount of oxygen carried by the blood. As the oxygen saturation decreases, the amount of oxygen carried by the hemoglobin decreases drastically. For example, an S_aO_2 drop from 100% to 90% corresponds to P_aO_2 drop from 100 mmHg (13.3 kPa) to 60 mmHg (8.0 kPa); at this S_aO_2 level the 10% decrement in saturation signals a 40% reduction in the blood's oxygen-carrying capacity.

Continuous pulse oximetry, now widely regarded as the standard of care for prehospital transport of critically injured patients [1], was reported useful in the prehospital setting as early as 1988 [2]. Subsequent experiences have confirmed the utility of prehospital pulse oximetry in prehospital programs worldwide [3–5]. In all patients, the ability to identify hypoxia allows prehospital care providers to act early to secure the airway or to

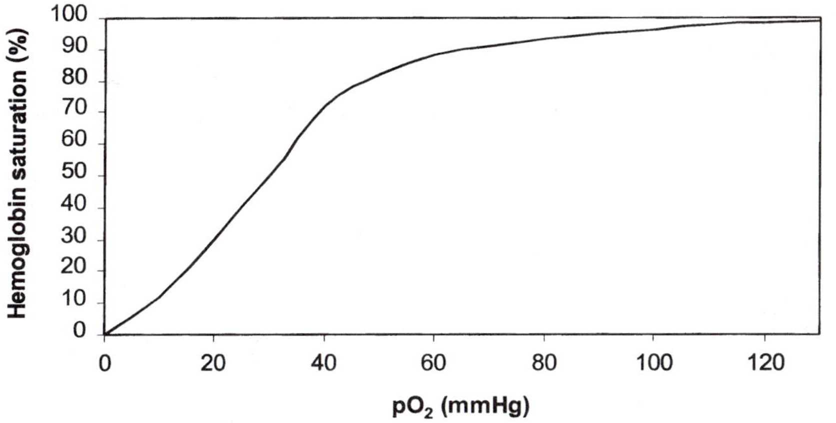

Figure 1 Hemoglobin oxygen dissociation curve.

increase oxygenation by other means, thus preventing health care providers from reacting only when—and if—hypoxia subsequently becomes clinically obvious. The pulse oximeter has been shown to be particularly useful for early identification of hypoxia in susceptible patients, such as those with chest or head injuries [3].

There are instances in which continuous reliable pulse oximetry is difficult to obtain, and many of these circumstances are particularly likely to be encountered in the prehospital setting (see Table 2). Reports on pulse oximetry have generally been quite favorable to its application in the out-of-hospital environment, demonstrating its ability to detect clinically occult hypoxia [6,7]. Pulse oximeters may fail, however, (due to hypoperfusion or difficulty in assessing the capillary bed), in patients who are hypothermic or profoundly hypotensive, or in burn or cardiac arrest patients. If carbon monoxide exposure or any dyshemoglobinemia is present, pulse oximetry can fail to identify hypoxemia. In either case the abnormal hemoglobin may absorb light in much the same way as oxyhemoglobin, thereby causing oximetry to show falsely high (normal) values. When the studies thus far are considered, however, occasional pulse oximetry failure has not detracted from the effective employment of this technology in the prehospital setting. Prehospital pulse oximetry is highly useful, as long as caregivers understand the effects of hypoperfusion and other factors that may give inadequate or false values. In clinical practice, pulse oximetry data displayed in the absence of an adequate wave form should be considered uninterpretable. In fact, the absence of a consistent pulse wave from the pulse oximeter probe can be used as clinical evidence of localized (at least) hypoperfusion unless there are physical reasons (e.g., dark nail polish) for lack of transcapillary signal transmission.

Table 2 Circumstances in Which Pulse Oximetry May Not Be Reliable

Hypoperfusion (e.g., shock, cardiac arrest)
Hypothermia, including localized (e.g., digital) hypothermia
Hypotension
Burns involving skin overlying capillary beds to be assessed
Dyshemoglobinemia

In summary, pulse oximetry has a consistent track record of utility in the prehospital arena. Given the demonstrated incidence of clinically occult hypoxia, this technology should be employed for all patients in whom there is any question of the development of hypoxia, and prehospital care providers should consider pulse oximetry as a standard of care (a "fifth vital sign") for all critical patients.

III. VENTILATION AND CO_2 MONITORING

Whereas early detection of hypoxia has long been a priority for prehospital care providers, identification of hypercapnia as an indicator of poor ventilation has received somewhat less attention. Much of this relative neglect doubtless results from a longstanding technology gap between pulse oximetry and its corresponding assessor of ventilation: continuous carbon dioxide (CO_2) monitoring. Continuous CO_2 monitors have been in use in the operating room for years, but until recently their size and expense relegated these devices to infrequent use in the emergency department and prehospital settings [4]. In recent years, however, enhanced stability of solid state electronics and computer technology has allowed these devices to become not only portable, but handheld (Fig. 2).

A. Respiratory (CO_2) Physiology

Before discussing CO_2 monitoring, a brief review of the underlying physiology is appropriate. With normal pressure and temperature, CO_2 is a colorless and odorless gas. Its concentration in air—0.03%—is so low that the atmospheric pCO_2 can, for our purposes, be considered zero. At rest, the average adult produces approximately 2.5 mg/kg/min of

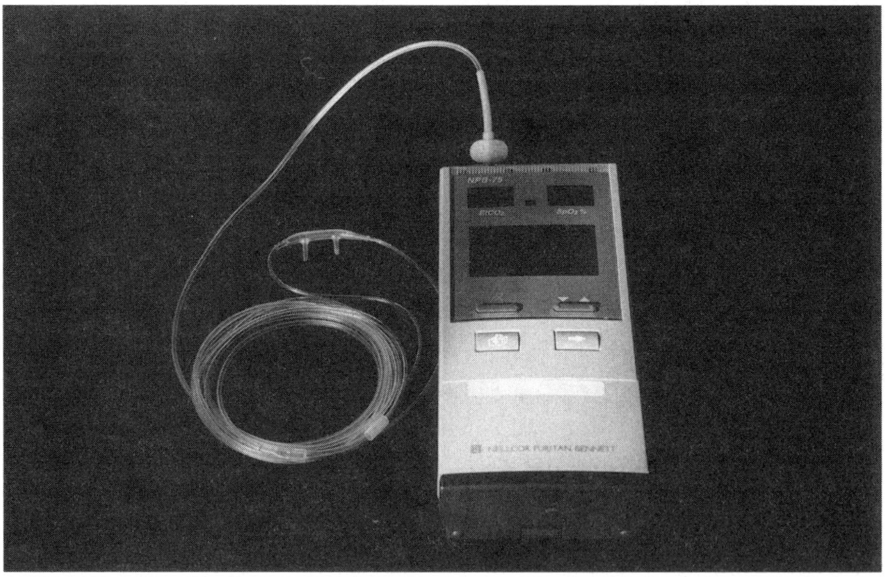

Figure 2 Continuous CO_2 monitor. Unlike most CO_2 monitors, which are used in intubated patients, this monitor's nasal cannula sensing system is designed for use in nonintubated patients. Other CO_2 monitors may be incorporated into multifunction monitoring systems.

CO_2. This CO_2 is then transported via the blood—in one of three forms—to the lungs, where it is excreted via alveolar ventilation. The majority of the CO_2 (60–70%) is transported via the bicarbonate ion, after conversion by red blood cell carbonic anhydrase. The next 20–30% of CO_2 is bound to plasma proteins as carbamino compounds. The remaining 5–10% is transported in physical solution in the plasma. This physically dissolved CO_2 represents the partial pressure or pCO_2. Once the CO_2 is transported to the lungs via the blood, it is reconstituted and diffuses into the alveoli. The driving mechanism for this diffusion is the partial pressure difference between the CO_2 in the pulmonary capillaries and the alveoli. Under normal conditions, this equilibrium is reached in less than 0.5 sec, although the time may be prolonged with some pulmonary pathologies.

The partial pressure of CO_2 in the arterial blood (P_aCO_2) therefore becomes a measure of the efficiency of ventilation. Further, because of the need for CO_2 transport via the blood, CO_2 excretion may be an indirect measure of cardiac output. Just as the measurement of arterial CO_2 is termed P_aCO_2, so is the measurement of end-exhalation levels of CO_2 termed end-tidal CO_2 ($ETCO_2$). Based upon physiologic considerations in the ideal situation, it follows that the $ETCO_2$ should provide a reflection of the P_aCO_2. There are important limitations to this assumption that warrant specific mention, however.

In healthy patients, the difference between $ETCO_2$ and P_aCO_2 is roughly 5 to 6 mmHg (just under 1 kPa). Patients undergoing transport, however, are often critically ill and therefore have a number of reasons to have suboptimal pulmonary function. Such alterations in pulmonary function have direct consequences limiting extrapolation of P_aCO_2 from $ETCO_2$. Clinically, the most important factor is ventilation-perfusion mismatching. In the presence of increased dead-space ventilation (e.g., pulmonary embolism, diminished cardiac output) the measured $ETCO_2$ underestimates P_aCO_2 due to the admixture of dead-space (non-CO_2-containing) air with exhaled air. Another factor that can affect $ETCO_2$–P_aCO_2 differences are CO_2 ''sampling'' errors related to tachypnea and/or shallow respirations; in these situations the CO_2 detected by the sampling device does not truly reflect alveolar CO_2. The importance of the preceding situations is that clinically the $ETCO_2$ should be used more for trend analysis than for absolute determination of P_aCO_2.

B. CO_2 Monitoring Devices

In CO_2 monitoring devices used in the prehospital setting the measurement is accomplished by the use of infrared, Raman spectrometer, or mass spectrometer technology. The sample is obtained either by a ''sidestream system'' (in which the sample is pulled from the source [i.e., the patient's airway] and delivered to a distant analyzer), or by a ''mainstream'' system (in which the sensor is in line in the patient's breathing circuit).

The advantage of a mainstream system (see Table 3) is that there is less need for tubing, decreased dead space, and the theoretical ability to obtain a more accurate sample. The mainstream device also can be incorporated directly into the endotracheal tube, as near to the source (alveolar space) as possible. This ability to be incorporated into the airway circuit may obviate a measurement time delay that can occur with some sidestream systems.

The advantages of a sidestream system include easier monitoring of the nonintubated patient, possible reduction in equipment cost, and newer technologies that obviate some of the time delay in signal recognition.

Table 3 Mainstream vs. Sidestream CO_2 Sampling

Advantages of mainstream sampling
Sampling device can be incorporated into the endotracheal tube.
Less need for tubing (which can be cumbersome in prehospital setting).
Decreased dead space since sampling device is closer to alveolar air.
Direct sampling results in theoretically more accurate measurement.
Lack of measurement time delay that can occur with sidestream sampling.
Advantages of sidestream sampling
Relatively easy monitoring of nonintubated patients.
Possible reduction in equipment costs.
Newer technologies are improving performance and minimizing problems associated with sampling time delays.

C. Use of CO_2 Monitoring

There are two types of data obtainable by prehospital CO_2 monitors. The *capnograph* is the measurement and numerical display of end-tidal CO_2 or the partial pressure of CO_2 appearing in the patient's airway during the entire respiratory cycle. This term also refers to the graphic display of the CO_2 concentration or partial pressure in a ''waveform'' format (Fig. 3). If the capnograph display is properly calibrated, capnography includes *capnometry*, which is a numerical display of $ETCO_2$ intended to reflect alveolar ventilation. As compared with capnometry, capnography provides the means to assess not only alveolar ventilation, but also the integrity of the airway, proper functioning of the respiratory delivery system, ventilator function, cardiopulmonary function, subtleties of rebreathing, and other fine points in the respiratory cycle (see Figs. 4–6) [8]. The ability to follow this additional respiratory information may be especially useful in the prehospital environment, in which auscultation may be limited by extraneous noise or other environmental conditions.

The information provided by the capnograph can be best analyzed by a systematic approach based on understanding both the goals and the role of capnography as a diagnos-

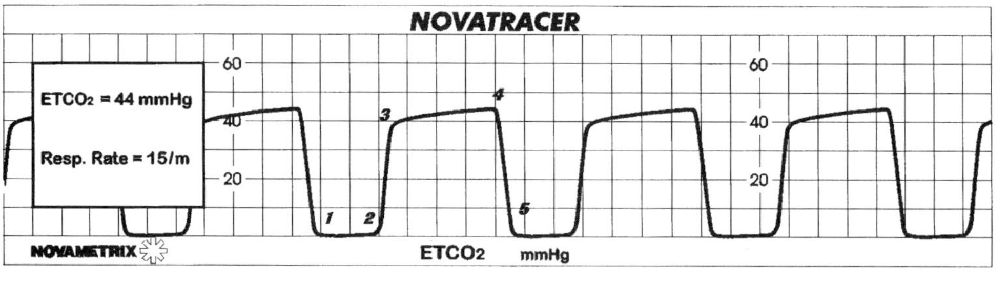

Figure 3 Normal capnogram, with single breath represented by numbers 1 through 5. The 1–2 segment represents early exhalation, with minimal CO_2 present in the gas from tracheal dead space. The 2–3 segment is usually sharp and contains a mixture of alveolar and dead space gas (washout of dead space gas). The 3–4 segment is the plateau phase (alveolar plateau), with point 4 representing end-tidal CO_2. The 4–5 segment represents inspiration with little CO_2 reentering the airway. (Conversion note: 7.5 mmHg = 1kPa). (Capnograph figures courtesy of Novametrix Medical Systems Inc., Wallingford, CT.)

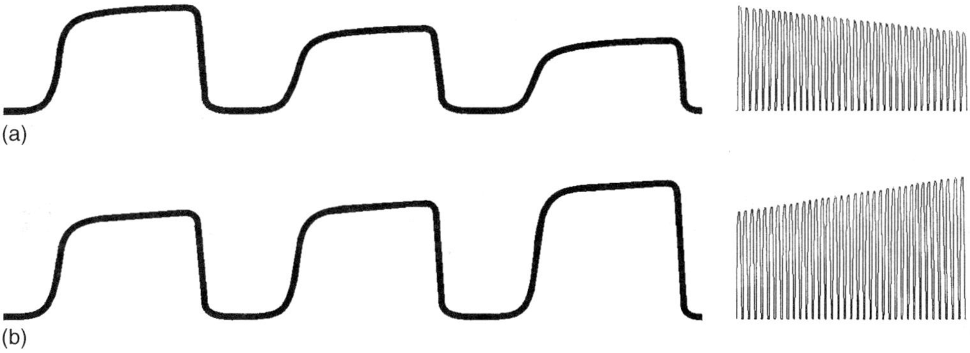

Figure 4 Capnogram tracings used as monitors of trends in hyperventilation and hypoventilation. In a and b, the left portion of the diagram is depicted on a time scale similar to that of Fig. 3, while the right portion of each tracing is time-compressed. Time compression allows for easier determination of trends in $ETCO_2$ (reflected by the peaks on the tracing) from hyperventilation (a) or hypoventilation (b). (Capnograph figures courtesy of Novametrix Medical Systems Inc., Wallingford, CT.)

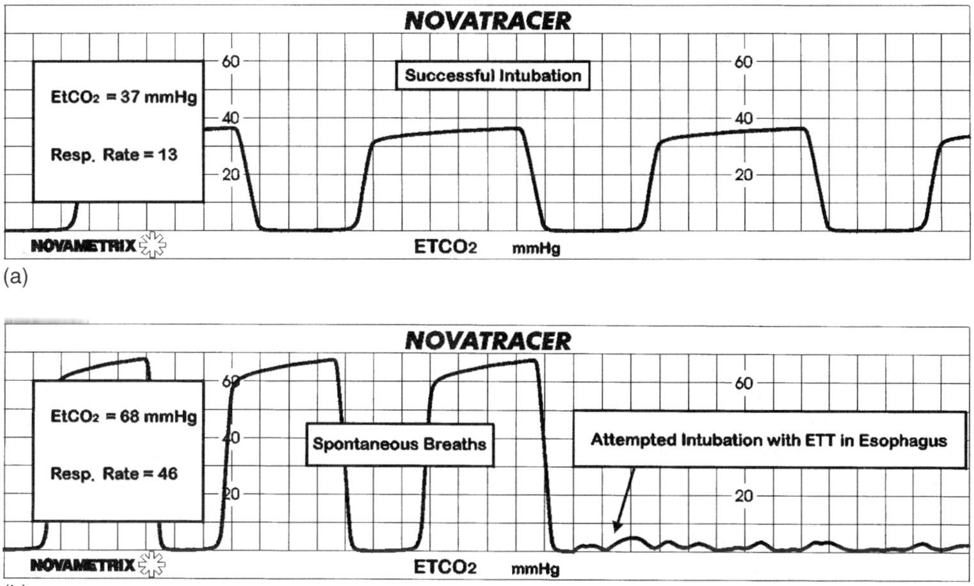

Figure 5 Capnogram tracings in patients undergoing successful (a) and unsuccessful (b) endotracheal intubation. The patient represented in (a) was spontaneously breathing prior to intubation, which was successful and resulted in continued normal appearance of the capnograph; (b) depicts an esophageal intubation occurring in a patient intubated for impending respiratory failure and hypoventilation (note the high end-tidal $ETCO_2$ value); the postintubation tracing shows no resemblance to expected normal capnography. (Conversion note: 7.5 mmHg = 1kPa). (Capnograph figures courtesy of Novametrix Medical Systems Inc., Wallingford, CT.)

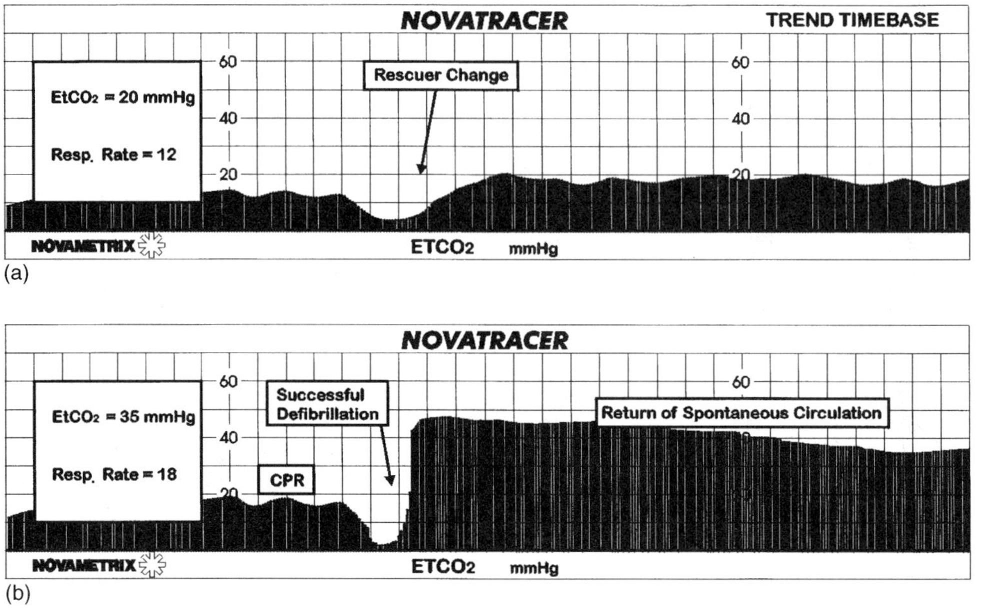

Figure 6 Capnography in the setting of cardiopulmonary resuscitation. The capnographs are time-compressed to allow easier determination of end-tidal CO_2 trends. (a) depicts the utility of capnography in assessing adequacy of chest compressions; improvement in $ETCO_2$ is noted when the tired rescuer is relieved. (b) shows the capnograph of a patient undergoing successful resuscitation as demonstrated by increased $ETCO_2$ readings. When perfusion is restored, a normal tracing and $ETCO_2$ return. (Conversion note: 7.5 mmHg = 1kPa). (Capnograph figures courtesy of Novametrix Medical Systems Inc., Wallingford, CT.)

tic tool. This discussion will focus on developing such an approach as relates to the role of prehospital capnography, addressing two primary issues related to CO_2 monitoring: (1) determination as to whether or not CO_2 is present, and (2) analysis and clinical interpretation of the appearance of the capnograph.

The first question to be addressed in reviewing CO_2 monitoring information is if exhaled CO_2 is present. If there is no CO_2 production, and there is no circuit disconnect or mechanical explanation, then critical failure exists in either ventilation or circulation. Clinically this means there may be an esophageal intubation (see Fig. 5), total airway obstruction, apnea, cardiac arrest, or failure to restore cardiopulmonary function with external compressions (see Fig. 6). No other device or technique has proven more effective at the detection of esophageal intubation or in documenting the failure to restore cardiopulmonary function [9–11].

Capnography is particularly well suited for field use in rapidly detecting whether successful endotracheal tube placement has occurred or whether adequate compressions are being performed during CPR (see Figs. 5 and 6). Given the primary importance of airway management in the prehospital setting, this niche alone would appear to justify widespread utilization of field CO_2 monitoring as the technology becomes cheaper. In fact, a form of CO_2 monitoring—the colorimetric CO_2 indicator (Fig. 7)—has long been proven to be of utility in the prehospital setting. The simplest of these detectors, attached to the proximal end of an endotracheal tube (Fig. 7), exhibits a color change in the presence

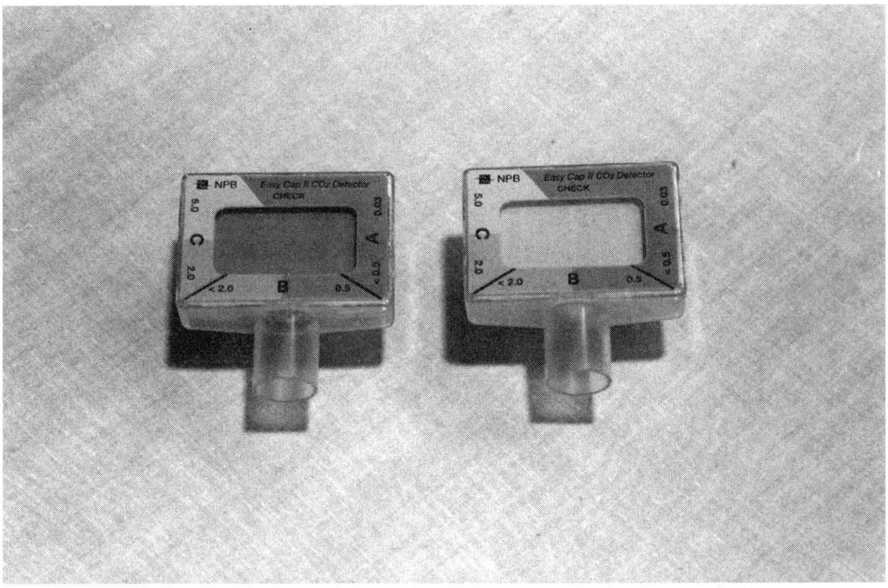

Figure 7 Though the photo is in black and white, the figure is representative of the clear change in indicator color from dark (purple in true color, device on left) to light (yellow in true color, device on right) in the presence of CO_2.

of exhaled carbon dioxide. Newer colorimetric CO_2 devices (Fig. 7) serve as quantitative capnometers, with four distinct color shades allowing delineation of varying levels of CO_2.

Colorimetric CO_2 indicators have been demonstrated to work well in nonarrest patients in the field [13,14]. There are limitations to the colorimetric devices, however. In an arrest setting, failure of CO_2 generation by the body can result in a negative colorimetric reading despite appropriate endotracheal intubation. False-positive readings are less of a problem, but can occur when color change occurs as a result of reflux of acidic gastric secretions or when intragastric CO_2 is released into the esophagus after the ingestion of carbonated beverages.

While colorimetric CO_2 monitors can answer the question "Is there CO_2 present?" and can begin to quantify the amount of CO_2 in exhaled gases, the capnograph can go further. As there are now handheld devices allowing field capnography, more detailed discussion of the capnograph is indicated as prehospital ventilatory monitoring increases in sophistication. The additional clinical information provided by the capnograph lies in the appearance of its displayed segments (see Figs. 3–6). The portions of the capnograph to be examined are the baseline segment, expiratory upstroke segment, and end-tidal CO_2 measurement. For the following discussion, the reader is referred to the capnograph in Figure 3.

The most likely clinically significant change in the baseline segment (between points 1 and 2 on the capnograph in Fig. 3) is an increase in the height of this segment, representing an increased inspiratory baseline CO_2 level. The most common cause is partial rebreathing secondary to inadequate ventilation or low gas flow. Other causes may be an incompetent expiratory valve and its effect on the tidal volume.

The next capnograph segment, the expiratory upstroke (between points 2 and 3 in

Table 4 Causes of Hypercapnia and Hypocapnia

Causes of hypercapnia [CO_2 > 45 mmHg (6 kPa)]
Alveolar hypoventilation
CO_2 rebreathing (e.g., obstruction or other problem with mechanical ventilation)
Increase in CO_2 delivery (e.g., exogenous HCO_3 administration)
Causes of hypocapnia [CO_2 < 35 mmHg (4.7 kPa)]
Alveolar hyperventilation (e.g., overaggressive manual ventilation)
Decreased CO_2 delivery (e.g., hypothermia, decreased cardiac output)
Increased arterial-to-exhaled CO_2 difference (e.g., V/Q mismatch from pulmonary embolism, mucous plugging, or mainstem intubation)

Fig. 3) may become slanted (prolonged) when gas flow is obstructed. The obstruction may be in either the breathing system (e.g., kinked endotracheal tube or mucous plug) or the patient's airway (e.g., during bronchospasm).

The final point on the capnograph (point 3 in Fig. 3) represents the end-tidal CO_2. Clinically important changes in the $ETCO_2$ can occur in either direction (see Fig. 4).

Causes of hypercapnia (increase in exhaled CO_2 > 45 mmHg [6 kPa]; see Table 4) are grouped into (1) alveolar hypoventilation, (2) CO_2 rebreathing, and (3) an increase in CO_2 delivery. Causes of CO_2 rebreathing include poor mechanical ventilation or failure, system leaks, inadequate fresh gas flow, disconnection, or obstruction. Increased delivery is usually secondary to exogenous (e.g., HCO_3 administration) or endogenous CO_2 production (e.g., fever, stress, muscle activity, malignant hyperthermia).

Causes of hypocapnia (decrease in exhaled CO_2 < 35 mmHg [4.7 kPa]; see Table 4) are categorized as (1) alveolar hyperventilation (e.g., aggressive ventilation), (2) decreased CO_2 delivery (e.g., hypothermia, decreased cardiac output) and, (3) increased arterial-to-exhaled CO_2 difference (e.g., V/Q mismatching secondary to pulmonary embolism, anesthesia, trauma, mucous plugging, or main stem intubation).

Uses of CO_2 monitoring (see Table 5) specific to the continuous CO_2 devices considered at this time are: (1) continuous monitoring of the airway, and thus endotracheal tube placement, during transport, (2) ventilatory control during transport of the patient with a potential head injury, (3) facilitation of controlled hypercapnia (such as in critical care transports involving severe pulmonary disease), and (4) assessment of the severity of ventilatory fatigue (CO_2 retention).

A scenario likely to be encountered in the prehospital setting, and one in which continuous CO_2 monitoring has been reported useful by aeromedical programs [14] would be a head-injured patient in whom controlled ventilation is employed to prevent development of hypercarbia. (See more on this controversial topic in the head injury chapter.) Those with head injuries comprise one of many groups of ill or injured patients in whom pretransport assessment of arterial blood gases (ABGs) can be useful to establish baseline

Table 5 Uses of CO_2 Monitoring in the Prehospital Setting

Intratransport monitoring of airway patency
Continuous monitoring of correct endotracheal tube positioning
Optimization of ventilatory control (e.g., in head-injured patients)
Facilitation of controlled hypercapnia (e.g., in patients with severe pulmonary disease)
Continuous monitoring for early signs of ventilatory fatigue and early respiratory depression
Monitoring for signs of effective cardiopulmonary resuscitation

information and correlate the ABG-indicated arterial CO_2 with the exhaled CO_2 level indicated by the transport capnometer.

An additional use of CO_2 monitoring is based on the fact that when pulmonary ventilation is constant, changes in cardiac output are accompanied by parallel changes in exhaled CO_2 [11,15,16]. This translates into potential uses of CO_2 monitoring in the assessment of resuscitation status and even prediction of death in patients with pulseless electrical activity [11,15,17]. In the setting of resuscitation assessment, CO_2 monitoring allows the tracking of production of CO_2 as an index of cellular metabolic activity and tissue perfusion with subsequent transport of CO_2 to the lungs. When the endotracheal tube is appropriately placed in the airway, a lack of CO_2 detection represents evidence of lack of functional perfusion and circulation. In patients with pulseless electrical activity, such a lack of perfusion bodes poorly for chances at successful resuscitation.

Besides the obvious advantages associated with early identification of respiratory embarrassment, there is a final important but as yet unproven use of capnometry in the nonintubated trauma patient receiving opioid analgesics in the field. In preliminary report [18,19] of prehospital use of the potent opioid fentanyl for trauma analgesia in nonintubated patients, the authors acknowledge that occult hypoventilation could occur due to fentanyl-induced respiratory depression. Such hypoventilation is particularly dangerous in prehospital patients, many of whom have possible head injury. Noninvasive CO_2 monitoring (Fig. 2), with proven utility in detecting occult hypoventilation in E.D. patients receiving fentany [20], is currently undergoing evaluation in the prehospital setting. If early (as yet unpublished) experience at one air transport program is confirmed by longer-term demonstration of this system's reliability and effectiveness, noninvasive CO_2 monitoring technology could assist prehospital care providers in their efforts to safely administer field analgesia to nonintubated trauma patients.

In summary, CO_2 monitoring in the prehospital setting has demonstrated utility with in-line monitors used in intubated patients [4,21]. Based on these reports and the increasing comfort with continuous CO_2 monitoring technology, the use of continuous capnography in intubated patients is expected to increase with the passage of time. Monitoring CO_2 in nonintubated patients, still in its infancy in the prehospital environment, may well prove beneficial in future studies of this technology's use in the field. Finally, while electronic CO_2 monitoring (e.g., capnography) devices represent the future state of the art in prehospital monitoring, preliminary investigation [22] has recently advocated use of the colorimetric devices as a surrogate for in-line capnometry when the latter technology is unavailable. The utility of colorimetric CO_2 monitoring devices remains unproven in this setting, but the relatively low cost and ease of use of these devices may translate into their wider use in the future for indications (e.g., monitoring of manual ventilation with semiquantitative capnometry) other than simple confirmation of endotracheal tube position.

Prehospital CO_2 monitoring provides the advanced emergency medical services provider with real data to make diagnostic and therapeutic decisions previously made based largely on guesswork. The use of CO_2 monitoring devices represents another step in the extension of the intensive care unit level of care to the prehospital setting.

IV. CONFIRMATION OF ENDOTRACHEAL TUBE PLACEMENT AND TUBE STABILIZATION

The first and most important aspect of monitoring that must occur after intubation is confirmation of the correct placement of the tube in the trachea. This is discussed in detail in the chapter on airway management, but it is worth reminding the reader that the assessment of endotracheal tube placement is an ongoing process that continues throughout transport. Endotracheal tube dislodgments do occur and are to some degree unavoidable, so prehospital care providers must always have an eye on monitoring the correct intratracheal position of the tube.

The devices mentioned in this chapter for monitoring oxygenation and ventilation are also useful as indicators of correct endotracheal tube positioning. Pulse oximetry and CO_2 monitoring—in all of its forms—provide clinicians with supportive means for continuous assessment of airway positioning and patency.

Prehospital practitioners, as part of securing oxygenation and ventilation, should take all reasonable precautions against endotracheal tube dislodgment (accidental extubation). While this problem has been reported to be rare in the air transport setting [23] there are few data available for ground transports. Given the fact that reintubation may be relatively difficult in the transport setting, however, special care should be given to pretransport airway stabilization. Even when accidental extubation does not occur, inappropriate mobility of the endotracheal tube may result in tracheal damage or induction of a gag or cough with a resultant rise in intracranial pressure [23]. Investigators have reported the utility of various devices (Fig. 8) designed to securely immobilize the endotracheal tube for prehospital transport, and it is recommended that all prehospital care providers consider using commercial endotracheal tube stabilizers, which provide more reliable tube stabilization than tape [23].

V. MANUAL VERSUS MECHANICAL VENTILATION

Once the endotracheal tube is confirmed to be in the trachea and oxygenation is initially secured, a decision must be made as to whether patients in the prehospital setting should undergo manual (i.e., bag-valve-mask) or mechanical ventilation. The choice of ventilatory method is sometimes difficult. The advantages and disadvantages of each ventilatory method (see Table 6) must be carefully considered in the light of the unique setting of prehospital care. This section discusses the general advantages and disadvantages of manual versus mechanical ventilation, while the final section addresses mechanical ventilation techniques in detail.

A. Manual Ventilation

The advantages of manual ventilation include ease of use and the ''feel'' of bagging. On the other hand, even the simplest transport ventilators require a certain amount of time investment to set up. They also may have settings, monitors, and tubes with which the prehospital team must deal. In addition, there is a loss of the feel of compliance obtained with manual ventilation. Experienced providers of manual ventilation note that the sense of compliance afforded by bag-valve-mask ventilation provides important clinical feedback in an environment in which many standard clinical monitoring parameters (e.g., auscultation) may fail. The feel of manual ventilation is reported to allow prehospital care providers to monitor for marked changes in compliance due to the development of tension pneumothorax or endotracheal tube obstruction or dislodgment [24].

B. Mechanical Ventilation

In favor of mechanical ventilation, extensive literature in the critical care arena suggests that manual ventilation, no matter how expert the provider, often results in unintentional

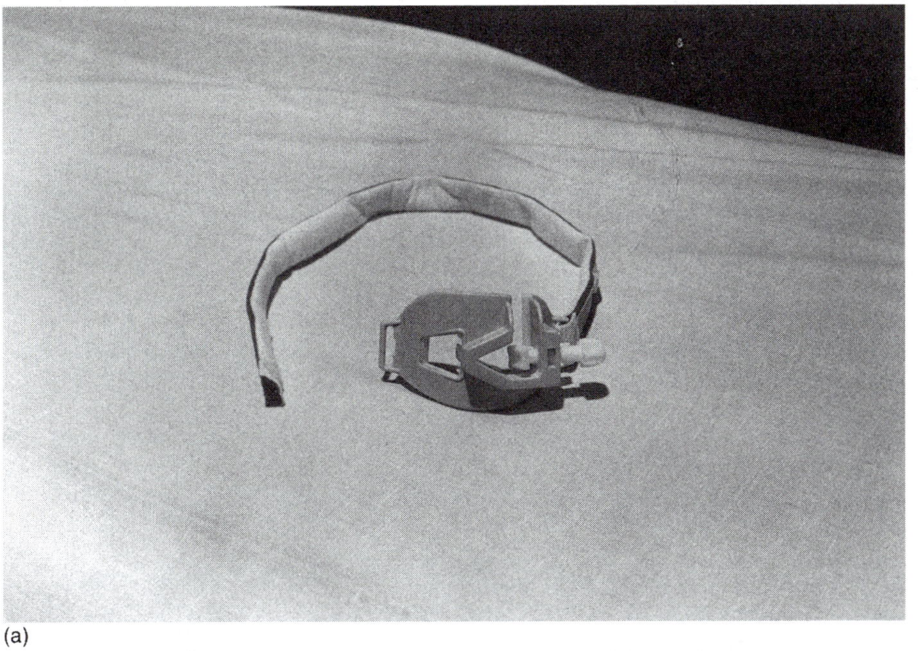

(a)

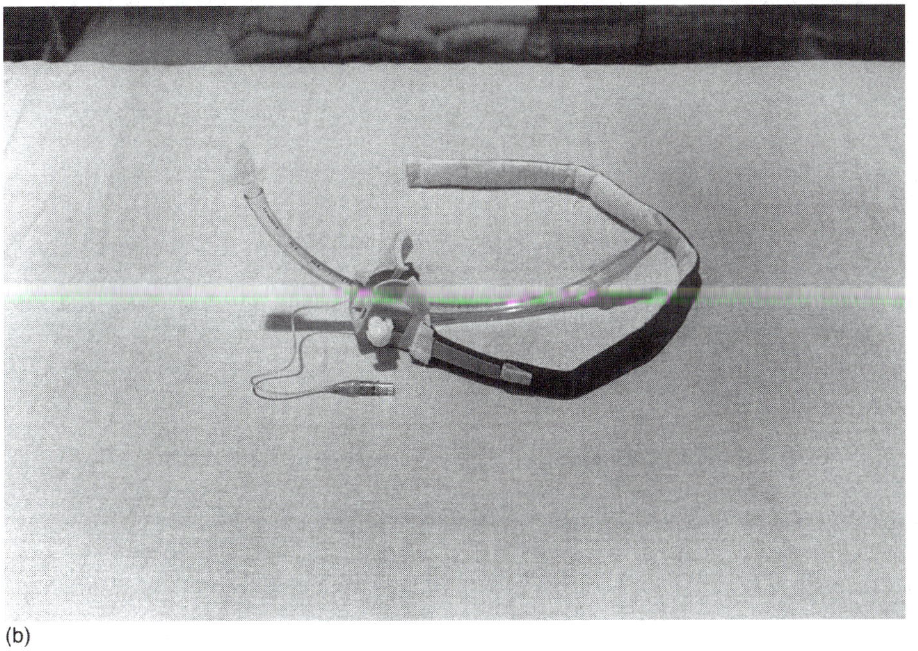

(b)

Figure 8 Device for securing endotracheal tube in place during transport. (a) The device is composed of a strap that passes circumferentially about the neck, a plastic fitting with a V-shaped channel (''pointing'' left) through which the endotracheal tube (ETT) passes, and a (white) screw mechanism (protruding on the right side of the figure) allowing snug fitting of the ETT. (b) Depiction of the ETT-securing device with ETT in place.

Table 6 Manual vs. Mechanical Ventilation

Advantages of manual ventilation
Ease of initiation (no hookups or ventilators to manage).
Not technically demanding.
Affords the crew tactile means to monitor compliance (''feel'' of bagging).
Experienced providers of manual ventilation can follow changes in perceived compliance as indicators of deterioration (e.g., tension pneumothorax).
Minute ventilation can be controlled with use of respirometry to follow minute volume.
Capnometry may allow manual ventilation with control of CO_2 in desirable range.
Advantages of mechanical ventilation
Compared to manual ventilation, less risk of overaggressive ventilation with respiratory alkalosis.
Extra setup time results in more crew-member freedom, as one provider is not occupied by performing manual ventilation at all times.
Overall, better control of respiratory parameters, with more consistence in tidal volume and respiratory rate.
''Feel'' of bagging is replaced by ventilator monitoring of parameters such as compliance, which allows detection of respiratory deterioration.
Avoids risk of fatigue associated with crew-member-provided manual ventilations.

or excessive hyperventilation, respiratory alkalosis, cardiac dysrhythmia, and hypotension [25–27]. The papers in the critical care transport literature suggest that manual ventilation can only be appropriate if respirometry is used to carefully follow minute volume. In addition, there are data suggesting that with capnometry in use prehospital manual ventilation can be provided with maintenance of the desired pCO_2 ranges in head-injured patients [28]. Given the limited number of health care providers in the prehospital setting, however, the extra time required for the institution of mechanical ventilation may be offset by the ''freeing'' up of another pair of hands for intratransport patient care. This ''release of hands'' advantage is particularly valuable for the transport of high acuity patients or for transports of long duration.

In addition to the release of one prehospital care provider from providing labor-intensive manual ventilation, the advantages of mechanical ventilation lie in the improved control of ventilation afforded by even the most basic transport ventilators. The abilities of different transport ventilators are discussed below, but it is clear that in general patients benefit from the better control of respiratory parameters provided by mechanical ventilation. Finally, especially for longer transports, mechanical ventilation has an additional advantage of providing more consistent ventilatory support and tidal volume than does manual ventilation.

In summary, then, mechanical ventilators provide improved control of ventilation, at a small cost of increased initial setup time. There may be a potential loss of the ''monitoring'' capabilities provided by the compliance feedback noted during provision of manual ventilation, but related information is obtainable from gauges on the transport ventilator (see below). For short scene transports, there may be little net benefit to utilizing mechanical ventilation, but this remains an area of controversy. As transport times or patient acuity increase, especially for interfacility transports, the improved control effected with mechanical ventilation offsets the disadvantages associated with this technique.

VI. TRANSPORT VENTILATORS

Mechanical ventilation's advantages over manual ventilation lie primarily in the improved control and consistency of tidal volume, respiratory frequency, and positive end-expiratory pressure (PEEP). Using mechanical ventilators will stabilize ventilation and oxygenation, and as has been mentioned, frees one member of the transport team for other patient care functions. Manual ventilation during long transports may also be fatiguing, and thus in these cases, manual techniques provide ventilation that is neither practical nor predictable. This section will consider some major issues relevant to the provision of mechanical ventilation in the transport setting.

Several criteria should be considered when selecting an appropriate transport ventilator (see Table 7). *Pressure-limited time-cycled ventilation* is most frequently used in critically ill newborns and small pediatric patients, whereas *volume-cycled ventilation* is more commonly utilized in adults, thus if the transport program will be transporting neonatal, pediatric, and adult patients, it is desirable to have a ventilator capable of supporting all patient populations—a ventilator capable of high variability in both tidal-volume delivery and frequency of ventilation as well as the ability to pressure-limit ventilation.

If chronic and acute ventilator-dependent patients will be transported, it is desirable to have multiple ventilatory modes available during transport, including *pressure support, intermittent mandatory ventilation* (SIMV), *assist-control*, and *pressure-limited* modes. As the transport population's variability in age and acuity increases, there is a concomitant decrease in the available options in selecting an appropriate transport ventilator.

The ideal transport ventilator is able to deliver a preset tidal volume with a peak inspiratory pressure-limiting valve that can be adjusted to the patient needs. Excess airway pressure is prevented by a preset blow-off valve. Furthermore, the transport ventilator should provide consistent tidal volume in the face of changing lung compliance. Ventilators that allow tidal volume to be determined by setting inspiratory and expiratory times along with flow rates are preferable. This characteristic allows a varying inspiratory/expiratory (I/E) ratio, and if necessary, a reverse (or inverse) I/E ratio. The reverse I/E ratio involves provision of an inspiratory time that exceeds the expiratory phase duration. This type of ventilation, historically used in the neonatal intensive care setting to improve

Table 7 Characteristics Desirable in a Transport Ventilator

Reliably delivers preset tidal volumes in the presence of possibly changing compliance.
Peak inspiratory pressure-limiting valve adjustable to patient needs.
Preset "blow-off" valve to vent excess airway pressure.
Tidal volumes can be set by changing inspiratory and expiratory times, as well as flow rates (i.e., inverse inspiratory/expiratory time ratios are allowed).
Variable positive end-expiratory pressure (PEEP) control.
Visual (as well as audible) alarms.
Release capability, light weight, and portability so ventilator can accompany patient into receiving hospitals.
Oxygen consumption rate is commensurate to oxygen-carrying capabilities (e.g., cylinders, liquid oxygen) of the particular transport program.
Ability to run off of batteries during patient transport between EMS vehicle and receiving hospital.

oxygenation and minimize barotrauma, may be useful in some adult patients, such as those with adult respiratory distress syndrome.

A variable PEEP control is also desirable. PEEP is intended to prevent alveolar collapse during exhalation by providing continuous positive pressure throughout the respiratory cycle. PEEP may be critical to maintaining oxygenation in patients with severe respiratory failure.

Finally, transport ventilators, especially those used in the air medical environment, must have appropriate visual as well as audible alarm systems (which may not be heard by crews in the noisy helicopter environment) to alert medical personnel to inappropriate volume or pressure changes. As altitude changes, Boyle's law becomes relevant. this law delineates the inverse relationship between pressure and volume; as pressure decreases with increasing altitude, there is a commensurate increase in the volume occupied by a given amount of a gas. Critical care transport personnel in the air medical environment therefore must have a working knowledge of altitude physiology and be proficient in manipulating a mechanical ventilator with changing altitudes. Frequent tidal volume assessment and continuous peak inspiratory pressure monitoring is necessary, as flow rates may have to be modified during air transport in order to guarantee appropriate ventilation. Many of these altitude physiology issues become relevant in ground transports that involve a significant change in altitude.

In the transport (especially air medical) environment, weight and space are limited and mounting; the weight and portability of the transport ventilator must be considered. Transport ventilators require secure mounting in a location that allows the crew ease of accessibility. The mounting device should have a release capability, allowing the ventilator to be transported into both sending and receiving facilities.

Ventilator oxygen consumption rates should also be considered when selecting a transport ventilator. Several transport ventilators use oxygen under pressure as the method for powering the internal ventilator component function. Such ventilators consume large amounts of oxygen, and most likely will require a liquid oxygen system in the transport vehicle in order to avoid multiple oxygen tank changes during patient transport.

Electrically powered transport ventilators are also available. These can be operated from a helicopter or ambulance invertor. Additionally, portable batteries will provide continuous power for 3 to 4 h, eliminating ventilator circuit interruptions during critical periods of the patient transport.

Patients with significant respiratory dysfunction should be placed on a transport ventilator at the sending facility and patient stability should then be adequately reassessed prior to transport. This practice allows flight crew members to observe and troubleshoot the patient while being ventilated by the transport ventilator, but also allows for continued access to a standard mechanical ventilator if necessary.

VII. SUMMARY AND KEY POINTS

The appropriate monitoring of oxygenation and ventilation are vital to optimal prehospital care, and the provision of mechanical ventilatory support is important to the function of air or ground critical care transport services. While the same basic ventilatory principles applicable to hospital-based ventilation are in effect in the prehospital setting, prehospital care providers must also mind the additional issues discussed above, which must be considered if optimal patient ventilation is to occur in the out-of-hospital setting. Some key points regarding oxygenation, ventilation, and airway monitoring in the prehospital setting include the following:

Assurance of adequate oxygenation and ventilation are especially important in the potentially critical patients transported by prehospital care providers.

Pulse oximetry represents the primary means of assessing oxygenation in the prehospital setting, but prehospital care providers should be familiar with its problems in application.

Compared to pulse oximetry, monitoring ventilation allows for more sensitive detection of respiratory depression.

Ventilatory monitoring in the prehospital setting is currently accomplished with CO_2 monitoring, which takes many forms and continues to evolve.

Continuous CO_2 monitoring (*capnometry*) and graphic output (*capnography*), currently in use primarily in intubated patients, provide important information with regard to the adequacy of systemic metabolic function and perfusion.

Given the patient transfers and potential environmental instability of the prehospital care environment, the risk of endotracheal tube dislodgment must be minimized with reliable means to secure tubes in place in the airway.

For short transports, especially those from trauma scenes, manual ventilation is usually preferred, as it affords an improved sense of compliance by the prehospital care provider providing ventilatory support. The primary risk of manual ventilation is that it is commonly associated with overvigorous ventilation and hypocapnia.

For longer transports or patients requiring careful control of ventilation, mechanical ventilation is preferable. Placement of patients on mechanical ventilators also "frees up" the hands of the prehospital care provider who otherwise would be absorbed with provision of manual ventilation.

Pressure-cycled mechanical ventilators are used most commonly in newborns and young pediatric patients, with volume-cycled ventilators usually employed in older patients. In either case, careful assessment of minute volume and constant monitoring of alarms are necessary, as altitude-related pressure-volume changes may alter ventilator function and minute ventilation.

REFERENCES

1. RE Fromm, RP Dellinger. Transport of critically ill patients. J Intens Care Med 7:223–233, 1992.
2. TJ McGuire, JE Pointer. Evaluation of a pulse oximeter in the prehospital setting. Ann Emerg Med 17:1058–1062, 1988.
3. M Helm, J Hauke, M Esser, L Lampl, KH Bock. Diagnosis of blunt thoracic trauma in emergency care: Use of continuous pulse oximetry monitoring. Chirurg 68:606–612, 1997.
4. AP Morley. Prehospital monitoring of trauma patients: Experience of a helicopter emergency medical service. Brit J Anaesth 76:726–730, 1996.
5. L Short, RB Hecker, RE Middaugh, EJ Menk. A comparison of pulse oximeters during helicopter flight. J Emer Med 7:639–643, 1989.
6. GW Bota, BH Rowe. Continuous monitoring of oxygen saturation in prehospital patients with severe illness: The problem of unrecognized hypoxemia. J Emerg Med 13:305–311, 1995.
7. JD Melton, MB Heller, R Kaplan, K Klein. Occult hypoxemia during aeromedical transport: Detection by pulse oximetry. Prehosp Disas Med 4:115–121, 1989.

8. DB Swedlow. Capnometry and capnography: The anesthesia disaster early warning system. Semin Anesth 3:194–200, 1996.
9. ST Sum Ping, MP Mehta, JM Anderton. A comparative study of methods of detection of esophageal intubation. Anesth Analg 69:627–632, 1989.
10. AB Sanders, KB Kern, CW Otto, MM Milander, GA Ewy. End-tidal carbon dioxide monitoring during cardiopulmonary resuscitation. JAMA 262:1347–1351, 1989.
11. MA Wayne, RL Levine, CC Miller. Use of end-tidal carbon dioxide to predict outcome in prehospital cardiac arrest. Ann Emerg Med 25:762–766, 1995.
12. SR Hayden, J Sciammerella, P Viccellio. Colorimetric end-tidal carbon dioxide detector for verification of endotracheal tube placement in out-of-hospital cardiac arrest. Acad Emerg Med 2:499–502, 1995.
13. RC Campbell, CR Boyd, RO Shields. Evaluation of an end-tidal carbon dioxide detector in the aeromedical setting. J Air Med Trans 9:13–15, 1990.
14. SE Martin, WE Agudelo, MG Ochsner. Monitoring hyperventilation in patients with closed head injury during air transport. Air Med J 16:15–18, 1997.
15. RL Levine, MA Wayne, CC Miller. End-tidal carbon dioxide and outcome of out-of-hospital cardiac arrest. New Eng J Med 337:301–306, 1997.
16. MH Well, J Bisera, I Trevino, EC Rackow. Cardiac output and end-tidal carbon dioxide. Crit Care Med 13:907–909, 1985.
17. S Isserles, PH Breen. Can changes in end-tidal carbon dioxide measure changes in cardiac output? Anesth Analg 73:808–814, 1991.
18. P DeVellis, SH Thomas, SK Wedel. Prehospital fentanyl analgesia in air-transported pediatric trauma patients. Pediat Emerg Care 14:321–323, 1998.
19. P DeVellis, SH Thomas, SK Wedel. Prehospital and E.D. analgesia for air transported patients with fractures. Prehosp Emerg Care 2:293–296, 1998.
20. LS Hart, SD Berns, CS Houck, DA Boenning. The value of end-tidal carbon dioxide monitoring when comparing three methods of conscious sedation for children undergoing painful procedures in the emergency department. Pediat Emerg Care 3:189–193, 1997.
21. CJ Erler, WF Rutherford, A Fiege, DR Nelson, A Stahl. Monitored arterial and end-tidal carbon dioxide during in-flight mechanical ventilation. Air Med J 15:171–176, 1996.
22. GA Petroianu, WH Maleck, WF Bergler, S Altmannsberger, R Rufer. Preliminary observations on the Colibri CO_2-indicator. Amer J Emerg Med 16:677–680, 1998.
23. AC Zecca, DR Carlascio, WJ Marshall, DJ Dries. Endotracheal tube stabilization in the air medical setting. J Air Med Transport March:7–10, 1991.
24. MJ Rouse, R Branson, R Semonin-Holleran. Mechanical ventilation during air medical transport: Techniques and devices. J Air Med Trans April:5–8, 1992.
25. S Braman, SM Dunn, CA Amico, RP Millman. Complications of intrahospital transport in critically ill patients. Ann Int Med 107:469–473, 1987.
26. JM Hurst, K Davis, RD Branson, JA Johannigman. Comparison of blood gases during transport using two methods of ventilatory support. J Trauma 29:1637–1640, 1989.
27. HW Gervais, B Eberle, D Konietzke, HJ Hennes, W Dick. Comparison of blood gases of ventilated patients during transport. Crit Care Med 15:761–763, 1987.
28. M Morris, S Kinkade. The effect of capnometry on manual ventilation technique. Air Med J 14:79–82, 1995.

15

Traumatic and Hemorrhagic Shock: Basic Pathophysiology and Treatment

RICHARD P. DUTTON

R Adams Cowley Shock Trauma Center, University of Maryland Medical System, Baltimore, Maryland

I. DEFINITION

Shock is a clinical syndrome characterized by cellular ischemia in multiple organ systems. Shock may be caused by a failure of oxygen delivery (due to hemorrhage, hypovolemia, cardiac failure, or hypoxia) or by intrinsic failure of the cell to take up and utilize oxygen (septic shock, cyanide poisoning). In a description in 1872, Gross described shock as ''a rude unhinging of the machinery of life'' [1]. Although shock may be caused by a wide variety of conditions, it produces predictable effects on the body. If unchecked, shock of any variety can produce a rapidly fatal downward spiral. Even when treated aggressively, a single episode of shock can cause permanent organ system injury.

II. HISTORY

The term shock was first used by the English surgeon George James Guthrie in 1815 to describe the pathophysiology occurring after injury [2], but it was not until the end of the First World War that organized scientific studies of shock first took place. Crile attributed the hemodynamic collapse seen in injured soldiers to a dysfunction of the central nervous system produced by pain and fatigue [3]. Cannon, summarizing medical experience during the war, was the first to link the syndrome of shock with the loss of circulating blood volume and advocate its treatment with hemostasis and transfusion [4]. This theory was much debated in the early years of the last century, and it was not until the scientific work of Blalock, published in 1940, that hemorrhage was recognized as the principal cause of shock following trauma [5]. Transfusion therapy became the mainstay of shock treatment during the middle years of World War II, as promulgated by Churchill [6] and Beeche [7].

The concept of an irreversible deficit in oxygen delivery was first proposed in the early 1940s by Wiggers, who observed that many patients successfully treated for shock later of died complications [8]. Moye et al. [9] and McClelland et al. [10] in the 1950s and 1960s elaborated the role of aggressive crystalloid infusion in the early support of shock patients. More recent scientific work has focused on the treatment and prevention of late complications of shock, including renal failure, sepsis, and adult respiratory distress syndrome, with a renewed interest in identifying the circulating inflammatory mediators of shock [11].

III. TYPES OF SHOCK

Table 1 is a summary of the different etiologies of cellular ischemia. Treatment of shock in the clinical environment depends on recognition and early correction of its cause. The shock produced by traumatic injury is distinct from the hemorrhagic shock produced in carefully controlled laboratory models. *Hemorrhagic shock* results from a single etiology, which can be easily standardized for research purposes. *Traumatic shock* most commonly begins with hemorrhage, but is frequently complicated by cardiac ischemia, hypoxia, neurologic injury, pain, and the effects of drugs and alcohol. Traumatic shock is what we observe clinically in the victims of accidents and injury, and is nearly always a multifactorial process.

IV. STAGES OF TRAUMATIC SHOCK

Hemorrhagic shock is described in the Advanced Trauma Life Support (ATLS™) manual as occurring in four stages (Table 2), based on a rough estimate of the amount of blood lost and its impact on normal adult physiology [12]. In clinical practice these indicators provide only a poor estimate of the amount of hemorrhage the patient has suffered. Different patients respond to blood loss differently, and not all signs are present in all patients.

Young patients may experience significant hemorrhage with little change in their vital signs, particularly if the hemorrhage is associated with significant pain. Elderly patients tend to become hypotensive with less hemorrhage, may have little or no change in their heart rate, and may even suffer from organ system ischemia without any visible change in vital signs [13].

Table 1 Causes of Cellular Ischemia

Cause	Clinical example
Decreased oxygen uptake in the lung	COPD, pulmonary edema
Decreased oxygen-carrying capacity	Anemia, carbon monoxide poisoning
Decreased intravascular fluid volume	Hemorrhage, capillary leak, tissue edema
Decreased venous tone	Spinal cord injury, anesthetic overdose
Diminished cardiac function	Tension pneumothorax, tamponade, cardiac ischemia, contusion, anesthetic overdose, CNS injury, sepsis
Failure of cellular metabolism	Sepsis, advanced shock of any cause

Table 2 Stages of Shock

I.	Blood loss up to 15% of the blood volume. Normal pulse and blood pressure. Mild anxiety.
II.	Blood loss up to 30% of the blood volume. Tachycardic, with normal blood pressure. Increased respirations, decreased urine output. Anxious.
III.	Blood loss up to 40% of the blood volume. Tachycardic and hypotensive. Tachypneic. Oliguric. Anxious and confused.
IV.	Blood loss greater than 40% of the blood volume. Tachycardic and hypotensive. Tachypneic. Anuric. Confused and lethargic.

Source: Ref. 12.

Although the patient's vital signs may not change exactly as described above, the body's progression through the clinical stages of traumatic shock is predictable and is based on the severity of the shock insult and the timeliness of medical intervention. The stages of traumatic shock are shown in Figure 1 and Table 3.

In *compensated traumatic shock* (curve A in Fig. 1) the body has adjusted to hemorrhage by diminishing blood flow to regions of the vascular tree that are ischemia-tolerant. An increase in the heart rate and the vasoconstriction of nonessential vascular beds protect those organs that are more sensitive to ischemia, allowing time for correction of the underlying problem. If hemostasis is established and fluid therapy initiated, compensated traumatic shock should be readily reversible with little long-term impact.

Decompensated traumatic shock (curve B), also known as "progressive shock," occurs when the failure to deliver oxygen begins to overwhelm the body's ability to protect its vital organs. This is a clinically dynamic stage, characterized by significant changes in vital signs; the patient whose hemorrhage has proceeded to

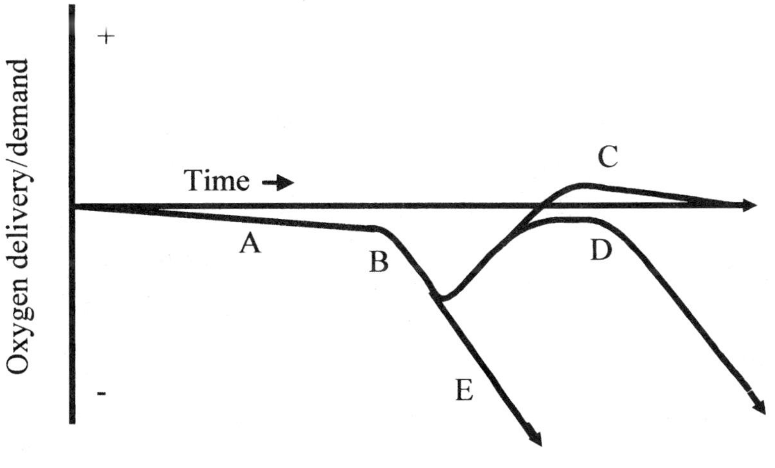

Figure 1 Outcomes from acute traumatic shock. Early shock (A) is caused by a decrease in oxygen delivery to the body. Shock that persists beyond the body's ability to compensate (B), can have one of three outcomes: the patient can recover (C), hemorrhage can be controlled, but the patient can die of organ failure (D), or the patient can die acutely from hemorrhage (E).

Table 3 Characteristics of the Time Course of Traumatic Shock

Stage	Vital signs	Hemorrhage	Organ failure	Death
Compensated	Normal	Active	No	No
Decompensated	Abnormal	Active	Maybe	Maybe
Subacute, reversible	Normalized	Controlled	Yes—treatable	No
Subacute, irreversible	Normalized	Controlled	Yes—not treatable	Yes
Acute, irreversible	Abnormal	Active	Acute	Yes

this point represents a surgical and metabolic emergency. Decompensated shock is also a transitory state, in which the lack of perfusion to certain tissues is building up an "oxygen debt" that will have to be reversed if the cell is to survive. Anaerobic metabolism is possible for a time, but causes an accumulation of lactic acid and other metabolic by-products that will produce a toxic effect on the organism when perfusion is reestablished. Shock is reversible at this stage (curve C), up to the theoretical point at which the oxygen debt becomes too great for the body to repay. Clinically this is the unstable patient who responds to initial fluid therapy but then becomes rapidly hypotensive again.

Subacute irreversible shock (curve D) occurs when the patient has suffered enough ischemia that fatal organ system failure becomes inevitable, even if the inciting event (typically hemorrhage) has been corrected. The patient's vital signs can be restored and bleeding stopped, but the patient will succumb at a later time to multiple organ system failure as a result of the cumulative toxic effects of ischemia and reperfusion. There is currently no good clinical marker for the point at which shock becomes irreversible, emphasizing the need for early and aggressive treatment of all patients.

Finally, *acute irreversible shock* (curve E) is the condition of ongoing hemorrhage, acidosis, and coagulopathy that leads to the immediate death of the patient. Ischemia is so profound that acute organ system failure occurs: the heart fails, coagulopathy cannot be reversed, inappropriate vasodilatation sets in, and the patient expires. In a modern hospital with advanced resuscitation equipment this may occur despite massive blood transfusions and correction of all surgical hemorrhage.

V. THE BODY'S RESPONSE TO SHOCK

The stages of traumatic shock are directly related to the body's response to hemorrhage. The initial responses of compensated shock are on the macrocirculatory level, and are mediated by the neuroendocrine system. Decreased blood pressure and/or pain lead to vasoconstriction and catecholamine release. Heart and brain blood flow is preserved, while other regional beds are constricted. Pain, hemorrhage, and cortical perception of traumatic injuries lead to the release of a number of hormones, including renin-angiotensin, vasopressin, antidiuretic hormone, growth hormone, glucagon, cortisol, epinephrine and norepinephrine [14]. This response sets the stage for the microcirculatory responses that will ultimately determine the patient's outcome.

On the cellular level the body responds to hemorrhage by taking up interstitial fluid, causing cells to swell [15]. This may obstruct adjacent capillaries, resulting in the "no-

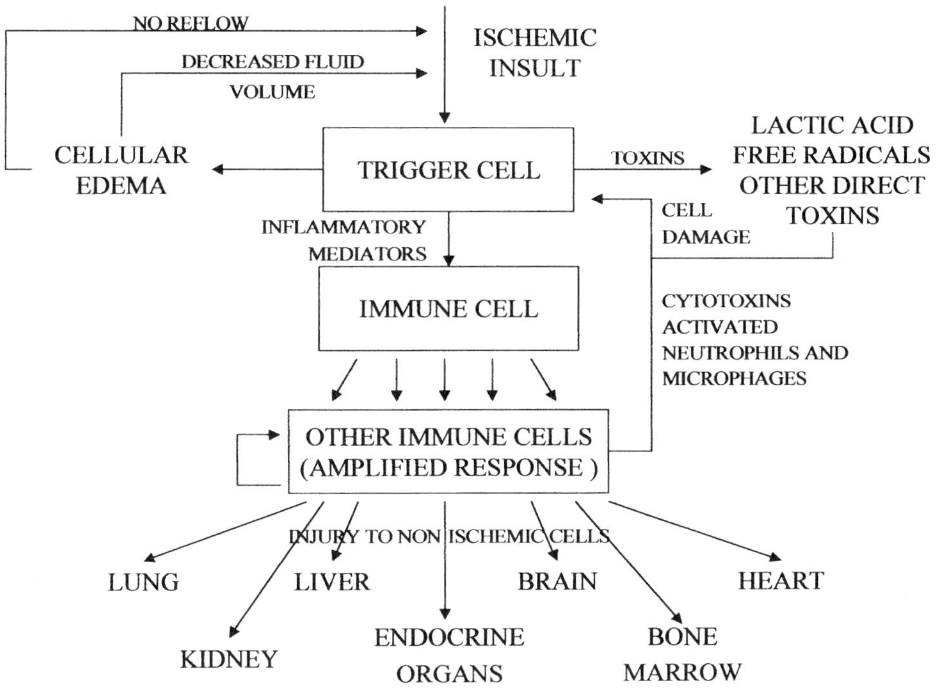

Figure 2 The inflammatory cascade of acute traumatic shock.

reflow'' phenomenon that prevents the reversal of ischemia even in the presence of adequate macroflow [16]. Ischemic cells produce lactate and free radicals, which are not cleared by the circulation. These compounds cause direct damage to the cell in which they are created, and may damage other cells and organ systems as well, when perfusion is reestablished. The ischemic cell will also produce and release a variety of inflammatory factors: prostacyclin, thromboxane, prostaglandins, leukotrienes, endothelin, complement, and inflammatory and anti-inflammatory cytokines [17]. Many of these factors act in turn to stimulate nonischemic cells of the immune system to accumulate and release their own factors, some of which are directly toxic to the cell (Fig. 2). These are the ingredients of acute and subacute irreversible shock. Space does not allow a complete listing of the dozens of chemicals known to be implicated in the inflammatory cascade, which would already be obsolete by the time this chapter is published. Suffice it to say that identification and modulation of this response is the single most active area in shock research, with the greatest potential to improve patient outcomes.

VI. ORGAN SYSTEM RESPONSES TO TRAUMATIC SHOCK

Specific organ systems respond to traumatic shock in specific ways, as shown in Table 4.

The central nervous system (CNS) is the prime trigger of the neuroendocrine response to shock, which acts to maintain perfusion to the heart and brain at the expense of other tissues [18]. Regional glucose uptake in the brain changes during shock [19]. Reflex activity and cortical electrical activity are both depressed during hypotension. These changes are reversible with mild hypoperfusion, but become permanent with prolonged ischemia.

Table 4 Effects of Traumatic Shock on Different Organ Systems

System	Effect
Central nervous	Lethargy, decreased reflexes; increased glucose uptake
Cardiovascular	Vasoconstriction, increased inotropy (early); vasodilatation, decreased inotropy (late)
Pulmonary	ARDS (late)
Hepatic	Reperfusion injury, ''no reflow''; loss of glucose regulation; loss of synthetic function
Gastrointestinal	Reperfusion injury; translocation of bacteria
Renal	Oliguria, acute tubular necrosis
Endocrine	Release of ''stress hormones''
Musculoskeletal	Production of lactic acid; uptake of free fluid
Immune	Early impairment; systemic inflammatory response

Failure to recover preinjury neurologic function—as measured by the Glasgow coma score—once hemorrhage has been controlled is a marker for subacute irreversible shock (and poor long-term outcome), even if the patient's hemodynamic functions are normal [20].

The *kidney* and *adrenal glands* respond to the neuroendocrine changes of shock, producing renin, angiotensin, aldosterone, cortisol, erythropoietin, and catecholamine [21]. The kidney itself maintains glomerular filtration in the face of hypotension by selective vasoconstriction and concentration of blood flow in the medulla and deep cortical area. Prolonged hypotension leads to decreased cellular energy and an inability to concentrate urine, followed by patchy cell death, tubular epithelial necrosis, and renal failure [18,22].

The *heart* is relatively preserved from ischemia during shock, due to maintenance or even an increase of nutrient blood flow, and cardiac function is generally well preserved until the late stages [18,21]. Lactate, free radicals, and other humoral factors released by ischemic cells all act as negative inotropes, however, and in the decompensated patient may produce cardiac dysfunction as the terminal event in the shock spiral [23].

The *lung*, which cannot itself become ischemic, is nonetheless the ''downstream filter'' for the inflammatory by-products of the ischemic body. The lung is often the sentinel organ for the development of multiple organ system failure (MOSF) [4,24]. Immune complex and cellular factors accumulate in the capillaries of the lung, leading to neutrophil and platelet aggregation, increased capillary permeability, destruction of lung architecture, and adult respiratory distress syndrome (ARDS) [25,26]. The pulmonary response to traumatic shock is the leading evidence that this disease is not just a disorder of hemodynamics; pure hemorrhage in the absence of hypoperfusion does not produce pulmonary dysfunction [24,27].

The *gut* is one of the earliest organs affected by hypoperfusion and may be one of the primary triggers of MOSF. Clinical measurement of pH in the stomach (gastric tonometry) has been proposed as a marker for adequacy of resuscitation, since acidosis has been shown to correlate well with ischemia throughout the body [28]. Intense vasoconstriction occurs early, and frequently leads to a ''no-reflow'' phenomenon even when the macrocirculation is restored [29]. Intestinal cell death causes a breakdown in the barrier function of the gut, which results in increased translocation of bacteria to the liver and lung [30]. The impact of this on the development of MOSF is controversial at present; studies of selective decontamination of the gut in trauma patients have not conclusively demonstrated a benefit to this therapy [31].

The *liver* has a complex microcirculation, and has been demonstrated to suffer reperfusion injury in recovery from shock [32]. Hepatic cells are also metabolically active, and contribute substantially to the inflammatory response to decompensated shock. Irregularities in blood glucose levels following shock are attributable to hepatic ischemia [33]. Failure of the synthetic function of the liver following shock is almost always lethal.

Skeletal muscle is not metabolically active during shock, and tolerates ischemia better than other organs. The large mass of skeletal muscle makes it important in the generation of lactate and free radicals from ischemic cells. The classic cellular response to shock of increasing intracellular sodium and free water were first elucidated in skeletal muscle cells [34].

The *immune system* is impaired by any ischemic injury, and this may contribute to the early development of sepsis in patients resuscitated from traumatic shock. Multiple blood transfusions, hypothermia, aspiration, gut translocation of bacteria, multiple invasive procedures, and breakdown of the integument are all stressors of the immune system.

VII. DIAGNOSIS OF TRAUMATIC SHOCK

To be effectively treated, shock must be recognized at the earliest possible moment. There is no direct measure available for cellular ischemia; the medical practitioner must rely instead on a number of indirect signs of inadequate perfusion, as summarized in Table 2. The most common marker for shock is a change in the patient's ''vital signs:'' blood pressure, heart rate, and respiratory rate, with a drop in blood pressure being the most important. Hypotension associated with a traumatic mechanism of injury and evidence of internal or external bleeding indicates at least some degree of shock. More subtle measures of inadequate perfusion, such as an elevated serum lactate level, will seldom be available to the prehospital care provider. These markers are useful at the level of definitive care (the receiving hospital) for identifying patients with mild or atypical shock and for monitoring the adequacy of resuscitation once it is begun.

As was indicated above, traumatic shock is most commonly caused by loss of blood. Hypoperfusion of at least some organ systems is likely in any patient who has lost more than 10% of his or her blood volume, and [illegible] than 20%. At a 30% blood loss the average patient will be decompensated and at high risk, and at 40% he or she will be near death. The diagnosis of traumatic shock therefore hinges on the diagnosis of hemorrhage.

VIII. PREHOSPITAL MANAGEMENT OF SHOCK

The advanced trauma life support (ATLS) course of the American College of Surgeons [12] teaches recognition and early treatment of traumatic shock in a systematized way that will be familiar to practitioners throughout the United States and in many other parts of the world. Diagnosis and treatment will vary from patient to patient and institution to institution, but the general course of patient care will proceed as described.

When a patient presents with clinical signs of shock, the first imperative must be to determine the etiology and eliminate it if possible. Table 5 shows the principal contributors to shock in acute trauma patients, and the recommended management for each. Once steps have been taken to eliminate obvious mechanical causes of shock (loss of airway or breathing, pneumothorax, tamponade, etc.) the prehospital care provider will be left with three main possibilities: hemorrhagic, neurogenic, or cardiogenic. Shock resulting

Table 5 Causes and Treatments of Traumatic Shock

Cause	Treatment
Hypoxia	Intubation, mechanical ventilation
Tension pneumothorax	Pleural decompression, tube thoracostomy
Cardiac tamponade	Surgical drainage
Cardiac contusion	Inotropic support, treatment of dysrhythmias
Spinal cord injury	Fluid administration, vasopressors
Hypovolemia	Correction of hemorrhage, fluid resuscitation

from trauma will be further aggravated by ''third-space'' loss of fluid into injured tissues due to capillary leak and edema. Traumatic shock may be triggered by any combination of these factors, including all three together.

Hemorrhage is by far the leading trigger of shock in trauma patients, to the point at which the ATLS protocol recommends presumptive treatment for hemorrhage in any hypotensive trauma patient. Hemorrhage sufficient to cause shock in a normal adult can occur into one of five compartments: the chest, the abdomen, the retroperitoneum, long bone fractures, or out of the body (''the street''). Diagnosis of significant hemorrhage is made by a number of means, ranging from simple examination of the patient (the primary and secondary surveys) through a variety of radiologic exams all the way to surgical exploration. Table 6 summarizes the most likely sites for hemorrhage and the available diagnostic modalities in the definitive care setting. The importance of physical examination cannot be underestimated in the field. Observing bleeding wounds or limb deformities is obvious. Auscultation and percussion of the chest can provide evidence of hemothorax, particularly in the presence of chest wall tenderness. Peritoneal signs, including distention, guarding, and rebound tenderness, are indicators of intra-abdominal trauma. Retroperitoneal hemorrhage is the hardest to diagnose in the field, especially in the absence of pelvic ring instability.

Treatment of hemorrhage is rightly given a high priority in the ATLS protocol, as unchecked hemorrhage is uniformly fatal. While fluid therapy will be dealt with at length in the next chapter, it should first be recognized that fluid resuscitation is *not* the primary treatment for hemorrhagic shock. Numerous animal studies [35–38] and one human trial [39] have shown that early aggressive administration of fluids may decrease survival in

Table 6 Options for the Diagnosis and Treatment of Traumatic Hemorrhage

Location of bleeding	Diagnostic modalities	Treatment options
Chest	Physical exam; chest X ray; thoracostomy tube output; chest CT scan	Observation; surgery
Abdomen	Physical exam; ultrasound exam (FAST); abdominal CT; peritoneal lavage	Surgical ligation; angiography; observation
Retroperitoneum	Physical exam?; CT scan; angiography	Angiography; pelvic fixation; surgical ligation
Long bones	Physical exam; plain X rays	Fracture fixation; surgical ligation
Outside the body	Physical exam	Direct pressure; surgical ligation

the actively hemorrhaging patient. Instead, all efforts should be made to *control the hemorrhage first*, while resuscitating only as needed to preserve minimally acceptable vital signs.

Control of hemorrhage may be achieved by direct pressure on the wound, by closure of a laceration, by angiographic embolization, by fixation of fractures, by exploratory surgery, or by tamponade and time. Pneumatic antishock garments (PASG or MAST) have not been shown to improve survival from hemorrhagic trauma, but may provide valuable fracture stabilization (especially of the pelvis) if a long transport to definitive care is anticipated.

Fluid resuscitation should begin as soon as shock is recognized, but should be limited to the minimum necessary until such time as active hemorrhage is controlled. Defining the ''minimum necessary'' is the focus of current human and animal research, as there are presently no good laboratory markers or monitors to indicate when subacute shock is approaching the threshold of irreversibility. Indeed, even young patients may require invasive hemodynamic monitoring to distinguish adequate from inadequate fluid resuscitation [40]. Table 7 outlines the short-term and long-term goals for fluid resuscitation from traumatic shock.

Cardiogenic shock in the trauma patient is a difficult diagnosis to make, but important because of the implications for fluid management. Cardiogenic traumatic shock may be due to pre-existing conditions (e.g., the patient suffered a myocardial infarction that resulted in a motor vehicle accident), triggered conditions (e.g., stress and pain have caused myocardial dysfunction), or direct injury (e.g., cardiac contusion leading to edema and ischemia of the myocardium). Cardiogenic traumatic shock is more common in elderly patients.

Diagnosis of cardiogenic traumatic shock in the field may be made by evidence of characteristic anginal symptoms (especially chest pain), acute ischemia on 12-lead electrocardiography, or the new onset of dysrhythmias in the presence of a suspicious premorbid history or mechanism of injury. Shock due to hemorrhage must still be excluded. Ventricular ectopy is common following cardiac contusion and should be closely monitored and aggressively treated. Lidocaine (1 mg/kg) should be administered for repeated ventricular couplets or ventricular tachycardia. Field transmission of ECG to the emergency depart-

Table 7 Goals for Early and Late Resuscitation from Hemorrhagic Shock

Parameter	Early	Late
Mental status	Normal	Normal
Systolic blood pressure	80 mmHg (low target)	>100 mmHg
Heart rate	<120	<100
Arterial oxygen saturation	>96%	>96%
Arterial pH	>7.20	Normal (7.40)
Hematocrit	>25%	>20%
Serum lactate	<6	<2.5 mm/l
Base deficit	>8	Normal (0)
Pulmonary artery occlusion pressure	Not available	>18 mmHg
Tissue oxygen delivery (derived from PA catheter data)	Not available	>550 m/min/m^2
Urine output	>15 cc/kg/hr	>30 cc/kg/hr

Note: Early resuscitation occurs while the patient is still actively bleeding; late resuscitation begins once bleeding has been controlled.

ment, followed by radiotelephone consultation, is invaluable in the field management of cardiogenic shock.

Cardiac function in relation to filling pressures can only be guessed at in the field, leaving the practitioner with little recourse but to administer fluids and observe the clinical response. No improvement in blood pressure following a fluid bolus—in the absence of signs of hemorrhage—raises the strong possibility of cardiac dysfunction. The presence of rales, distended neck veins, or cardiac murmurs may also indicate a failure of pump function. Inotropic therapy may enhance cardiac function if the gain in contractility increases oxygen delivery to the heart itself enough to outweigh an increase in oxygen consumption. Epinephrine is the normal first-line therapy in the field, but should be reserved for use only in patients who are severely hypotensive. One-half to 1 mg intravenously will restore blood pressure in almost any patient in cardiogenic shock for a period of 10 to 15 min.

Neurogenic shock is the result of injury to the spinal cord or brain resulting in an interruption of sympathetic outflow, a loss of vascular tone, and inappropriate vasodilatation. Loss of sympathetic innervation above T-2 will also cause a loss of chronotropic and inotropic stimulation of the heart, resulting in a combined cardiogenic/neurogenic etiology for shock. Neurogenic traumatic shock should be suspected whenever the patient has a clinically evident neurologic deficit and/or significantly depressed level of consciousness.

Intracranial pathology may significantly impact fluid management, as underresuscitation will lead to an inappropriately low mean arterial pressure, with dire consequences for cerebral perfusion. Therapy must be directed at maintenance of the cerebral perfusion pressure (CPP)—defined as the mean arterial pressure minus the higher of intracranial pressure (ICP) or central venous pressure (CVP)—in the normal to high range (70–80 mmHg). Determination of CPP on an ongoing basis requires invasive hemodynamic and intracranial pressure monitoring; in the field, the practitioner should focus on maintaining a mean arterial blood pressure of at least 80 mmHg. Fluid therapy may be further complicated by the early development of disseminated intravascular coagulopathy caused by breakdown of the blood–brain barrier leading to activation of the coagulation cascade by tissue thromboplastin.

Treatment of shock in the presence of spinal cord pathology focuses on the restoration of normal vascular tone early in the course of fluid resuscitation by infusion of pressor or inotropic/chronotropic drugs. Since high spinal cord injuries are characterized by both loss of vascular tone and loss of cardiac function, dopamine at 5 to 20 μg/kg/min is the usual first-line therapy in the hospital. In the prehospital environment the spinal-cord–injured patient may be hypotensive and bradycardic, but not usually to extreme levels. A systolic blood pressure of 80 mmHg in the field is typical. Lower pressures raise the strong possibility of hemorrhage in addition to spinal shock, and should be treated with aggressive fluid infusion.

IX. GOALS FOR RESUSCITATION

Once the diagnosis of shock has been made and the triggering etiologies identified and addressed, resuscitation should proceed until it is clear that normal oxygen delivery and utilization have been restored. Clinical markers for this state are summarized in Table 7. It is clear from numerous studies that patients who are going to survive traumatic shock maximize their tissue oxygen delivery (D-O_2) and oxygen onsumption (V-O_2) in the early postresuscitative phase and normalize their serum lactate levels more quickly than those who will not survive [41,42].

The question of whether or not forcing the patient into this hyperdynamic state with aggressive volume administration and inotropic infusions can improve survival is still controversial, however. One study in trauma patients showed a benefit of this approach [42] but a contemporaneous protocol showed no improvement in outcome from inotropes beyond that provided by adequate fluid administration [43]. Our current approach is to monitor the patient to ensure that we are providing enough fluid volume but not to use inotropic support unless the patient is clearly underperfused.

Reliance on conventional vital signs and traditional clinical measures of end-organ perfusion does not reflect the optimal degree of volume replacement in the early postinjury period. At the roadside, this may be all the practitioner has available, which can make it difficult to determine the optimal amount of fluid to administer. This is especially true in the elderly and in patients with underlying pathology of the heart, lungs, liver, or kidneys. In general, a stable or rising blood pressure, a decrease of elevated heart rate, a working pulse oximeter, good color, appropriate mentation, and control of visible hemorrhage are the goals for resuscitation in the prehospital phase. Once these conditions have been achieved, fluid administration should be slowed until in-hospital diagnostic technologies can be applied.

X. ADJUVANT THERAPIES FOR SHOCK

Position: The patient's ability to constrict his or her vascular space in the face of hemorrhage and preserve flow only to vital organs can be augmented by elevation of the legs above the level of the heart. This "autotransfusion" can redirect as much as a liter of blood volume from the periphery to the central circulation. This may be a valuable temporizing measure in shock management, particularly in austere environments and prior to the initiation of fluid therapy. Elevating blood pressure may exacerbate bleeding, so this therapy should be reserved for hypoten- [illegible] fying the source of shock; elevation of the lower extremities will benefit patients who have hemorrhaged or who are inappropriately vasodilated, but will elevate intracranial pressure and may acutely exacerbate cardiogenic shock. The reverse Trendelenberg position will benefit patients in spinal shock but must be accomplished while preserving full spinal immobilization.

Military antishock trousers (MAST) or pneumatic antishock garments (PASG): This device is placed around the legs and pelvis of the trauma victim, then inflated by a foot pump to externally pressurize the lower extremities. As with positional therapy, fluid is shifted from the periphery to the central vascular compartment. In practice, MASTs may actually worsen outcome in the average trauma patient due to increased hemorrhage, and their use has been abandoned in many jurisdictions [44]. Specific indications for MASTs include rapid stabilization of long bone and pelvic fractures, austere environments, and patients who will have a long transport time to the trauma center.

Both positional therapy and MASTs pose an additional risk to the patient when they are reversed, as intravascular volume will leave the central circulation and

Table 8 Benefits and Detriments of Deliberate Mild Hypothermic Management of Trauma Patients (33–34°C)

Benefits	Detriments
Improved functional outcome of some closed head injuries	Decreased immune function
Reduced metabolic demand for oxygen	Potential for cardiac dysrhythmias
Facilitated shunting of blood to vital organs	Impaired coagulation
	Need for active rewarming—shivering will increase metabolic load markedly
	Decreased survival seen in hypothermic patients [46]

return to the legs and pelvis once pressure is removed. Repositioning the patient or deflating the MASTs should be undertaken in gradual steps after initiation of fluid therapy.

Deliberate hypothermia: This technique has been shown to be beneficial in the management of some intracranial injuries [45] and is known to reduce the degree of tissue ischemia associated with cardiac bypass procedures. Animal models of traumatic shock have shown improved outcome with deliberate mild hypothermia during the resuscitative period, but human studies are not yet underway. Issues that must still be addressed include the impairment of coagulation caused by hypothermia and the metabolic debt that must be repaid when the hypothermic patient is rewarmed. Table 8 summarizes the benefits and detriments of deliberate hypothermic management.

Accidental hypothermia commonly results from a combination of patient exposure, environmental conditions, and iatrogenic factors. For the reasons listed above it is preferential at this time to maintain patient temperature in the normal range whenever possible. The environment should be warm and dry, the patient should be covered, and all administered fluids should be warmed to body temperature prior to infusion. While it is understandable that these things can be difficult to accomplish at the scene of a prolonged extrication from a motor vehicle crash (for example), they are nonetheless goals that the prehospital care provider should strive to achieve. It is far easier to keep a patient warm than it is to rewarm him or her once the core body temperature has fallen.

XI. FUTURE INITIATIVES IN SHOCK MANAGEMENT

Although still investigational at this time, several new drugs and therapies are now under study that will impact the way in which traumatic shock is managed in the coming decades.

Deliberate hypotension is the subject of at least one ongoing trial in resuscitation from hemorrhagic shock. As was indicated above, there is substantial evidence in animal models of uncontrolled blood loss that targeting a lower than normal mean blood pressure will improve short-term survival. It is not known, however, what the long-term effects of deliberate hypotension will be; converting acute irreversible shock to subacute irreversible shock (controlling hemorrhage only at the expense of perfusion) would not be a satisfactory result. It is more hopeful that over time this research will identify better clinical markers for resuscitation than blood pressure and provide the field practitioner a more clearly defined target for immediate resuscitation.

Blood substitutes, particularly hemoglobin-based oxygen carriers (HBOCs), are currently undergoing phase III trials at a number of trauma centers. Multiple products are under investigation, derived from outdated human blood, bovine hemoglobin, or recombinant technology. While specifics vary from product to product, each of these compounds shares the same essential nature: a noninfectious, noncellular capacity to transport oxygen with similar loading and unloading characteristics to native red blood cells. With a plasma half-life of several days, HBOCs can serve as a ''bridge to transfusion'' that will sharply reduce the banked blood requirements of acute trauma patients. The way in which these products interact with the shock state has not been fully elucidated; perhaps due to vasoconstriction from nitric oxide scavenging, the frequently described hypertensive response to HBOCs may improve perfusion or may worsen hemorrhage. Even low doses of HBOCs are theoretically beneficial in the delivery of oxygen to ischemic tissue [47], but their use in the trauma patient population has not yet been adequately studied.

Vasopressors and inotropes were studied in a hemorrhage model by Shaftan [48]. Vasopressors were found to exacerbate bleeding without improving perfusion, and have never found a place in resuscitation from hemorrhage (although they may be useful in resuscitation from spinal shock). Inotropic agents are currently used only in extremis or in patients in whom close hemodynamic monitoring is available.

Specific treatment of reperfusion injury has been studied extensively in patients receiving solid organ transplants. Various ''cocktails'' developed for minimizing tissue ischemia in isolated organs may some day be viable for total-body preservation in traumatic shock. Research is also underway to develop specific blocking agents for the active by-products of the shock cycle released during reperfusion. The goal is to allow the lowest possible blood pressure during the initial assessment and hemodynamic control of hemorrhage while avoiding or minimizing the metabolic consequences of organ ischemia.

XII. CONCLUSION

Traumatic shock is a disease of tissue ischemia. Hemorrhage is the leading cause, but cardiac or neurologic impairment may also contribute.

Shock is a disease of the entire body, with effects on every organ system.

Control of hemorrhage and restoration of adequate tissue oxygen delivery are the keys to clinical treatment of the patient in shock.

The future will see new techniques added to the treatment of shock, including ways to manage reperfusion injury, the inflammatory cascade, and the ''no-reflow'' phenomenon.

REFERENCES

1. SG Gross. A System of Surgery: Pathological, Diagnostic, Therapeutic, and Operative. Philadelphia: Lea & Febiger, 1872.

2. GJ Guthrie. On Gunshot Wounds of the Extremities. London: Longman, 1815.
3. GW Crile. A Physical Interpretation of Shock, Exhaustion, and Restoration. London: Henry Frowde, Oxford University Press, 1921.
4. WB Cannon, J Fraser, EM Cowell. The preventive treatment of wound shock. JAMA 70:618, 1918.
5. A Blalock. Principles of Surgical Care, Shock, and Other Problems. St. Louis: Mosby, 1940.
6. ED Churchill. Surgeon to Soldiers. Philadelphia: Lippincott, 1972.
7. HK Beecher. Resuscitation and Anesthesia for Wounded Men. Springfield, IL: Charles C. Thomas, 1949.
8. CJ Wiggers. Physiology of Shock. New York: Commonwealth Fund, 1950.
9. CA Moyer. Burns, Shock, and Plasma Volume Regulation. St. Louis: Mosby, 1967.
10. RN McClelland, GT Shires, CR Baxter, et al. Balanced salt solution in the treatment of hemorrhagic shock. JAMA 199:166, 1967.
11. R Demling, C Lalonde, P Saldinger, J Knox. Multiple organ dysfunction in the surgical patient: Pathophysiology, prevention, and treatment. Curr Prob Surg 30:345–424, 1993.
12. Committee on Trauma, American College of Surgeon. Advanced Trauma Life Support: Program for Physicians. Chicago: American College of Surgeons, 1993.
13. CW Schwab, DR Kauder. Trauma in the geriatric patient. Arch Surg 127:701, 1992.
14. AB Peitzman. Hypovolemic shock. In: MR Pinsky, JFA Dhainaut, eds. Pathophysiologic Foundations of Critical Care. Baltimore: Williams and Wilkins, 1993, pp. 161–169.
15. GT Shires, N Cunningham, CRF Baker, et al. Alterations in cellular membrane function during hemorrhagic shock in primates. Ann Surg 176:288–295, 1972.
16. GT Shires, D Coln, J Carrico, et al. Fluid therapy in hemorrhagic shock. Arch Surg 88:688–693, 1964.
17. AB Peitzman, TR Billiar, BG Harbrecht, et al. Hemorrhagic shock. Curr Prob Surg 32:929–1002, 1995.
18. WB Runciman, GA Sjowronski. Pathophysiology of haemorrhagic shock. Anaesth Intens Care 12:193–205, 1984.
19. MM Bronshvag. Cerebral pathophysiology in haemorrhagic shock: Nuclide scan data, flourescence microscopy, and anatomic correlations. Stroke 11:50–59, 1980.
20. CG Peterson, FP Haugen. Hemorrhagic shock and the nervous system. Amer J Surg 106:233–238, 1963.
21. JA Collins. The pathophysiology of hemorrhagic shock. Prog Clin Bio Res 108:5–29, 1982.
22. DA Troyer. Models of ischemic acute renal failure: Do they reflect events in human renal failure? J Lab Clin Med 110:379–380, 1987.
23. AM Lefer, J Martin. Origin of a myocardial depressant factor in shock. Amer J Physiol 218: 1423–1427, 1970.
24. JH Horovitz, CJ Carrico, GT Shires. Pulmonary response to major injury. Arch Surg 108: 349–355, 1974.
25. J Thorne, S Blomquist, O Elmer. Polymorphonuclear leukocyte sequestration in the lung and liver following soft tissue trauma: An in vivo study. J Trauma 29:451–456, 1989.
26. BA Martin, R Dahlby, I Nicholls, JC Hogg. Platelet sequestration in lungs with hemorrhagic shock and reinfusion in dogs. J Appl Physiol 50:1306–1312, 1981.
27. RL Fulton, AVS Raynor, C Jones. Analysis of factors leading to posttraumatic pulmonary insufficiency. Ann Thor Surg 25:500–509, 1978.
28. G Gutierrez, F Palizas, G Doglio, et al. Gastric intramucosal pH as a therapeutic index of tissue oxygenation in critically ill patients. Lancet 339:195, 1992.
29. PM Reilly, GB Bulkley. Vasoactive mediators and splanchnic perfusion. Crit Care Med 21: S55–S68, 1993.
30. JA Redan, BF Rush, JN McCullogh, et al. Organ distribution of radiolabeled enteric Escherichia coli during and after hemorrhagic shock. Ann Surg 211:663–668, 1990.
31. AM Korinek, MJ Laisne, NH Nicholas, et al. Selective decontamination of the digestive tract

in neurosurgical intensive care patients: A double-blind, randomized, placebo-controlled study. Crit Care Med 21:1466–1473, 1993.

32. K Chun, J Zhang, J Biewer, et al. Microcirculatory failure determines lethal hepatocyte injury in ischemic-reperfused rat livers. Shock 1:3–9, 1994.
33. SR Maitra, ER Geller, W Pan, et al. Altered cellular calcium regulation and hepatic glucose production during hemorrhagic shock. Circ Shock 38:14–24, 1992.
34. AB Peitzman, WA Corbett, GT Shires III, H Illner, et al. Cellular function in liver and muscle during hemorrhagic shock in primates. Surg Gyn Ob 161:419–424, 1985.
35. A Capone, P Safar, S Tisherman, et al. Treatment of uncontrolled haemorrhagic shock: Improved outcome with fluid restriction. J Trauma 35:984, 1993.
36. JC Sakles, MJ Sena, DA Knight, JM Davis. Effect of immediate fluid resuscitation on the rate, volume, and duration of pulmonary vascular hemorrhage in a sheep model of penetrating thoracic trauma. Ann Emer Med 29:392–399, 1997.
37. A Stern, SC Dronen, P Birrer, X Wang. Effect of blood pressure on haemorrhagic volume in a near-fatal haemorrhage model incorporating a vascular injury. Ann Emer Med 22:155–163, 1993.
38. WC Shoemaker, AB Peitzman, R Bellamy, et al. Resuscitation from severe hemorrhage. Crit Care Med 24:S12–S23, 1996.
39. WH Bickell, MJ Wall, PE Pepe, et al. Immediate versus delayed resuscitation for hypotensive patients with penetrating torso injuries. NEJM 331:1105–1109, 1994.
40. B Abou-Khalil, TM Scalea, SZ Trooskin, et al. Hemodynamic responses to shock in young trauma patients: Need for invasive monitoring. Crit Care Med 22:633, 1994.
41. D Abramson, TM Scalea, R Hitchock, et al. Lactate clearance and survival following injury. J Trauma 35:584–589, 1993.
42. MH Bishop, WC Shoemaker, PL Appel, et al. Prospective, randomized trial of survivor values of cardiac index, oxygen delivery, and oxygen consumption as resuscitation endpoints in severe trauma. J Trauma 38:780–787, 1995.
43. RM Durham, K Neunaber, JE Mazuski, et al. The use of oxygen consumption and delivery as endpoints for resuscitation in critically ill patients. J Trauma 41:32–40, 1996.
44. KL Mattox, W Bickell, PE Pepe, et al. Prospective MAST study in 911 patients. J Trauma 29:1104, 1989.
45. DW Marion, LE Penrod, SF Kelsey, et al. Treatment of traumatic brain injury with moderate hypothermia. NEJM 336:540–546, 1997.
46. GJ Jurkovich, WB Greiser, A Luterman, et al. Hypothermia in trauma victims: An ominous predictor of survival. J Trauma 27:903, 1987.
47. F Panico, RP Dutton, MR Gastonguay, J McManigle, A Manalaysay. Can stroma-free hemoglobin improve oxygen extraction in ischemic tissue? Anesth Analg 80(suppl.):S5, 1995.
48. GW Shaftan, C Chiu, C Dennis, B Harris. Fundamentals of physiologic control of arterial hemorrhage. Surgery 58:851–856, 1965.

16

Prehospital Vascular Access for the Trauma Patient

THOMAS A. SWEENEY

Christiana Care Health Systems, Wilmington, Delaware

ANTONIO MARQUES

Hospital Geral de Santo Antonio, Porto, Portugal

Vascular access is a key intervention provided to victims of sudden illness or injury cared for by prehospital emergency medical service (EMS) advanced providers. Fluid resuscitation and most emergent pharmacologic therapies require adequate venous access. A number of controversies surround intravenous (IV) therapy established in the field. Intravenous access can potentially delay transportation to definitive care. There is a risk to prehospital care providers carrying out the procedure and a risk of subsequent IV site infections. In addition, there are alternatives to simple peripheral IV catheters such as intraosseous infusion and central venous access.

I. IV THERAPY: A DELAY TO DEFINITIVE CARE?

Intravenous access remains a controversial prehospital intervention because of concerns that obtaining venous access may delay patient transport. The benefits from IV access such as the ability to resuscitate with IV fluids, give medications, and draw blood samples may be outweighed by associated delays in achieving more definitive care [1]. Concern developed after McSwain et al. [2] noted that average on-scene times were 12.2 min longer for victims of cardiac arrest for whom paramedics attempted IV lines than for those victims who had no IV attempted. Several groups have now completed prospective studies that found that the actual time to obtain IV access is much less.

Pons et al. [3] conducted a prospective on-scene analysis using a nonparamedic observer to determine the time for IV access in the Denver, Colorado, EMS system, consisting of 75 full-time ambulance paramedics. Lines were successfully begun in 51 trauma patients with first attempt success in 46 (90.2%). It took an average of 2.20 ± 0.20 min to start the first IV line and obtain a 30-cc blood sample. Trauma scene times were 11.0 ± 0.79 min for patients who had IV lines initiated in the field versus 9.40 ± 0.70 min for patients who had no field procedures performed. The authors stress the importance of medical direction and ongoing quality assurance aimed at minimizing the time spent in the field.

Jones et al. [4] also used independent observers on paramedic units in Los Angeles County, California, to measure the time required for IV access. Twenty-six of the 97 patients were trauma victims. The time for an IV line attempt averaged 2.8 min, with the 93 successful IV lines averaging 2.5 min and the 9 IV line failures averaging 6.3 min. On-scene and en route starting times for trauma patients were identical and averaged 2.2 min. On-scene times averaged 17 min for trauma patients. The authors recommended that IV lines be started en route, with the only exception being when definitive or resuscitative medical therapy is available.

Spaite et al. [5] used one observer to gather prospective data on 58 patients who underwent an IV attempt in 20 EMS agencies throughout Arizona. Fifty-seven patients had at least one IV line successfully started. Fifteen were victims of trauma and had their IV lines started in a mean time of 1.0 ± 0.4 min. For all patients, IVs were started more rapidly on the scene (1.3 ± 1.0) then during transport (2.0 ± 2.3). Ninety-five percent of IV line procedure intervals were less than 4 min. No differences were noted between urban and nonurban EMS personnel, leading the authors to conclude that skills retention was being maintained through training, continuing education, and practice even among nonurban EMS personnel encountering relatively fewer patients than their urban colleagues.

O'Gorman et al. [6] reviewed 350 patients in Vermont, 86 suffering from traumatic injury. Following an IV protocol designed to limit scene time, 74% of the patients had their IVs attempted while en route to the hospital. The success rates noted for on-scene versus en route IV placement (77% vs. 81%) was essentially identical. The presence of hypotension did not statistically impact the ability of the EMTs to gain intravenous access. The average time to start the on-scene IV lines was 3.8 min, while lines begun en route required an average of 4.1 min. Sixty-five percent of the EMTs placing IVs in this study were volunteers.

Slovis et al. [7] looked retrospectively at the success of Grady Memorial Hospital paramedics in Atlanta, Georgia, in attempting IV access in a moving ambulance. By policy, IVs were to be started en route rather than delaying transport. At least one IV line was successfully placed in 218 of 237 trauma patients (92%). Intravenous access was obtained in 95% of the 79 trauma patients who had a systolic blood pressure below 90 mmHg. The average on-scene time for hypotensive trauma patients was 11.64 ± 6.26 min. It was concluded that IV access should be established en route unless scene IV drug administration might provide definitive care.

These studies indicate that IV access can be initiated by EMS personnel within 3 min in most cases, and can be successfully accomplished while en route to the hospital. Volunteer personnel and those EMTs serving rural areas appear to be able to accomplish IV insertion rapidly despite caring for fewer patients than paramedics in urban settings. The presence of hypotension does not reduce intravenous success rates.

Although controversy may rage about the utility of fluid resuscitation in the trauma patient, IV access and early blood sampling is certainly of benefit should transfusion or pharmacologic therapy such as rapid sequence intubation become necessary. As long as the establishment of IV access accounts for none of the time a patient spends in the field (if started en route) or only a very small percentage of the time spent in the field (if started at the scene), it should be considered.

II. A THREAT TO FIELD PROVIDERS: CONTAMINATED NEEDLE STICKS

Emergency medical service providers are put at direct risk by accidental needle stick for the transmission of a number of blood-borne infectious diseases, including HIV, hepatitis B, and hepatitis C. The often chaotic prehospital work environment and the necessity to begin IVs in a moving ambulance to speed the patient's arrival to the hospital contribute to this risk. Conventional measures used to decrease needle sticks have included educational programs emphasizing the danger of needle recapping, the introduction of rigid sharps containers, and the institution of universal precautions. The effectiveness of these measures is debated [8].

One relatively recent development that appears to reduce accidental needle sticks is the self-capping IV catheter (see Fig. 1). In order for the catheter to be inserted after

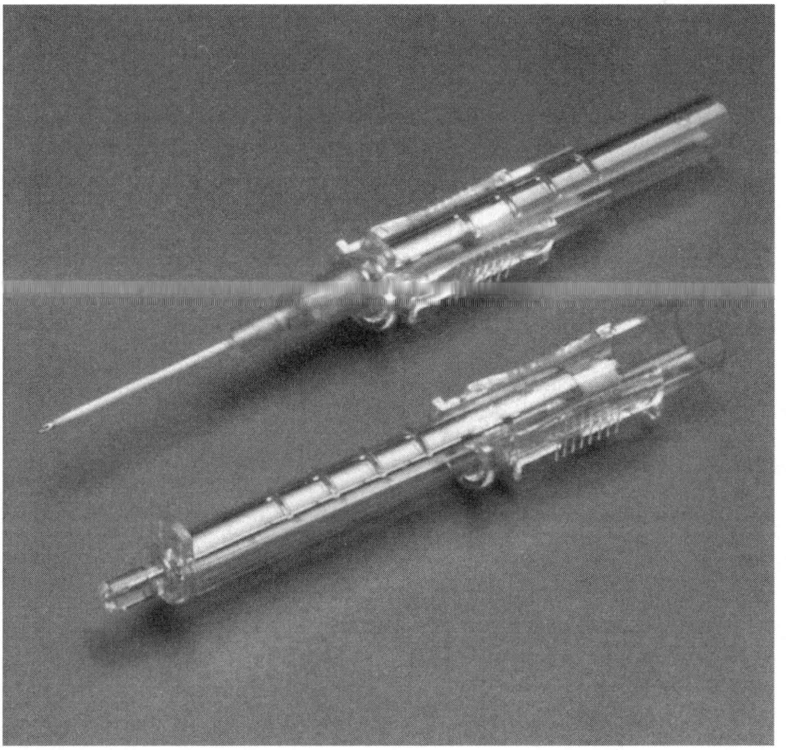

Figure 1 The top example depicts the catheter prior to use and the lower example depicts the needle assembly following catheter insertion. (From Ref. 9.)

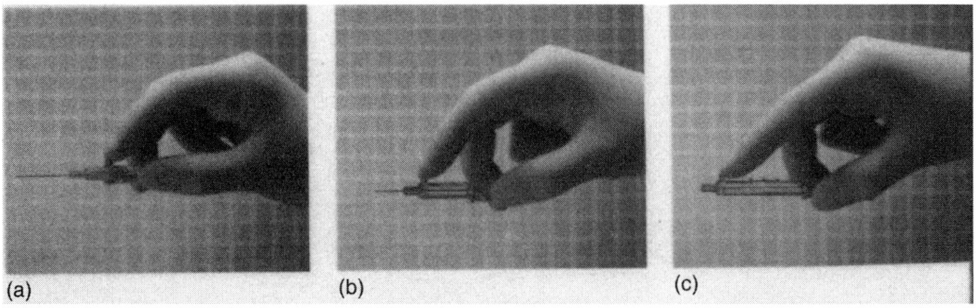

Figure 2 After puncturing the vein and visualizing a blood flash (a) the operator advances the catheter over the needle until the vein is cannulated (b), and the needle locks in place (c). The catheter has been removed from b and c to enhance the demonstration. (From Ref. 9.)

entrance into the vein, a protective plastic sleeve must be advanced over the contaminated needle to force the catheter forward. A plastic sleeve pushes the catheter completely off the needle and then locks in place to serve as a needle cap (see Fig. 2). Once the needle is so capped, it cannot be uncapped and may be safely discarded.

O'Connor et al. [9] compared the needle stick rate with conventional IV needles and then with a self-sheathing IV catheter in approximately 6500 patients requiring prehospital IV access. Eleven contaminated needle sticks were reported using conventional catheters and none was reported after the introduction of the self-capping catheter. Although the paramedics were initially displeased with the new concept, as they felt that its use would impair their ability to achieve IV catheterization, their IV success rate increased from 88 to 90%, a statistically insignificant change between the two study periods.

In addition to education about universal precautions and the threat of blood-borne contagions, EMS system should carefully consider the utility of technologies such as the self-capping IV catheter.

III. IV SITE INFECTIONS

Site infection is a potential complication of IV therapy. Should significantly more infections result from prehospital IV procedures as compared to those conducted within the hospital, this would argue against these procedures being done routinely by EMS.

This possibility was raised in 1988 by Lawrence and Lauro [10], who reviewed 191 patients admitted to Charity Hospital in New Orleans, 82 with prehospital IV therapy and 109 with emergency department (ED) IV therapy. They found that 34% of the prehospital patients developed phlebitis, a 4.65 times higher rate than for patients who had IV lines placed in the ED. Unexplained fever was noted in 22% of cases, a rate 5.58 times higher than in the ED group. Seventeen EMT-paramedics (EMT-P) and EMT intermediates (EMT-I) started the prehospital IVs, and all had similar complication rates, with the exception of one who was noted to have signs of phlebitis in over two-thirds of his cases. This EMT was subsequently counseled to improve his aseptic technique.

Lawrence and Lauro felt that IV therapy started in the prehospital setting presents a greater risk of complications than does IV therapy started in the ED. They stressed continuing education for skill maintenance, aseptic technique using hand cleanser or gloves, changing prehospital IV lines on admission (which was already common practice in their ICUs), and the risks posed by catheter movement. They speculated whether or not the short time intervals within which prehospital IV lines are begun in some systems allow for proper decontamination.

In 1995, Levine et al. [11] reviewed 859 prehospital IV lines and noted one infection (0.12%) compared to 2,326 hospital-started IV lines with four infections (0.17%). No attempt was made to assess fever or other systemic signs of infection.

The major difference between this study and that of Lawrence and Lauro is the definition used for complication. The former study considered phlebitis to be a complication, whereas the latter study utilized Center for Disease Control and Prevention guidelines for identifying nosocomial skin and soft tissue infections, which require evidence of purulence at the wound site or isolation of an infecting organism. Only a small proportion of patients with infusion-related phlebitis actually have an IV line infection.

It would be desirable to document the IV complication rate in various EMS systems. Given the large sample size and meticulous, multidisciplinary surveillance methods of Levine et al., however, it appears that IV therapy can be safely initiated in the prehospital setting.

IV. INTRAOSSEOUS INFUSION

Intravenous access is significantly more difficult in children, especially for those under six years of age [12]. Intraosseous (IO) infusion is a technique readily adopted by prehospital personnel (see Fig. 3). Seigler et al. [13] demonstrated that 100 full-time paramedics could successfully be taught the technique during a 3-hr course. They went on to place 16 IO infusion lines in 17 patients over the next year. The majority of the infusions were established within 1 min of the decision to undertake the procedure. They noted that bone marrow aspirate was obtained from only 2 of the 16 IO sites. Subsequent training stressed fluid administration under pressure with observation to exclude infiltration as the preferred technique to confirm placement.

Glaeser et al. [14] reviewed the experience on 144 Milwaukee paramedics over 5 years. Seventy-six percent of 152 patients had an IO line established successfully. Success rates varied by patient age (see Table 1); however, no significant differences were noted between the two busiest paramedic units, which placed 54% percent of the lines, and the other 9 paramedic units. No skill degradation was appreciated over the 5 years, despite a lack of any additional formal training. Although not formally assessed, the authors reported that the procedure was generally accomplished within 1 min.

Twelve percent of the 115 patients who underwent successful IO infusion line placement subsequently were noted to have infiltration into subcutaneous tissue. None of the patients with this sequela survived more than 48 hr, due to the underlying illness. Needle bending and error in site identification (one needle was placed into a patella) were noted as the most identified causes of failed attempts.

Tibial IO access is not feasible in adults because of the thickness of the cortex. The adult sternum has a relatively thin cortex and a very vascular marrow space. Sternal IO devices are now available, and encouraging prehospital data [15] are just beginning to appear, indicating that this may be a viable technique in adult patients for whom peripheral access is not possible.

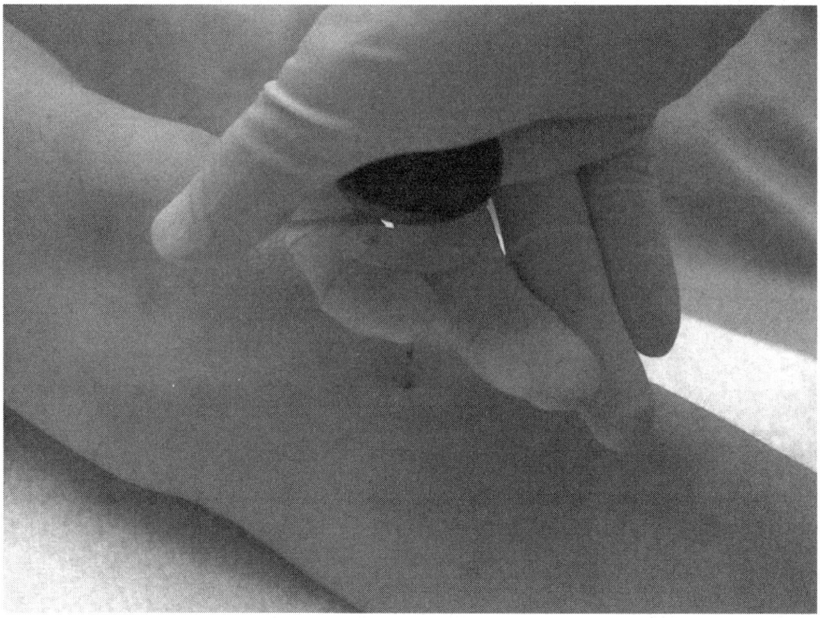

Figure 3 Intraosseous (IO) insertion is undertaken on the flat, anteromedial aspect of the proximal tibia 1 to 3 cm below the tibial tuberosity. The leg is supported above and below the insertion site, and the hand should not be placed behind the proximal tibia to avoid accidental needle stick. The needle hub is held firmly in the palm and a rotary motion is applied with steady, moderate pressure until the cortex is penetrated. The needle should be directed perpendicular to the tibia or slightly caudad to avoid injury to the growth plate. Care must be taken to avoid exerting so much force that the needle bends or pushes through the opposite side of the bone. Once in place, the stylet is removed and aspiration is attempted. This may be unsuccessful, especially in cases of cardiac arrest. Other methods to assess placement include evaluating the stability of the IO needle in the bone and whether or not fluids can be infused without evidence of swelling or extravasation.

Table 1 Patient Age and Intraosseous Infusion Line Success Rates

	Patient Age				
	0–11 Months	1–2 Years	3–9 Years	≥10	Total
Number of patients	109	20	9	14	152
Number of attempts	118	22	11	14	165
Success rate per patient (%)	78	85	67	50	76
Success rate per attempt (%)	72	77	70	50	70

Source: Ref. 14.

V. CENTRAL VENOUS ACCESS

Peripheral IV placement is preferred for prehospital trauma victims, given the speed of placement under most circumstances and the minimal complications encountered. Given Poiseuille's law, which states that the rate of flow is proportional to the fourth power of the radius of the cannula and is inversely related to its length, the central venous catheter (CVC) provides little benefit over two large-bore peripheral IV lines for volume resuscitation. Dutky et al. [16] compared flow rates through a number of devices, including the 4 1/4 in., 8.5 French central IV catheter and the 2 1/4 in., 14-gauge (g) peripheral IV. Two 14-g or 16-g peripheral IV cannulae were comparable to a 8.5 French central IV cannula. Tubing size had a significant impact on the flow rate (see Table 2).

Although central venous access appears to offer clinically insignificant advantage over peripheral access when delivering drugs in normal perfusion states [17], in low flow states such as cardiac arrest, a central venous access appears to be superior to peripheral access [18]. It may be possible, however, to significantly reduce the delay in transit to the central circulation associated with peripheral venous drug administration by using a 0.5-ml/kg postinfusion saline bolus under pressure.

When the transport time is extended (longer than 30 min) and peripheral IV establishment is impossible due to issues such as severe burns, gross obesity, very significant multiple extremity trauma, history of IV drug abuse, severe edema, or scar tissue, then CVC might salvage a dire situation if the patient requires emergent volume expansion. Patient entrapment might also conceivably preclude the establishment of a peripheral IV and make central access necessary.

Any medical technique is only feasible if the care provider is well versed in the technique and confident of his or her ability to carry it out. This constitutes a major factor in any discussion of the utility of CVC placement in the prehospital setting in countries in which EMS systems rely solely on paramedics. Placement can be regarded as just a sequence of technical steps and therefore could potentially be taught to paramedic personnel; however, the rare need for CVC placement in the prehospital setting, the complexity of the procedure, the seriousness of the potential complications, and the immediate need to detect and treat these complications dictate that as a general rule CVC placement should be reserved for the experienced physician. When done by experienced personnel the complication rate is low [19], but can rise with inexperienced doctors [20].

In some European EMS systems, prehospital physician involvement (often with anesthesia/intensive care physician and nurse teams) is the norm, and expertise and equipment is not an issue. In those cases in which CVC lines are placed, the potential benefits

Table 2 Effect of Tubing Size on Flow Rates of Crystalloids (25 °C) Using Common Intravenous Cannulae (cc/min)

	Regular IV tubing	Blood tubing	Trauma tubing
18-gauge	87	108	117
16-gauge	125	193	247
14-gauge	147	268	417
8.5 French	160	316	805

Source: Ref. 16.

of line placement must be weighed against the risks of prolonging scene time and delaying hospital arrival.

There are several possible approaches to CVC placement, each associated with possible complications. As a general rule, the IV access site should be chosen keeping the traumatized anatomy in mind. A patient suffering a pneumothorax should not have a CVC attempted that might endanger the contralateral thorax and risk bilateral pneumothorax. As most trauma victims will be at risk for abdominal injury, a sole access below the level of the diaphragm may be ineffective [21]. Air embolism is a threat in hypovolaemic patients with any CVC approach [22].

The external jugular (EJ) approach can be used for either a simple IV or CVC and is a relatively safe and reliable alternative [23]. Hemorrhage is easier to control and the risk of carotid or pleural puncture is minimal in comparison to the internal jugular (IJ) route. The major disadvantage in the blunt trauma patient is the need to immobilize the cervical spine. Neck access is complicated by the cervical collar and lateral head immobilization devices [21]. In situations involving cardiopulmonary resuscitation, however, it represents the best alternative to the antecubital vein.

The basilic and cephalic arm veins can be used to gain central access, but in trauma, these routes are excellent for short, thick catheters rather than as a route for central access. The introduction of a 8.5 French catheter (over a guide wire inserted through a 20-g catheter) can be considered, and with a pressure infusion bag can deliver up to a liter of crystalloid a minute [16,23].

More conventional CVC approaches include the IJ, the subclavian (SC), and the femoral vein (FV). In general, rather than a central line with a small lumen, the use of the 8.5 French introducer sheath as a stand-alone catheter should be considered, as it is capable of high flow rates up to twice as fast as through a 14-g catheter [16,23].

The right-sided IJ approach is preferred, as there is no risk of thoracic duct injury and the pleural space is lower in the chest than on the left [23]. Carotid puncture is a definite risk (2–10% of cases) [24], and hematoma formation might put the airway at risk. In case of hemorrhage one should never attempt access on the contralateral jugular [21,25]. Neck immobilization may hinder placement and will impair site inspection and detection of complications.

The SC approach is perhaps easier access than IJ in the patient with possible cervical spinal trauma. It is associated with complications such as hemothorax or pneumothorax, which occur in 1–5% of all cases [19]. Given the decrease in atmospheric pressure during flight, a life-threatening tension pneumothorax might conceivably result [26]. In case of thoracic trauma, the SC insertion should be attempted on the traumatized side [23] to avoid iatrogenic pneumothorax on the opposite intact side.

The FV is accessible, allows for concurrent airway management, has fewer than 10% immediate complications, and is easily compressed to control hemorrhage [21]. Infection may be a significant complication later in the hospital course but this risk can be minimized if alternative routes are attained and the femoral line removed in 48 to 72 hr [27].

Given that peripheral IV access is usually possible, CVC utilization in the prehospital setting is difficult to justify even with a skilled medical team on site. If extremity peripheral access is impossible, the EJ route should be considered using a simple IV catheter. Given an extended transport time, inability to obtain IV access, progressive hypovolemic shock, and the presence of a competent clinician, the CVC might be considered in the prehospital setting.

VI. CONCLUSIONS

Trauma patients should have venous access established while en route to the hospital. Exceptions might include entrapped patients or patients with concomitant medical conditions, such as severe hypoglycemia, which could be definitively treated in the field.

Contaminated needle sticks pose a real threat to EMS personnel that may be reduced through proper precautions, including the utilization of self-capping IV catheters.

Prehospital IVs can be started routinely without exposing patients to an increased risk of IV site infections. Intravenous site infection rates should be monitored from time to time by individual EMS services.

Intraosseous infusion should be rapidly utilized if conventional peripheral IV access is difficult in critically ill or injured children.

Central access offers little if any benefit in the prehospital arena when compared to two conventional large-bore peripheral cannulae.

Efforts to increase the rate of fluid resuscitation should focus first on improvements gained by utilizing larger-diameter IV tubing.

REFERENCES

1. JS Sampalis, H Tamim, R Denis, S Boukas, R Sebastien-Abel, A Nikolis, A Lavoie, D Fleiszer, R Brown, D Mulder, JI Williams. Ineffectiveness of on-site intravenous lines: Is prehospital time the culprit? J Trauma 43:608–617, 1997.
2. GR McSwain, WB Garrison, CR Artz. Evaluation of resuscitation from cardiopulmonary arrest by paramedics. Ann Emerg Med 9:341–345, 1980.
3. P Pons, E Moore, J Cusick, M Brunko, B Antuna, L Owens. Prehospital venous access in an urban paramedic system—A prospective on scene analysis. J Trauma 28:1460–1463, 1988.
4. SE Jones, TP Nesper. Alcouloumre E: Prehospital intravenous line placement: A prospective study. Ann Emerg Med 18:244–246, 1989.
5. DW Spaite, TD Valenzuela, EA Criss, HW Meislin, P Hinsberg. A prospective in-field comparison of intravenous line placement by urban and nonurban emergency medical services personnel. Ann Emerg Med 24:209–214, 1994.
6. M O'Gorman, P Trabulsy, DB Pilcher. Zero time prehospital IVs. J Trauma [illegible], 1989.
7. CM Slovis, EW Herr, D Londof, TD Little, BR Alexander, RJ Guthmann. Success rates for initiation of intravenous therapy en route by prehospital care providers. Am J Emerg Med 8: 305–307, 1990.
8. CC Linnemann, C Cannon, M DeRonde, B Lanphear. Effect of educational programs, rigid sharps containers, and universal precautions on reported needlestick injuries in healthcare workers. Infec Con Hosp Epid 12:214–219, 1991.
9. RE O'Connor, SP Krall, RE Megargel, LE Tan, JE Bouzoukis. Reducing the rate of paramedic needlesticks in emergency medical services: The role of self-capping intravenous catheters. Acad Emerg Med 3:668–674, 1996.
10. DW Lawrence, AJ Lauro. Complicatins from IV therapy: Results from field-started and emergency department-started IVs compared. Ann Emerg Med 17:314–317, 1988.
11. R Levine, DW Spaite, TD Valenzuela, EA Criss, AL Wright, HW Meislin. Comparison of clinically significant infection rates among prehospital-versus in-hospital-initiated IV lines. Ann Emerg Med 25:502–506, 1995.
12. KA Lillis, DM Jaffe. Prehospital intravenous access in children. Ann Emerg Med 21:1430–1434, 1992.
13. RS Seigler, FW Tecklenburg, R Shealy. Prehospital intraosseous infusion by emergency medical services personnel: A prospective study. Pediatrics 84:173–177, 1989.

14. PW Glaeser, TR Hellmich, D Szewczuga, JD Losek, DS Smith. Five-year experience in prehospital intraosseous infusions in children and adults. Ann Emer Med 22:1119–1124, 1993.
15. BT Horwood, J Adams, BR Tiffany, CV Pollack, B Adams, R Scalzi, M Sucher. Prehospital use of a sternal intraosseous infusion device (abstract). Ann Emerg Med 34(part 2):S65–S66, 1999.
16. PA Dutky, SL Stevens, KI Maull. Factors affecting rapid fluid resuscitation with large-bore introducer catheters. J Trauma 29:856–860, 1989.
17. WG Barsan, JR Hedges, H Nishiyama, ST Lukes. Differences in drug delivery with peripheral and central venous injections: Normal perfusion. Am J Emerg Med 4:1–3, 1986.
18. JR Hedges, WB Barsan, LA Doan, SM Joyce, SJ Lukes, WC Dalsey, H Nishiyama. Central versus peripheral intravenous routes in cardiopulmonary resuscitation. Am J Emerg Med 2: 385–390, 1984.
19. ET Simpson, MB Aitch. Percutaneous infraclavicular subclavian vein catheterization in shocked patients: A prospective study in 12 patients. J Trauma 22:781–784, 1982.
20. JI Sznajder, FR Zveibil, H Bitterman, et al. Central vein catheterization: Failure and complication rate by percutaneous approaches. Arch Int Med 46:259–261, 1986.
21. MN Sweeney. Vascular access in trauma: Options, risks, benefits, and complications. In: CM Grande, CE Smith, eds. Anesthesiology Clinics of North America: Trauma. Philadelphia: Saunders, March 1999, pp. 97–106.
22. W Bickell, RE Pepe, KL Mattox. Complications of resuscitation. In: KL Mattox, ed. Complication of Trauma. New York: Churchill Livingstone, 1994.
23. MA Berk. Vascular access. In: JE Tintinalli, E Ruiz, RL Krome, eds. Emergency Medicine: A Comprehensive Study Guide. 4th ed. New York: McGraw-Hill, 1996, pp. 50–57.
24. MG Seneff. Central venous catheterization: A comprehensive review. part 2. Intensive Care Med 2:218–232, 1987.
25. RJ De Falque. Percutaneous catheterization of the internal jugular vein. Anesth Analg 53:116, 1974.
26. T Martin, HD Rodenberg. Clinical considerations in transport of the ill and injured. In: Aeromedical Transportation: A Clinical Guide. Hants: Burlington, VT, 1996, pp. 131–196.
27. MG Seneff. Central venous catheterization: A comprehensive review. part 1. Intensive Care Med 2:218–232, 1987.

17

Fluid Resuscitation and Circulatory Support: Fluids—When, What, and How Much?

HENGO HALJAMÄE

Sahlgrenska University Hospital, Göteborg, Sweden

MAUREEN McCUNN

R Adams Cowley Shock Trauma Center, University of Maryland Medical System, Baltimore, Maryland

I. INTRODUCTION

Fluid resuscitation of trauma patients presenting with hemorrhagic hypotension is an integral, mandatory component of the restoration of normal organ physiology. In the initial prehospital management it is important to consider the severity of the condition, the possibilities to stop or reduce blood loss, and the urgency with which to start fluid resuscitation. The following aspects of prehospital fluid resuscitation of trauma patients are fundamental (Fig. 1):

When?	Indications for start of fluid therapy
What?	Choice of fluid
How much?	Monitoring and goals for the fluid resuscitation

II. WHEN? INDICATIONS FOR START OF FLUID THERAPY

A. General Aspects

Aggressive therapeutic measures during the first ''golden hour'' following trauma are usually considered vital for the outcome of trauma patients. In the case of a short transport

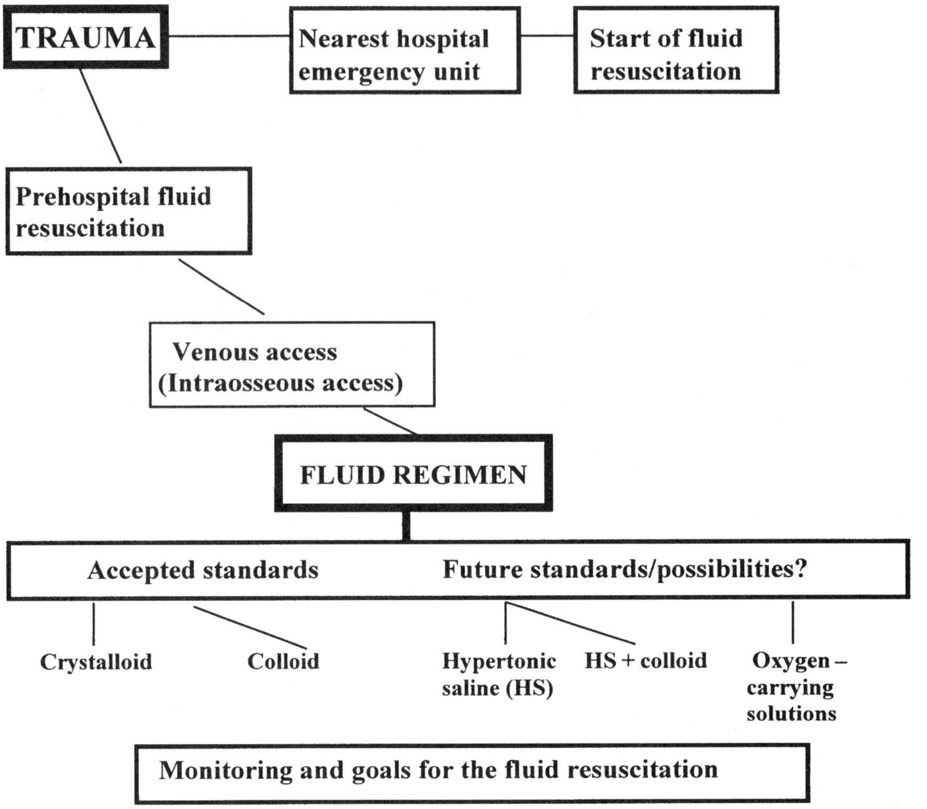

Figure 1 Strategies and alternative possibilities in prehospital fluid resuscitation.

time to the nearest hospital emergency department however, the necessity of intravenous access and start of fluid resuscitation in the field may be questioned. It may be more important for survival to get the patient to the emergency department rather than delay transportation by attempts to start fluid therapy. The facilities of a hospital emergency department allow not only better resuscitation conditions but also more advanced diagnostic modalities and more prompt surgical intervention for the reduction of blood loss. In most trauma situations, however, establishing IV access and the initiation of fluid infusion as early as possible in the clinical course (i.e., in the prehospital setting) is considered essential (Fig. 1). Venous cannulation is certainly easier to perform in the early posttraumatic phase before severe hypovolemia develops than in established hypovolemic shock. In late shock, peripheral venous cutdown or central venous cannulation may be the only remaining access alternatives. Whenever possible, at least one—but preferably more than one—large-bore IV line should be established and safely secured in trauma patients, and fluid therapy should be started.

In pediatric patients venous access is usually more difficult than in adults. This is especially true in the prehospital setting, in which the establishment of a venous line may be all too time-consuming. In pediatric trauma patients insertion of an intraosseous needle for fluid infusion as well as for the administration of drugs may be a lifesaving alternative.

In adults the value of intraosseous infusions in trauma resuscitation is less obvious and the clinical experience more limited, although recent clinical trials have shown promise.

B. Trauma-Induced Internal Fluid Fluxes

Trauma is commonly accompanied by major disturbances of the fluid homeostasis between the different fluid spaces of the body [1]. In addition to direct blood and plasma losses there will be major internal fluid redistributions in response to trauma-induced endogenous blood volume supporting defense mechanisms.

It is important to consider that two-thirds of the fluid content of the body (i.e., about 28 liters in a 70-kg individual) is normally within the intracellular space (Fig. 2). The interstitial and intravascular spaces contain most of the remaining fluid (about 14 liters), and the ratio of the interstitial and intravascular fluid volumes is approximately 4/1.

In response to the neuroendocrine activation induced by trauma and hemorrhage, about 1.0 liter of fluid can be transferred from the intracellular and interstitial spaces into the intravascular compartment in an adult (Fig. 2). The main components of this endogenous plasma volume-supporting defense mechanism (transcapillary refill) are the following:

Glucose-osmotic fluid mobilization [2]: Trauma-induced hyperglycemia will increase plasma osmolality, whereby about 2 to 3 liters of fluid is mobilized from the intracellular compartment into the intersititial space. Of this fluid about 0.5 liters will reach the intravascular compartment and support blood volume. Trauma-induced insulin resistance will facilitate this fluid flux.

Resetting the pre- to postcapillary resistance ratio [2]: Capillary hydrostatic pressure is reduced by resetting the pre- to postcapillary resistance ratio. The equilibrium of the transcapillary Starling exchange process is consequently altered in favor of net fluid reabsorption from extravascular sources. About 0.5 liters of fluid can

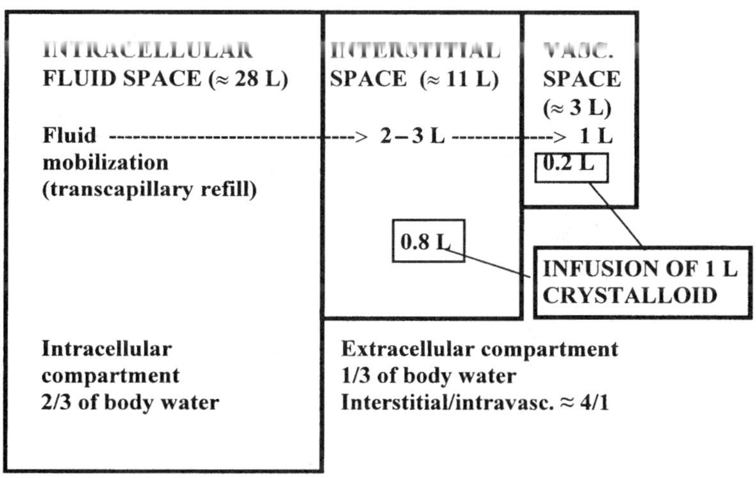

Figure 2 Fluid spaces, shock- and trauma-induced transcapillary refill, and the plasma volume supporting effect of crystalloid resuscitation fluid.

be mobilized into the intravascular compartment by this compensatory mechanism in the hypovolemic trauma patient.

In addition to direct fluid losses and internal compensatory fluid shifts, there may be additional generalized internal fluid losses in the trauma patient. These fluid losses are caused by a trauma-induced activation of the cascade systems, evoking a systemic inflammatory response syndrome (SIRS) influencing endothelial cell function and thereby capillary permeability [3,4]. This more generalized increase of capillary permeability will further enhance the hypovolemia and contribute to the redistribution of blood flow to central vital organs at the expense of the perfusion of the splanchnic vascular bed, the kidneys, skeletal muscle, and skin.

In order to achieve normovolemia and hemodynamic stability and reestablish fluid homeostasis in trauma patients, it is obvious that not only direct blood losses but also all of these internal fluid fluxes have to be compensated for during fluid resuscitation [4]. Furthermore, the maintenance of an adequate plasma colloid osmotic pressure (COP) may be of importance for improving the microvascular blood flow [4]. Prevention of cascade system activation and trauma-induced increase in blood coagulability are additional factors to be considered at the resuscitation of trauma patients.

Primary Goals of Fluid Resuscitation
The primary goals of fluid resuscitation of trauma patients are [4] as follows:
Re-establish normovolemia and hemodynamic stability
Compensate for the internal fluid fluxes from the interstitial and intracellular compartments
Maintain an adequate plasma colloid osmotic pressure (COP)
Improve microvascular blood flow
Prevent cascade system activation and trauma-induced increase in blood coagulability
Normalize oxygen delivery to tissue cells and thereby cellular metabolism and organ function
Prevent reperfusion type of injury

III. WHAT? CHOICE OF FLUID THERAPY

A. Initial Resuscitation With Crystalloid or Colloid?

The optimal fluid regimen (i.e., the use of crystalloids or colloids) for resuscitation of trauma patients has remained a matter of controversy [4]. It has even been claimed that colloid resuscitation is associated with increased mortality (Table 1). On the basis of systematic reviews (meta-analyses) of randomized controlled studies it has been suggested that colloid administration may deletoriously influence the outcome of trauma patients

Table 1 Comparative Mortality Figures from Two Systematic Meta-Analytic Assessments of Mortality of Trauma Patients Resuscitated With Crystalloid or Colloid

Reference	Crystalloids	Colloids
Velanovich [5]	12.3% lower mortality	Increased mortality vs. crystalloids
Schierhout and Roberts [6]	Mortality 44/301 patients	Mortality 82/335 patients; relative risk vs. crystalloids 1.30 (0.95–1.77)

Table 2 Advantages and Disadvantages of Crystalloid as Compared to Colloid Fluid Regimens in Trauma Resuscitation

	Advantages	Disadvantages
Crystalloid	Balanced electrolyte composition	Poor plasma volume support
	Buffering capacity (lactate/acetate)	Large quantities needed
	Easy to administer	Risk of overhydration
	No risk of adverse reactions	Risk of hypothermia
	No disturbance of hemostasis	Reduced plasma COP
	Promoting diuresis	Risk of edema formation
	Inexpensive	
Colloid	Good intravascular persistence	Risk of volume overload
	Reduced resuscitation time	Adverse effects on hemostasis
	Moderate volume required	Tissue accumulation
	Enhancing microvascular flow	Adverse effects on renal function
	Plasma COP moderately altered	Risk of anaphylactoid reactions
	Minor risk of tissue edema	More expensive than crystalloid
	Moderation of SIRS	

Source: Ref. 4.

[5,6]. In his meta-analysis assessment of the influence of crystalloid and colloid resuscitation on outcome published in 1989, Velanovich [5] included eight clinical studies of trauma resuscitation. Of the studies considered for inclusion in the meta-analysis, a reduced mortality of 12.3% in favor of crystalloid resuscitation was observed (Table 1).

A meta-analysis published in 1998 [6] was based on a systematic review of 26 published randomized studies comparing mortality (of all reasons) in critically ill patients receiving fluid therapy with either colloids or crystalloids. Of the reviewed studies, seven dealt with trauma patients. The review indicated that the relative risk of death for trauma patients treated with colloid was 1.30, compared to patients receiving crystalloid. It was therefore suggested that as colloids are not associated with improved survival and are considerably more expensive than crystalloids, it is hard to see how their continued use outside randomized controlled trials in subsets of patients of particular concern can be justified [6].

It should be noted, however, that in 14 out of the 26 studies the colloids infused were albumin or plasma protein fraction, and in three of the trauma studies hypertonic (7.5%) saline was used rather than conventional crystalloids as the fluid treatment regimen. The reported association [7] between human albumin administration in critically ill patients and increased mortality could influence the outcome following trauma resuscitation.

Another important question to consider is the clinical relevance of data obtained from meta-analyses of ''historical'' studies for the present practice of trauma care. The original publications included in the meta-analysis of Velanovich in 1989 [5] were published between 1977 to 1984. The report by the *Cochrane Injuries Group Albumin Reviewers* [7] was based on a systematic review of controlled studies published over the past 23 years. During this long time period many basic therapeutic procedures in trauma resuscitation in addition to the choice of fluid regimen have changed considerably and do not really reflect present practice. Furthermore, in a recent study of the outcome after hemorrhagic shock in trauma patients Heckbert et al. [8] demonstrated a highly significant association between increasing volume of crystalloids infused in the first 24 hr and increased mortality.

Although a more recent meta-analysis [9] also indicates a lower mortality in trauma patients resuscitated with crystalloids, it still cannot be overlooked that due to their specific characteristics, artificial colloids may play an important role in the treatment of trauma patients [4,10].

B. Characteristics of Crystalloid- and Colloid-Based Fluid Regimens

In the prehospital setting initial infusion of crystalloid is more commonly chosen than infusion of colloid. The advantages and disadvantages of crystalloid and colloid-based fluid regimens in the initial fluid management of trauma patients are summarized in Table 2.

1. Crystalloids

With infusion of a crystalloid the initial volume-supporting effect is reasonably adequate. Balanced salt solutions will freely cross the capillary membrane, however, and consequently equilibrate within the whole extracellular fluid space. The intravascular retention of a crystalloid is poor, and for prolonged volume support large quantities—that is, four to five times the actual intravascular volume deficit (Fig. 2)—have to be infused in order to achieve normovolemia in shock and trauma states [4]. Distribution throughout the whole extracellular space and leakage into cells explains an intravascular volume-supporting efficacy of only about 0.15 to 0.20 liter per liter of crystalloid infused. Crystalloid infusion for achievement of normovolemia is consequently associated with an obvious risk of hypothermia in the trauma patient unless the fluid is properly heated. If hypothermia is induced, blood coagulation will be impaired. In conjunction with the consequences of direct dilution of coagulation factors, this may enhance blood losses.

Since large quantities of crystalloid are needed for the restoration of hemodynamic stability in hypovolemic trauma patients, it is necessary to choose a ''balanced'' crystalloid with an electrolyte composition similar to that of plasma (i.e., a Ringer's type of solution) to avoid acute disturbances of serum electrolyte levels.

Commonly used crystalloid resuscitation fluids also have a ''buffering capacity.'' This is achieved by a content of either lactate or acetate. When the lactate or acetate ions are metabolized by tissue cells, bicarbonate ions are produced, and a buffer effect is achieved. Acetate-containing Ringer's solutions seem more advantageous than lactate-containing ones since the capacity of the body to metabolize acetate is less reduced in shock than the capacity to metabolize lactate [4]. A lactate-containing solution may therefore even aggravate an already existing lactic acidosis since the metabolic capacity of the two main lactate-clearing organs (i.e., the liver and the kidney) is disturbed in severe shock. Acetate, on the other hand, can be metabolized by most tissue cells of the body. Ringer's solutions containing acetate therefore seem more advantagous for shock treatment than those containing lactate [4].

A crystalloid-based resuscitation will always result in tissue edema formation since 75–80% of the infused volume will lodge in the extravascular compartments [4]. Fluid will accumulate mainly in tissues with a high compliance, such as skin and connective tissue. It is usually considered that this type of peripheral edema, resulting from excessive crystalloid resuscitation, is mainly of cosmetic and not of functional importance. Generalized edema may, however, disturb the transport of oxygen and nutrients to tissue cells and contribute to the development of multiple organ failure. Iatrogenic tissue edema caused by crystalloid resuscitation is reflected by a significant weight gain and has been considered to result in a prolonged need for mechanical ventilation, impaired wound healing, and prolonged ICU stays [4]. Increased extravascular lung water, influencing lung function, on the other hand, does not seem a common problem associated with crystalloid resuscitation [11].

2. Colloids

Even in low concentrations, colloids will considerably reduce the fluid volume requirements for the proper resuscitation of a patient in shock [4]. The larger, oncotically active colloid molecules will not easily cross capillary membranes. The greater capacity of colloids to remain within the intravascular space results in a more efficient intravascular plasma volume support/expansion without a risk of fluid overload of extravascular tissues (Table 2). The better intravascular persistance of a colloid will significantly reduce the resuscitation time, (i.e., the time needed to normalize the hemodynamics of shock and trauma patients). The choice of a colloid will also make it possible to maintain a better hemodynamic stability after the initial resuscitation period.

It has been repeatedly shown that colloid resuscitation will improve oxygen transport (DO2) to tissues, thereby enhancing tissue oxygen metabolism (VO2) more effectively than crystalloid fluid resuscitation [12]. There is, therefore, considerable clinical support for the concept that in the resuscitation of trauma patients the therapeutic goals should be adequate expansion of the plasma volume to enhance tissue perfusion, oxygen delivery (DO2), and oxygen consumption (VO2). Such a response can be achieved most effectively when a colloid resuscitation regime is chosen [4].

The volume and concentration of a colloid solution (i.e., the dose of colloid infused) has in experimental shock been shown to be of major importance for intravascular volume support and for survival [4]. It seems that 2–3% colloid solutions are optimal for a balanced normalization of the shock-induced disturbances of the fluid equilibrium between the different fluid spaces of the body. The plasma volume is rather rapidly normalized by such a colloid concentration, and enough fluid will reach out into the extravascular and intracellular spaces to compensate for the above considered endogenous fluid fluxes that occur initially in response to the traumatic stress on the body. The risk of fluid overload out into the tissues during resuscitation with colloids is reduced since major reduction of COP (as seen following resuscitation with crystalloids) does not occur.

Artificial (synthetic) as well as natural colloids have been commonly used in the initial resuscitation of trauma patients (Table 3). The dominating groups of artificial col-

Table 3 Relative Efficacies of Commonly Used Colloids for Plasma Volume Support, Cascade System Modulation, and Hemorheology in Trauma Patients

	Plasma volume support	Intravascular persistance	Prevention of cascade system activation	Hemorheologic effects
Artificial colloids				
Dextran	+++	+++	++	+++
HES, pentastarch	+++	+++	+	++
Gelatin, polygeline	+	+	(+)	+
Natural colloids				
Plasma	++	++	−	+
Albumin	++	++	+	++

Effects: +++ = good; ++ = moderate; + = poor; (+) = insignificant; − = nonbeneficial.
Source: Refs. 4, 10.

loids are dextrans, gelatins, and different hydroxyethyl starch preparations. Plasma as well as albumin solutions of different concentrations are the main natural colloid preparations for plasma volume expansion. Colloid characteristics such as plasma volume supporting capacity, intravascular persistance of the macromolecules, modulating effects on cascade system activation, hemorheological influences on microvascular blood flow, and colloid safety are important for the choice of colloid [4,10].

In spite of the well-documented beneficial effects of colloid-containing resuscitation fluids in trauma resuscitation, it still seems that common practice is to add colloid at a later stage in the resuscitation, usually during the continued in-hospital treatment of the trauma patient rather than in the prehospital trauma environment. It should be noted, however, that the presently ongoing crystalloid versus colloid controversy, based on meta-analyses of randomized controlled studies [5,6,9], may challenge such a resuscitation routine.

C. Small-Volume Hypertonic Saline Resuscitation

Initial prehospital hypertonic saline (HS) resuscitation in hypovolaemic shock is a new therapeutic approach that is considered advantageous since HS has been shown experimentally as well as clinically to increase systemic blood pressure, cardiac output, peripheral tissue perfusion, and survival rates [4,13]. Most commonly a 7.5% NaCl (2,400 mOsm/L) solution (with or without colloid) is used. The volumes infused in the treatment of hypovolemia are small, usually about 4 ml/kg body weight. This ''small-volume'' principle should be compared to the large fluid volume requirements of about four to five times the blood-volume deficit that have to be infused when isotonic crystalloid solutions are used in the treatment of hypovolemia and shock.

The advantages and disadvantages of HS and HS+colloid resuscitation are summarized in Table 4. The central hemodynamic support induced by HS is the result of a rapid

Table 4 Advantages and Disadvantages of Prehospital Hypertonic Saline (Without or With Colloid) Resuscitation in Trauma

	Advantages	Disadvantages
Hypertonic saline (HS)	Small volume needed	Local pain on infusion
	Rapid volume support	Increased sodium load
	Reduced cardiac afterload	Negative inotropic effects
	Increased cardiac output	Risk of cardiac arrhythmias
	Enhanced capillary blood flow	Risk of increased bleeding
	Reduction of tissue edema	Short duration of volume support
	Promoting diuresis	
HS + colloid	Small volume needed	Local pain on infusion
	Prolonged plasma volume support	Increased sodium load
	Reduced cardiac afterload	Negative inotropic effects
	Increased cardiac output	Risk of cardiac arrhythmias
	Enhanced capillary blood flow	Risk of increased bleeding
	Reduction of tissue edema	Colloid associated reactions
	Promoting diuresis	

Source: Refs. 4, 13.

mobilization of fluid from the extra- and intracellular compartments into the vascular compartment. This dynamic fluid redistribution, caused by an osmotic gradient, is similar to the previously discussed endogenous transcapillary fluid mobilization that is induced by the initial hyperglycemic response to shock and trauma [2]. The circulatory effect induced by 7.5% HS, however, is much more pronounced.

It has been well documented that the treatment of hypovolemic conditions with HS solutions improves cardiac output. The direct effects of HS on myocardial performance may, however, be slightly depressant rather than stimulatory. It is therefore likely that other physiological mechanisms may be involved in the cardiovascular stimulatory actions induced by HS treatment. Central sympathetic activity seems enhanced by increased sodium levels. Hypertonic saline therapy also promotes diuresis, which may be of importance for prevention of renal failure in the trauma patient.

The hemodilution that follows the HS-induced dynamic fluid redistribution offers hemorheological advantages. As a result, blood flow through the terminal vascular bed is improved and venous return is enhanced. There is an efficient restitution of organ perfusion following HS infusion, especially when a hypertonic–hyperoncotic fluid combination is chosen rather than HS alone. The beneficial effects of HS on microvascular blood flow are probably multifactorial. A deswelling of blood cells and vascular endothelial cells will occur following infusion of HS in addition to the direct vasodilatory effects of HS (Table 4).

There are several potential disadvantages of HS therapy (Table 4). In addition to local pain at the site of infusion and transient negative effects on cardiac function, a risk of increased bleeding due to vasodilatory effects has been suggested.

1. HS Therapy and Clinical Outcome

A meta-analysis of the efficacy of prehospital or initial intrahospital treatment of trauma patients with hypertonic 7.5% saline in combination with 6% dextran (Table 5) indicates that the HS–dextran combination is superior to HS alone or the usual standard of care [13], especially in trauma patients with head injuries. Survival to hospital discharge has been found to be significantly increased (from 16–32%).

Although small volume (about 1 ml/kg) prehospital trauma resuscitation with hypertonic saline in combination with colloid presently is the standard prehospital fluid regimen in only a few countries in the world, it still seems a promising fluid regimen that may in the future become the standard of care worldwide.

Table 5 Outcome Data of Small Volume (250 ml) Hypertonic Saline (HS) and HS + Dextran (HSD) Resuscitation as Compared to Isotonic Fluid Standard of Care (SOC) Resuscitation of Hypotensive Trauma Patients

Fluid therapy	Number of trauma patients	Discharge survival
HS	340	69.1%
Isotonic (SOC)	379	69.7%
HSD	615	74.6%
Isotonic (SOC)	618	71.0%

Source: Refs. 4, 13.

D. Artificial Oxygen Carriers—the Future?

Initial fluid therapy with oxygen-carrying solutions is another possible future resuscitation regimen in trauma [14]. Two major types of oxygen carriers—modified hemoglobin solutions and fluorocarbon emulsions—have for years been experimentally tested and are under development as potential clinical volume expanders in emergency situations.

1. Hemoglobin Solutions

Two different types of hemoglobin preparations are being tested: solutions containing modified hemoglobin molecules or liposome-encapsulated hemoglobin. The source of stroma-free hemoglobin is outdated human blood, bovine hemoglobin, or human recombinant hemoglobin. The hemoglobin preparations are modified to optimize the oxygen-carrying capacity (CaO2) and oxygen unloading in the tissues. By polymerization or encapsulation a colloidal plasma volume-supporting capacity is also achieved. The oxygen-carrying characteristics of modified hemoglobin solutions are similar to those of red blood cells; that is, a sigmoidal oxygen dissociation curve is achieved. High inspiratory oxygen concentration is therefore not mandatory for efficient oxygen transport.

In experimental studies, hemoglobin solutions have been found to restore circulating blood volume in hemorrhagic hypotensive states and provide adequate tissue oxygenation. A problem associated with some of the hemoglobin solutions has been vasoconstriction influencing systemic as well as pulmonary vessels. The suggested mechanism has been interference with the normal nitric oxide (NO) levels due to the binding of NO to free hemoglobin molecules. Clinical phase II and III studies are in progress and hemoglobin solutions may in the near future be the fluid of choice in prehospital trauma resuscitation.

2. Perfluorocarbons

Carbon–fluorine compounds are characterized by a high gas-dissolving capacity, low viscosity, and chemical and biological inertness [14]. Fluosol-DA, originally developed in Japan, was considered years ago as a potentially valuable oxygen-carrying emulsion. It appeared, however, to have a potential to cause anaphylactoid reactions and to be unstable at room temperature. Several new generations of fluorocarbon emulsions have appeared and are well tolerated, except by patients with egg allergy, since egg-yolk phospholipids are used as emulsifiers.

The oxygen-transporting capacity of fluorocarbon emulsions is not as great as that of hemoglobin solutions. There is a linear relationship between oxygen partial pressure and oxygen content; that is, high (100%) inspired oxygen is necessary for a good oxygen transport. Since perfluorocarbon emulsions are rather rapidly eliminated, they may become of considerable value as oxygen carriers in the initial prehospital phase of trauma resuscitation.

IV. HOW MUCH? MONITORING AND GOALS OF FLUID THERAPY

A. Monitoring

Regardless of the fluid used for resuscitation, it is imperative to use reliable physiologic endpoints to gauge the initial response to treatment and to adjust the therapy to meet the individual needs of the patient. The variables usually monitored during the prehospital

Table 6 Monitoring of Prehospital Fluid Therapy in Trauma Patients

The "clinical eye"	Pulse, skin color, vascular filling, capillary blood flow, mental state, etc.
Hemodynamic variables	Heart rate, ECG, blood pressure, pulse oximetry
Tissue perfusion	Skeletal muscle pO2
Tissue perfusion/metabolism	Intramucosal tonometry of CO2, blood lactate, acid-base status
Renal function	Diuresis

care, in addition to those appreciated by the "experienced clinical eye," are blood pressure, heart rate, ECG, and pulse oximetry (Table 6). The "clinical impression" is of major importance for recognition of valuable information about respiration, ongoing blood losses, signs of hypovolemia (vascular filling, capillary blood flow, anemia), mental state, and so on. Added to these, the monitored variables are helpful for assessing the severity of the condition and the efficacy of the fluid resuscitation.

The basic management principle is to first *stop the bleeding* and to then replace the volume lost. Management is directed toward providing adequate oxygenation at the cellular level. In hypoperfusion shock syndromes, reduced oxygen delivery (DO2) results in a fall in oxygen consumption (VO2), resulting in an oxygen deficit (oxygen debt). There appears to be a critical rate of oxygen debt accrual *and* an absolute level beyond which probability increases sharply; an exponential relationship between oxygen debt and mortality has been demonstrated in both animal and human studies [15,16]. Inadequately perfused and oxygenated cells initially compensate by shifting to anaerobic metabolism, resulting in the formation of lactate and the development of lactic acidosis. If shock is prolonged and substrate delivery for the generation of ATP is inadequate, the cellular membrane loses its ability to maintain its integrity and cellular functional disturbances ensue.

1. Traditional Variables

No single endpoint is sufficient by itself, and any endpoint must be considered concurrently with other hemodynamic and metabolic vital signs. The stress response to hypovolemia, with endogenous catecholamines and neural mechanisms (the transcapillary refill process), tends to maintain arterial pressure in the face of decreasing flow for a variable time. Criteria for the severity of shock are frequently based on crude measurements, such as blood pressure and heart rate. Used alone, however, blood pressure and heart rate may be poor predictors of the severity of shock or the adequacy of resuscitation. In a study comparing blood pressure and heart rate to cardiac index during resuscitation from traumatic injury [16] patients were found to have persistent tachycardia that was not related to corresponding cardiac index; that is, there was *no* correlation between heart rate and cardiac index. The cardiac output in both survivors and nonsurvivors was initially high but subsequently decreased in nonsurvivors. Blood pressure was not found to correlate with cardiac index; a decrease in mean arterial pressure often lagged behind the decrease in cardiac index, and with fluid resuscitation, an increase in mean pressure often preceded an increase in cardiac index. Relying on hypotension as an early warning sign of impending circulatory shock and relying on normal blood pressure values as a measure of the adequacy of fluid resuscitation or presence of satisfactory tissue perfusion may thus be questioned.

It is difficult to accurately estimate the blood volume lost in severely traumatized and hemodynamically stable patients. It is often impossible to monitor blood volume, cardiac index, and oxygen delivery before and during administration of large volumes of fluids in severely traumatized patients in the field, the admitting area of the emergency room, or the operating room. Fluid resuscitation must thus often begin based on global physiologic responses to hypovolemia and continue based on hemodynamic responses to therapy (Table 6). Even so, how does one know when the patient has been adequately resuscitated? Assessment of the adequacy of intravascular volume has been attempted by evaluating arterial blood pressure, peripheral pulses, mental status, and urine output (Table 6). Unfortunately, normal values of heart rate, blood pressure, and urine output may be inappropriate as resuscitation goals. Heart rate and blood pressure measurements may remain normal despite significant blood loss, and these variables do not reflect what is truly of interest: the situation at a cellular-metabolic level [17].

More invasive monitoring to guide aggressive therapy has been shown to improve mortality from trauma in geriatric patients [18], but the usefulness of central venous pressure, pulmonary artery occlusion pressure, and arterial blood gas monitoring as therapeutic endpoints has also been questioned, since the mean values of these variables may be similar in surviving and nonsurviving trauma patients [15]. Recent investigations in trauma patients have shown that the right ventricular end-diastolic volume index (RVEDI) may be a better indicator of preload in the critically injured patient [19,20].

Resuscitation endpoints of survivor (''supranormal'') values of cardiac index, oxygen delivery, and oxygen consumption studied in a prospective trial demonstrated decreased morality compared with conventional therapy. In order to achieve these goal indices, protocol patients received significantly more colloid solutions following admission and were given more blood products and total fluids intraoperatively and in the intensive care unit [21]. The time frame in which the survivor values are reached appears to be as important as the values themselves, likely due to the avoidance of development of an ''irreversible oxygen debt.'' Although of considerable value, such aggressive, invasive monitoring is usually postponed until the in-hospital phase of trauma resuscitation.

2. Perfusion-Related Variables

Monitoring perfusion-related variables such as arterial–venous oxygen content difference, mixed venous pH, arterial base deficit, or lactate levels can predict survival and help to assess the adequacy of resuscitation. In a canine model of hemorrhagic, hypovolemic shock, both lactic acidosis and base excess were independent variables that predicted the probability of death [15].

Lactate levels are a measure of anaerobic metabolism secondary to inadequate oxygen delivery to the tissues. Once DO2 decreases to a critical level an oxygen debt develops; VO2 then decreases linearly. When DO2 is restored to the tissues, VO2 increases to a level above which no further increase in DO2 results in increases in VO2. This is known as non-flow-dependent VO2. Patients suffering multiple traumatic injuries who achieved non-flow-dependent oxygen consumption have been shown to achieve 100% survival if lactate is normalized in 24 hr, but only 75% survival if it takes 48 hr to clear lactate [22].

3. Technical Aspects

Invasive monitoring, to determine whether flow-dependent consumption is present is not generally feasible during the initial resuscitation of injured patients in the field.

A minimally invasive technique that can be used during acute trauma is tissue oxygen monitoring. Skeletal muscle blood flow decreases early in the course of shock and is restored late during resuscitation, making skeletal muscle pO2 a sensitive indicator of low flow. By observing the effects of increased inspired oxygen on tissue pO2 during acute trauma resuscitation, flow-dependent consumption may be detected [23]. When flow dependency was not present, there was always a positive response in tissue pO2 to oxygen challenge.

B. Goals of Fluid Therapy

1. Hypervolemic Versus Normovolemic Resuscitation ("Delayed" Resuscitation)

Restoration of intravascular volume and increases in blood pressure before hemorrhage is controlled may increase bleeding or worsen outcome [24]. The benefit of early fluid resuscitation is being questioned in both blunt and penetrating trauma.

A current concept is that of ''damage control'': stop bleeding as quickly as possible and *then* institute full resuscitation. In a hemorrhage model that incorporates a vascular injury [25] attempts to restore blood pressure to normal with rapidly infused crystalloid had the undesirable effects of accentuating hemorrhage volume and mortality.

In a comparison of saline resuscitation to mean arterial pressures of 40 mmHg, 60 mmHg, or 80 mmHg following hemorrhage, animals severely underresuscitated (40 mmHg) experienced the least intraperitoneal hemorrhage volume and lowest mortality, but as demonstrated by a marked metabolic acidosis and significantly decreased oxygen delivery, at the expense of tissue perfusion. Moderate underresuscitation (60 mmHg) resulted in only a minimal increase in hemorrhage and mortality, with markedly improved tissue perfusion. Attempts to restore blood pressure to a normotensive state increased intraoperative hemorrhage volume and mortality.

The benefits and risks of early aggressive prehospital fluid resuscitation in trauma are summarized in Table 7. Aggressive resuscitation with crystalloid may lead to an early, sharp increase in pulse pressure at a time when blood viscosity is decreased greatly and the clot associated with the vascular injury has had little time to stabilize. Significant decreases in blood viscosity, which occur with crystalloid resuscitation, may result in an increased blood flow through and around an unstable clot.

Investigators have attempted to define the optimal *timing* of fluid resuscitation and the optimal *rate* of infusion, as they effect blood loss and mortality. In an animal model

Table 7 Benefits and Risks of Early Aggressive Prehospital Fluid Resuscitation in Trauma

Benefits	Risks
Rapidly increased plasma volume	Rebleeding due to increased blood pressure
Increased cardiac output	Increased loss of blood
Increased systemic blood flow	Impaired hemostatic competence
Enhanced microvascular perfusion	Increased losses of RBCs
Improved oxygen delivery to tissue cells	More pronounced anaerobiosis at arrival
Prevention of major oxygen debt	Increased oxygen dept
Reduced risk of MODS	Impaired survival

Source: Refs. 24–29.

of uncontrolled hemorrhage (designed to mimic the clinical scenario of severe shock caused by a major abdominal vascular injury following a stab wound or low-velocity gunshot wound), moderate posttraumatic hypotension has been found to cause little disturbance in tissue perfusion as measured by base deficit, and has a tendency for rapid spontaneous correction [26]. In contrast, severe hypotension did require early fluid resuscitation in order to avoid excess mortality. When the time interval from injury to resuscitation was short, blood loss was greater. If the time to resuscitation following injury was increased, blood loss decreased. At higher infusion rates, blood loss also increased.

The potential risk of inducing recurrent hemorrhage from major blood vessels prior to surgical control could be reduced by avoiding too fast an infusion rate in the early stage after the injury.

2. Arterial Versus Venous Hemorrhage

The doctrine of an increase in blood loss with aggressive fluid resuscitation following *arterial* injury has now been extended into the low-pressure *venous* system. In a sheep model of uncontrolled pulmonary vascular hemorrhage [27] a significant increase in the rate, volume, and duration of hemorrhage occurred with immediate fluid resuscitation compared to unresuscitated controls. Despite the fact that the fluid resuscitation group had a higher blood pressure and improved blood flow, oxygen delivery was similar in both groups during the infusion because the improved blood flow was offset by a marked reduction in hematocrit.

3. Blunt Versus Penetrating Injury

Penetrating injuries are readily reproducible in the laboratory setting, but extrapolating these data to blunt traumatic injury is difficult. Investigators therefore have induced parenchymal injury to the liver in an uncontrolled hemorrhage model to evaluate the effects of various fluids used for resuscitation [28]. Increases in mean arterial pressure were seen following both large-volume (24 cc/kg) and HS (4 cc/kg) infusions that were greater than the increases seen following small-volume infusions (4 cc/kg) or no resuscitation. Similar volumes moved from the extravascular to the intravascular space in all groups. There was significantly more intraperitoneal blood in animals resuscitated with large-volume crystalloid or HS. Despite this, HS significantly reduced mortality, possibly due to a greater percentage remaining in the intravascular space during the first hour following hemorrhage.

The concept of ''delayed resuscitation'' or ''controlled underresuscitation'' may be of considerable practical importance in the early prehospital resuscitation of trauma patients [29]. Victims of penetrating torso injury showed improved survival if fluid administration was delayed until surgical hemostasis in the operating room [24]. At least in the case of short prehospital times and short admission-to-operation times, ''immediate'' aggressive resuscitation in the prehospital phase may not be beneficial. The major argument against immediate resuscitation in this setting is that it reverses vasoconstriction of injured blood vessels, dislodges early thrombus, and when given in large volume, dilutes coagulation factors and changes viscosity due to the resistance to flow.

4. The Trauma Patient With Head Injury

Delay in resuscitation becomes a problem in unconscious patients who may have sustained a traumatic brain injury. The combination of hemorrhagic shock with traumatic brain injury dramatically increases mortality rate compared with head injury alone [30]. The outcome from closed head injury is determined primarily by the severity of the injury and the age of the patient. Important cofactors are the presence of hypoxia and hypotension. It is critical to maintain cerebral perfusion pressure >70 mmHg [31]. Fluid resuscitation in the case of combined hemorrhagic shock and head injury should be directed toward this goal.

C. Massive Fluid Resuscitation

Limitations in massive fluid resuscitation include hemodilution (and a resultant decrease in oxygen delivery), coagulopathy, and hypothermia. ''Massive transfusion'' is usually defined as the administration of fluids and blood products, equal to the patient's blood volume, within a 24-hr period

A dilutional coagulopathy may develop secondary to a decrease in coagulation components. All coagulation factors are stable in stored blood, with the exception of factors V and VIII, but deficiencies of these factors are rarely severe enough to account for clinical bleeding. Thrombocytopenia may occur in proportion to the volume transfused, or bleeding may occur with a normal platelet count secondary to dysfunctional platelets. Prolongation of the prothrombin and partial thromboplastin time have not been found to be predictive of bleeding unless levels are 1.5 to 1.8 times the control value [32]. Disseminated intravascular coagulation is a pathologic process that can be seen in the setting of massive trauma when extensive tissue injury leads to thromboplastin release in the face of hypotension and acidosis.

REFERENCES

1. H Haljamäe. Pathophysiology of shock-induced disturbances in tissue homeostasis. Acta Anaesth Scand 29, suppl. 82:38–44, 1985.
2. H Haljamäe. Interstitial fluid response. Clin Surg Internat 9:44–60, 1984.
3. AE Baue. Multiple organ failure, multiple organ dysfunction syndrome, and the systemic inflammatory response syndrome—Where do we stand? Shock 6:385–397, 1994.
4. H Haljamäe. Use of fluids in trauma. Internat J Intensive Care 6:20–30, 1999.
5. V Velanovich. Crystalloid versus colloid fluid resuscitation: A meta-analysis of mortality. Surgery 105:65–71, 1989.
6. G Schierhout, I Roberts. Fluid resuscitation with colloid or crystalloid solutions in critically ill patients: A systematic review of randomised trials. BMJ 316:961–964, 1998.
7. Cochrane Injuries Group Albumin Reviewers. Human albumin administration in critically ill patients: Systemic review of randomised controlled trials. BMJ 317:235–240, 1998.
8. SR Heckbert, NB Vedder, W Hoffman, et al. Outcome after hemorrhagic shock in trauma patients. J Trauma 45:545–549, 1998.
9. PT-L Choi, G Yip, LG Quinonez, DJ Cook. Crystalloids vs. colloids in fluid resuscitation: A systematic review. Crit Care Med 27:200–210, 1999.
10. H Haljamäe, M Dahlqvist, F Walentin. Artificial colloids in clinical practice: Pros and cons. Baillière's Clin Anaesth 11:49–79, 1997.
11. WH Bickell, SM Barrett, M Romine-Jenkins, SS Hull Jr, GT Kinasewitz. Resuscitation of canine hemorrhagic hypotension with large-volume isotonic crystalloid: Impact on lung water, venous admixture, and systemic arterial oxygen tension. Am J Emerg Med 12:36–42, 1984.
12. WC Shoemaker. Hemodynamic and oxygen transport effects of crystalloids and colloids in critically ill patients. Curr Stud Hem Blood Transf 53:155–176, 1986.
13. CE Wade, GC Kramer, JJ Grady, TC Fabian, RN Younes. Efficacy of hypertonic 7.5% saline and 6% dextran-70 in treating trauma: A meta-analysis of controlled clinical studies. Surgery 122:609–616, 1997.

14. NM Dietz, MJ Joyner, MA Warner. Blood substitutes: Fluids, drugs, or miracle solutions? Anesth Analg 82:390–405, 1996.
15. CM Dunham, JH Siegal, L Weireter, et al. Oxygen debt and metabolic acidemia as quantitative predictors of mortality and the severity of the ischemic insult in hemorrhagic shock. Crit Care Med 19:231–243, 1991.
16. CCJ Wo, WC Shoemaker, PL Appel, et al. Unreliability of blood pressure and heart rate to evaluate cardiac output in emergency resuscitation and critical illness. Crit Care Med 21:218–223, 1987.
17. MH Bishop, WC Shoemaker, PL Appel, et al. Relationship between supranormal circulatory values, time delays and outcome in severely traumatized patients. Crit Care Med 21:56–63, 1993.
18. TM Scalea, HM Simon, AO Duncan, et al. Geriatric blunt multiple trauma: Improved outcome with early invasive monitoring. J Trauma 30:129–134, 1990.
19. L Diebel, RF Wilson, J Heins, et al. End-diastolic volume versus pulmonary artery wedge pressure in evaluating cardiac preload in trauma patients. J Trauma 37:950–955, 1994.
20. MC Chang, JW Meredith. Occult hypovolemia and subsequent splanchnic ischemia in globally resuscitation trauma patients is associated with multiple organ failure and mortality. J Trauma 41:192, 1996.
21. MH Bishop, WC Shoemaker, DL Appel, et al. Prospective, randomized trial of survivor values of cardiac index, oxygen delivery and oxygen consumption as resuscitation endpoints in severe trauma. J Trauma 38:780–787, 1995.
22. D Abramson, TM Scalea, R Hitchcock, et al. Lactate clearance and survival following injury. J Trauma 35:584–588, 1993.
23. K Waxman, C Annas, K Daughters, GT Tominaga, G Scannell. A method to determine the adequacy of resuscitation using tissue oxygen monitoring. J Trauma 36:852–856, 1994.
24. WH Bickell, MJ Wall Jr, PE Pepe, et al. Immediate versus delayed fluid resuscitation for hypotensive patients with penetrating torso injuries. New Eng J Med 331:1105–1109, 1994.
25. SA Stern, SC Dronen, P Birrer, X Wang. Effect of blood pressure on hemorrhagic volume and survival in a near-fatal hemorrhage model incorporating a vascular injury. Ann Emerg Med 22:155–163, 1993.
26. A Leppaniemi, R Soltero, D Burris, et al. Fluid resuscitation in a model of uncontrolled hemorrhage: Too much too early or too little too late? J Surg Res 63:413–418, 1996.
27. JC Sakles, MJ Sena, DA Knight, JM Davis. Effect of immediate fluid resuscitation on rate, volume and duration of pulmonary vascular hemorrhage in a sheep model of penetrating thoracic trauma. Ann Emerg Med 29:392–399, 1997.
28. T Matsouka, J Hildreth, DH Wisner. Uncontrolled hemorrhage from parenchymal injury: Is resuscitation helpful? J Trauma 40:915–921, 1996.
29. JL Falk, JF O'Brien, R Kerr. Fluid resuscitation in traumatic hemorrhagic shock. Crit Care Clin 8:323–340, 1992.
30. JH Siegel, DR Gens, T Mamantoy, et al. Effect of associated injuries and blood volume replacement on death, rehabilitation needs, and disability in blunt traumatic brain injury. Crit Care Med 19:1252–1265, 1991.
31. SM Hamilton, P Breakey. Fluid resuscitation of the trauma patient: How much is enough? Can J Surg 39:11–16, 1996.
32. D Ciavarella, RL Reed, RB Counts, et al. Clotting factor levels and the risk of diffuse microvascular bleeding in the massively transfused patient. Brit J Haem 67:365–368, 1987.

APPENDIX: GUIDELINES FOR PREHOSPITAL FLUID RESUSCITATION/SUMMARY

1. To start or not to start fluid resuscitation
   A. Short transit time to nearest hospital, wait—do not delay transport.
   B. In most trauma situations prehospital fluid resuscitation is indicated.
2. Establish vascular access
   A. One (preferably 2) venous lines.
   B. Intraosseous access (e.g., pediatric trauma patients) after two failed attempts.
3. Start fluid infusion
   A. First choice—crystalloid with buffering capacity (lactate or acetate content) *but in case of major volume requirements*: consider addition of a colloid, since colloid even in low concentrations will markedly reduce the fluid volume requirements at the resuscitation. (Do not forget to consider heating the infusions to avoid hypothermia.).
   B. Hypertonic saline + colloid (second choice, if available); small-volume HS in combination with a colloid seems promising in trauma resuscitation and may be superior to the usual standard of care, especially in trauma patients with head injuries.
   C. Artificial oxygen carriers—future alternative?.
4. Monitoring
   A. "Clinical impression" and blood pressure, heart rate, ECG, pulse oximetry, urine output (not adequate indicators of the efficacy of the resuscitation).
   B. Perfusion-related variables (arterial base deficit, blood lactate, tissue pO2, intramucosal pCO2, pHi).
5. Goals for fluid resuscitation
   A. Overall goals:
      1. Reestablishment of normovolemia and hemodynamic stability.
      2. Compensation for the trauma-induced internal fluid fluxes from the interstitial and intracellular compartments.
      3. Maintenance of an adequate plasma colloid osmotic pressure (COP).
      4. Improvement of the microvascular blood flow.
      5. Prevention of cascade system activation and trauma-induced increase in blood coagulability.
      6. Normalization of oxygen delivery to tissue cells and thereby cellular metabolism and organ function.
      7. Prevention of reperfusion type of cellular injury.
   B. Consider delayed resuscitation or "controlled underresuscitation" in victims of traumatic injury until bleeding is controlled.

18

Fluid Resuscitation and Circulatory Support: Use of Pneumatic Antishock Garment

NELSON TANG

The Johns Hopkins University School of Medicine, Baltimore, Maryland

RICHARD D. ZANE

Brigham and Women's Hospital and Harvard Medical School, Boston, Massachusetts

The prehospital phase of acute trauma management remains at the forefront of intense scientific investigation and critical evaluation. With rapid advances in the practice of Emergency Medical Services (EMS), advanced life support (ALS) interventions in the field are increasingly being weighed against the goal of rapid transport to appropriate trauma centers and definitive care. Interventions whose benefits are merely speculative or anecdotal at best are no longer acceptable when considered at the expense of increased out-of-hospital time. Within this context, the prehospital use of the pneumatic antishock garment (PASG) continues to be the focus of long-standing medical controversy.

Since its introduction to battlefield medicine during the Vietnam-era conflicts for the treatment of hemorrhagic shock, the PASG (also referred to as military antishock trousers, or MAST) enjoyed widespread initial civilian EMS implementation, but this use has been followed by progressive general disfavor. In fact, the use of PASG has been subject of some of the greatest debates in modern EMS. The medical literature is voluminous with regard to clinical evaluation of the device. Despite this, the leadership of prehospital care and EMS medical directors remain undecided regarding the efficacy and role of the PASG.

I. PNEUMATIC ANTISHOCK GARMENT

The PASG is a noninvasive suit device constructed of synthetic fabric in the overall shape of a pair of trousers. It has three individual circumferential compartments, two each for the legs and one for the lower abdomen. Each compartment is secured in the closed configuration with hook-and-loop-type fasteners. Inflation of the device is accomplished through a foot pump, and some variations of the device have gauges that allow visualization of inflation pressures. The inflatable compartments are equipped with pressure-release valves, designed to allow full inflation to 100 mmHg. When uninflated, the PASG is compact, foldable, and easily stored aboard most EMS transport vehicles. With proper training in its use, application of the device in the prehospital setting can be done relatively quickly and without difficulty.

II. PHYSIOLOGIC EFFECTS

The hemodynamic effects of the PASG have been widely reported [1]. The principal effect of the device is that of increasing peripheral vascular resistance (PVR), or afterload. With the initial inflation of the PASG, venous return, stroke volume, and cardiac output are transiently increased. This is accompanied by a rise in peripheral vascular resistance [2–4]. Over time the effects on venous return, preload, and cardiac output decrease, and the effects on maintaining blood pressure of PVR and afterload predominate [2,3,5].

The concept of autotransfusion, or shifting of blood into the central circulation, was felt to be a significant effect of the PASG. The effect of autotransfusion has been shown to occur only when venous pooling in the peripheral circulation occurs and is independent of changes in PVR [6,7]. Additionally, the blood volume shifted centrally with PASG inflation is less than originally thought [6–8]. Autotransfusion is likely to be even less contributory in hypovolemic trauma patients.

III. CRITICAL EVALUATION

In the United States, EMS implementation of the PASG was widely recommended in the 1970s, and field application was nearly universal. Despite widespread reports of the apparent benefits of the PASG, there remained a paucity of clinical evidence to support the efficacy the device. In the 1980s scientific evaluation regarding the PASG and its role in prehospital trauma care intensified. In two early studies, Bickell et al. found no improvement in trauma scores and survival rates when the PASG was applied to patients with blunt and penetrating trauma and resultant hypotension [9,10].

In what is regarded as a landmark study, Mattox and his colleagues in Houston, Texas, conducted a large prospective randomized study of the PASG in urban trauma patients and demonstrated a significant (5%) increase in mortality with its use [11]. The study population was primarily victims of penetrating trauma (87%). Of particular note, a subgroup of the study population with systolic blood pressure less than 50 mmHg appeared to have an increased survival rate [11]. Although the small size of this particular subgroup did not enable statistical significance, the improved survival with PASG use was subsequently reported in a large retrospective review of trauma patients with profound hypotension [12]. Additional prospective studies have not been done.

Developed throughout the last 25 years, the body of medical literature regarding the application of the PASG in trauma care is extensive. The numbers of reports notwithstanding, the number of studies that support its efficacy with adequate scientific basis remains limited. In 1997, the National Association of EMS Physicians (NAEMSP) in the United States published a position paper that addressed this issue [13]. In this document, the authors critically examined the cumulative literature regarding the PASG and formulated recommendations for its use based on the American Heart Association (AHA) Emergency Cardiac Care Committee classification system (Table 1). Of particular note is that the only Class I (usually indicated, useful, and effective) application suggested by this classification scheme is for the treatment of hypotension due to a ruptured abdominal aortic aneurysm [13].

Table 1 Clinical Indications for PASG Use

Class I:	Usually indicated, useful, and effective
	Hypotension due to ruptured AAA
Class IIa:	Acceptable, uncertain efficacy, weight of evidence favors usefulness and efficacy
	Hypotension due to suspected pelvic fracture
	Anaphylactic shock (unresponsive to standard therapy)[a]
	Otherwise uncontrollable lower extremity fracture[a]
	Severe traumatic hypotension (palpable pulse, blood pressure not obtainable)[a]
Class IIb:	Acceptable, uncertain efficacy, may be helpful, probably not harmful
	Elderly
	History of congestive heart failure
	Penetrating abdominal injury
	Paroxysmal supraventricular tachycardia (PSVT)
	Gynecologic hemorrhage (otherwise uncontrolled)[a]
	Hypothermia-induced hypotension[a]
	Lower-extremity hemorrhage (otherwise uncontrolled)[a]
	Pelvic fracture without hypotension[a]
	Ruptured ectopic pregnancy[a]
	Septic shock[a]
	Spinal shock[a]
	Urologic hemorrhage (otherwise uncontrolled)[a]
	Assist intravenous cannulation [a]
Class III:	Inappropriate option, not indicated, may be harmful
	Adjunct to CPR
	Diaphragmatic rupture
	Penetrating thoracic injury
	Pulmonary edema
	To splint fractures of the lower extremities
	Extremity fracture
	Abdominal evisceration
	Acute myocardial infarction
	Cardiac tamponade
	Cardiogenic shock
	Gravid uterus

[a] Data from controlled trial not available. Recommendations based on other evidence.
Source: NAEMSP Position Paper: Use of the Pneumatic Antishock Garment (PASG). Courtesy of National Association of EMS Physicians.

IV. CLINICAL APPLICATIONS

In the prehospital management of the acutely traumatized patient, there may be specific indications for the use of the PASG. Its use may be especially useful in rural EMS systems or when transport times to definitive care in trauma centers are prolonged.

There is considerable evidence in animal models of all types of hemorrhages that mean arterial pressure is improved with the application of the PASG. Additionally, if the hemorrhage is directly compressed by the PASG, decreased blood loss and improved survival is achieved [1]. Studies in human subjects, however, are less conclusive. At present, the potential benefit of PASG use appears to be greatest in cases of profound traumatic hypotension. Several studies have reported increased mortality with PASG use in cases of penetrating trauma, particularly thoracic injuries [11,14]. Application of the device is thus relatively contraindicated in patients with penetrating thoracic, and possibly abdominal, trauma. The use of the PASG for control of extremity hemorrhage by direct compression has been described and appears to be an effective intervention for otherwise uncontrolled bleeding.

Retroperitoneal hemorrhage and resultant hypotension due to severe pelvic fractures may represent another scenario in which the PASG is beneficial. By inflation of the abdominal compartment of the device, the functional volume of the pelvis is reduced by the apposition of fracture fragments, thereby producing retroperitoneal tamponade [15]. Its use as a temporizing measure for pelvic stabilization until definitive orthopedic fixation can occur has been described [16–19].

There are several potential contraindications to PASG use that deserve mention. Due to its demonstrated effects of increasing peripheral vascular resistance, ventricular workload, and pulmonary capillary wedge pressure, use of the PASG should be avoided in patients with pulmonary edema and diminished cardiac reserves [20,21]. Although potentially effective in gynecologic causes of hemorrhage, inflation of the abdominal compartment in gravid females is generally contraindicated. Although elevation of intracranial pressure is a theoretical concern of PASG use on patients with closed head injury, this effect has not been demonstrated in the literature. Use of the PASG has been associated with extremity compartment syndromes, and prolonged application at high pressures must be performed with caution [22–25].

V. CURRENT PRACTICE

Despite awareness that the effectiveness of the PASG may be less than was previously believed, its use remains a widely available adjunct in prehospital trauma care. Education and training in its use remains very much a part of modern EMS curricula [26]. The National Registry of Emergency Medical Technician (NREMT), the central certifying body for ALS providers in the United States, still requires proficiency in use of the device. Although de-emphasized, application of the PASG is taught to emergency physicians and trauma surgeons through the Advanced Trauma Life Support (ATLS™) program of the American College of Surgeons [27]. Although many EMS systems have variably limited use of the device, it still is not uncommon to see patients arrive in emergency departments or trauma centers today with the PASG in place, if not inflated.

The PASG continues to be a most intriguing device. That a relatively simple and noninvasive intervention may be of potential utility in critically injured trauma victims has sustained decades of medical interest in its use. As many of the conventional paradigms in EMS and prehospital care become challenged by current evidence-based approaches to clinical practice, EMS physicians must develop a rational approach to the applications of the PASG. Review of the available literature in many ways prompts more questions than provides answers. The current consensus is that the clinical efficacy of the PASG may be far less than was previously thought.

REFERENCES

1. RE O'Connor, RM Domeier. An evaluation of the pneumatic anti-shock garment (PASG) in various clinical settings. Prehosp Emerg Care 1:36–44, 1997.
2. J Ali, K Duke. Timing and interpretation of the hemodynamic effects of the pneumatic anti-shock garment. Ann Emerg Med 20:1183–1187, 1991.
3. SR Goldsmith. Comparative hemodynamic effects of anti-shock suit and volume expansion in normal human beings, Ann Emerg Med 12(6):348–350, 1983.
4. J Ali, B Vanderby, C Purcell. The effect of the pneumatic anti-shock garment (PASG) on hemodynamics, hemorrhage, and survival in penetrating thoracic aortic injury. J Trauma 31: 846–851, 1991.
5. M Hauswald, ER Greene. Aortic blood flow during sequential MAST inflation. Ann Emerg Med 15:1297–1299, 1986.
6. FA Gaffney, ER Thal, WF Taylor, BC Bastian, JA Weigelt, JM Atkins, CG Blomqvist. Hemodynamic effects of medical anti-shock trousers (MAST Garment). J Trauma 21:931–937, 1981.
7. HG Bivins, R Knopp, C Tiernan, PA dos Santos, G Kallsen. Blood volume displacement with inflation of anti-shock trousers. Ann Emerg Med 11:409–412, 1982.
8. TJ Jennings, JF Seaworth, LL Howell, LD Tripp, CD Goodyear. The effects of various anti-shock trouser inflation sequences on hemodynamics in normovolemic subjects. Ann Emerg Med 15:1193–1197, 1986.
9. WH Bickell, PE Pepe, CH Wyatt, WR Dedo, DJ Applebaum, CT Black, KL Mattox. Effect of antishock trousers on the trauma score: a prospective analysis in the urban setting. Ann Emerg Med 14:218–222, 1985.
10. WH Bickell, PE Pepe, ML Bailey, CH Wyatt, KL Mattox. Randomized trial of pneumatic antishock garments in the prehospital management of penetrating abdominal injuries. Ann Emerg Med 16:653–658, 1987.
11. KL Mattox, W Bickell, PE Pepe, J Burch, D Feliciano. Prospective MAST study in 911 patients. J Trauma 29:1104–1112, 1989.
12. CG Cayten, BM Berendt, DW Byrne, JG Murphy, FH Moy. A study of pneumatic antishock garments in severely hypotensive trauma patients. J Trauma 34:728–735, 1993.
13. RM Domeier, RE O'Connor, TR Delbridge, RC Hunt. Use of the pneumatic anti-shock garment (PASG). Prehosp Emerg Care 1:32–35, 1997.
14. B Honigman, SR Lowenstein, EE Moore, K Roweder, P Pons. The role of pneumatic anti-shock garments in penetrating cardiac wounds. JAMA 266:2398–2401, 1991.
15. TH Blackwell. Prehospital Care. In: JA Marx, ed. Advances in Trauma. Emerg Med Clin North Am 11:1–14, 1993.
16. LM Flint, A Brown, JD Richardson, HC Polk. Definitive control of bleeding from severe pelvic fractures. Ann Surg 189:709–716, 1979.
17. JD Richardson, J Harty, M Amin, LM Flint. Open pelvic fractures. J Trauma 22:533–538, 1982.
18. BM Evers, HM Cryer, FB Miller. Pelvic fracture hemorrhage: Priorities in management. Arch Surg 124:422–424, 1989.
19. L Flint, G Babikian, M Anders, J Rodriguez, S Steinberg. Definitive control of mortality from severe pelvic fractures. Ann Surg 221:703–706, 1990.

20. JA Savino, I Jabbour, N Agarwal, D Byme. Overinflation of pneumatic antishock garments in the elderly. Am J Surg 155:572–577, 1988.
21. BJ Rubal, MR Geer, WH Bickell. Effect of pneumatic antishock garment inflation in normovolemic subjects. J Appl Physiol 67:339–345, 1989.
22. KS Christensen. Pneumatic antishock garments (PASG): Do they precipitate lower-extremity compartment syndromes? J Trauma 26:1102–1105, 1986.
23. D Templeman, R Lange, B Harms. Lower-extremity compartment syndromes associated with use of pneumatic antishock garments. J Trauma 27:79–81, 1987.
24. C Aprahamian, G Gessert, DF Bandyk, L Sell, J Stiehl, DW Olson. MAST-associated compartment syndrome (MACS): A review. J Trauma 29:549–555, 1989.
25. MH Vahedi, A Ayuyao, MH Parsa, HP Freeman. Pneumatic antishock garment-associated compartment syndrome in uninjured lower extremities. J Trauma 38:616–618, 1995.
26. National Highway Traffic Safety Administration. Emergency Medical Technician Paramedic: National Standard Curriculum. Washington, DC: U.S. Department of Transportation, 1998.
27. American College of Surgeons Committee on Trauma. Advanced Trauma Life Support. Chicago: American College of Surgeons, 1997.

19

Surgical Procedures

STEPHEN R. HAYDEN and GARY M. VILKE

University of California San Diego Medical Center, San Diego, California

TOM SILFVAST

Helsinki University Hospital and Helsinki Area HEMS, Helsinki, Finland

CHARLES D. DEAKIN

Southampton General Hospital, Southampton, United Kingdom

I. PREHOSPITAL NEEDLE THORACOSTOMY VS. TUBE THORACOSTOMY

A. Indications

Many prehospital systems have debated the utility and indications of needle thoracostomy and tube thoracostomy in the field. Indications (see Table 1) will vary based on many factors, including transport time, mode of transport, patient status, and individual prehospital personnel. Candidates for field needle thoracostomy include all patients who may be suffering from a tension pneumothorax. Both medical and trauma patients can deteriorate quickly into full arrest if a tension pneumothorax is not treated promptly.

Patients with underlying pulmonary disease and patients who suffered chest trauma are at risk for developing tension pneumothorax. The signs and symptoms of tension pneumothorax include a combination of increasing respiratory distress, unilateral decrease in breath sounds, hypotension, and hypoxia. This physiology must have definitive treatment initiated. Cyanosis and tracheal deviation are late findings in tension pneumothorax,

Table 1 Prehospital Tube Thoracostomy

Indications	
	Tension pneumothorax
	Hemopneumothorax in hemodynamically unstable patients
	Prophylaxis for prolonged transport
Contraindications	
	Known or suspected pulmonary adhesions
	Bleeding dyscrasias
Complications	
	Infection
	Bleeding
	Failure to penetrate pleura
	Visceral trauma
	Increased scene time

and often do not occur. Tension pneumothorax is in the differential diagnosis of pulseless electrical activity (PEA), but the rest of the presenting history and exam must support the diagnosis. Tension physiology will frequently manifest itself after the initiation of positive pressure ventilation (typical after recent endotracheal intubation), during which a simple traumatic pneumothorax may expand into a tension pneumothorax.

Field tube thoracostomy should be considered in unstable patients who suffered thoracic trauma with probable pneumothorax or hemothorax. Needle thoracostomy is a quick but temporary treatment for tension pneumothorax. A chest tube should be placed in any patient who will have prolonged transport, who is at risk for reaccumulation from decreased atmospheric pressure when the patient flies at altitude, or if the symptoms of tension pneumothorax recur after treatment with a needle thoracostomy.

Another option in the field that has been described is use of a simple thoracostomy (i.e., incision but no tube) in ventilated patients to provide rapid decompression of a tension pneumothorax [1]. Under positive pressure ventilation it is not necessary to use a tube, as the skin edges act as a one-way valve and the positive pressure expels air through the incision. This technique is much quicker because it avoids the additional time needed to insert the tube.

A stable patient being transported by ground does not necessarily require field intervention in cases of suspected simple traumatic or spontaneous pneumothorax, but personnel should be prepared to treat if tension physiology develops. Again, care should be taken to closely watch patients for deterioration after intubating, and some would advocate prophylactic tube thoracostomy for simple pneumothorax if a patient does require intubation. A more practical approach, however, is to be prepared to treat with needle thoracostomy if the patient deteriorates. Aeromedical crews flying at altitude must consider that decreased barometric pressure will cause a pneumothorax to expand, potentially causing patient deterioration. Patients in these situations are best treated with prophylactic tube thoracostomy to avoid this complication.

B. Contraindications

There are no field contraindications to needle thoracostomy for patients with suspected tension pneumothorax. Contraindications to field tube thoracostomy include patients with known pulmonary adhesions or those at risk for them from previous transthoracic procedures, and patients with bleeding dyscrasias. Age is not a contraindication if the clinical scenario warrants emergent therapy [2].

C. Necessary Equipment

For needle thoracentesis all that is required is a large-bore catheter over a needle, antiseptic solution, and a tape or suture to secure it (see Table 2). Most prehospital provider units will have a prepackaged *tube thoracostomy kit* that includes local anesthetic, sterile drapes, scalpel, Kocher clamps, curved Mayo scissors, one-way flutter valves and collection system, towel clamps, #2 or larger suture material with a curved needle, and petroleum gauze. Size 16–38 French chest tubes should be available.

D. Procedure: Needle Thoracostomy

There are two locations for placement of the catheter in a needle thoracostomy. First and most often used is the second intercostal space in the midclavicular line (see Fig. 1). This is the most easily accessible region, especially if a patient is in PEA with chest compressions or requiring intubation or other procedures simultaneously.

The other location is the fifth intercostal space at the anterior axillary line (the same location as tube thoracostomy placement). The advantage to this location is that it avoids the often very large pectoral muscles anteriorly. It also affords the need to prepare the site only once if a chest tube is going to be placed after needle decompression.

Prepare the site with Betadine or a similar antiseptic. Insert the catheter over the needle in a perpendicular direction to the skin surface, pushing with slow and steady pressure until a pop is heard (associated with a rush of air). Remove the needle and leave the catheter in place. Remember to keep monitoring the patient for signs of reaccumulation of the tension pneumothorax, especially if a chest tube is not subsequently placed.

Table 2 Necessary Equipment—Tube Thoracostomy

Betadine preparation
Lidocaine 1% anesthetic (at least 10 cc)
10-cc syringe
21-g 1.5-in. needle
#10 blade scalpel
Sterile fenestrated drape
Sterile gloves
Curved Mayo scissors
Kocher clamps [2]
Towel clamp
Petroleum-based gauze
4 × 4 gauze sponges [6]
Chest tube
28 to 36 F (for adults)
16 to 24 F (for children)
Flutter valve
Sterile collection system

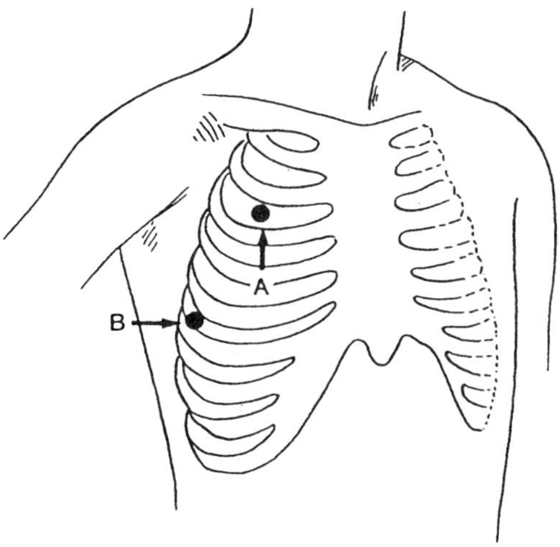

Figure 1 Standard sites for tube thoracostomy. A, The second intercostal space, midclavicular line. B, The fourth or fifth intercostal space, midaxillary line. Most clinicians prefer midaxillary line placement for all chest tubes, regardless of pathology. Note that placing the tube too far posteriorly will not allow the patient to lie down comfortably. (Courtesy of W.B. Saunders Co.)

E. Procedure: Tube Thoracostomy

The patient should be positioned supine with the ipsilateral arm placed behind the patient's head. This gives better exposure to the lateral chest wall and spreads open the intercostal spaces. The site of incision should be determined at the fifth intercostal space at the middle to anterior axillary line. This avoids the large chest muscles anteriorly and back muscles posteriorly. The fifth intercostal space can be quickly estimated by moving laterally from the nipple in the male patient and the inframammary line in the female patient.

The appropriately sized chest tube should be selected for the size of the patient. Use as large a tube as possible. If only a pneumothorax is suspected, a smaller-diameter chest tube can be used. If the patient suffered blunt or penetrating chest trauma, however, a larger tube should be used in the anticipation of bleeding so that the tube does not become obstructed by a clot. The chest tube should be cross-clamped on the distal end with one Kocher clamp and clamped longitudinally on the proximal end (with ports) with the other Kocher clamp. Many thoracostomy tube sets in Europe and the United Kingdom come with a metal stilette that can be used as an alternative to the proximal end clamp. The tube also can be fed with the fingers. Chest tubes with sharp trochars for chest wall puncture should not be used, as they increase the risk of pulmonary injury.

The area should be prepared in sterile fashion, and if practical, a fenestrated drape may be placed. In the awake patient, local anesthetic should be used and systemic analgesia should be considered. Inject up to 10 cc of lidocaine 1% using the 22-gauge needle and 10-cc syringe. An initial wheal should be raised at the incision site about 2 to 3 cm in length following the rib contour over the top of the sixth rib. Deeper injection should be performed at this time as well into the fifth intercostal space. Be liberal with the use of the lidocaine.

An incision should be made over the site of anesthesia following the contour of the ribs on the middle to upper aspect of the sixth rib. Care should be taken to avoid the

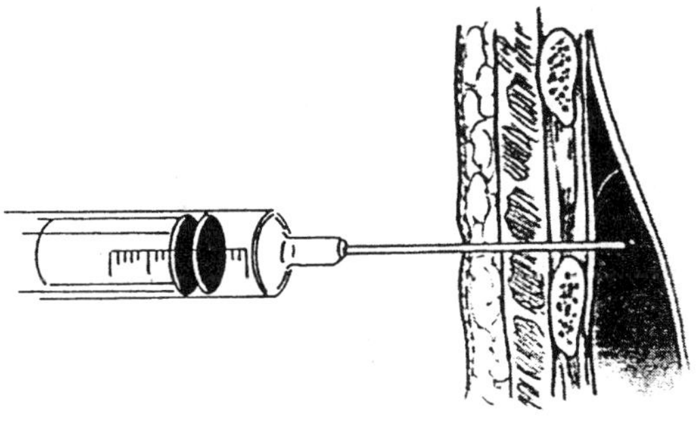

Figure 2 Use of the anesthetic needle to puncture the parietal pleura and establish the presence of blood or air in the pleural space. This procedure not only is diagnostic, but also may be a temporary therapeutic maneuver in a patient with tension pneumothorax.

inferior aspect of the ribs where the neurovascular bundle is located. In the awake patient, additional lidocaine can be injected into the incision to anesthetize the pleura, the most sensitive tissue in the procedure. Even if the pleural space is entered during injection, this is not a problem, as a large chest tube is about to be placed through the same location (Fig. 2).

Next, the closed Mayo scissors or curved clamp should be directed into the incision to slide just over the sixth rib and into the chest cavity (Fig. 3). Care should be taken to

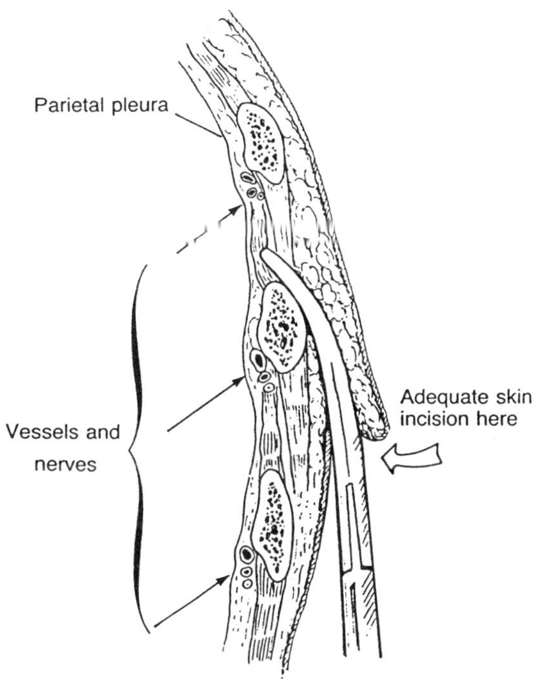

Figure 3 Location of the intercostal neurovascular bundle, running interiorly and slightly medial to the rib. (From Ref. 2a.)

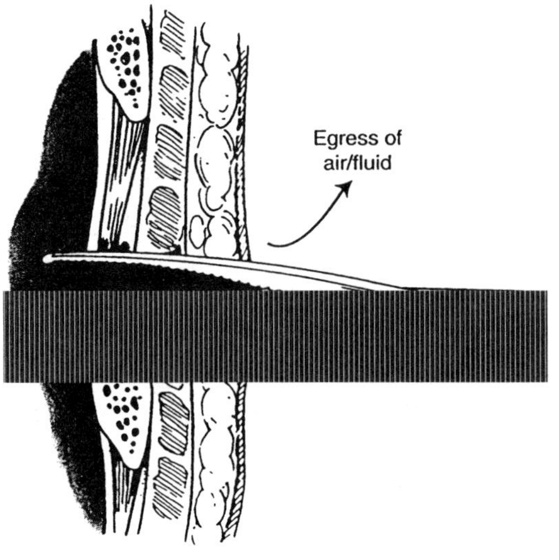

Figure 4 One accomplishes blunt dissection by forcing the closed points of the clamp forward and then spreading the tips and pulling back with the points spread. A rush of air or fluid signifies penetration into the pleural space. (From Ref. 2b.)

maintain control of the scissors' or clamps' tip with the nondominant hand while applying gradual but steady pressure with the dominant hand. A significant amount of pressure may be needed to penetrate the pleura, especially in younger patients. Once through, the scissors or clamp are opened wide and pulled out (Fig. 4). This is to widen the hole in the pleura. A finger should be placed into the hole and swept circumferentially to confirm

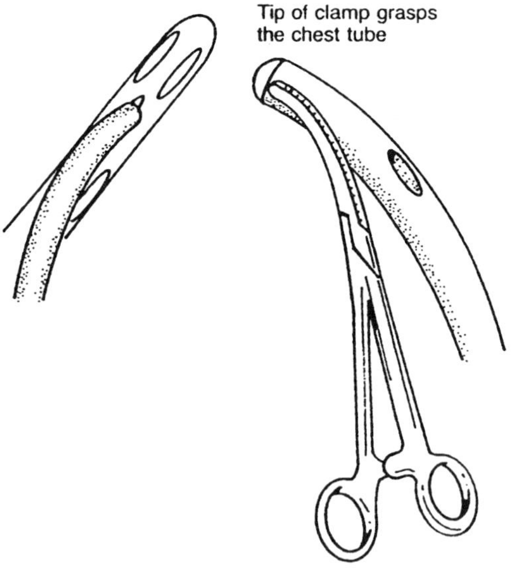

Figure 5 The tube is grasped with the curved clamp with the tube tip protruding from the jaws. (Courtesy of W.B. Saunders Co.)

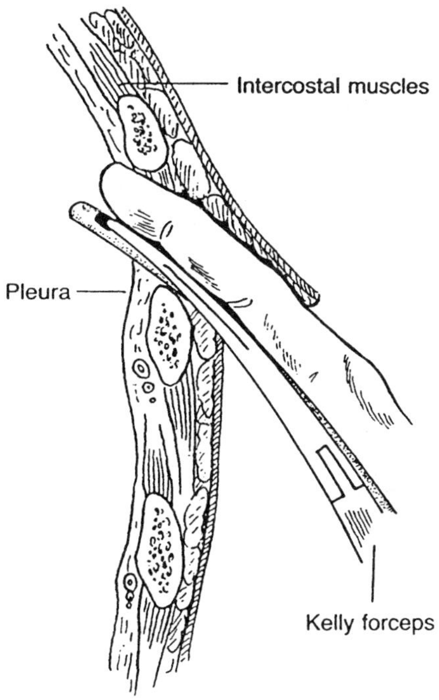

Figure 6 Using the finger as a guide to ensure entry into the pleural cavity, one places the tip of the tube into the pleural cavity. It is surprisingly easy to advance a chest tube subcutaneously, entirely missing the pleural space. (From Ref. 2a.)

appropriate pleural placement and to make sure there are no adhesions. If abdominal organs are encountered, the tube should not be placed.

The chest tube should be directed into the incision using the Kocher clamp or guided with a finger, and once inside the clamp should be released while advancing the tube in a posterior and cephalad direction (Figs. 5 and 6). If resistance is met, care should be taken not to force the tube, as it may be in a fissure. It can be backed out and redirected. The tube must go in far enough to cover all the ports.

The tube can be secured temporarily by using a towel clamp to hold the incision closed and sticking the tube through the clamp finger holes while making sure not to pierce the chest tube. It may also be secured with tape and gauze, as depicted in Fig. 7. Alternately, a purse string suture may be used to seal the site (Fig. 8). Petroleum-based gauze should be wrapped around the incision to seal the site (Fig. 9). The distal clamp should be released from the chest tube once a one-way flutter valve and collection system is in place. If a hemothorax is encountered, the one-way flutter valve should be omitted and a blood collection system connected.

F. Complications

Complications of needle thoracostomy include infection and bleeding, which has been documented to be fairly significant with an intercostal artery laceration when appropriate needle placement is not followed. Failure to penetrate the pleura is occasionally encoun-

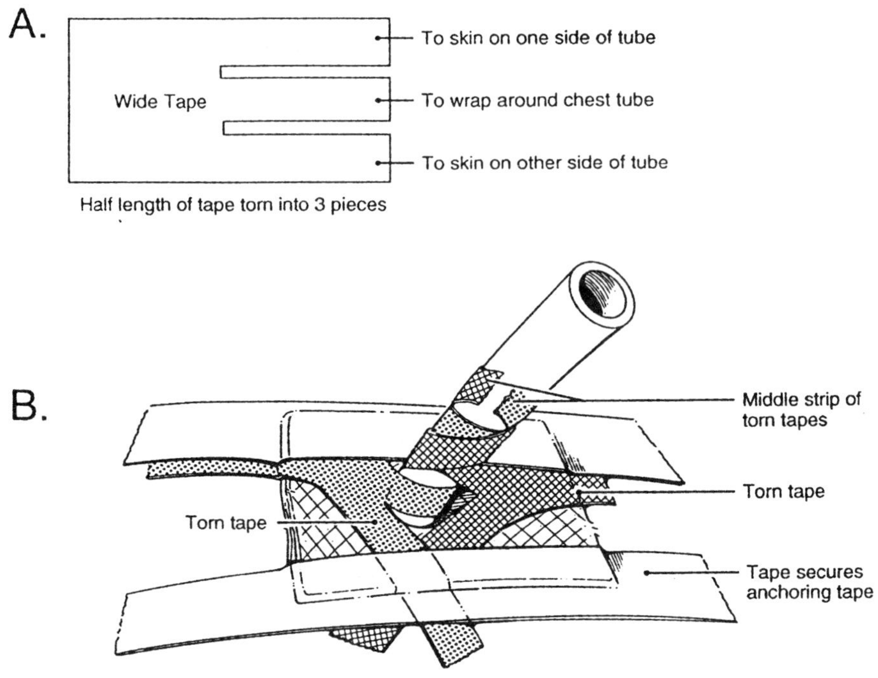

Figure 7 (A) The distal half of a wide piece of tape is longitudinally split into three pieces. The two outside pieces are placed on the skin on either side of the tube, and the center strip is wrapped around the chest tube itself. (B) This process may be repeated with a similar piece of tape placed at a 90° angle. The tape is securely anchored to the skin (benzoin is optional, but the skin must be clean and dry), and the torn tape is wrapped around the tube. Each anchoring piece is covered by another piece of tape. (Courtesy of W.B. Saunders Co.)

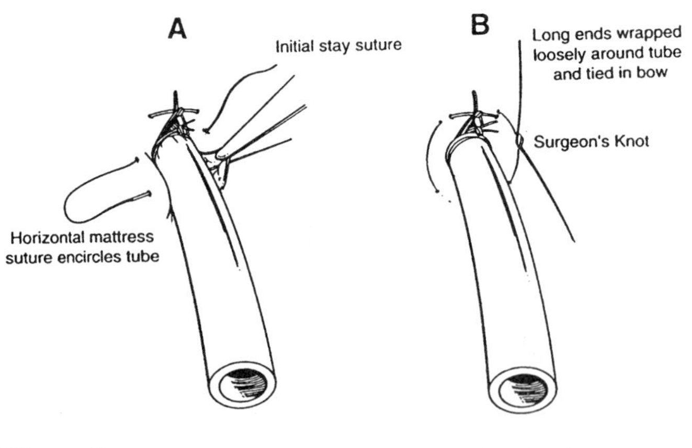

Figure 8 (A) A horizontal mattress suture is placed around (above) the tube and is held only with a surgeon's knot. (B) The loose ends also are wrapped around the tube and are tied loosely in a bow to identify the suture. This suture will be untied and used to close the skin incision after tube removal. (Courtesy of W.B. Saunders Co.)

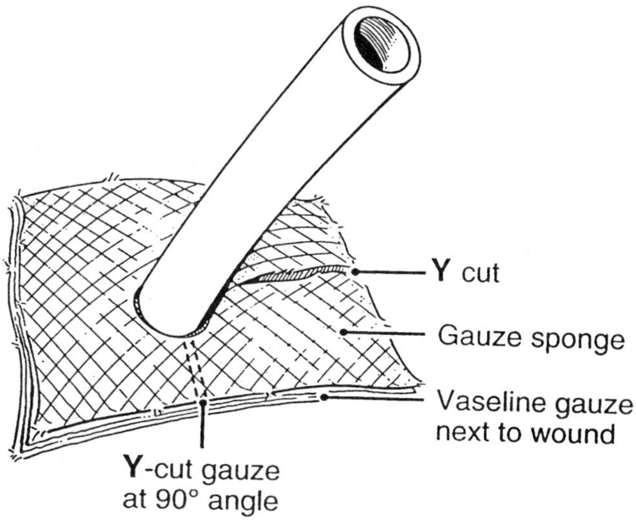

Figure 9 A dressing consisting of petrolatum-impregnated gauze and gauze sponges with a Y cut is applied to the entry site to provide an airtight seal. Two pieces are placed at angles. (Courtesy of W.B. Saunders Co.)

tered, and the creation of an iatrogenic pneumothorax, when none was felt to have been present initially, has also been reported [3].

As tube thoracostomy is more invasive and technically more challenging, more complications are associated with this procedure [4], with prehospital complication rates of up to 21% reported [5]. Complications of tube thoracostomy include bleeding and infection, which range from simple skin infections to empyemas. The tube can be placed into the wrong tissue plane, especially in obese patients, and thus never enter the thoracic cavity. Failure to relieve the pneumothorax can occur, requiring a second chest tube placement. If overzealous pressure is placed, visceral trauma can result, including pulmonary lacerations, diaphragmatic perforation with injury to underlying organs, and mediastinal compression, including vascular compression. If a vascular injury with tamponading of the bleeding by the thoracic wall, had occurred from the initial trauma, and a chest tube is placed, the tamponade can be released with the tube's introduction, thus causing continued significant bleeding. Increased scene time has been reported with prehospital tube thoracostomy compared to needle thoracostomy [5].

G. Postprocedure Management

The patient's respiratory and hemodynamic status should be monitored closely. Observe for the development of air leaks. If the respiratory status does not improve, a second chest tube must occasionally be placed. In the case of significant hemothorax, autotransfusion of blood may be performed. (See later section in this chapter.) Transport the patient to the nearest hospital immediately.

H. Options for Obtaining Necessary Procedural Experience

Clearly, only qualified personnel should perform the procedures. Prehospital needle thoracostomies are performed by paramedics and flight nurses in many programs [6]. Tube thoracostomy is a skill that is less widely used in the prehospital setting [7], and is usually restricted to flight nurses and physicians [8]. The needle thoracostomy can be taught fairly easily to paramedics and flight nurses with didactic lessons. A cadaver or animal lab is ideal for gaining comfort with the procedure and the ''feel'' of penetrating the pleura. If need be, after didactics the operator could be talked through the procedure on a radio by a qualified physician.

Tube thoracostomy is a technically more difficult procedure and has potentially more serious complications, and thus requires formal training, including cadaver or animal lab training. This procedure also requires frequent use to keep skills current. If the operator is not placing chest tubes several times a year into patients, then cadaver or animal lab refreshers are required. With appropriate training, studies have suggested that tube thoracostomy can be performed by aeromedical crews without increased risks to the patients [5,7].

Several papers have been written on the topic of prophylactic antibiotics for field tube thoracostomies, but no consensus has been attained. Several small prospective studies [9] and a meta-analysis [10] support the use of antibiotics, while others report that antibiotics are not necessary [5,8]. Since definitive improvement in outcome has not been demonstrated, it is not appropriate to administer antibiotics in the field setting, and should be considered by the admitting service once the patient has been taken to the hospital.

II. PREHOSPITAL SURGICAL AIRWAY

A. Indications

Airway obstruction has been estimated as contributing to death in as many as 85% of patients who die before reaching the hospital [11]. Aggressive prehospital airway management is therefore important in reducing morbidity and mortality from airway obstruction. Brantigan and Grow first described surgical cricothyroidotomy in 1976, and since then it has been adopted worldwide and has saved many thousands of lives. It is an important procedure that those providing prehospital care need to be capable of performing.

In the prehospital setting, the only indication for cricothyroidotomy is an inability to intubate the trachea in patients with actual or impending airway obstruction. In the trauma patient, this is usually due to facial trauma causing upper airway hemorrhage, airway burns, vomiting, tissue debris, or anatomical disruption preventing nasal and/or oral intubation. It is also indicated when intubation is impossible due to patient position during entrapment [12]. Prehospital cricothyroidotomy is performed in 2.6–7.7% patients with major trauma [13].

B. Contraindications

If the airway is obstructed, there are few contraindications to establishment of a surgical airway. Cricothyroidotomy is generally contraindicated below 6 years of age because the cricoid ring is the narrowest part of the airway, and edema or reactive granuloma at this site may cause serious airway obstruction. Needle cricothyroidotomy and surgical tracheostomy are better alternatives in these patients.

No studies have examined the effect of cricothyroidotomy on cervical spine movement. Optimum positioning for the procedure involves extension of the neck, which is likely to cause distraction of unstable cervical spine vertebrae. Performing the procedure with the neck in a more neutral position is likely to increase the risk of complications.

C. Necessary Equipment

Relatively little equipment is needed to perform a surgical cricothyroidotomy. Successful attempts have been reported using just a pen knife and biro tubing. Optimal equipment includes a scalpel, gauze swabs, tracheal dilators, gum elastic bougie, and a range of cuffed endotracheal or cricothyroidotomy tubes.

D. Patient Preparation

Cricoid and thyroid landmarks are most prominent if the neck is extended, but this may not be appropriate if cervical spine trauma is suspected. Since this procedure is usually performed in a life-threatening situation, there is usually little time to prepare a sterile field.

E. Performance of Procedure

The cricothyroid membrane is identified (Fig. 10). A 2–3 cm vertical or horizontal incision is made into the skin covering the membrane until the membrane is pierced. Although the final cosmetic result is better with a horizontal incision, in a life-threatening situation an initial vertical incision in the midline is preferred. This potentially avoids vascular structures, and the incision may be extended cephalad or caudad easily if the cricothyroid membrane is not immediately below the initial incision site. An exception to this may be if the operator has significant experience with a horizontal incision and performs the procedure regularly. The tracheal dilators are then used to enlarge the hole if necessary. This can also be performed by placing the blunt end of a scalpel in the cricoid ring and turning the handle 90°. Failure to make an incision and tract of sufficient size to allow entry of the endotracheal or cricothyroidotomy tube is a common cause of failure of a surgical airway. It may be difficult to clearly identify the tract into which the cricothyroidotomy tube is to be inserted. A tracheal hook may be used to hook under the distal portion of the thyroid cartilage and elevate it to assist passage of the tube. This may be a particular problem in patients with a fat neck or those in whom the neck cannot be extended. In these patients, insertion of a gum elastic bougie through the cricothyroid membrane to guide a cricothyroidotomy tube may make the procedure easier [14].

Both endotracheal or cricothyroidotomy tubes are suitable. Cuffed tubes allow isolation of the airway from blood and debris. Care must be taken when using a standard endotracheal tube to avoid right main bronchus intubation.

Cricothyroidotomy kits are available that involve transfixing the cricothyroid membrane with a large-bore needle through which a guidewire is then introduced (Seldinger technique). A dilator is then placed over the wire, which allows subsequent introduction of a 4.0-mm tube through the cricothyroid membrane. This is of insufficient diameter to enable spontaneous respiration, but is adequate for mechanical ventilation for short periods of time.

Alternately, translaryngeal jet ventilation (TTV) may be performed in children less than 6 years old or if cricothyroidotomy is not felt to be appropriate for the situation. Translaryngeal jet ventilation does not provide a definitive airway or secure adequate

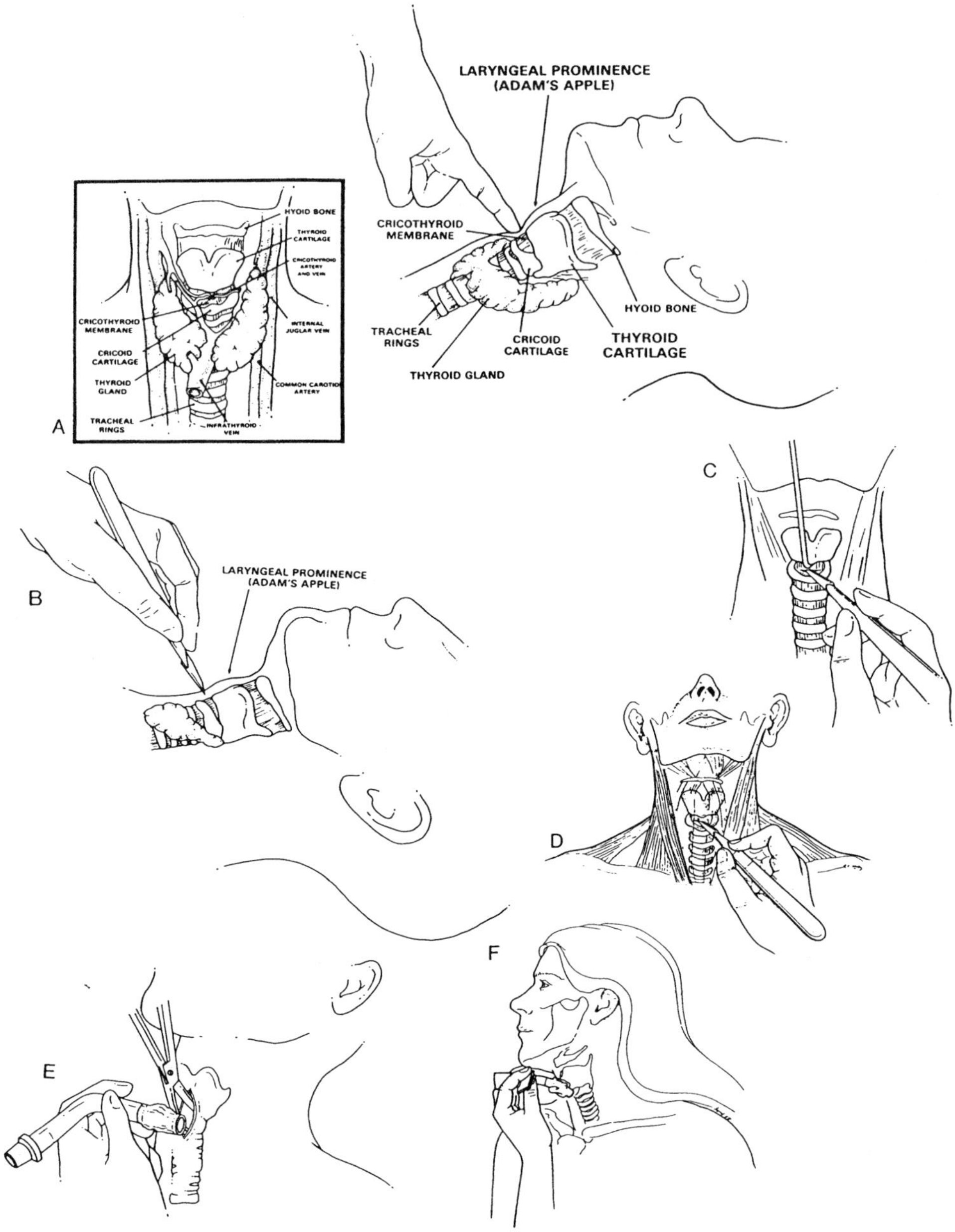

Figure 10 Prehospital surgical airway. (A) The cricothyroid membrane is identified. (B) A 2–3 cm longitudinal skin incision is made to expose the membrane. (C, D) A transverse incision is made through the cricothyroid membrane and the hole is enlarged with a tracheal dilator or blunt end of the scalpel blade. A tracheal hook may be inserted. (E) A properly sized cuffed tracheostomy or endotracheal tube is guided through the hole in a caudal direction. (F) The tube should be checked for proper placement, cuff inflated, and secured in place. (Courtesy of W.B. Saunders Co.)

Table 4 Cricothroidotomy—Necessary Equipment

Minimum
Scalpel blade
Tubing
Optimum
Betadine preparation
#11 blade scalpel
Tracheal dilator
Tracheal hook
Cuffed endotracheal or tracheostomy tubes

the result of a stab wound to the heart [22], with approximately 80–90% of such stab wounds producing tamponade [22,23]. Only about 20% of gunshot wounds demonstrate acute hemopericardium [23]. Blunt chest trauma rarely results in cardiac tamponade, though severe deceleration injury may cause aortic dissection and hemopericardium.

The pericardial sac normally contains 25 to 35 cc of serous fluid [24]. Eighty to 120 cc more blood can be accommodated acutely, but the next 20 to 40 cc cause a significant rise in intrapericardial pressure, which can lead to sudden hemodynamic compromise [25]. Withdrawing a given volume of fluid or blood from the pericardium drops intrapericardial pressure more than its addition originally raised it, a phenomenon known as ''hysteresis'' [26]. It is this effect that led to the observation that withdrawing even a small amount of blood in acute hemopericardium can significantly improve the hemodynamic status of the patient.

The diagnosis of cardiac tamponade can be difficult in the prehospital trauma patient. The triad of elevated venous pressure, decreased arterial pressure, and muffled heart sounds described by Beck in 1935 is present in less than one-third of major trauma victims [27,28]. Patients should be suspected of having acute hemopericardium with tamponade if any of the following are present:

- Stab wound to the chest
- Beck's triad (decreased blood pressure, muffled heart tones, distended neck veins)
- Kussmaul's sign (a rise in venous pressure with normal inspiration)
- Pulsus paradoxus of greater than 10 mmHg (exaggerated drop in systolic blood pressure with inspiration)
- Pulseless electrical activity in the absense of hypovolemia or tension pneumothorax

If any of the above are present in a hemodynamically unstable patient, pericardiocentesis should be considered.

B. Contraindications

Pericardiocentesis may be misleading in acute hemopericardium. Blood in the pericardium often clots, leading to false negative pericardiocentesis or no relief of compromised cardiac output. Furthermore, blood frequently will reaccumulate despite leaving a catheter in place, therefore pericardiocentesis is not considered definitive therapy for acute hemopericardium. Pericardiocentesis is contraindicated if emergent open thoracotomy is necessary or if the treating health care provider is unfamiliar with the procedure or does not have the appropriate equipment.

C. Necessary Equipment

There are several techniques described for pericardiocentesis, each requiring somewhat different equipment. Remember, pericardiocentesis in a major trauma patient is performed as an emergent procedure to temporarily relieve cardiac temponade. Time is of the essence, and the most rapid and least complicated approach is best under these circumstances. While several options for performing the procedure will be presented, the simplest—and recommended—approach is blind xiphosternal puncture with an over-the-needle catheter [29]. Other acceptable approaches are a spinal needle with ECG chest (V) lead attached, and the Seldinger technique [30].

D. Patient Preparation

If possible, patients should be sitting upright at a 45° angle to bring the heart more anterior. Most trauma patients, however, are in full C-spine precautions, supine, and this is not possible. Patients should have their airways managed appropriately, be placed on supplemental oxygen, have adequate vascular access, and be attached to a continuous cardiac monitor (12-lead ECG if available). A defibrillator should be ready for use if dysrhythmia occurs. Most trauma patients receiving pericardiocentesis are obtunded or unresponsive, but if the patient is cognizant, adequate sedation and local anesthesia should be used. If the patient's stomach is distended, a nasogastric tube should be placed prior to performing pericardiocentesis (if time permits).

E. Performing the Procedure

1. Recommended Method for Emergent Pericardiocentesis (Catheter-Over-Needle)

For a depiction of this procedure see Figure 12.

1. Monitor the patient's vital signs and cardiac rhythm (ECG if available) continuously.
2. Prepare xiphoid/subxiphoid area with surgical antiseptic.
3. Administer local anesthesia if necessary.
4. Assess the patient for possible mediastinal shift.
5. Xiphosternal approach is perferred.
6. Insert needle between xiphoid process and costal margin 1 to 2 cm inferior and to the left of xiphochondral junction.
7. Needle should be angulated 30° to 45° to the skin and cephalad.
8. Recommendations vary as to how to direct the needle from tip left scapula to the right shoulder. A reasonable approach is to direct needle cephalad toward the sternal notch initially and modify directions as needed for subsequent attempts.
9. Advance the needle slowly, aspirating while proceeding. The pericardium should be entered approximately 6 to 8 cm below the skin in most adults, 5 cm in children [24].
10. If the needle is advanced too far into the epicardium, myocardium, or ventricle, an injury pattern or PVC is usually noted on the ECG. Withdraw the needle a few millimeters until a baseline ECG pattern is restored.

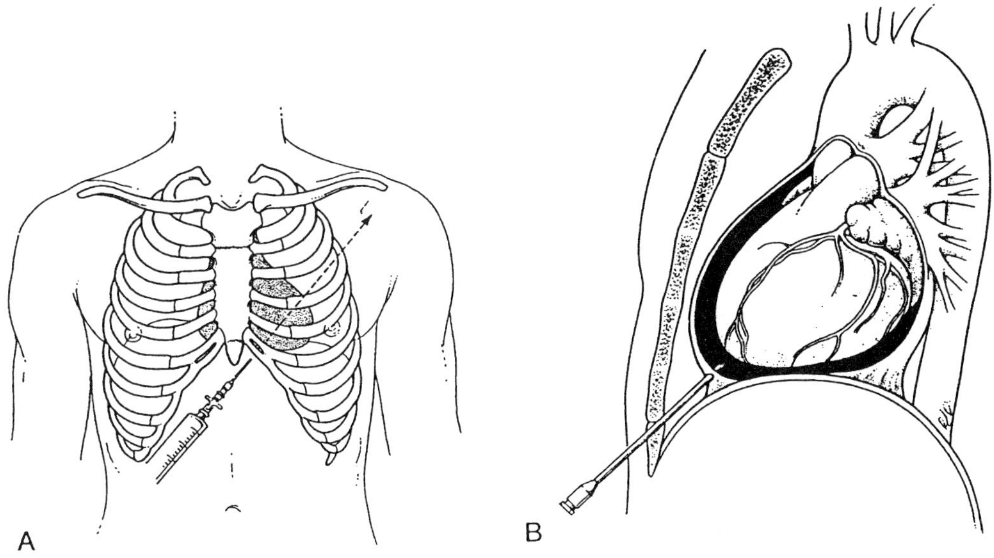

Figure 12 Recommended method for pericardiocentesis: catheter-over-needle. (A) The sub-xiphoid approach with needle directed toward tip of left clavicle. (B) Catheter left in position within the pericardial space. (Courtesy of W.B. Saunders Co.)

11. When the needle tip enters the blood-filled pericardium withdraw as much blood as possible. Watch the ECG/cardiac monitor. As the pericardial sac collapses, an injury pattern may recur, requiring withdrawal of the needle another millimeter or two.
12. Nonclotting blood is indicative of a pericardial aspirate; however, pericardial fluid with a large amount of blood in it may clot and thus is not indicative of ventricular over pericardial blood.
13. When aspiration is complete, withdraw the needle and secure the catheter in place with suture or tape.
14. Attach a three-way stopcock for further aspiration if necessary.

2. Use of Spinal Needle and Attached ECG Lead (Time Permitting)

1. The technique is the same as described above, except a metal spinal needle is used.
2. After the skin is punctured but before the pericardial sac is entered, attach one end of an alligator clamp to the needle near the hub and the other end to one of the chest or V leads of an ECG monitor.
3. The V lead is recorded as the tip of the needle now becomes an ECG electrode.
4. Advance the needle as above in 6.5.1 while aspirating. If the needle touches the epicardium/myocardium ST segment elevation or PVCs will occur and the needle should be withdrawn 1 to 2 millimeters.
5. The needle should be within the pericardial space, and attempts to aspirate blood should be made.
6. Once aspiration is complete, the needle should not be left in the pericardial space. It should either be withdrawn, or a guide wire of appropriate size may be passed so that an indwelling plastic catheter may be placed using the Seldinger technique.

3. Seldinger Technique

1. The initial steps of either procedure above are the same.
2. Use an appropriately sized needle or prepackaged kit so that a J wire may be passed through the needle
3. When aspiration of pericardial blood is complete, pass the J wire into the pericardial sac and remove the needle.
4. A flexible plastic catheter is guided over the wire in the standard Seldinger technique and secured in place. A dilator may be used to create a tract through skin and subcutaneous tissues, but do not pass a dilator into the pericardial sac.
5. Attach a three-way stopcock to the catheter.

There are alternate approaches to the xiphosternal site that have been described. These include puncture in the left fifth intercostal space medial to the border of cardiac dullness and the apical approach, in which the needle puncture site is 1 cm outside the palpable apex beat and the intercostal space below is aimed toward the right shoulder. The alternate approaches, however, are associated with a greater risk of pneumothorax and other complications and generally are less desirable than the xiphosternal approach [26,31].

F. Complications

For a list of complications see Table 5.

G. Postprocedure Patient Management

Pericardiocentesis is a temporizing procedure done only to alleviate acute hemopericardium that is compromising cardiac output. The definitive treatment for cardiac tamponade is open thoracotomy and pericardectomy, or subxiphoid pericardiotomy done via a pericardial window. Patients must be transported or transferred to a trauma center at which definitive management can be performed (Table 6).

The catheter in the pericardium must be secured and the patient constantly reassessed for reaccumulation of hemopericardium. If the patient's hemodynamic status changes, connect a syringe to the stopcock and attempt aspiration again. General principles of trauma resuscitation should be ongoing simultaneously.

Table 5 Pericardiocentesis

Indications
Acute cardiac tamponade/hemopericardium in prehospital trauma patient
Contraindications
Need for emergent open thoracotomy
Complications
Injury to ventricle epicardium/myocardium
Laceration of coronary artery or vein
Iatrogenic hemopericardium
Pneumothorax
Puncture of great vessel or other organ (esophagus, stomach, etc.)
Air embolism

Table 6 Pericardiocentesis—Necessary Equipment

Catheter-over-needle approach (recommended for emergent pericardiocentesis)
Surgical antiseptic (povidone-iodine)
Local anesthetic if necessary
#16-to-#18-gauge, 15-cm (6-in.) over the needle catheter
60-cc syringe
Three-way stopcock
Spinal needle connected to ECG lead
Surgical antiseptic (povidone-iodine)
Local anesthetic if necessary
#18-gauge spinal needle
Alligator clamp connected to V lead of ECG device
60-cc syringe
Three-way stopcock
Seldinger technique
Surgical antiseptic (povidone-iodine)
Local anesthetic if necessary
#14-to-#16-gauge catheter over J wire kit
Three-way stopcock

H. Options for Obtaining Procedural Experience

Besides actual patient encounters, there are currently few controlled training situations that adequately recreate the physiologic state of cardiac tamponade. As of this writing there are no satisfactory manikins or simulations for training in this particular procedure. Human cadavar models are not applicable for pericardiocentesis. It is possible to design an animal model for training. A pig or primate model is preferable due to similarities with human chest anatomy. An open thoracotomy is first performed, then a small pericardiotomy is done with a catheter placed inside the pericardial space and secured with a purse-string suture. Saline can then be injected into the pericardial sac, and attempts at pericardiocentesis can be performed using the xiphosternal approach until saline is withdrawn. A similar procedure could be done on newly deceased patients if informed consent can be obtained from family members.

IV. PREHOSPITAL THORACOTOMY

Cardiac arrest due to trauma carries a poor prognosis. In trauma to the chest, death is usually caused by irreversible injuries, such as rupture of the heart or great vessels. In some instances, however, death is caused by cardiac tamponade, which per se is a reversible condition. Because control of bleeding due to other causes is extremely difficult to achieve (at least not in the prehospital setting) and requires skills not possessed by emergency physicians, prehospital thoracotomy is indicated in the presence of a strong suspicion of cardiac tamponade.

A. Indications

Prehospital emergency thoracotomy can be performed in patients with perforating chest trauma whose vital signs deteriorate into lifelessness in the presence of the treating physi-

Table 7 Prehospital Thoracotomy

Indications for prehospital thoracotomy
Penetrating chest trauma with suspicion of cardiac tamponade
Fewer than 4 lesions
Cardiac arrest in the presence of EMS team (or PEA as initial rhythm on arrival of EMS team)
Surgical facility more than 10 min away with cardiopulmonary bypass
No other lethal injuries
Contraindications for prehospital thoracotomy
Blunt trauma
More than 3 lesions
Unwitnessed cardiac arrest, asystole
Immediate complications
Visceral organ injury (lung, spleen)
Excessive bleeding
Injury to the phrenic nerve

cian (see Table 7). Patients who are encountered lifeless but who still have electrical activity in the heart are also candidates for the procedure if the onset of cardiac arrest can be counted in minutes. An alternate procedure when hemopericardium is suspected is pericardiocentesis, discussed in an earlier section. A facility with the capacity to perform instantaneous emergency thoracotomy should be more than 10 min away, including transfer of the patient to the vehicle and transportation to the hospital. In all instances, possible concomitant injuries must be compatible with survival.

1. Penetrating Trauma

Penetrating trauma to the chest is most often caused by stabbing or by gunshot. The resulting injury depends on the path of the perforating violence, with lesions to the heart or great vessels being most dangerous. The cause of cardiac arrest in these patients is often cardiac tamponade. Perforation of adjacent vessels, causing exsanguination, is also possible, especially if the patient has suffered several hits. A patient with a solitary injury is therefore more likely to benefit from thoracotomy than a patient who has suffered multiple stabs or has been shot several times. Injuries caused by low-caliber handguns are more likely to be isolated than injuries caused by high-velocity rifles or shotguns.

Because lesions of the great vessels are extremely difficult to deal with in the prehospital environment, the main indication for prehospital thoracotomy is suspicion of cardiac tamponade in the absence of other lethal trauma.

2. Blunt Trauma

In blunt thoracic trauma, the cause of cardiac arrest is often massive injuries to the intrathoracic organs. There are several studies showing that resuscitative thoracotomy is not indicated in patients developing cardiac arrest due to blunt trauma.

B. Contraindications

In perforating thoracic trauma, thoracotomy is not indicated if the patient has numerous wounds in his central thorax. High-velocity gunshot wounds to the chest are also likely to cause injuries such that survival is not possible. Patients with blunt trauma are not candidates for thoracotomy in the field. Whichever the cause, a patient whose cardiac

Table 8 Prehospital Thoracotomy—Necessary Equipment

Rib retractor
Regular (Mayo) scissors
Long scissors
Long regular forceps
Criles/mosquitos
Suture set
Suctioning tip
Also needed
Sterile gloves for two persons
Disinfectant
Dressings
Scalpel

arrest is not witnessed by the treating team and whose initial cardiac rhythm is asystole is not likely to be saved by thoracotomy.

C. Necessary Equipment

A sterile set for thoracotomy should be available. It should contain the equipment listed in Table 8.

D. Patient Preparation

After the primary survey and a determination if appropriate indication exists, the patient is immediately intubated and an attempt at vascular access established via at least two large-bore cannulae (see Fig. 13). As soon as the patient is intubated and the tube fixed, he or she is tilted to his or her right side by placing, for example, a cushion under the left scapula. The thorax is exposed and disinfectant poured on the skin, although it is unclear if this truly provides sufficient sterility to this procedure.

E. Performance of the Procedure

With the patient positioned, a left lateral thoracotomy incision is performed beginning two centimeters left from the sternum to the midaxillary line along the fourth or fifth rib under the left breast (see Fig. 14). In female patients, the incision is made along the inframammary fold. The incision is performed through all tissue layers to the pleura. If it is anticipated that exposure of the right side of the heart will be needed, an alternative incision extends from the left axilla, across the sternum to the right axilla. Large Mayo scissors can be used to cut across the sternum.

On entering the pleural cavity, the bag is disconnected from the endotracheal tube to enable the lung to collapse. The pleura is then opened using the scissors. The rib cage is widened using the retractor, with the handle facing laterally. The lung is pulled to the left and the pericardial sac visualized. In case the pericardium is filled with blood, it looks dark blue or red and distended. Identify the phrenic nerve coursing longitudinally along the pericardial sac, and the pericardium is opened using the scissors to make a small hole at the sternal part of the pericardium anterior to, and avoiding, the phrenic nerve. A finger

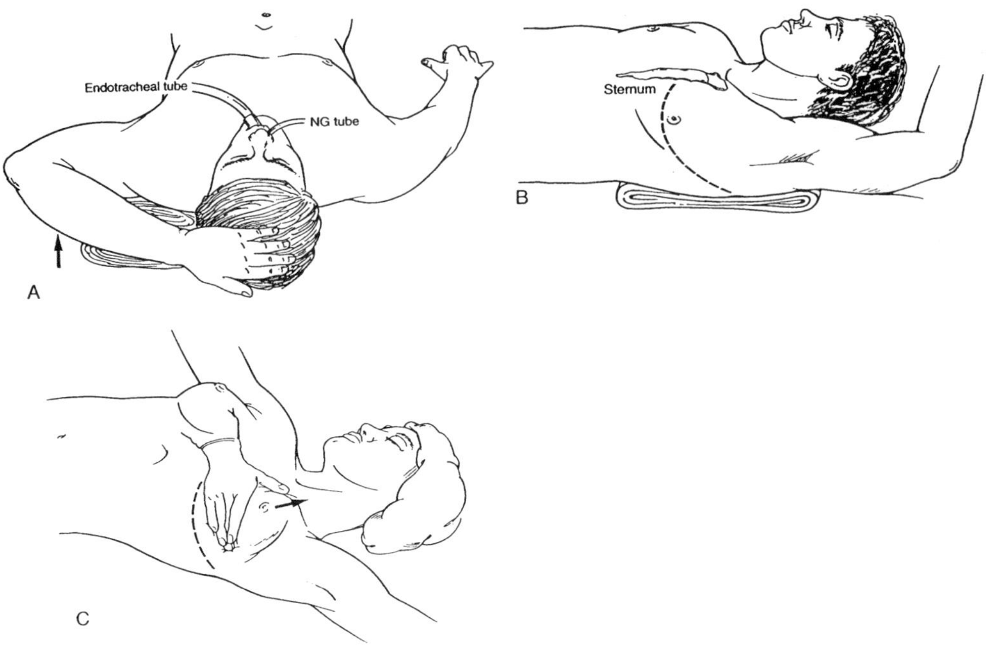

Figure 13 Left anterolateral thoracotomy. (A) Several towels of sandbags are placed under the left scapula and the arm is raised above the head. The patient should be intubated. A nasogastric tube can be inserted to facilitate differentiation of the esophagus from the aorta. (B) The left anterolateral submammary incision is the suggested initial approach. Ideally, the incision is made between the fourth and fifth ribs. Generally, the incision is just inferior to the nipple (male) or along the inframammary fold (female). The incision begins on the sternum and extends to the posterior axillary line, where it should be deep enough to partially transect the latissimus dorsi muscle. (C) Dashes indicate the incision site of the inframammary fold in women. (Courtesy of W.B. Saunders Co.)

is inserted into the pericardial sac and the hole distended in a cephalocaudal direction in order not to injure the phrenic nerve in the mediastinal pleura.

Typically, if tamponade is present, the clot and blood are expunged. The heart may spontaneously resume beating when the constricting obstacle is removed. If the heart does not beat, the hole in the pericardium is enlarged and manual compression of the heart is begun. If there is enough room, the apex of the heart is placed between the palms and the heart is squeezed to provide forward flow. Alternately, the right hand is inserted dorsal to the heart, which may be gently squeezed against the dorsal surface of the sternum. Care should be taken not to tilt the heart or compress the atrial parts.

If the heart resumes beating, blood usually starts to flow from the wound(s). To control bleeding, a finger is inserted through the hole into the heart. At this time, the patient may show signs of an increasing level of consciousness. This is best dealt with by inducing anesthesia, using ketamine, or administering repeated small doses of diazepam and opioid.

The descending aorta can be cross-clamped using a large vascular clamp or by manually compressing it against the anterior surface of the vertebral bodies.

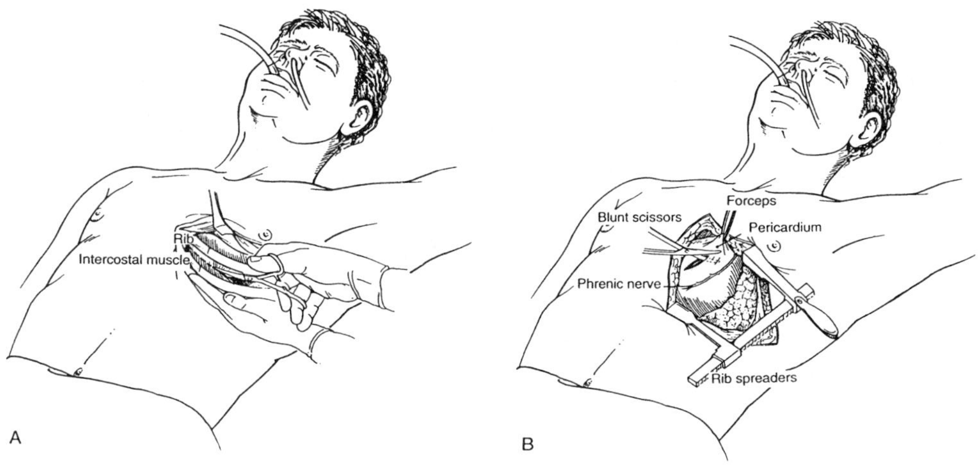

Figure 14 (A) entering the pleural cavity, it is important to make the incision on top of the rib to avoid the intercostal vessels. Once a hole has been made into the pleural space, the incision is widened with blunt scissors by cutting the intercostal muscles. The fourth and fifth fingers of the operator's free hand are inserted into the pleural space to fend off the lung as the scissors divide the intercostal muscle. Momentary cessation of ventilation will collapse the lung. Alternatively, the right mainstem bronchus can be intubated, which permits continuous ventilation and oxygenation without inflating the left lung into the operating field. (B) The incision must always be carried to the posterior axillary line to maximize exposure. The rib spreader should be placed with the handle laterally. Because it can be difficult to determine if tamponade has occurred using visual inspection alone, the pericardium must be opened to definitively determine if tamponade is present. Using tissue pickups with teeth, the operator must press hard against the pericardium to engage it within the tissue pickups. The incision is started near the diaphragm and anterior to the phrenic nerve, which is easily identified as a thick tendonlike structure. Using blunt scissors, the incision is carried to the root of the aorta. (Courtesy of W.B. Saunders Co.)

F. Postprocedure Management

After relieving the tamponade, preparations for immediate transportation are begun. Since the filling of the heart can be manually felt, an empty heart requires aggressive fluid administration. If the heart beats, the finger is kept in the cardiac wound until the wound can be closed. Closure can be accomplished by placing a large horizontal mattress suture across the open wound through which a vascular catheter can be inserted or by quickly stapling it. Alternately, an appropriately sized Foley/urinary catheter can be inserted into the wound and the balloon can be inflated to impede the extravasation of blood (Fig. 15). Crystalloid fluid can be administered through this catheter. The myocardial wound should be sealed in some manner before transporting the patient.

G. Complications

Lesions to the lung are possible during the initial incision. The phrenic nerve in the mediastinal pleura may be injured while opening the pericardial sac. Failure to control bleeding after pericardiotomy may result in massive bleeding.

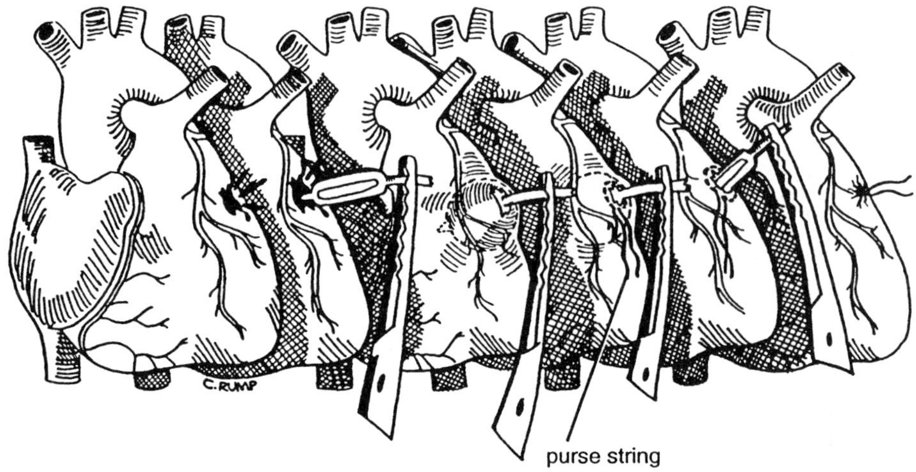

Figure 15 Serial illustration. Gentle traction on an inflated Foley catheter will control hemorrhage and allow easy repair. The balloon is inflated with saline, and care is taken to avoid rupturing the balloon with the suture needle. This technique is particularly useful with injuries of the inferior cavoatrial junction, with posterior wounds, and during cardiac massage. Volume loading can be obtained by infusion of blood or crystalloid solutions through the lumen of the catheter. Care should be taken to avoid an air embolus through the lumen of the catheter during placement. (Courtesy of W.B. Saunders Co.)

H. Options for Obtaining Necessary Procedural Experience

If thoracotomy is not part of the daily work of a given hospital, basic and topographic anatomy of the thoracic cavity is best examined and learned at autopsy. At least two visits to the autopsy department are well advised. When the relevant structures are familiar, the next step is participating in elective thoracotomy under the guidance of a surgeon who knows the objective of the participation. The various structures are identified, and depending on the surgeon, making the incision, applying the retractor, and exposing the pericardium are of benefit for further needs. When training is completed, orientation of the prehospital team and presentation of indications is accomplished. The team members are taught the procedures step by step, and the instruments are presented. A ''standard operational procedure'' algorithm should be created.

Alternately, similar experience can be gained in the laboratory setting. If local restrictions permit, performing the procedure on live, anesthetized animals provides a more realistic experience in managing cardiac wounds. If such a model is considered, the thorax of a pig is similar enough to a human thorax to provide worthwhile training. Finally, human cadavers can provide practice with the relevant anatomical landmarks.

V. PREHOSPITAL EMERGENCY CESAREAN SECTION

Cardiac arrest during pregnancy carries a poor prognosis compared with outcome from cardiac arrest in nonpregnant patients. With increasing gestational age, the impact of the enlarged uterus on aortocaval blood flow becomes of greater importance. Venous return is decreased in the supine position, with a concomitant decrease in cardiac output, and consequently, also placental blood flow. During resuscitation, these unfavorable hemodynamic changes are accentuated, and at the end of the third trimester, delivery by cesarean section may be the only way to restore normal blood flow.

Despite the desperate situation, survival of both mother and child has been reported. Survival of the mother requires the physician to be well trained in performing cesarean section, a condition that is not usually met in the out-of-hospital environment. Cesarean section in the prehospital environment is therefore mainly considered in those situations in which the life of the mother is no longer salvageable but the baby may survive.

A. Indications

Prehospital emergency cesarean section (perimortem cesarean section) is performed in women who are pregnant in their thirtieth week or later (see Table 9). The mother should have suffered a witnessed cardiac/traumatic arrest refractory to conventional resuscitative measures of no more than 5 min duration before the procedure. Furthermore, the mother's illness or injuries are considered lethal.

B. Contraindications

Contraindications include a pregnancy of shorter duration than 30 weeks, unwitnessed cardiac/traumatic arrest, or duration of arrest more than five min. Depending on the skill of the physician, witnessed arrest which is potentially reversible.

C. Necessary Equipment

A sterile set for the procedure should be available (see Table 10).

D. Patient Preparation

With ongoing CPR to ensure placental blood flow, after the primary survey and a determination if appropriate indication exists, the mother is immediately intubated to ensure optimal ventilation with 100% oxygen. Vascular access may be established if performed without delay.

Table 9 Prehospital Cesarean Section

Indications for prehospital emergency cesarean section.
All four of the following criteria must be fulfilled:
Pregnancy >30 weeks
Mother's cardiac arrest in the presence of the EMS team
CPR preceding cesarean section of no more than 5 min
Mother's irreversible cause of death
Contraindications for prehospital emergency cesarean section include the following:
Pregnancy <30 weeks
Duration of cardiac arrest of more than 5 min
Mother's survival probable
Complications include the following:
Injury to visceral organs
Amniotic fluid or air embolism
Excessive bleeding

Table 10 Prehospital Cesarean Section—Necessary Equipment

Scissors
Forceps
Criles/mosquitos
Suture set
Suctioning tip
Also needed
Sterile gloves
Disinfectant
Dressings
Scalpel

At the same time, if not already done, the patient is tilted 20° to 30° to her left by placing a cushion under her right flank. The abdomen is exposed and disinfectant poured on the skin.

E. Performance of the Procedure

With the patient positioned, a lower midline incision is performed from the umbilicus to the symphysis. The incision is performed through the skin and muscle layers to the peritoneum. An opening is made with the scissors in the peritoneum and the opening is vertically cut larger. The skin is manually retracted and the crest of the urinary bladder identified. The bladder crest is pulled in caudal direction and a transversal incision on the uterine wall is performed immediately above it. The incision is manually distended laterally, and one hand is inserted in the uterus. The assistant places his hands on the fundus and forces the baby down toward the operator, and the baby is assisted out. The airways of the baby are immediately suctioned and an assessment of vital signs begun. The umbilical cord is clamped, tied, and cut. As soon as the baby's vital signs are secured, it is dried and protected against the cold. The placenta is removed from the uterine cavity.

F. Postprocedure Management

Cardiopulmonary resuscitation of the mother may be continued after delivery, depending on the indication of the procedure. If CPR is terminated, the uterine and abdominal incisions are closed with a few stitches. If return of spontaneous circulation occurs, the placenta is removed from the uterus. The uterine wall should be sutured to ensure that hemostasis and oxytocin may be given intravenously.

The baby may need immediate intubation and suctioning, depending on its respiratory status and other indications of postdelivery status (i.e., Apgar score). Heat loss must be prevented by wrapping the baby in blankets.

G. Complications

Lesions to the intestines may occur if the initial incision is too deep and there are intestines between the uterus and the peritoneum. The bladder may be incised. Amniotic fluid or air embolism may ensue due to the rich vascular supply of the pregnant uterus. Extensive bleeding may occur from incised uterine vessels and the placenta. Lesions to the ureters are also a risk.

H. Options for Obtaining Necessary Procedural Experience

Participating in elective cesarean section as well several emergency sections is desirable.

VI. PREHOSPITAL AUTOTRANSFUSION

A. Indications

All victims of major trauma can be considered potential candidates for autologous blood transfusion. In the prehospital setting, however, this will mostly be limited to victims of blunt or penetrating chest trauma in cases in which a thoracostomy tube is placed for significant (>500 ml) hemothorax. In addition, autotransfusion of blood in the field should be reserved for patients who are hypotensive from class III or IV hemorrhage.

B. Contraindications

The procedure should not be accomplished if significant delay in transport to definitive care will result from setup or performance. Furthermore, Reul et al. [32] identify other relative contraindications, including the presence of known malignant lesions in the area of traumatic blood accumulation, known renal or hepatic insufficiency, wounds older than 4 to 6 hr, or gross contamination of pooled or collected blood.

C. Necessary Equipment

There are numerous commercial devices available to perform autotransfusion (see Fig. 16). Most of them have these components in common: some sort of sterile blood collection bag or bottle, in-line blood filter, and use of an anticoagulant (acid citrate dextrose [ACD], citrate phosphate dextrose [CPD], etc.). A number of commercial products require the use of vacuum suction, often in the form of an electric aspirator and battery. These products can be used in the prehospital setting [33], although some authors have described amplified techniques using gravity alone and a chest tube connected to a sterile bag via a micropore filter [34,35]. Cell savers are costly and complex devices and have no role in autotransfusion in the field.

D. Patient Preparation

The key to patient preparation in the prehospital setting is to maintain strict aseptic technique throughout the entire procedure to reduce the risk of contamination of blood products. Second, it is important to minimize the time of air–blood contact to reduce hemolysis. Finally, a properly placed chest tube is a prerequisite for autotransfusion in the field.

E. Performance of Autotransfusion

There are two phases for autotransfusion: blood collection and reinfusion. Any of the commercially available products or a simple chest tube bottle can be used connected to a chest tube. Once the collection of blood is complete, blood may be reinfused through a micropore blood filter. Blood flow may be increased by gravity, manual squeezing, pressure pumps, and the like to improve reinfusion. Blood collection may be continued

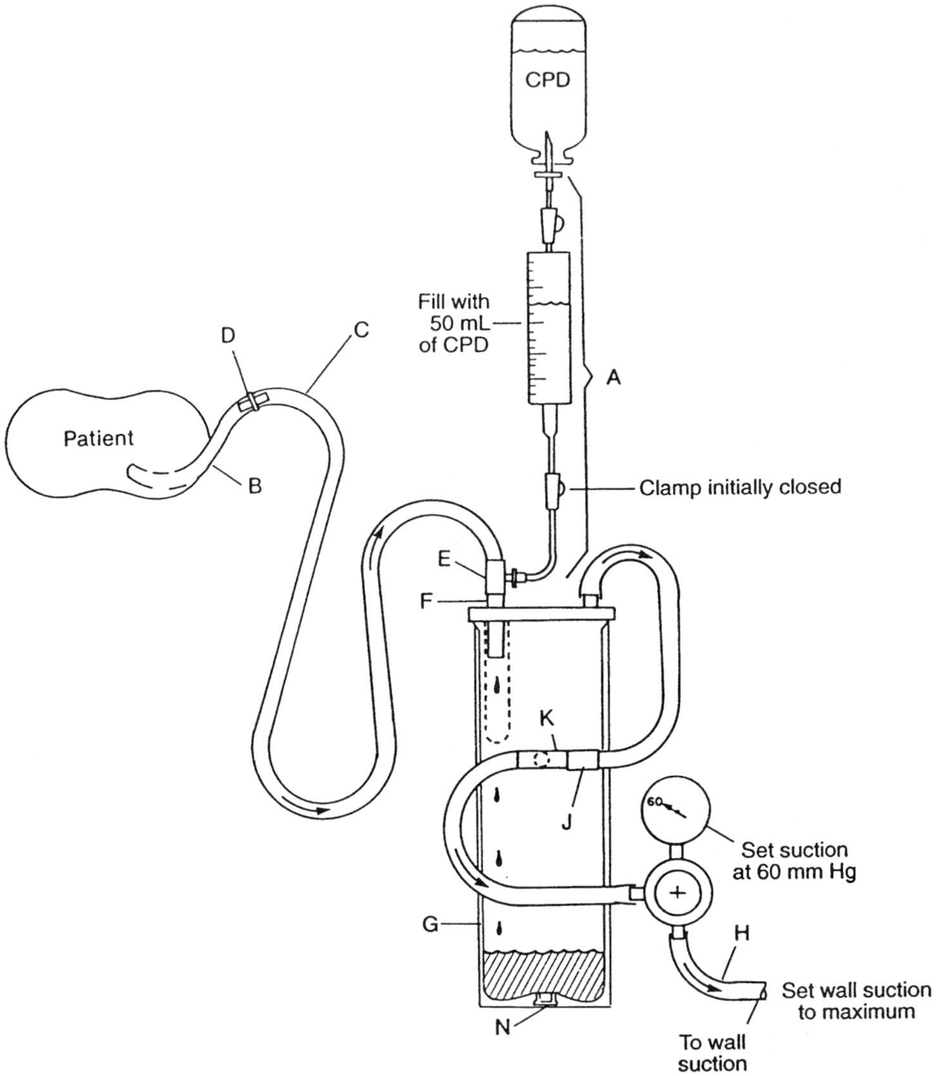

Figure 16 Abbott receptal disposable collection apparatus. A, Anticoagulant volume-control burette (fill with 50 mL of CPD anticoagulant); B, Chest tube; C, Latex drainage tubing; D, Male-to-male connector; E, End of drainage tubing with side port; F, Inlet port of red liner cap attached to collection canister; G, Collection liner bag; H, Downstream suction hose (do not exceed 60 mmHg of suction); J, Liner lid tubing connector; K, Canister tee; N, Liner stem with protective cap. (Modified from Ref. 35a, reproduced by permission.)

during reinfusion by using another bag or bottle. Use each bag or bottle only once. Reinfusion should begin immediately after collection is complete. Do not let blood stand for a significant time period (4 hr or more). If collected blood becomes clotted it should be discarded. Change the blood filter after each 1000- to 2000-ml transfusion.

F. Complications

Complications can be divided into two main groups: hematologic and nonhematologic (Table 11).

Thrombocytopenia is most common, followed by hypofibrinogenemia and hemolysis [36,35], although these are not generally clinically significant. Of the nonhematologic complications, sepsis is a concern, as is microemboli and subsequent development of ARDS. In general the benefits gained exceed these potential risks.

G. Options for Obtaining Necessary Procedural Experience

Autotransfusion is a common practice in most hospital trauma units or emergency departments. Participation in the routine operation of these units and becoming familiar with the equipment and its use in this setting should be adequate preparation for using this technique in the field.

VII. SUMMARY

Field tube thoracostomy should be considered in unstable patients who suffered thoracic trauma with probable pneumothorax or hemothorax. Needle thoracos-

Table 11 Prehospital Autotransfusion

- Indications
  - Placement of thoracostomy tube for blunt or penetrating chest trauma
  - Hypotensive patients (class III or IV hemorrhagic shock)
- Contraindications
  - If autotransfusion results in delay in transport
  - Known chest malignancy
  - Known renal or hepatic insufficiency
  - Wounds more than 4–6 hr old
  - Gross contamination of blood
- Potential Complications of Autotransfusion
  - Hematologic
    - Decreased platelet count
    - Decreased fibrinogen level
    - Increased fibrin split products
    - Prolonged prothrombin time
    - Prolonged partial thromboplastin time
    - Red blood cell hemolysis
    - Elevated plasma-free hemoglobin
    - Decreased hematocrit
  - Nonhematologic
    - Bacteremia
    - Sepsis
    - Microembolism
    - Air embolism

tomy is a rapid, temporary means of decompressing a tension pneumothorax that may be performed prior to chest tube insertion.

In intubated patients ventilated with positive pressure, simple thoracostomy (incision without a tube) is an alternative to tube or needle thoracostomy.

An autotransfusion apparatus may be successfully used in the prehospital setting for massive hemothorax.

In the prehospital setting, the only indication for cricothyroidotomy is the inability to intubate the trachea in patients with actual or impending airway obstruction.

Field thoracotomy should only be performed under the following circumstances: properly trained personnel present, suspicion of cardiac tamponade, less than four penetrating wounds, loss of vital signs in the presence of EMS, no other lethal injuries, and a definitive care facility less than 10 min away.

Cesarean section in the field is a measure to be performed only as a last resort to save a potentially viable baby. Indications include gestation more than 30 weeks, witnessed arrested no more than 5 min duration, and maternal injuries considered to be fatal.

Pericardiocentesis using a subxiphoid approach is a method to attempt relieving hemopericardium in the field prior to thoracotomy.

REFERENCES

1. CD Deakin, G Davies, A Wilson. Simple thoracostomy avoids chest drain insertion in prehospital trauma. J Trauma 39:373–374, 1995.
2. I Inci, C Ozcelik, O Nizam, N Eren, G Ozgen. Penetrating chest injuries in children: A review of 94 cases. J Pediat Surg 44:673–676, 1996.
2a. JS Millikan, EE Moore, E Steiner. Complications of tube thoracostomy for acute trauma. Am J Surg 140:739, 1980.
2b. DL Bricker. Safe, effective tube thoracostomy. ER Rep 2:49, 1981.
3. M Eckstein, D Suyehara. Needle thoracostomy in the prehospital setting. Prehosp Emerg Care 64:132–135, 1998.
4. T Moskal, K Liscum, K Mattox. Subclavian artery obstruction by tube thoracostomy. J Trauma 64:368–369, 1997.
5. ED Barton, M Epperson, DB Hoyt, D Fortlage, P Rosen. Prehospital needle aspiration and tube thoracostomy in trauma victims: A six-year experience with aeromedical crews. J Emerg Med 13:155–163, 1995.
6. R Westfal. Paramedic protocols. In: RE W, ed. Paramedic Protocols. New York: McGraw Hill, 1997, pp. 86–105.
7. D York, L Dudek, R Larson, W Marshall, D Dries. A comparison study of tube thoracostomy: Aeromedical crews vs. in hospital trauma service. J Air Med Trans 10:69, 1991.
8. U Schmidt, M Stalp, T Gerich, M Blauth, KI Maull, H Tscherne. Chest tube decompression of blunt chest injuries by physicians in the field: Effectiveness and complications. J Trauma. 44:98–101, 1998.
9. R Gonzalez, M Holevar. Role of prophylactic antibiotics for tube thoracostomy in chest trauma. Am Surg 64:617–620, 1998.
10. J Evans, J Green, P Carlin, L Barrett. Meta-analysis of antibiotics in tube thoracostomy. Am Surg 64:215–219, 1995.
11. L Hussain, A Redmond. Are pre-hospital deaths from accidental injury preventable? Brit Med J 308:1077–1080, 1994.
12. NS Xeropotamos, TJ Coats, AW Wilson. Prehospital surgical airway management: 1 year's experience from the Helicopter Emergency Medical Service. Injury 24:222–224, 1993.

13. S Norwood, MB Myers, TJ Butler. The safety of emergency neuromuscular blockade and orotracheal intubation in the acutely injured trauma patient. J Am Coll Surg 179:646–652, 1994.
14. A Morris, D Lockey, T Coats. Fat necks: Modification of a standard surgical airway protocol in the pre-hospital environment. Resuscitation 35:253–254, 1997.
15. JH Isaacs Jr, AD Pedersen. Emergency cricothyroidotomy. Amer Surg 63:346–349, 1997.
16. CK Salvino, D Dries, R Gamelli, M Murphy-Macabobby, W Marshall. Emergency cricothyroidotomy in trauma victims. J Trauma 34:503–505, 1993.
17. B Esses, B Jafek. Cricothyroidotomy: A decade of experience in Denver. Ann Otol Rhin Laryn 96:519–524, 1987.
18. D Spaite, M Joseph. Prehospital cricothyrotomy: An investigation of indications, technique, complications and patient outcome. Ann Emerg Med 19:279–285, 1990.
19. L Calder. Primary survey in major trauma. Brit Med J 300:1652, 1990.
20. G DeLaurier, M Hawkins, R Treat, A Mansberger. Acute airway management: Role of cricothyroidotomy. Am Surg 56:12–15, 1990.
21. D Leibovici, B Fredman, O Gofrit, J Shemer, A Blumenfeld, S Shapira. Prehospital cricothyroidotomy by physicians. Am J Emerg Med 15:91–93, 1997.
22. P Symbas, N Harlafhs, W Waldo. Penetrating cardiac wounds: A comparison of different therapeutic methods. Ann Surg 183:377, 1976.
23. A Borja, A Lansing, H Randal. Immediate operative treatment for stab wounds of the heart. J Thor Cardiovasc Surg 59:662, 1970.
24. A Baue, W Blakemore. The pericardium. Ann Thor Surg 14:81, 1972.
25. R Shabetai, N Fowler, W Guntheroth. The hemodynamics of cardiac tamponade and constrictive pericarditis. Am J Cardiol 26:480, 1970.
26. W Pories, A Gaudiani. Cardiac tamponade. Surg Clin North Amer 55:573, 1975.
27. W Shoemaker, S Carey, S Yao. Hemodynamic monitoring for physiologic evaluation, diagnosis, and therapy of acute hemopericardial tamponade from penetrating wounds. J Trauma 13: 36, 1973.
28. J Dipasquale, JR. P. Penetrating wounds of the heart and cardiac tamponade. Postgrad Med 49:114, 1971.
29. DW Moores, SW Dziuban Jr. Pericardial drainage procedures. Chest Surg Clin North Am 5: 359–373, 1995.
30. K Liu, W Liu, X Li, et al. Pericardiocentesis and drainage by a silicon rubber line without echocardiographic guidance: Experience in 55 consecutive patients. Jpn Heart J 35:751–756, 1994.
31. T Treasure, L Cotter. Practical procedures: How to aspirate the pericardium. Brit J Hosp Med 24:488, 1980.
32. G Reul, R Solis, S Greenberg. Experience with autotransfusion in the surgical management of trauma. Surgery 76:546, 1974.
33. P Lassiae, F Sztark, M Petitjean. Autotransfusion, with blood drained from a hemothorax, using the constavac device. Annales Franc D Anethes et de Reanim. 13:781–784, 1994.
34. E Schweitzer, J Hauer, K Swan. Use of the Heimlich valve in a compact autotransfusion device. J Trauma 27:537, 1987.
35. P Barriot, B Riou, P Viars. Prehospital autotransfusion in life-threatening hemothorax. Chest 93:522, 1988.
35a. GP Young, TB Purcell. Emergency autotransfusion. Ann Emerg Med 12:180, 1983.
36. K Mattox. Autotransfusion in the emergency department. JACEP 4:218, 1975.

BIBLIOGRAPHY

Durham LA, et al. Emergency center thoracotomy: Impact of prehospital resuscitation. J Trauma 32:775–779, 1992.

Keogh SR, Wilson AW. Survival following pre-hospital arrest with on-scene thoracotomy for a stabbed heart. Injury 27:525–527, 1996.
Lanoix R, et al. Perimortem cesarean section: Case reports and recommendations. Acad Emerg Med 2:1063–1067, 1995.
Lorentz PH, et al. Emergency thoracotomy: Survival correlates with physiologic status. J Trauma 32:780–788, 1992.
Mauer DK, et al. Cardiopulmonary resuscitation (CPR) during pregnancy. Eur J Anaesth 10:437–440, 1993.
Morris JA, et al. Infant survival after cesarean section for trauma. Ann Surg 223:481–488, 1996.
Ordog GJ. Emergency thoracotomy. Am J Emerg Med 5:312–316, 1987.

20

Hypothermia: Prevention and Treatment

MATTHIAS HELM, JENS HAUKE, and LORENZ A. LAMPL

Federal Armed Forces Medical Center Ulm, Ulm, Germany

I. INTRODUCTION

Accidental hypothermia, which is defined as a core body temperature of less than 36°C, commonly results from an injury in a cold environment, submersion in cold water, or a prolonged exposure to low temperatures without adequate protective clothing [1].

Beside these classical reasons, however, accidental hypothermia is a frequent phenomenon in trauma patients. Recent studies have shown that even at the scene of accident—independent from the season of the year—and even in temperate climate zones, nearly every second trauma victim is affected by accidental hypothermia [2]. Hypothermia affects the function of all organ systems and may lead to pathological changes, which in turn additionally complicate the trauma (e.g., relevant increase of blood loss caused by hypothermia-induced coagulation disorders and increased rate of wound infection in hypothermic trauma victims) [3,4]. Hypothermia may therefore increase posttraumatic morbidity and mortality [5–7]. In a study of Ferrara et al. [5] multisystem trauma patients with a core body temperature of <34°C showed a mortality rate of 50% compared to 13% in those who had been normothermic (identical ISS in both groups); Luna et al. [7] found a significant correlation between the stage of hypothermia and mortality in trauma victims.

Accidental hypothermia therefore poses a relevant but highly underdiagnosed phenomenon in the prehospital treatment of traumatized patients, and requires a rapid response with properly trained personnel and techniques.

II. PATHOPHYSIOLOGY

Body temperature is neither homogeneous nor constant. Core body temperature varies as much as ±0.7°C from 37.0°C from diurnal variation, exercise, and ambient temperature stress [8]. At typical ambient conditions, a temperature gradient exists from skin temperature to core body areas [9]. This temperature gradient is larger in colder ambient conditions and smaller in warmer ones. The temperature of local tissues is a balance between heat production and heat elimination [10]. Maintenance of homeostasis is achieved through a complex interaction between thermoreceptors throughout the body and the preoptic area of the hypothalamus as a temperature control center that affects the response to changes sensed by these cells [11]. These responses include shivering and nonshivering thermogenesis, cutaneous vasoconstriction, or vasodilation and sweating.

A. Mechanisms of Heat Loss

Heat loss from the human body occurs by four mechanisms [12,13] (Fig. 1): radiation, convection, evaporation, and conduction. *Radiant heat loss* occurs whenever exposed skin and viscera are warmer than the surrounding environment [14]. Radiant heat loss is proportional to the temperature difference between the patient and the environment and accounts for 40–50% of total heat loss. *Convective heat loss* is accelerated or increased by whatever air currents are present because of the continual removal of warmed air by the skin or viscera [14]. Heat loss via convection is mainly determined by ambient temperature, air velocity, and surface area, and accounts for 25–35% of total heat loss [15].

In the prehospital setting, *heat loss via evaporation* is mainly caused by insensible perspiration, including evaporation from the respiratory tract [15]. The infusion of large amounts of cool fluids and a cold stretcher are the main causes for *heat loss via conduction* in the prehospital setting. Evaporation and conduction account for 15% of total heat loss.

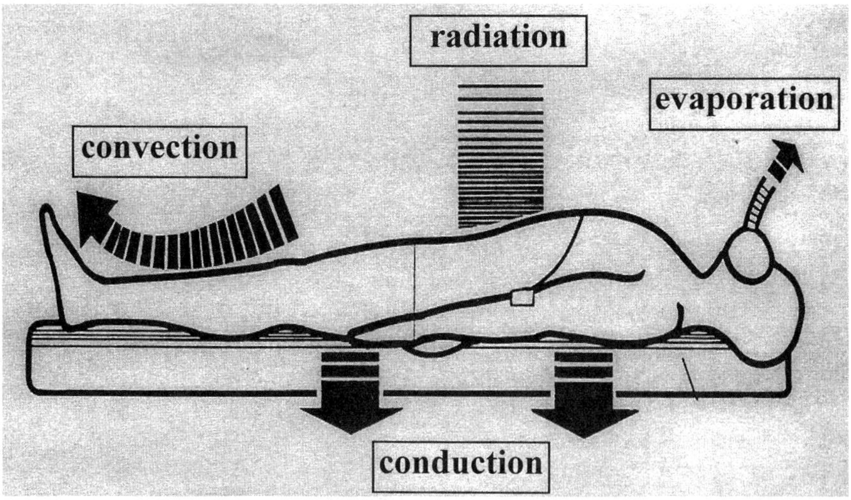

Figure 1 Mechanisms of heat loss: *radiation*: heat loss via electromagnetic waves; *convection*: heat loss as a result of moving air, exposed tissue, and cold ambient environment; *evaporation*: heat loss during vaporization of water or other solutions (e.g., cleaning agents); *conduction*: heat loss by direct contact between objects (e.g., cold backboard).

There are numerous factors favoring the development of posttraumatic accidental hypothermia, including the following:

Exposure: Low ambient temperature, high wind speed (''windchill factor''), and a long exposure time as well as inadequate clothing are important factors predisposing accidental hypothermia [2,16,17]. Another factor is submersion in cold water, which can cool the core body temperature much more rapidly than exposure to cold air, because thermal conductivity of water is 32 times greater than that of air [18].

Extremes of age: The very young and the very old are most susceptible to hypothermia [19–21]. In infants, core body temperature will cool more quickly than in adults, as infants have poor thermal insulation and a larger ratio of surface area to body weight than adults, allowing greater heat loss. Infants cannot generate as much heat as adults. Elderly people have a lower metabolic rate than the young, thus it is more difficult for them to maintain a normal body temperature when the ambient temperature drops. Aging seems to be accompanied by changes in the ability to detect temperature changes; older people may not seek enough shelter to avoid becoming hypothermic [1].

Substance abuse: Alcohol consumption as well as drug ingestion (especially barbiturates) increases the risk of acquiring or aggravating hypothermia. Alcohol causes cutaneous vasodilation, impairment of shivering mechanism, hypothalamic dysfunction, and a decrease in awareness of environmental conditions [22]. Drugs cause hypothermia through their action on the central nervous system [23,24].

Injury Cofactors: Various injuries seem to increase the risk of acquiring or aggravating posttraumatic hypothermia, especially head injury by dysfunction of central thermoregulation mechanisms and severe injuries to the extremities by extended heat loss due to open wounds and an unfavorable surface/mass index [25,26].

Hypoxia: Hypoxia, a high degree of injury severity, and a long prehospital intervention time are found to aggravate the degree of posttraumatic hypothermia [16].

Anesthetic effects: The implementation of general anaesthesia in the traumatized patient in the field (normally performed as a total intravenous anaesthesia [TIVA]) may aggravate hypothermia by various mechanisms: depression of the thermoregulatory centers, abolished shivering by muscle relaxants, altered sweating, and peripheral vasodilation [27].

Comorbidity: Pre-existing medical conditions such as hypothyroidism, hypoadrenalism, circulatory failure, central nervous system disorders, and protein malnutrition also cause hypothermia [12].

There is a considerable increase in the risk of acquiring and aggravating posttraumatic hypothermia in situations in which several of the above-mentioned factors coincide. Exemplary in this context is ''entrapment trauma'' (Fig. 2); it combines a high degree of injury severity and a high percentage of associated head injury, as well as injuries to the extremities and a prolonged prehospital intervention time resulting from technical extrication maneuvers [2].

B. Classification and Clinical Features of Accidental Hypothermia

Numerous different classifications of accidental hypothermia have been described. The most established and the most widely accepted is the classification of accidental hypothermia into the following three stages:

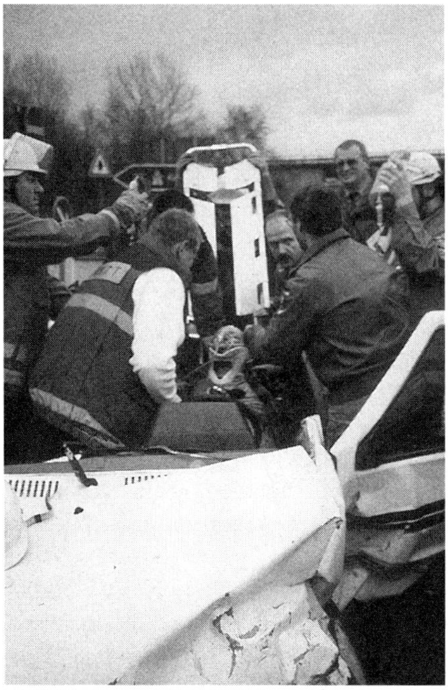

Figure 2 Entrapment trauma: 35-year-old multisystem trauma victim trapped in his car after a motor vehicle accident; situation at the scene during prehospital treatment by the medical team of the Helicopter Emergency Medical Service (HEMS) Christoph 22, Ulm, Germany. Core body temperature at the scene: 34.2°C (IRED tympanon thermometer).

Mild hypothermia: Core body temperature 36.0–34.0°C; the so-called *response phase*.

Moderate hypothermia: Core body temperature 34.0–30.0°C; the so-called *adynamic phase*

Severe hypothermia: Core body temperature <30.0°C; the so-called *slowing phase*

The clinical signs of hypothermia (Table 1) vary not only with core body temperature but also with the speed of cooling, coexisting disorders, and associated injuries. Characteristic for the classical course of accidental hypothermia is that a phase of increased body function activity (response phase) is followed by two phases of more or less attenuation of body function activity (''adynamic'' and ''paralytic phase'').

Mild hypothermia is characterized by an attempt on the part of the patient to maintain body temperature. The most important cause of increased heat production is skeletal muscle ''shivering.'' This leads to a relevant increase in oxygen consumption. Thermoregulatory peripheral vasoconstriction helps preserve the core body temperature by preventing cooling of blood in the extremeties that subsequently returns to the core [1]. This results in pale and cold skin. At this stage of hypothermia, patients are conscious but agitated and confused [18,21,28]. Normally the patients complain about pain in the joints. Ventilation is increased as the body counteracts cooling through an increase in basal metabolic rate, parallel to an increase in pulse rate, blood pressure, central venous pressure, and cardiac output [17].

Table 1 Clinical Symptoms of Accidental Hypothermia by Stage

Mild hypothermia (CBT: 36.0–34.0°C)
Patient awake, but agitated and confused
''Shivering''
Pale and cold skin
Cold extremities
Tachypnea
Increased BMR; increased pulse rate, blood pressure, CVP, and CO
Moderate hypothermia (CBT: 34.0–30.0°C)
Impaired consciousness
Increasing stiffness of muscles and joints
Bradypnea
Decreased BMR; decreased pulse rate and blood pressure, CVP, and VO2
Cardiac arrhythmias/occurrence of J wave (Osbsorn wave)
Severe hypothermia (CBT: <30°C)
Patient unconscious/coma
Further increase of muscle stiffness
Areflexia
Dilated, nonreacting pupils
Extreme bradypnea
Extreme bradycardia/bradyarrhythmia/ventricular fibrillation
Cardiac arrest

Note: Core body temperature: CBT; basal metabolic rate: BMR; central venous pressure: CVP; cardiac output: CO; oxygen consumption: VO2.

With the transition from mild to *moderate hypothermia* (from response phase to adynamic phase), muscle shivering is replaced by an increasing stiffness of muscles and joints. Consciousness is impaired. Ventilation is reduced concomitantly with oxygen consumption and cell metabolism, resulting in bradypnea [17]. Parallel to a decrease in pulse rate, blood pressure, central venous pressure, and cardiac output, the risk of cardiac arrhythmias (common is atrial fibrillation, but virtually any atrial, junctional, or ventricular arrhythmias can occur) is significantly increased [1]. In 80% of the patients at this stage of hypothermia the J wave (Osborn wave), which is prominent in lead V_3 or V_4 in the ECG, occurs [29] (Fig. 3).

Severe hypothermia (slowing phase) is characterized by a further increase of muscle stiffness. Tendon reflexes are absent. The vital functions are extremely reduced; unconsciousness, extreme bradycardia, and brady-arrhythmias, as well as ventricular fibrillation and extreme bradypnea occurs. At this stage, the hypothermic patient may appear clinically dead (without palpable pulse, blood pressure, or respiration), but may still be successfully resuscitated with little or no neurological sequelae if proper and aggressive management is instituted [1].

C. Incidence of Accidental Hypothermia in Trauma Victims

Accidental hypothermia is a frequent phenomenon in trauma patients. We have shown that already at the scene of accident and independent from the season of the year (even in temperature climate zones), every second trauma victim is affected by accidental hypo-

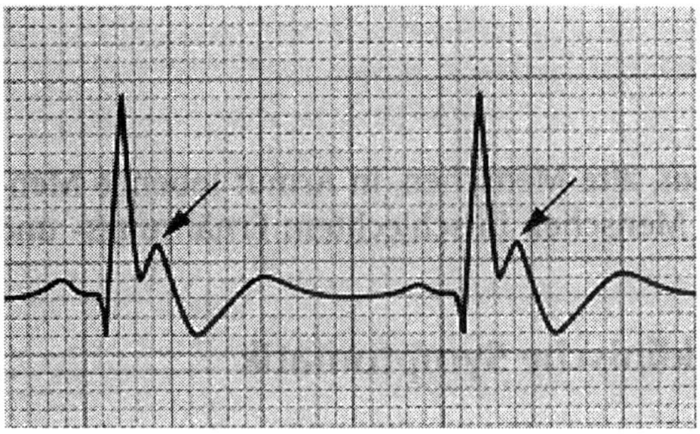

Figure 3 The J wave (Osborn wave), which is most prominent in lead V_3 or V_4, occurs in 80% of hypothermic patients and increases in size with decreasing core body temperature.

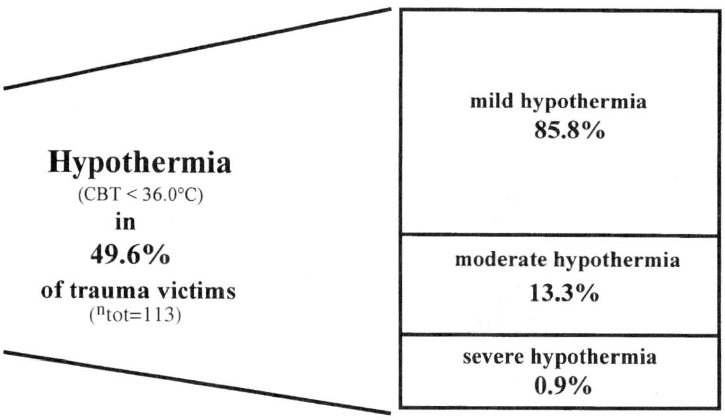

Figure 4 Incidence and stage of accidental hypothermia in trauma victims [2]. Note: Core body temperature, CBT.

Table 2 Entrapment Trauma as a Predisposing Factor of Accidental Hypothermia

The *incidence* of accidental hypothermia is significantly increased in patients with entrapment trauma (ET):

98.1% in patients with ET vs. 34.5% in patients without ET; $P < 0.001$.

100% in *elderly* ET patients vs. 58.8% in younger ET patients; $P < 0.001$.

The *stage* of accidental hypothermia is higher in patients with ET:

29.6% of moderate and severe hypothermia cases in patients with ET vs. 0.0% in patients without ET; $P < 0.001$.

Source: Ref. 1.

thermia [1] (Fig. 4). There is a considerable risk of acquiring or aggravating posttraumatic hypothermia in situations in which ''predisposing'' factors coincide. An example of this is entrapment trauma (Table 2). We found a statistically significant higher percentage of posttraumatic hypothermia in patients with entrapment trauma (98.1% vs. 34.5% P <0.001). If entrapment trauma was combined with high age (>60 years), all patients were hypothermic (100% vs. 58.8%; $P <0.001$) [1]. Not only the incidence but the stage of hypothermia was increased in patients with entrapment trauma. We found a higher percentage of moderate and severe hypothermia cases (29.6% vs. 0.0% in patients without entrapment trauma; $P < 0.001$) [1].

III. DIAGNOSIS OF HYPOTHERMIA IN TRAUMA PATIENTS

With typical clinical symptoms not only can the diagnosis of accidental hypothermia be made, but ideally the stage of the hypothermia can be stated more precisely. The variability or total absence of clinical symptoms in cases of mild hypothermia (e.g., shivering in less than 5% of these patients [1]) and the ambiguity of clinical symptoms in cases of moderate and severe hypothermia (e.g., arrhythmias, hypotension, and respiratory dysfunction), as well as the masking of clinical symptoms of hypothermia by more dramatic symptoms of associated injuries (e.g., severe head injury) underlines the necessity for *prehospital monitoring of core body temperature*. Only the measurement of core body temperature enables both–the definite diagnosis of accidental hypothermia in the trauma victim and a determination of the stage of hypothermia.

The temperature of the arterial blood perfusing the preoptic area of the hypothalamus (or temperature control center) dictates the body's physiologic response to temperature stresses in maintaining homeostasis [9], therefore body sites at which the temperature most closely approximates and changes with that of the hypothalamus provide the most accurate temperature information on which physiologic responses are based. Although estimates of body temperature can be obtained with traditional thermometers by equilibrating with oral, rectal, bladder, or vascular tissues, these sites are subject to multiple influences that make them inaccurate in assessing hypothalamic temperature [30] Benzinger

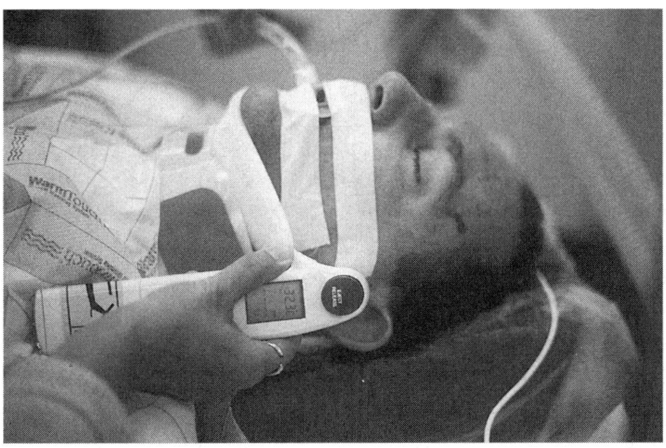

Figure 5 Monitoring of core body temperature by IRED tympanic thermometry in a 24-year-old severely hypothermic trauma victim with associated head injury.

showed that the tympanic membrane temperature is the most reliable measurement of core body temperature [31], therefore the prehospital measurement of core body temperature by infrared emission detection (IRED) tympanic thermometers [30,32] (Fig. 5) is highly recommended (because it is easy to use, fast, and accurate).

IV. PREVENTION AND TREATMENT OF HYPOTHERMIA IN TRAUMA PATIENTS

As pointed out above, accidental hypothermia is a frequent but a highly underdiagnosed phenomenon in traumatized patients. On the other hand, only early recognition of hypothermia and rapid response with properly trained personnel and techniques maximize survival [1]. Procedures to prevent and/or treat hypothermia in the trauma victim therefore must be integrated into the prehospital treatment algorithm of the traumatized patient on a routine basis.

First of all, prehospital emergency personnel must maintain a high index of suspicion of hypothermia in any traumatized patient independent from the season of the year, even in temperate climate zones [1,2,32].

Ideally, the prehospital monitoring of core body temperature in any trauma victim should be performed on a routine basis. For this purpose, thermometers registering temperatures of 30°C or less must be utilized; IRED tympanic thermometers are highly recommended because they are easy to use, fast, and accurate.

Factors that increase the risk of acquiring or aggravating posttraumatic hypothermia (see Sec.II.A) must be recognized by prehospital emergency personnel.

All (prehospital) procedures must be directed at avoiding further core temperature loss. (Remember: up to 85% of heat loss occurs by radiation and convection.) The ''hypothermia treatment algorithm'' (Fig. 6) therefore starts with a number of procedures that must be performed on any trauma patient (''mandatory actions''), including the following:

- *Careful removal of wet garments* (only in warm surroundings).
- *Protection against heat loss and windchill.*
  - Heat the ambulance; keep the doors closed.
  - Immobilization and insulation of the patient (recommended order: place the trauma victim on a vacuum mattress that is covered by a [single-use] insulation blanket; cover the trauma victim with another [single-use] insulation blanket; Fig. 7).
  - Maintainance of horizontal position.
  - Avoidance of rough movements as well as excess activity to minimize the risk of orthostatic blood pressure drop due to cold-induced cardiovascular reflex impairment and occurence of cardiac arrhythmias.
  - Use of HME (heat and moisture exchanger) filters in intubated/ventilated trauma victims on a routine basis.
- *Continuous monitoring of vital functions* (especially ECG for early diagnosis of cardiac arrhythmias, blood pressure, oxygen saturation).
- *Initiation of a peripheral IV line* (ideally warmed IV fluids) and *administration of oxygen* (e.g., via a face mask).

In the prehospital setting *passive rewarming* methods are preferred [2,17]; *active core rewarming* techniques are the in-hospital primary therapeutic modality in hypothermic trauma patients with severe hypothermia or victims in cardiac arrest [1].

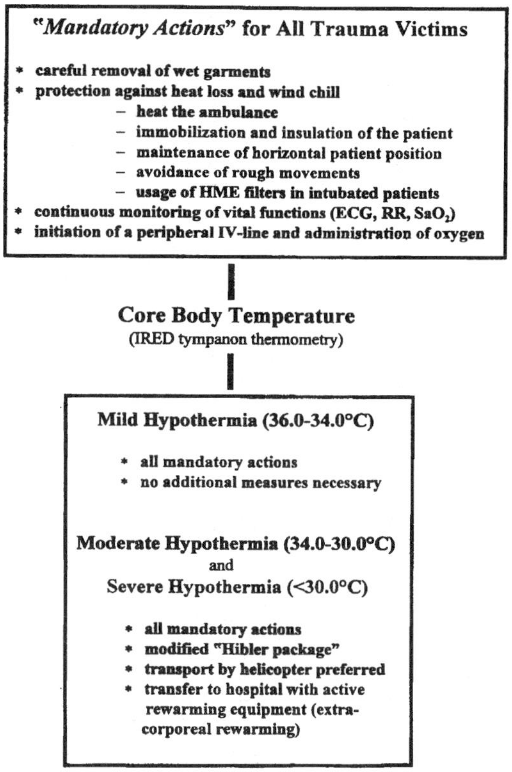

Figure 6 "Hypothermia Treatment Algorithm" for trauma victims. Only passive rewarming techniques in the prehospital setting. Active core rewarming techniques are the inhospital primary therapeutic modality.

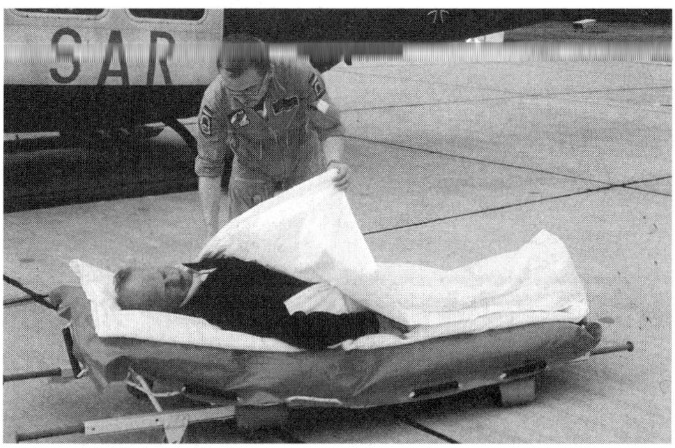

Figure 7 Standardized immobilization and insulation of trauma victims (recommended order at the HEMS Christoph 22, Ulm, Germany). The patient is placed on a vacuum mattress, which is covered by a single-use insulation blanket and is covered with another single-use insulation blanket (demonstration).

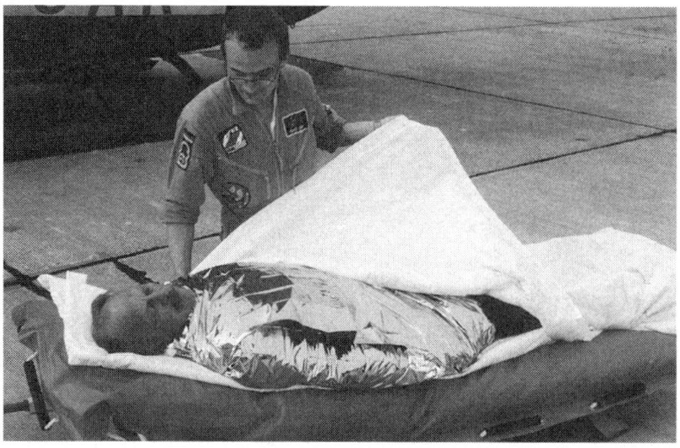

(a)

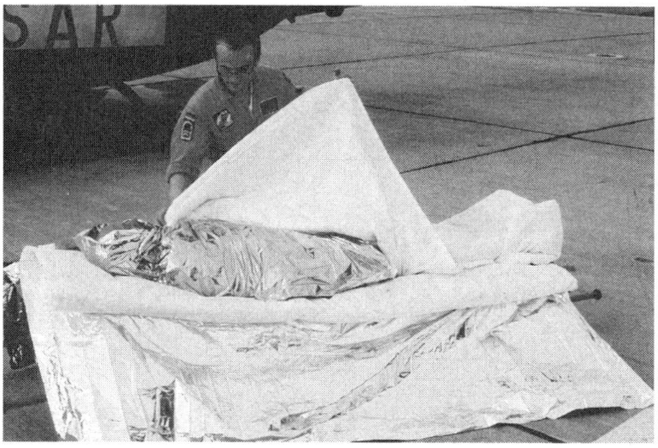

(b)

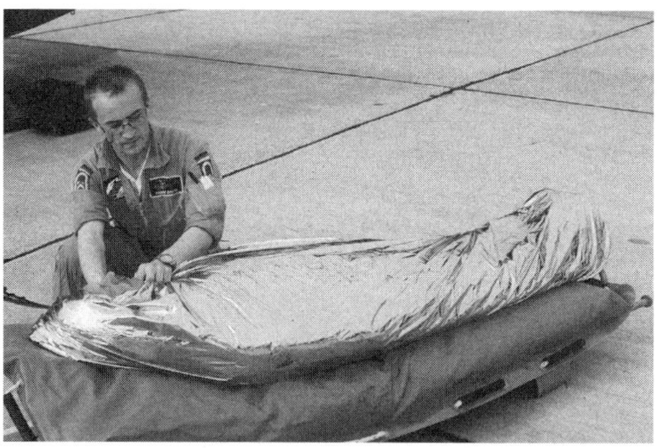

(c)

Figure 8 Modified Hibler package. Standardized immobilization and insulation procedure is expanded by using additional heat-reflecting aluminium foil around the truncal area only (a) and/or the whole body (b, c).

Patients with *mild hypothermia* have a good prognosis [18,28]. Prehospital treatment should include all the basic measures (mandatory actions) of the hypothermia treatment algorithm (Fig. 6).

In patients with *moderate and severe hypothermia*, the basic measures may be supplemented by a modified ''Hibler package'' (Fig. 8) using additional heat-reflecting aluminium foil placed around either just the truncal areas or the whole body [2,16]. In these patients transportation to the hospital should be performed as gently as possible in order to avoid precipitating ventricular fibrillation, and the patients should be moved in the horizontal position to avoid afterdrop. Especially in the case of longer transport distances, transportation should be performed by helicopter.

There is no generally binding recommendation for severely hypothermic trauma victims in cardiac arrest at the scene. Schou [17] recommends starting CPR at the scene only in younger patients without serious underlying diseases. Also, the degree of injury severity, the kind of underlying injury, and the injury pattern must be included in the decision of whether or not to initiate CPR at the scene. If there are any doubts, CPR might be initiated and the patient should be transported under continuous CPR to a hospital with extracorporeal rewarming equipment.

As pointed out previously, *passive core rewarming* techniques are preferred in the prehospital setting, but a new technique of *active core rewarming* may play an important role in the (prehospital) treatment of accidental hypothermia in the future. This technique combines the application of subatmospheric pressure and heat to a single forearm and hand [33]. The first results of recent studies [33,34] have shown that not only does this technique seem to be very effective and fast in restoring core body temperature, but it also seems to be safe. (Afterdrop was not observed.) To determine the full potential as well as the potential risks of this new active rewarming technique, studies with a larger number of colder patients are needed.

V. SUMMARY

Accidental hypothermia (core body temperature <36°C) poses a relevant but highly underdiagnosed phenomenon in trauma victims (nearly 50% of traumatized patients are hypothermic), which in turn additionally complicates the trauma and may increase posttraumatic morbidity and mortality.

Heat loss occurs in different ways; whereas radiation and convection count for 85%, evaporation and conduction count for 15% of heat loss. Numerous factors favor the development of posttraumatic accidental hypothermia. (See Sec. II.A.)

Situations in which several such factors coincide increase the risk of acquiring and/or aggravating posttraumatic hypothermia.

Three stages of hypothermia are classified: mild (36.0–34.0°C), moderate (34.0–30.0°C), and severe (<30°C). The variability or total absence of clinical symptoms in cases of mild hypothermia (e.g., shivering in less than 5% of these patients) and the ambiguity of clinical symptoms in cases of moderate and severe hypothermia (e.g., arrhythmias, hypotension, and respiratory dysfunction), as well as the masking of clinical symptoms of hypothermia by more dramatic symptoms of associated injuries (e.g., severe head injury) underline the necessity for prehospital monitoring of core body temperature.

Only the measurement of core body temperature enables one to make a definite diagnosis of an accidental hypothermia in the trauma victim as well as to determine the stage of hypothermia.

IRED tympanic thermometers are highly recommended for the prehospital measurement of core body temperature, because they are easy to use, fast, and accurate.

Procedures to prevent and/or treat hypothermia in the trauma victim must be integrated into the prehospital treatment algorithm of the traumatized patient on a routine basis. This hypothermia treatment algorithm starts with a number of procedures that have to be performed on any trauma patient (mandatory actions).

Also, depending on the stage of hypothermia, special passive rewarming methods have to be initiated (e.g., a modified Hibler package with aluminum foil). Active rewarming techniques are the primary in-hospital therapeutic modality.

REFERENCES

1. AD Weinberg. Hypothermia. Ann Emer Med 22:370–377, 1993.
2. M Helm, J Hauke, L Lampl, et al. Accidental hypothermia in trauma patients. Anästhesist 44: 101–107, 1995.
3. RC Valeri, G Cassidy, S Khuri, et al. Hypothermia induced reversible platelet dysfunction. Ann Surg 205:175–181, 1987.
4. RW Haley, DH Culver, WM Morgan, et al. Identifying patients at high risk of surgical wound infection: A simple multivariate index of patient susceptibility and wound contamination. Am J Epidem 121:206–215, 1985.
5. A Ferrara, JD MacArthur, KW Hastings, et al. Hypothermia and acidosis worsen coagulopathy in the patient requiring massive transfusion. Ann J Surg 160:1990.
6. GJ Jurkovich, WB Greiser, A Lutermann, et al. Hypothermia in trauma victims: An ominous predictor of survival. J Trauma 27:1019–1024, 1987.
7. GK Luna, RV Maier, EG Pavlin. Incidence and effect of hypothermia in seriously injured patients. J Trauma 27:1014–1018, 1987.
8. WI Cranston. Temperature regulation. Brit Med J 2:69–75, 1966.
9. TH Benzinger. Heat regulation: Homeostasis of central temperature in man. Physiol Rev 49: 671–759, 1969.
10. JN Hayward, MA Baker. Role of cerebral arterial blood in the regulation of brain temperature in a monkey. Am J Physiol 215:389–403, 1968.
11. FM Lyons, GM Hall. Thermal balance during anaesthesia. In: Weyland et al., eds. Perioperative Hypothermie. Ebelsbach, Germany: Aktiv Druck & Verlag, 1997, pp. 15–20.
12. MD Fallacaro, NA Fallacaro, TJ Radel. Inadvertent hypothermia: Etiology, effects and prevention. AORN J 44:54–61, 1986.
13. N Spampinato, P Stassano, C Gagliardi, et al. Massive air embolism during cardiopulmonary bypass: Successful treatment with immediate hypothermia and circulatory support. Ann Thor Surg 32:602–603, 1981.
14. ChE Smith, P Nileshkumar. Prevention and treatment of hypothermia in trauma patients. In: Hypothermia in Trauma—Deliberate or Accidental. Baltimore: 1997, pp. 11–16.
15. DL Bourke, H Wurm, M Rosenberg, et al. Intraoperative heat conservation using a reflective blanket. Anesthesiology 60:151–154, 1984.
16. M Helm, J Hauke, L Lampl. Accidental hypothermia in trauma patients. Acta Anaesth Scand 41(suppl. 111):44–46, 1997.
17. J Schou. Hypothermia. In: J Schou, ed. Prehospital Emergency Medicine. Amsterdam: Harwood Academic Publishers, 1997, pp. 271–277.
18. JB Reuler. Hypothermia: Pathophysiology, clinical settings and management. Ann Int Med 89:519–527, 1978.

19. RH Fox, PM Woodward, AN Exton-Smith, et al. Body temperature in the elderly: A national study of physiological, social and environmental conditions. Brit Med J 1:200–206, 1973.
20. A Goldmann, AN Exton-Smith, G Francis, et al. A pilot study of low body temperatures in old people admitted to hospital. J R Coll Physicians 11:291–306, 1977.
21. RF Edlich, KA Silloway, PS Feldmann, et al. Cold injuries and disorders. Curr Con Trauma Care 4–11, 1986.
22. AE Weymann, DM Greenbaum, WJ Grace, et al. Accidental hypothermia in an alcoholic population. Amer J Med 56:13, 1974.
23. SM Schneider. Hypothermia: From recognition to rewarming. Emer Med Rep 13:1–20, 1992.
24. JD White. Hypothermia: The Bellevue experience. Ann Emer Med 11:417–421, 1982.
25. B Hilka, P Kalbe. Polytrauma und Unterkühlung. Rettungsdienst 10:89–92, 1987.
26. I Linde, JS Kontokollias, A Klockgether-Radke. Die akzidentelle Hypothermie im Rettungsdienst. Rettungsdienst 11:678–680, 1988.
27. W Klingensmith. Inadvertent hypothermia during surgery. Tex Med 67:52–55, 1971.
28. RM Harnett, JR Pruitt, FR Sias. A review of the literature concerning resuscitation from hypothermia: I and II. Aviat Space Eviron Med 54:425–434, 487–495, 1983.
29. M Okada, F Nishimura, H Yoshino, et al. The J wave in accidental hypothermia. J Electrocardi 16:23–28, 1983.
30. TE Terndrup. An appraisal of temperature assessment by infrared emission detection tympanic thermometry. Ann Emer Med 21:1483–1492, 1992.
31. M Benzinger. Tympanic thermometry in surgery and anesthesia. JAMA 209:1207–1211, 1969.
32. M Helm, J Hauke, L Lampl, et al. Präklinische Messung der Körpertemperatur mit Hilfe der IRED Tympanon Thermometrie. Notarzt 11:78–82, 1995.
33. D Grahn, JG Brock-Utne, DE Watenpaugh, CH Heller. Recovery from mild hypothermia can be accelerated by mechanically distending blood vessels in the hand. J Appl Physiol 85(5): 1643–1648, 1998.
34. E Soreide, D Grahn, JG Brock-Utne, L Roden. A non-invasive means to effectively restore normothermia in cold stressed individuals: A preliminary report. J Emer Med 17(4):725–730, 1999.

21

Analgesia, Sedation, and Other Pharmacotherapy

AGNÈS RICARD-HIBON

Hôpital Beaujon, Clichy, France

JOHN SCHOU

Kreiskrankenhaus Lörrach, Lörrach, Germany

In emergency trauma care, drug therapy often plays a less prominent role than in other emergencies, which are only occasionally part of a scenario involving traumatic injury. Emergency medical services (EMS) personnel certainly encounter nontraumatic emergencies, but they are not discussed in this chapter, in accordance with the focus of this book. Moreover, the generally futile attempts to resuscitate a patient in cardiac arrest after having sustained an injury do not merit a special description here of the drugs used in cardiopulmonary resuscitation. What remains is a consideration of the drugs used for the following conditions or purposes:

Shock (see Chap. 15)
Anesthesia (see Chap. 13)
Analgesia and sedation (discussed in this chapter)
Antiemetics (discussed in this chapter)
Cranial and spinal injuries (glucocorticoids discussed in this chapter; see also Chap. 23)
Burns and electrical injuries (see Chap. 29)
Infections (discussed in this chapter)

In all cases, intravenous (IV) access (see Chap. 16) offers the ideal route for drug therapy. Some drugs initially may be injected intramuscularly (IM), either if no IV line is present or for the purpose of establishing an IV line (e.g., IM ketamine).

Apart from fluid resuscitation (see Chaps. 17, 18), it is generally overlooked that one purpose of an IV line is to make drug therapy possible. For example, IV administration of an anesthetic technique is highly recommended in most situations requiring prehospital endotracheal intubation and as a precondition for the use of military antishock trousers (MAST). If they are to be effective at all (discussed below), drugs that reduce focal or generalized edema (see Chaps. 31–34) should be given as early as possible, ideally in the prehospital arena. In general, patients may benefit more from analgesia and/or sedation than from any other prehospital measure.

I. CHOICE AND STORAGE OF PREHOSPITAL DRUGS

Many drugs compete to fulfill the aims of medical therapy, and it is certainly necessary to restrict the amount administered, as directed by the participating physicians. Medical therapy protocols must be devised with care, and they should be reviewed annually with respect to advances in pharmacology and new reports in the medical literature. Local storage problems may restrict the availability of some agents, particularly in hot areas. Other problems arise from concern about who can inject the drugs. For example, paramedics may not be allowed to carry and administer drugs with an abuse potential, and for that reason the drugs are not permitted for prehospital use by some national regulations. Finally, the choice of drugs available in prehospital trauma services should harmonize with those on hand for nontrauma emergencies that may be encountered by the same EMS. When possible, a drug should serve several purposes [1].

Certain characteristics (not necessarily possible to fulfill) influence the choice of drugs for prehospital use (Table 1). Any EMS crew that must be prepared for nontrauma emergencies will need a larger armamentarium of drugs than those listed in this chapter. The choice of drugs will also be influenced by differences in EMS personnel; paramedics are more limited than physicians in the kinds of drugs they can administer. The choice of drugs available for prehospital care is also affected by drugs' safety profiles.

Drugs used for shock, for burns, and for inducing anesthesia and muscle relaxation are discussed elsewhere in this text. In this chapter, we discuss the prehospital use of sedatives, analgesics, antiemetics, glucocorticoids, and antibiotics.

Table 1 Ideal Requirements for Selecting Prehospital Emergency Drugs

Ready for use; to employ rapidly
Resistant to temperature changes; for storage in the ambulance
No histamine-releasing effect; to avoid hypotension and respiratory distress
Controllable effect; to titrate desired properties
Known properties; to predict side effects
Parenteral preparations; to allow IV administration
Only one concentration; to avoid misdosing and mistakes
Restriction in purpose(s); for clear indications
Restriction in number; to minimize storage requirements and costs
No abuse potential; to minimize unauthorized use and theft
Agreement between doctors regarding selection and use

Source: Ref. 1.

II. SEDATIVES

Many drugs have sedative properties. In prehospital trauma care, it is difficult to find a superior alternative to the short-acting benzodazepine *midazolam*. This agent has the properties typical of its group; that is, inducing anxiolysis, sedation, and amnesia, and having an anticonvulsive effect. It is short acting, and has high, rapid bioavailability. *Midazolam* has become the first choice in the treatment of convulsions, which are usually of nontraumatic origin but are also encountered in prehospital trauma care. In case of overdose, the drug can be antagonized by *flumazenil*.

Indications for the use of sedative drugs in trauma patients are controversial. The following two principles can be identified for their use:

1. Beyond single use in patients who are anxious, upset, hyperventilating, or (rarely) convulsive, benzodiazepines (*midazolam* in particular) can be used to potentiate the properties of strong analgesic drugs; that is, effect so-called analgosedation (or sedoanalgesia). A question remains, however. How much is won when possible adverse opioid effects are potentiated by *midazolam*'s side effects?
2. Alternatively, the use of sedative drugs may be justified only when anxiety and agitation persist despite efficient analgesia. Indeed, agitation and anxiety are most often caused by acute pain, and the use of higher doses of opioids, possibly utilizing their sedative side effects, is usually sufficient to obtain analgesia and adequate sedation without the use of *midazolam*. Moreover, the combination of benzodiazepine and opioids can be extremely deleterious due to the potentiation of hemodynamic and respiratory side effects [2,3], particularly in elderly and hypovolemic patients [4]. In addition, the variability in individuals' responses to *midazolam* is extreme and unpredictable [5], therefore *midazolam* must be used with considerable caution and close patient monitoring.

Adult dosage: *Midazolam* by boluses of 1 to 2 mg IV; higher doses only in intubated patients. *Flumazenil* 0.2 to 0.5 mg IV (for iatrogenic overdose); 0.5 to 1.0 mg IV (for suicidal overdose of benzodiazepines).

III. ANALGESIA

Administration of analgesics is generally insufficient in the prehospital setting. Indeed, all studies performed on emergency patients (in the emergency room and in prehospital care) point out that "oligoanalgesia" is frequently observed [6–14]. The fear of adverse effects of analgesics or of the risk of masking a diagnosis has long dominated attitudes about the insufficient use of opioids in the prehospital setting. Difficulties in evaluating pain intensity have contributed to oligoanalgesia [12,13].

It is therefore necessary to define all situations in which there is a clear demand for analgesics for patients with acute (or chronic) pain. The indications must consider ethical reasons (imagine being the patient) as well as the direct adverse effects of pain on the cardiovascular and respiratory systems. Pain causes tachycardia, vasoconstriction, and increased oxygen consumption, and thus aggravates early shock, occasionally even worsening it through pain-restricted respiration. Conversely, alleviation of pain has become one of the primary tasks in prehospital care, and it can be one of the most satisfying procedures for both patients and care givers. Prehospital care providers cannot always save lives and prevent morbidity, but they should at least aim to reduce the pain being experienced by their patients.

Because physicians and nurses consistently underestimate acute pain intensity [11,15–17], pain should be evaluated by the patients themselves using pain scales such as a verbal rating scale, a numeric scale, or a visual analog scale [18–22]. Objectives of analgesia provided in the field have been defined and can be achieved [13]; a verbal rating scale score of less than 3 and/or a visual analog scale score of less than 30 mm are the thresholds that define relief in this context. Alleviation of pain must be done with attention to safety recommendations (e.g., a preserved level of consciousness with a Ramsay score less than 3, respiratory rate more than 12 breaths per min, and preserved hemodynamics).

Various levels of analgesia are described below. An analgesic algorithm is presented in Figure 1. Of course, drug therapy should not make other basic procedures superfluous (e.g., actions should be explained to the patient, fractures should be splinted, and hypothermia must be avoided).

A. Weak "Peripheral" Analgesics

In the emergency setting, the need for analgesia rarely calls for weak peripheral analgesics. Administration of *acetylsalicylic acid* (aspirin), which may be available for thrombolysis in certain nontrauma emergencies, is contraindicated in trauma because of its unpredictable effect on coagulation. Aspirin can aggravate bleeding and make locoregional anesthetic techniques impossible. The use of *nonsteroidal anti-inflammatory drugs* (NSAIDs) is also limited by their side effects (e.g., gastric bleeding, renal dysfunction, coagulation impairment, allergy). In addition, none of these drugs is universally available. *Ketoprophene* is available in some countries for IV administration.

Paracetamol is available for IV use in some countries. Side effects are rare and minor, and contraindications are limited to patients with severe hepatic disease and those allergic to the agent. It can (and must) be associated with other analgesics used in prehospital care to potentiate pain relief. Efficacy is achieved 20 to 30 min after IV administration. A better analgesia can be obtained with *metamizol*, which, when used IV, should be infused slowly rather than injected suddenly because of rare but serious side effects (e.g., disseminated intravascular coagulation).

Adult dosage: *Paracetamol*, 2 g in a 15-min infusion. *Metamizol*, 1 g in a 15-min infusion; ketoprophene, 100 mg in a 10-min infusion.

B. Nitrous Oxide in 50% Oxygen (Entonox)

A mixture of equal volumes of nitrous oxide and oxygen provides analgesia without an IV line and is therefore preferred in some EMS systems that do not rely on the prehospital participation of physicians [23,24]. This effective means of achieving analgesia has a very low risk of direct adverse cardiovascular or respiratory effects. In addition, the upper airway reflexes remain intact. The mixture can be self-administered, and is characterized by rapid onset and recovery after cessation. The risk of hypoxia after withdrawal justifies the administration of oxygen for at least 15 min.

Nitrous oxide can have indirect adverse effects, especially in trauma patients; the risk of fatal air cavities (e.g., pneumothorax and pneumoencephalon) is increased after inhalation of nitrous oxide. Attention must be given to the influence of low ambient temperature on the mixture fractions, causing inhomogeneity with a risk of low oxygen concentration inhalation. Entonox is therefore contraindicated at temperatures below 5°C.

Furthermore, the chance and effects of leakage of an anaesthetic into an ambulance compartment cannot be ignored.

C. Opioids

Physicians tend to be quite skilled in choosing one or more opioids, and it would not be wise to place restrictions on their preferences. In prehospital care, however, some substances are better avoided; for example, *buprenorphine* (which has long duration without being susceptible to the antagonistic effect of naloxone in case of overdose) and *pentazocine* (which can induce opioid σ-receptor stimulation, causing hallucinations and occasional direct cardiodepressive effects.)

Tramadol is an opioid μ agonist with weak action. It is generally insufficient alone for severe pain, but impressive results have been obtained when used in combination with metamizol, described above [25]. Adult dosage: 1.5 mg/kg (100 mg) IV.

Nalbuphine is primarily a κ agonist that causes sedation and analgesia. It causes only mild analgesia on the μ receptor, but a high affinity on this receptor causes antagonism if another opioid was bound to it previously. Its ceiling effect limits its analgesic effect but makes it safer in sole use; nevertheless, the respiratory depressant effect has been reported to be similar to that of morphine in equianalgesic doses [26].

The use of nalbuphine by paramedics has been evaluated with good results in terms of efficacy and safety [27,28]. The sedative effect of *nalbuphine* (κ-mediated) is stronger than that observed for agonists, and can be reversed by *naloxone*. Particularly strong synergism is found with *midazolam* [29]. This may account for the comparatively ''low'' ceiling effect of *nalbuphine* in comparison with other opioids, but caution is required for possible oversedation by this combination. If anesthesia is needed after admission, agonists are preferred to *nalbuphine* since they would otherwise only be weakly active in its presence.

Dosage: Adult, 0.3 mg/kg (20 mg) IV; children, 0.2 mg/kg IV or IM.

Morphine, the oldest existing purified opiate, is used widely for acute pain relief in both in-hospital care and the prehospital setting [13,30,31]. It is a strong μ agonist. Adverse effects are dose-dependent, but so is the analgesic action. Higher doses may be associated with pruritus, histamine liberation, respiratory depression, nausea, vomiting, and—particularly in hypovolaemic patients—hypotension. These side effects can be diminished by cautious, repetitive dosage until achievement of the best balance between adequate analgesia and minor side effects. Respiratory depressant effects do not exist in a patient who is still experiencing pain. Intravenous *morphine* has been validated in the prehospital setting for its efficacy and safety in this context [13,32].

Adult dosage: Bolus of 1 to 4 mg repeatedly IV.

Forty years in the service of anesthesia, *fentanyl* remains a unique drug in many respects, including uncertainty of its actual duration of action. It has been used by some EMS systems in spontaneously breathing patients [33], but has never been validated for this indication in the prehospital setting. *Fentanyl* is much stronger than morphine. It is not a potent histamine liberator, but (like all *fentanyl* derivatives) can induce thoracic rigidity. In hypovolemic patients, IV bolus of *fentanyl* induces systemic hypotension.

Adult dosage: 0.05–0.1 mg IV in spontaneously breathing patients.

Other *fentanyl* derivates may be interesting but have not yet been evaluated thoroughly for prehospital care. *Alfentanil* is an opioid with a very short duration of action (15–25 min), and—in contrast to fentanyl–without cumulative effects following repetitive use (dosage: 0.5–1.0 mg). *Sufentanil* is marked by less respiratory depressant than *fentanyl*

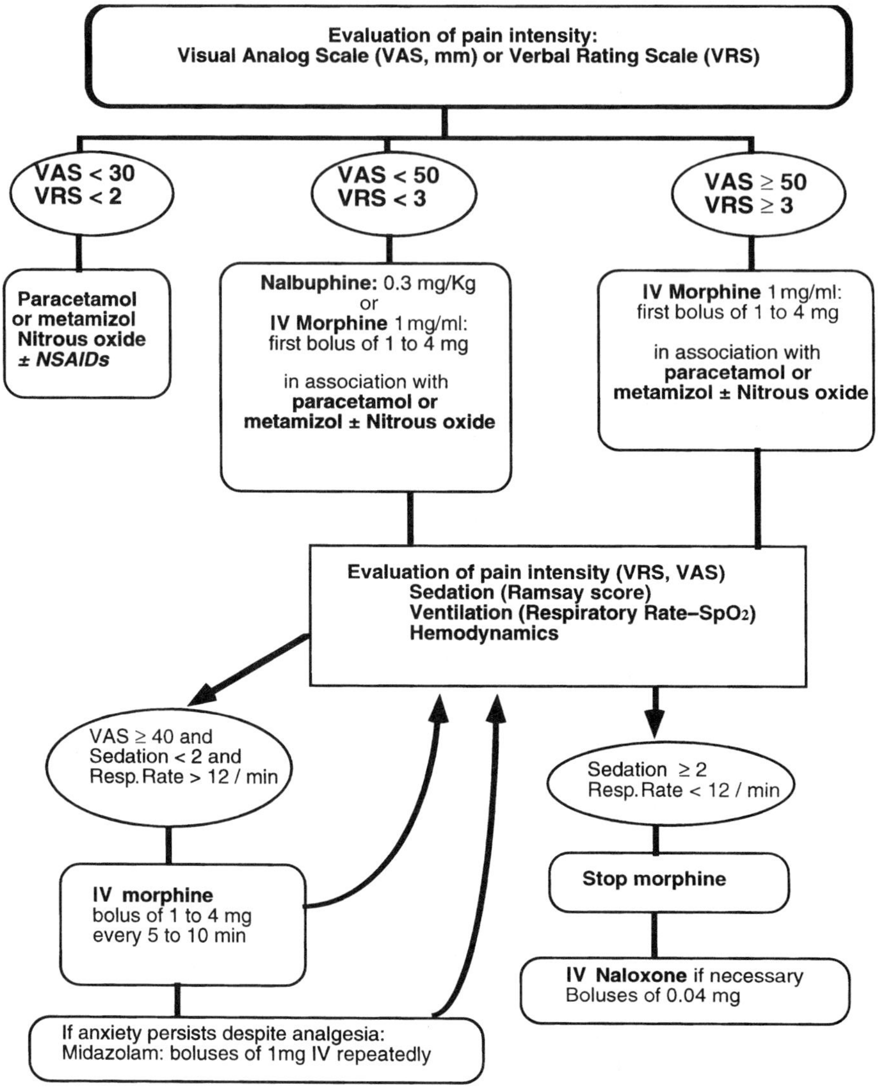

Figure 1 Algorithm for analgesia and sedation in prehospital care.

and its own sedative action (dosage: 10 μg IV), but it can induce vocal cord closure [34] (common to all *fentanyl* derivatives). *Remifentanil* is the shortest acting opioid, but because of problematic preparation, the need to administer via perfusion, and side effects (respiratory depressant effect for minimal change in dose), this drug is not recommended for prehospital care. According to some authorities *fentanyl* and/or *sufentanil* are not recommended for analgesia in spontaneous breathing patients and should be preferred for mechanically ventilated patients [31].

Naloxon is the antagonist to all the mentioned opioids (except *buprenorphine*) in case respiratory depression should occur. To maintain a certain analgesic level, it must be administered extremely cautiously (e.g., 0.04 mg repeatedly IV). Higher doses may cause a serious withdrawal effect [35,36]. *Nalbuphine* also can be used as an antagonist [37].

D. *Ketamine*

Ketamine can be given in analgesic doses (when the patient remains responsive), with gradual progress to virtual anesthesia. *Midazolam* can be added for potentiation and reduction of the hallucinogenic effects, but with great caution for the resulting synergism of side effects (sedation, respiratory depressant effect, etc.). The racemate s-(+)-*ketamine* is nearly twice as potent and is associated with less hallucinogenic effect [38].

Adult analgesic dosage: Ketamine, 10–25 mg (0.2–0.3 mg/kg) IV. S-(+)-*ketamine*, 5–10 mg (0.1–0.2 mg/kg IV).

In *burned patients* and those with caustic skin damage, simple rinsing with cool (not cold) water will serve both therapeutic and analgesic purposes. Because of skin damage and the possible beginning of shock, only the IV route of drug application should be considered.

E. Locoregional Techniques

Femoral nerve block is the only locoregional technique that can be used in the prehospital setting and that has been validated in the prehospital setting [39]. The use of these modalities is left to physicians, who are particularly skilled in these techniques.

Occasionally an utterly painful condition will call for nothing less than *general anaesthesia*. These are mostly the cases in which anesthesia would have been induced after admittance to an emergency room and those in which extending this procedure into the prehospital phase may provide further advantages in patient care (e.g., for setting multiple fractures).

IV. ANTIEMETICS

The use of antiemetics is [illegible] effects and to prophylactic dosage for air transport. Conversely, it is possible to dispense with these drugs in a ground rescue service.

Droperidol, a neuroleptic agent, is effective against emetic side effects to opioids, even in a very small adult dosage of 0.5 to 1.5 mg IV. In higher dosage, it has also been used in prehospital care for sedating combative patients [40], but it is not recommended here because of the potential side effects (in particular, hypotension by vasodilation). It should be noted, however, that this drug in itself may cause difficulty to register until questioning the patient long afterward. In addition, in higher doses, all neuroleptic drugs may cause parkinsonlike symptoms, and in rare cases, even irreversible dyskinesia.

Metoclopramid is a weak neuroleptic drug with predominant action on the stomach itself. It is less effective as an antiemetic drug but also has fewer side effects than droperidol. Adult dosage: 10–20 mg IV.

Selective $5HT_3$ antagonists, such as *odansetron* and later developments are void of neuroleptic side effects and are at least as potent antiemetics as droperidol. They are currently too expensive for regular prehospital use, however.

V. GLUCOCORTICOIDS

What makes glucocorticoids potentially interesting in trauma care is their antioxidant effect toward ischaemia-induced lipid peroxidation and cell-membrane destabilization. Since 1992, only one randomized study of their use has been published [41], while another randomized trial of 499 cases (NASCIS-3) [42] examined different dose regimens and compared them with another drug, tirizalid. The remaining 10 studies, all American, employed historical or occasional controls. They [41] felt it impossible to ignore the recommendations arising from the previous randomized trial, NASCIS-2 [43], although a generally negative approach to these recommendations was expressed.

NASCIS-2 [43] involved 487 patients who were randomly allocated to receive either *methylprednisolone* (MP) or naloxone (or a placebo) after blunt spinal cord injury. An analysis of the entire population failed to disclose any significant difference in effect associated with these drugs, but such difference was found when MP was administered within 8 hr after injury. The dosages used were a loading dose of 30 mg/kg of MP over 1 hr, followed by 5.4 mg/kg/hr for 23 hr. In the NASCIS-3 study, this dose was recommended for spinal trauma only when started within 3 hr after injury, whereas the maintenance dose was extended to 48 hr when treatment started 3 to 8 hr after injury.

Not surprisingly, this high dose of MP results in an increase of infectious problems in treated patients, influencing both mortality and the length of hospital stay. By restricting observations to penetrating spinal cord injury (primarily gunshot wounds), one group even found a worse outcome in treated patients [44]. Alternative drugs, such as the calcium antagonist *nimodipine* and *tirilazad mesylate*, as an MP inhibitor of lipid peroxidation, may offer some effect without yielding the adverse effects of glucocorticoids; this approach needs further evaluation.

In cranial trauma, there is currently little enthusiasm in the literature concerning a beneficial effect of drug therapy. This attitude may be of some indirect advantage, focusing the efforts on basic therapy: maintaining circulation of oxygenated blood and adequate intracranial perfusion pressure rather than compensating with drug therapy (essential for all neurotrauma).

In conclusion, the use of glucocorticoids as recommended by the NASCIS-3 study may be a valuable addition in blunt spinal trauma, but priority must be given to immobilization and general measures. There is currently no valid support for its use in cranial trauma.

VI. ANTIBIOTICS

Antibiotics are widely utilized for the prophylaxis of infections in trauma care. It is emphasized that they should be applied early, before an operation is carried out, to be of any use. So far, however, their prehospital use has not been validated. This may relate to a number of problems, including the following:

1. Antibiotics are seldom ready for use, and dissolving them implies increased on-scene time.
2. Adverse effects (e.g., allergic reactions) are prone to occur, and patient history information on allergy is generally unreliable.
3. Early use is associated with the development of resistance and the selection of insensitive bacteria.

4. In general, an infected port is cleaned surgically before antibiotics are considered; however, this does not exclude prophylactic use.

Still, it is reasonable to study the impact of certain well-tolerated antibiotics that are already given in the prehospital phase, on postoperative complications of certain injuries. At the moment, no recommendations can be given.

VII. CONCLUSION

The use of drugs for prehospital care is an absolute necessity and must be favored and developed in this setting. It implies, however, adequate training of prehospital teams and must be according to validated protocols and regularly reviewed according to medical and scientific progress. The use of drugs must be then evaluated to control the real applications of recommendations and make sure that no deviation exists, according to a quality control program methodology.

VIII. SUMMARY

The use of drugs in prehospital care is an absolute necessity. Many criteria influence the choice of drugs. Medical therapy protocols should be validated in the EMS and reviewed regularly.

The use of drugs by prehospital teams implies adequate training and an evaluation of the balance between benefit and risk.

Acute pain relief is often neglected in prehospital care, and more attention must given to analgesia and sedation in the prehospital setting.

The use of sedatives (with no analgesic effect) in spontaneous breathing trauma patients is controversial in this setting. *Midazolam* is preferred to others sedatives. It must be administered by small boluses to limit the risk of side effects.

Analgesics must be administered according to patients' evaluation of pain intensity by using pain scales.

Weak analgesics can be used for low or moderate pain or in association with strong analgesics for severe pain. Nitrous oxide is safe, efficient, and does not require an IV line.

Severe pain should be treated by opioids. *Nalbuphine* is interesting in this context, but analgesia is limited by a ceiling effect. Intravenous morphine is the only agonist recommended in spontaneously breathing patients. Its use is safe and efficient if administered in small boluses to control analgesia without the appearance of side effects. Precautions must be given to the use of opioids and benzodiazepines association because of the potentiation of side effects.

Ketamine is interesting, but needs further evaluation in this context.

Locoregional anesthesia is limited to femoral block nerve and requires well-trained physicians.

Antiemetics are used to treat emetic opioid side effects or to control air transport nausea.

The use of glucocorticoids has been proposed in blunt spinal trauma. There is no valid support for its use in cranial trauma.

The use of antibiotics in the prehospital setting has not been validated.

REFERENCES

1. J Schou. Selection of emergency drugs. In: J Schou, ed. Prehospital Emergency Therapy. 2nd ed. Harwood Academic, 1997, 371–379.
2. P Bailey, N Pace, M Ashburn, JW Moll, KA East, TH Stanley. Frequent hypoxemia and apnea after sedation with midazolam and fentanyl. Anesthesiology 73:826–830, 1990.
3. A Ricard-Hibon, J Marty. Anesthesia and analgesia in prehospital critical care medicine. JEUR 3:142–146, 1998.
4. P Adams, S Gelman, J Reves, DJ Greenblatt, M Alvis, E Bradley. Midazolam pharmacodynamics and pharmacokinetics during acute hypovolemia. Anesthesiology 63:140–146, 1985.
5. P Montravers, B Dureuil, J Desmonts. Effects of i.v. midazolam on upper airway resistance. Brit J Anaesth 68:27–31, 1992.
6. SM Selbst, M Clark. Analgesic use in the emergency department. Ann Emerg Med 19:99–102, 1990.
7. AS Fung, TM Bentley. Pre-operative analgesia for acute surgical patients: No place for complacency. Ann Royal Coll Surg Engl 76:11–12, 1994.
8. LM Lewis, LC Lasater, CB Brooks, and the St. Louis Physicians' Association Research Group. Are emergency physicians too stingy with analgesics? South Med J 87:7–9, 1994.
9. JE Wilson, JM Pendleton. Oligoanalgesia in the emergency department. Am J Emerg Med 7: 620–623, 1989.
10. R Morgan-Jones. Pre-operative analgesia after injury. Injury 27:539–541, 1996.
11. JK Whipple, KS Lewis, EJ Quebbeman, M Wolff, MS Gottlieb, M Medicus-Bringa, KR Hartnett, M Graf, RK Ausman. Analysis of pain management in critically ill patients. Pharmacotherapy 15:592–599, 1995.
12. A Ricard-Hibon, N Leroy, M Magne, A Leberre, C Chollet, J Marty. Evaluation of acute pain in pre-hospital emergency medicine. Ann Fr Anesth Rean 8:945–949, 1997.
13. A Ricard-Hibon, C Chollet, S Saada, B Loridant, J Marty. A quality control program for acute pain management in pre-hospital critical care medicine. Ann Emerg Med 34:738–744, 1999.
14. JA Chambers, HR Guly. The need for better pre-hospital analgesia. Arch Emerg Med 10:187–192, 1993.
15. CMP Mather, LB Ready. Management of acute pain. Brit J Hosp Med 51:85–88, 1994.
16. J Lander. Clinical judgments in pain management. Pain 42:15–22, 1990.
17. M Donovan, P Dillon, L McGuire. Incidence and characteristics of pain in a sample of medical-surgical inpatients. Pain 30:69–78, 1987.
18. EC Huskisson. Measurement of pain. Lancet ii:1127–1131, 1974.
19. F Boureau, M Luu. Les methodes d'evaluation de la douleur clinique. Doul et Analg 1:65–73, 1988.
20. MP Jensen, P Karoly, S Braver. The measurement of clinical pain intensity: A comparison of six methods. Pain 27:117–126, 1986.
21. EE Ohnhaus, R Adler. Methodological problems in the measurement of pain: A comparison between the verbal rating scale and the visual analog scale. Pain 1:379–384, 1975.
22. B Blettery, L Ebrahim, D Honnart, H Aude. Pain scale in an emergency care unit. Rean Urg 5:691–697, 1996.
23. PJF Baskett. Nitrous oxide in pre-hospital care. Acta Anaesth Scand 38:775–776, 1994.
24. BD Amey, JA Ballinger, EE Harrison. Pre-hospital administration of nitrous oxide for control of pain. Ann Emerg Med 10:247–251, 1981.
25. BM Ure, E Neugebauer, K Ullmann, R Driever, H Troid. Patientenkontrollierte Analgesie (PCA) zur postoperativen Schmerztherapie. Eine prospektive Beobachtungsstudie zur Technologiebewertung im Stationsbetrieb [Patient-controlled analgesia (PCA) for postoperative pain relief. A prospective observational study for evaluating the technology in a ward routine]. Chirurg 64:802–808, 1993.
26. T Gal, C Difazio, J Moscicki. Analgesic and respiratory depressant activity of nalbuphine: A comparison with morphine. Anesthesiology 57:367–374, 1982.

27. JK Stene, L Stofberg, G MacDonald, RA Myers, A Ramzy, B Bruns. Nalbuphine analgesia in the pre-hospital setting. Am J Emerg Med 6:634–639, 1988.
28. JA Chambers, HR Guly. Pre-hospital intravenous nalbuphine administered by paramedics. Resuscitation 27:153–158, 1994.
29. J Schou. Three techniques for prehospital emergency anaesthesia. JEUR 3:139–145, 1994.
30. M Chauvin. for a Consensus conference. Management of postoperative pain in adults and children. Ann Fr Anesth Rean 7:445–470, 1998.
31. JE De la Coussaye. for an Expert conference. Sedation and analgesia in out-of-hospital critical care medicine. Ann Fr Anesth Rean 19: 2000.
32. BM Bruns, R Dieckmann, C Shagoury, A Dingerson, C Swartzell. Safety of pre-hospital therapy with morphine sulfate. Am J Emerg Med 10:53–57, 1992.
33. C Martin. Sedation outside the hospital. JEUR 8:110–119, 1995.
34. JA Bennett, JT Abrams, DF Van Riper, JC Horrow. Difficult or impossible ventilation after sufentanil-induced anesthesia is caused primarily by vocal cord closure. Anesthesiology 87: 1070–1074, 1997.
35. FM Cuss, CB Colago, JH Baron. Cardiac arrest after reversal of opiates with naloxone. Brit Med J 288:363–364, 1984.
36. GM Gaddis, WA Watson. Naloxone-associated patient violence: An overlooked toxicity? Ann-Pharmacother 26:196–198, 1992.
37. J Schou, J Deklerk, M Scherb, J Kübler. Antagonism vs. ventilation in drug overdose. JEUR 8:136–139, 1995.
38. E Pfenninger, C Baier, S Claus, G Hege. Untersuchungen zu psychometrischen Veränderungen sowie zur analgetischen Wirkung und kardiovaskulären Nebenwirkungen von Ketamin-Razemat versus (S-(+)-Ketamin in subanästhetischer Dosierung. Anaesthesist 43(suppl. 2): S68–S75, 1994.
39. P Barriot, B Riou, L Ronchi, S Bellaiche. Femoral block nerve in prehospital management of fractured shaft of femur. JEUR 1:21–24, 1988.
40. CL Rosen, AF Ratliff, RE Wolfe, SW Branney, EJ Roe, PT Pons. The efficacy of intravenous droperidol in the prehospital setting. J Emerg Med 15:13–17, 1997.
41. ME Petijean, V Pointillart, F Dixmerias, L Wiart, F Sztark, P Lassie, M Thicoipe, P Dabadie. Traitement medicamenteux de la lesion medullaire traumatique au stade aigu. [Medical treatment of spinal cord injury in the acute stage]. Ann Fr Anesth Reani 17:114–122, 1998.
42. MB Bracken, MJ Shepard, TR Holford, L Leo-Summers, EF Aldrich, M Fazl, M Fehlings, DL Herr, PW Hitchon, LF Marshall, RP Nockels, V Pascale, PL Perot, J Piepmeier. Administration of methylprednisolone for 24 or 48 hours or tirilazad mesylate for 48 hours in the treatment of acute spinal cord injury. Results of the Third National Acute Spinal Cord Injury Randomized Controlled Trial. National Acute Spinal Cord Injury Study. JAMA 277:1597–1604, 1997.
43. MB Bracken, MJ Shepard, WF Collins, TR Holford, W Young, DS Baskin, HM Eisenberg, E Flamm, L Leo-Summers, J Maroon, LF Marshall, PI Perot, J Piepmeier, VKH Sonntag, FC Wagner, JE Willberger, HR Winn. A randomized controlled trial of methylprednisolone or naloxone in the treatment of acute spinal cord injury. N Eng J Med 322:1405–1411, 1990.
44. RF Heary, AR Vaccaro, JJ Mesa, BE Northrup, TJ Albert, RA Balderston, JM Cotler. Steroids and gunshot wounds to the spine. Neurosurgery 41:576–583, 1997.

22

Patients With Multiple Trauma, Including Head Injuries

GIUSEPPE NARDI

Friuli Venezia Giulia Regional Emergency Helicopter Medical Service, Udine, Italy; and S. Camillo Hospital, Rome, Italy

STEFANO DI BARTOLOMEO

Friuli Venezia Giulia Regional Emergency Helicopter Medical Service, Udine, Italy

PETER OAKLEY

North Staffordshire Hospital, Stoke-on-Trent, United Kingdom

I. EPIDEMIOLOGY OF MULTIPLE TRAUMA

According to the Global Burden of Disease Study (GBDS) [1] published by the Harvard School of Public Health in 1990, injuries were responsible for 5.1 million deaths worldwide, accounting for 10.1% of all deaths. The number of deaths is expected to increase further over the next 20 years. Vehicular injury is now by far the most important cause of injury-related death.

A high proportion of motor vehicle accidents (MVAs), as well as accidents that occur at work or in sports, cause injuries to more than one body region. According to Utstein-style [2] recommendations for uniform reporting of data following major trauma, multiple trauma (polytrauma) is defined as injury to two body cavities (head, thorax, or abdomen) or to one body cavity plus two long bone and/or pelvic fractures. A recent population-based study [3] demonstrated that two-thirds (68.9%) of patients with an injury severity score (ISS) >15 following vehicle, work, or sports accidents fall within the definition of polytrauma. Such patients have a high risk of secondary insults from hypotension or hypoxia and pose a major challenge to trauma care providers. Some are initially inaccessible or require extrication from car wreckage, leading to unavoidable delays and prolonged prehospital times.

Multiple trauma associated with MVAs is the leading cause of death and disability in young people in Europe, where 40,000 to 50,000 die, and up to 150,000 survive with serious disability every year. The figures may actually be higher as there are no nationwide trauma registries. A further significant number of deaths are caused by work and sports accidents, in which a third of those who die are under 24 years of age. In North America, a large proportion of trauma patients suffer from penetrating injuries (often involving a single body area). There, too, blunt trauma from MVAs still represents a major health problem, with over 40,000 deaths per year [4].

Mortality and morbidity following MVAs vary throughout the world, but given the differences in health care spending, the differences in outcome are often less than expected. In recent years, trauma has overtaken infectious diseases as the principle cause of death in the youthful population of many low- and middle-income countries in southern Asia and Africa. Vehicular injuries result in a proportionally greater death and disability toll in developing countries, despite a much lower number of vehicles. This may be due to the poor condition of the roads or failure to observe speed limits, but alcohol also plays an important role. The number of alcohol-related vehicular deaths in sub-Saharan Africa appears to be twice as great as in the established market economies [1]. The incidence of death from injury in childhood is also considerably higher in the less developed countries as a consequence of a lack of preventive measures, including helmets and vehicular restraint systems.

The number of road traffic deaths per million population is highest in South Africa and Malaysia, in spite of a vehicle/population ratio seven times lower than in the United States [5] (Table 1). The shortfall in medical personnel and available resources may have a contributory effect, as well as differences in the organization of the emergency system. A study from Mock et al. [6] compared the mortality for all seriously injured persons (ISS >9) in three nations with different economic status and trauma treatment capabilities. Overall survival increased with increasing economic status, from 36% in Ghana to 65% in the United States. The improvement in survival was primarily due to a decrease in

Table 1 Comparison of Road Traffic Deaths by Country

Country	Deaths per 100,000 population	Death per 10,000 vehicles	Vehicle per 1000 inhabitants
South Africa	30.5	24.8	123
Kuwait	27.1	6.7	408
Malaysia	23.9	21.5	111
New Zealand	21.1	3.9	545
Greece	21.1	12.0	176
United States	19.1	2.7	711
Australia	18.6	3.4	540
Canada	15.8	2.8	561
Germany	13.1	3.8	440
Norway	10.7	2.7	397
Japan	10.3	2.6	403
United Kingdom	10.3	3.2	322

Source: Adapted from Ref. 5.

prehospital deaths. In Ghana, 51% of trauma victims died in the field, compared with 40% in Mexico and 21% in Seattle.

A. From Hospital-Based to Population-Based Data

Despite its enormous impact in terms of death, years of productive life lost, and overall health and social costs, there are few population-based data to estimate the incidence and final outcome of patients with severe injuries. One of the major obstacles in collecting, interpreting, and comparing data is the lack of a clear, universally accepted definition of severe trauma. Most of the published studies use an ISS greater than 15 to define severe trauma, while others adopt a broader definition (e.g., ISS >12) or include patients on the basis of simple physiological criteria (e.g., GCS <9 or systolic blood pressure <90 mmHg).

In the United States, several large trauma data banks have been developed, but most of the data are restricted to patients who have been hospitalized. Accurate information on prehospital deaths is generally missing. Moreover, most of the data is not population-based and is prone to selection bias. In the rest of the world, fewer data are generally available, although some national trauma databases have now been established, such as that developed by the Trauma Audit and Research Network in the United Kingdom.

Many studies throughout the world have shown that a high percentage of the deaths and disabilities resulting from multiple trauma are preventable. In a recent analysis [7,8], 25–40% of trauma deaths were considered to be preventable, although lower figures have been reported from the United States. The characteristics of the admitting hospital have been considered to be a major influence on the number of preventable deaths, supporting the concept of trauma centers. A threefold increase in the preventable mortality rate following MVAs between small regional hospitals and a level 1 trauma center was observed in a quality assessment study from Australia [8].

Preventable prehospital deaths have seldom been investigated. Thirty-nine percent of prehospital trauma deaths were considered to be potentially preventable in a study performed by Hussain and Redmond [9], and similar results were obtained by Papadopoulos et al. in Greece (29–48%) [10]. For many years, efforts to improve trauma care have focused on treatment in the hospital. The most widely used prognostic indexes are based on the results of the Major Trauma Outcome Study [11] (MTOS). The MTOS database and most of the other large trauma data banks consider only those patients who are admitted to the hospital, however.

The lack of comprehensive population-based data and the use of different selection criteria make it difficult to identify weak links in the survival chain or to compare epidemiological data from different countries. In Canada, the Ontario Trauma Registry uses the trauma and injury severity score (TRISS) methodology to analyze outcome, but excludes patients who arrive at the hospital already sedated and intubated [12]. Should similar criteria be applied in northeast Italy, more than 80% of trauma patients with ISS >25 would be excluded from the analysis.

Very few studies have included data collected in the prehospital setting. In a large study in a population of over 3.2 million in Wales and northwest England, Gordman et al. [13] showed that most trauma deaths occur before hospital admission. This is consistent with the results of an audit of major trauma patients (ISS >15) who were still alive when first rescued in a population of over 1 million in northeast Italy [14]. According to the study, about 25% of all trauma deaths took place before arriving at the hospital.

In recent years considerable effort has been made to improve the quality of trauma care by implementing an integrated approach involving both the development of trauma centers and improvements in prehospital care.

A better understanding of the epidemiology of severe trauma is essential to identify the best management strategies. To improve the effectiveness of emergency medical services, we need to know which prehospital interventions affect mortality and morbidity and how many patients could potentially benefit from better treatment in the prehospital setting.

About 10% of the whole population seeks medical aid following injury each year. In northeast Italy, 1.2% per year are admitted to the hospital because of an injury [3]. Only 2–4% of those admitted are considered to have suffered severe trauma. The precise incidence of severe trauma has proved difficult to establish, in part due to the lack of clear definitions. In the Utstein-style recommendations, it is defined as an ISS >15 [2]. The same criteria were used by Gorman and colleagues, who reported an incidence of 1,088 patients per year in a population of 3.2 million people, or 340 per million per year. In an Italian study [14], which was limited to victims who were found alive in the field, the estimated incidence of severe trauma was 385 per million, with a mortality rate of 30.8%. The mortality is consistent with that reported by Spaite et al. in Arizona (32.6%) [15] and Demetriades et al. in California [16].

According to the available information on patients with an ISS >15, the expected mortality is about 30%, and a high percentage (25%–60%) of those who eventually die do so before they arrive at the hospital. It seems reasonable that these patients might benefit from enhanced supportive treatment in the prehospital setting. The trauma system should anticipate a total of 300 to 400 severely injured patients per million population per year. Some of these will be unsalvageable, dying before the first rescuers arrive from major brain, heart, or large vessel injuries (immediate deaths). Other less injured patients will need to be assessed by the advanced life support (ALS) providers, even if their eventual ISS <16, sacrificing specificity in order to achieve the sensitivity required to intervene promptly in the cases of those who need it. Given the uncertainty inherent in the initial scene information, many emergency services plan to send ALS providers on every ambulance. This in turn demands a much larger number of ALS providers, with more resources needed for their training. Moreover, each practitioner will then attend major trauma cases less frequently, and as a consequence receive less ongoing experience.

The percentage of trauma victims who die on the spot is highly influenced by the characteristics of the vehicles and the use of protective measures, such as air bags and seat belts. Our data [3] show a consistent relation between the number of trauma patients with ISS >15 found alive on the scene and those who die immediately. This ratio is approximately 2.5:1, and remained substantially unchanged during a 7-year time span. As there is no effective way for a dispatch system to differentiate people who are already dead from those who require immediate resuscitation, the trauma victims who die on the spot also ought to be included in the expected target for advanced prehospital care, bringing this figure up to at least 500 to 550 people per million per year.

B. Prevalence of Injuries and Common Combinations

A study on MVA deaths in Victoria, Australia [17], demonstrated that only 16% of the victims had injuries limited to one body region. Thirty-six percent of fatalities had injuries in three body regions, while 23% involved two regions and 20% affected four regions.

Head injury was the main cause of death in 63.5% of the cases. These data are consistent with the results of a recent epidemiological study in an Italian region with a population of 1.2 million people [3]. During 1 year, 166 trauma victims were found dead on the scene and 12 more died during prehospital stabilization or transport. Of 14,000 trauma patients admitted to any of the regional hospitals, 449 (3.3%) had major injuries (ISS >15, Fig. 1). More than two-thirds of these had multiple injuries, defined according to the Utstein-style recommendations. Two-thirds (68.3%) of major trauma victims had sustained a severe injury to the head (AIS ≥3). Head trauma occurred as an isolated injury in 35.3% of the cases, while in the remaining 64.7% it was associated with serious injuries (AIS ≥2) involving other body areas (Table 2). Among those with major trauma but no head injury, very few had an isolated injury to the thorax, abdomen, or pelvis. The majority had a combination of regional injuries.

In the Italian study, MVA was by far the most important cause of injury (80.7%), followed by work (6.7%), domestic accidents (5.3%), and sports accidents (1.8%). Falls were the principal mechanism in work, sports, and domestic accidents. Interpersonal violence was responsible for only 1.8% of major trauma cases (Table 3). Similar figures were recorded in the Netherlands in 723 patients with multiple injuries (Table 4) [18].

In the past there have been many descriptions of the pattern of injuries resulting from different types of road accidents [19]; an extensive review is beyond the scope of this chapter. A classic description of lesions in unrestrained front seat occupants can be found in Daffner's work [20]. Rear seat passengers have been shown to have similar injuries [21]. Ejection, entrapment, and lateral impact are all factors associated with higher

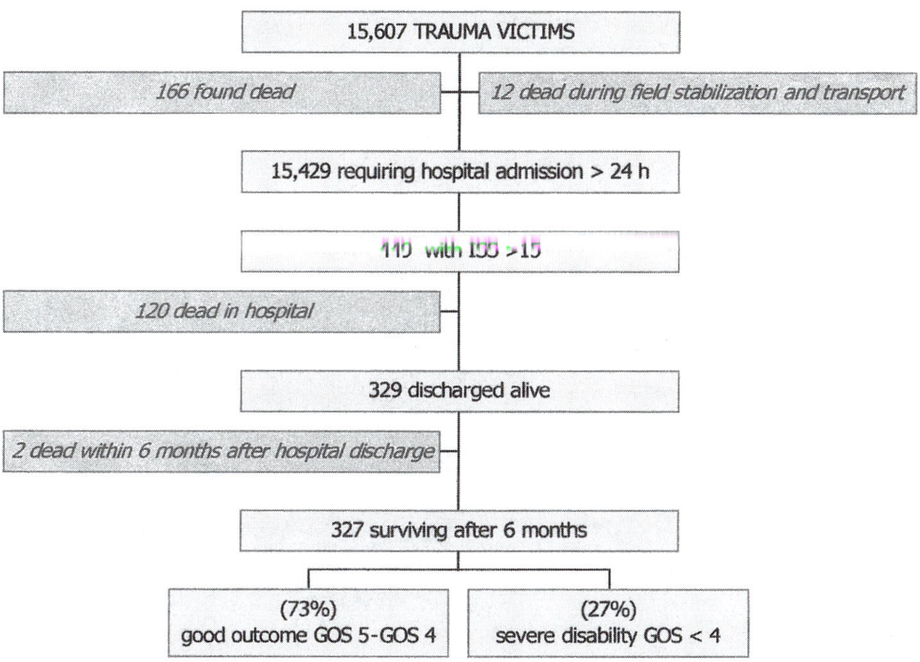

Figure 1 Incidence of major trauma in northeast Italy—prehospital mortality, hospital admissions, and final outcome (Friuli Venezia Giulia: 7,200 sq. km, 1,160,000 inhabitants). (From Friuli Venezia Giulia population-based study on major trauma.)

Table 2 Association of Extracranial Injuries (AIS ≥2) in Patients with Severe Head Trauma (AIS ≥3)

Body region	
Chest	36%
Abdomen	17%
Pelvis and/or limbs	43%
Spine (cervical, thoracic, lumbar)	14%
Face	27%
Isolated head trauma	35%

Source: Ref. 3.

Table 3 Causes of Major Trauma (ISS >15) in Italy

	Number of cases	Percent
MVA	506	80.7
Work accidents	42	6.7
Domestic accidents	33	5.3
Assaults	11	1.8
Sports accidents	11	1.8
Other causes	22	3.5
Overall	625	99.7
Not reported	2	0.3
Total	627	100.0

Table 4 Causes of Multiple Trauma

MVA	77.2%
Car	44.1%
Bicycle	21.7%
Pedestrian	15.4%
Moped	11.3%
Motorcycle	6.5%
Bus	0.5%
Trucks	0.5%
Domestic	9.3%
Work	6.2%
Sport	2.3%
Other causes	11.1%

Source: Ref. 18.

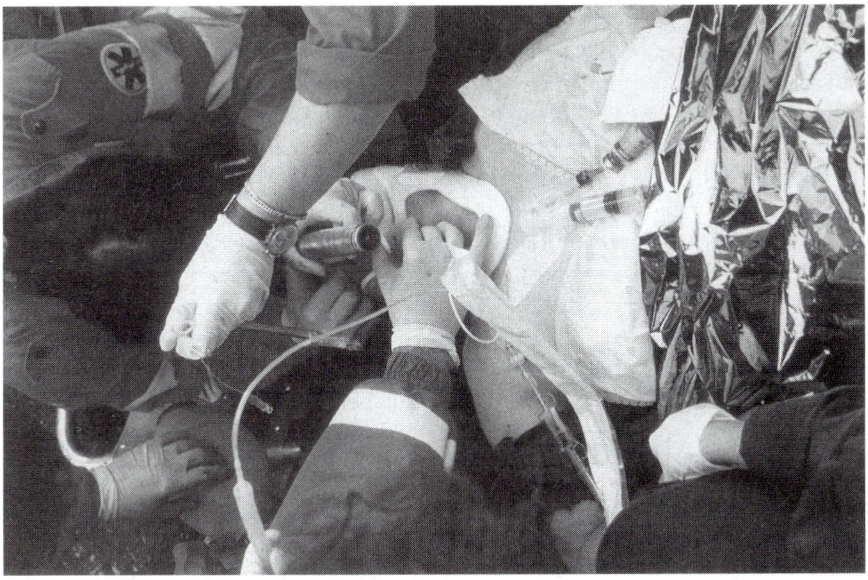

Figure 2 Vehicular entrapment requiring prolonged extrication.

severity [22,23]. Entrapment is a special challenge for prehospital rescue teams because its victims often need advanced maneuvers performed immediately, despite the difficult access and the delay incurred by their extrication [24] (Fig. 2). Restraint devices (seat belts and air bags) offer valuable protection and lead to a modified pattern of injuries [25,26]. Motorcycle [27] and pedestrian accidents have their own patterns of injuries, although some of the classic descriptions have recently been questioned [28].

Falls produce a different spectrum of injuries, although many of the general features are the same as in road accidents. For example, a combination of injuries to the head, pelvis, and lower extremities is very common. Suicidal and accidental falls differ. In the former, serious injuries (AIS > 3) most commonly involve the pelvis, while in the latter, serious head injuries are more frequent.

II. FIELD RESUSCITATION IN MULTIPLE TRAUMA

In performing advanced prehospital life support of the multiple trauma patient, the traditional ABCD scheme of assessment and intervention is followed. In the evolving situation, careful, continual re-evaluation is essential to detect any signs of deterioration. Although some injuries are more obvious than others (e.g., compound fractures with major bleeding or severe pain), they must not distract the care giver from following the prioritized ABCD scheme, which is specifically designed to identify and treat injuries in the order in which they tend to threaten life.

A. Airway and Cervical Spine Protection

Prevention and treatment of hypoxemia, hypercapnia, and inhalation is of major importance in the severely injured patient in order to limit secondary injuries. Securing the airway and ensuring adequate ventilation is one of the most important steps. Pfenninger and Lindner [29] were able to obtain a blood gas measurement from head trauma patients on the accident site, and they observed a very close correlation between the initial depth of unconsciousness and the degree of hypercapnia. A low Glasgow coma scale (GCS) was also associated with hypoxia, although the correlation was weaker. Both hypoxia and hypercapnia were effectively corrected by intubation and artificial ventilation, with significant improvement in blood gas parameters on hospital admission. Endotracheal intubation provides the best means of achieving airway control and assisted ventilation, but is an invasive procedure with potentially catastrophic complications. Persistent attempts can worsen the situation by causing local airway injury, raising intracranial pressure, or contributing to secondary hypoxic injury. Patients with injuries to the head, face, or neck may have distorted airway anatomy, as well as blood, vomit, or other debris in the lumen. Head and neck positioning is restricted by spinal injury considerations. Limited access to the patient makes prehospital intubation even more challenging. The decision of whether or not to intubate at the scene is clearly not straightforward.

Opponents of field intubation claim that it delays definitive care, increases intracranial pressure, and contributes to worsening shock by affecting preload during positive pressure ventilation [30]. In a study over 1000 comatose head injury patients, however, endotracheal intubation in the field was associated with significant improvements in the outcome of patients with a GCS <9 [31]. The lack of intubation was the main cause of preventable deaths in a regional audit [17].

The criteria for field intubation of trauma patients are still widely debated and depend on the patient's condition and the experience of the operator. While most authors agree that patients with a GCS <9 would benefit from prompt tracheal intubation and artificial ventilation, some regard this criterion as too stringent. Oswalt et al. [32] showed that a delay in intubating patients with a GCS <13 was associated with a higher mortality rate than that predicted by the TRISS method. In our experience, trauma patients with a GCS between 9 and 12 who were intubated on the scene before helicopter transport had fewer complications than those who were not, although the mortality rate was not significantly different [33]. There is little doubt that general anaesthesia is required for the intubation of a comatose or hypoxic patient, who may be combative with intact pharyngeal reflexes and at risk from intracranial hypertension. Greater skill is required by the rescue team than that needed to intubate an unconscious, reflex-free patient in cardiac arrest. Moreover, the need to minimize movement of the cervical spine adds to the technical difficulty.

Blind nasotracheal intubation without the use of anesthetic drugs was recommended as a technique up until a few years ago, but is gradually being replaced with rapid sequence induction (RSI) and orotracheal intubation [34]. Vilke et al. [35] compared field intubations by the nasotracheal route with awake orotracheal intubation and orotracheal intubation following rapid sequence induction. In this study, rapid sequence orotracheal intubation was associated with a higher success rate, fewer complications, and a better patient outcome.

Prehospital intubation under general anaesthesia in the multitraumatized patient has a high success rate and few complications in the right hands. While field intubation has been shown to be effective when performed by well-trained paramedics [36], the success rate is higher still when carried out by experienced physicians. A recent review of the Friuli Venezalia Giulia Helicopter Emergency Medical Service showed that in more than 900 attempted prehospital intubations in trauma cases, the flight anesthesiologist was successful in all but one case. The one patient who could not be intubated at the scene, despite three attempts, was uneventfully ventilated en route by face mask and subsequently intubated using fibroscopy. In one further case, there was severe injury to the face and the neck, exposing the trachea. This was treated by field tracheostomy in preference to orotracheal intubation.

The technique of field intubation in the road accident victim is difficult to standardize, as the best choice varies with the experience of the operator, the physical setting (e.g., entrapment), the clinical situation (e.g., shock or associated facial trauma), and the available equipment. A few general principles, though, must be adhered to. It is essential to minimize the risk of damaging the spinal cord in a potentially unstable spine by maintaining spinal precautions. Orotracheal intubation with manual online stabilization has been proved to be safe [37] and better than the nasotracheal route. Nasotracheal intubation, though contraindicated in basal skull fracture and less successful, is considered in cases in which access is limited and direct laryngoscopy is impossible (e.g., entrapment) [24].

Variants on the standard technique of orotracheal intubation have been described. It has been suggested that the left lateral decubitus position affords a more rapid intubation with better glottic visualization than the classic kneeling position [38]. Inverse intubation, also known as "intubation au piolet," has also been described as a useful alternative for the patient lying on the ground. Whichever technique is employed, an escape plan for failed intubation (e.g., cricothyroidotomy) must be considered in advance. Backup equipment must be immediately available, checked, and ready to use.

The primary aims of endotracheal intubation in the multitraumatized patient are to prevent hypoxia, hypercapnia, and aspiration of gastric contents. There is pressure on the operator to perform this maneuver as the first priority if the patient's airway is considered to be at risk. If the airway is initially patent—though at risk—and the breathing is adequate, minor delays to provide spinal immobilization, to preoxygenate, and to perform a brief evaluation of the cardiovascular system are acceptable. Recommendations for the timing of field intubation have been summarized by the Italian Resuscitation Council [39] (Tables 5 and 6).

Trauma patients must be intubated at step A (airway) in case of apnea or when a patent airway cannot be achieved by less invasive means. Intubation should be considered at step B (breathing) in the event of persistent hypoxia (SaO_2 <85%), despite receiving

Table 5 Timing of Tracheal Intubation and Technical Requirements

Step	Priority	Requirement	Monitor
A • Apnea • Complete airways obstruction	Immediate	• Cervical spine immobilization	None
B • Severe hypoxia ($SpO2$ <85%)	Time for • IV access • Drugs administration	• Cervical spine immobilization • Cervical collar	SpO_2
D • GCS ≤8 • (GCS <12)	Time for • Complete primary survey • IV access • Drugs administration	• Cervical spine immobilization • Cervical collar	• SpO_2 • Cardiac activity • Blood pressure

Table 6 Recommendations for Prehospital Intubation in Trauma Patients According to IRC

Orotracheal route
1. Ketamine 2 to 3 mg/kg (± low dosage benzodiazepine) + neuromuscular blocker (NB)
2. Fentanyl 2.5 to 5 μg/kg + midazolam 0.15 to 0.20 mg/kg (or diazepam 0.2–0.3 mg/kg) + NB
3. Thiopental 4 mg/kg + NB (to be reserved to isolated head trauma or seizures)
Nasotracheal route
Midazolam 0.15 to 0.20 mg/kg (or diazepam 0.2–0.3 mg/Kg) ± fentanyl 2 to 3 μg/Kg +

NB = neuromuscular blocking drug.
Source: Ref. 39.

a high concentration of oxygen. In the case of suspected pneumothorax, the decision whether to intubate before or after chest decompression should be made on the basis of the degree of respiratory distress. Intubation at step D (disability) is strongly recommended when the GCS is lower than 8. There is some evidence that field intubation is of benefit in trauma patients with a GCS between 9 and 12 [32,33], although these patients may be irritable or agitated and require a high level of skill.

A consensus has emerged that ''eager'' intubation without an anesthetic or appropriate sedation is no longer appropriate. Not only is it technically more difficult in all but the most obtunded of patients, it may cause the patient to gag and vomit, risking aspiration. In the shocked or unconscious patient, anesthetic and sedative drug doses should in general be reduced, but there is no evidence-based data to define the best choice of drugs for field intubation. Patients with trauma limited to the head may be safely intubated with a carefully judged dose of thiopental, making every effort to avoid hypotension. It should be used with extreme caution if there is a high risk of hypovolemia. The combination of fentanyl and a benzodiazepine is widely used, although these agents also carry a risk of unmasking hypovolemia or of causing dangerous hypotension [34]. Because of its marked vasodilatatory effect, propofol is not generally recommended as an induction agent in the prehospital setting, although its safe use has been reported by the London Helicopter Emergency Medical Service (HEMS). Ketamine is well established as a field anesthetic and is being used increasingly in Europe. For its ability to maintain the blood pressure, it has been recommended as the first choice for intubating hypotensive or potentially hypovolemic trauma patients in the field [39]. In a review of field intubations performed by flight anesthesiologists in Italy (Fig. 3), the proportion of trauma patients intubated with ketamine rose from 10% to over 90% over a 7-year time span. Whichever technique is chosen for prehospital intubation, an immutable rule is that in the hostile field environment, with its noise, confusion, restricted access, and limited resources, only fully trained professionals with ongoing experience of performing lifesaving procedures should be allowed to perform it.

B. Breathing

The second priority after airway control with cervical spine protection is assuring adequate ventilation. Many patients with chest trauma present with impaired ventilation and a low oxygen saturation (SaO_2) at the scene. In the face of severe hypoxia or dyspnoea, artificial ventilation should be instituted promptly, preferably by intubation and assisted ventilation.

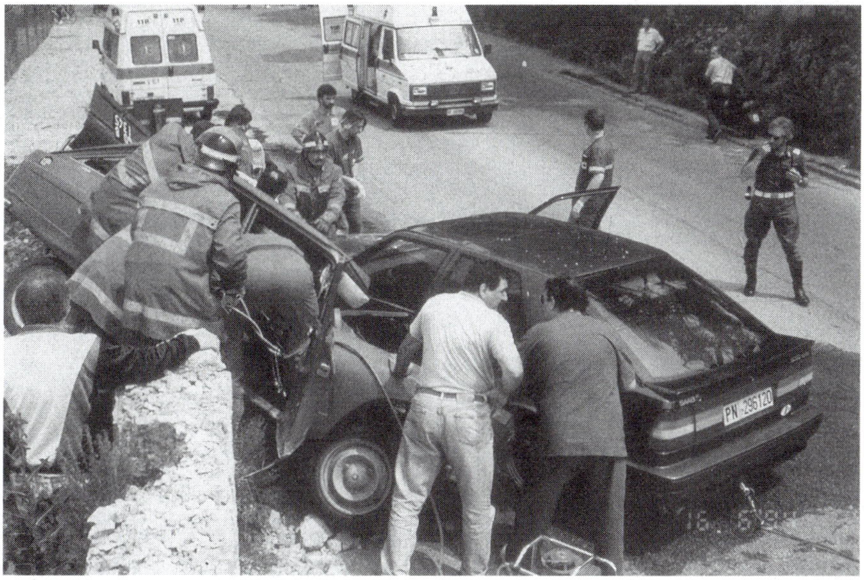

Figure 3 Field intubation with cervical collar and manual stabilization. (From G. Nardi et al., with permission.)

Although positive pressure ventilation will usually improve oxygenation, it can be extremely harmful if there is a concomitant pneumothorax. Pneumothorax remains one of the most frequent, life-threatening complications of injury to the chest and requires early recognition and treatment. Unrecognized tension pneumothorax is still an important cause of preventable death. A tension pneumothorax may develop before medical intervention or arise as a complication of artificial ventilation. It has been clearly established that the diagnosis of tension pneumothorax must be made on clinical grounds; emergency treatment should be immediate and not delayed until the patient reaches the hospital or undergoes radiological investigation.

Although the overall incidence of pneumothorax has not been well defined, its complication rate is sufficiently high to promote a high level of awareness. In an Italian population-based study, the incidence of traumatic pneumothorax was 81 per million population per year. About 20% of major trauma patients developed a unilateral (74%) or bilateral (26%) pneumothorax [40]. In patients with severe thoracic trauma (AIS ≥3), up to 50% may have a pneumothorax. Fifteen percent of all traumatic pneumothoraces were treated by early field decompression, and a further 38% required emergency treatment soon after arrival in the emergency room.

There is no doubt that emergency decompression of a tension pneumothorax is a lifesaving procedure. It is an essential skill for all prehospital ALS providers. Major differences exist, however, in the percentage of trauma patients who receive emergency thoracic decompression by different ALS services [41]. The use of tube thoracostomy in the treatment of a suspected tension pneumothorax in the field is controversial. Some authors report an increased risk of complications after prehospital chest tube insertion. A high rate of malposition has been reported, and organ injuries have occurred in up to 30% of cases [42]. Most of these complications follow the use of a trocar to insert the tube, a technique that has been outlawed by the ATLS course. Schmidt et al. [43] reported that in a group of 63 trauma patients in whom a prehospital chest tube was inserted using blunt dissection, there were no pleural infections and no intraparenchymal tube placements. In 24% of these patients, neither pneumothorax nor hemothorax were confirmed following the procedure; tube thoracostomy turned out to be nontherapeutic. In this study, indications for on-scene chest decompression included decreased breath sounds, chest wall instability, subcutaneous emphysema, and penetrating injuries to the chest. The protocol did not include needle decompression or exploratory thoracentesis to confirm a suspected pneumothorax before thoracostomy.

Tube thoracostomy is the standard treatment of pneumothorax and hemothorax in the hospital. Although not difficult to learn in the hospital, the technique requires considerable judgment and skill to be performed safely at the scene. Some degree of cleanliness and sterility is required at the scene, despite the logistical difficulties; the tube is likely to remain in situ for at least 48 hr, during which time most severely injured patients are effectively immunosuppressed. In an interesting study, the HEMS group at the Royal London Hospital reported that 216 out of 3,113 trauma patients required roadside decompression of at least one pneumothorax [44]. They suggest that a simple thoracotomy (without insertion of a drain) in patients receiving positive pressure ventilation is quick, simple, and effective.

According to the Italian Resuscitation Council's (IRC) guidelines [39] for trauma care, patients presenting with hypoxemia, hypotension, and either subcutaneous emphysema or severe unilateral hypoventilation are submitted to an exploratory thoracentesis on scene. If release of air under tension is noted, then thoracic decompression is performed.

The prehospital use of a small-diameter (2.2-mm) drain, introduced through a large-bore needle, has been used for several years to provide chest decompression in the field. Although the procedure has been considered to be quick and safe in experienced hands, such a small drainage strategy may not be adequate to treat a pneumothorax caused by a large pleural laceration with a massive air leak (and will certainly be of no use in draining blood from a hemothorax; Fig. 4).

Recently the simple thoracostomy technique suggested by the London group has been successfully introduced in clinical practice in northeast Italy. Although it too requires significant training, it is intrinsically simpler to perform at roadside than the insertion of a chest tube. Delaying chest tube insertion until the patient arrives in the hospital saves time and reduces risk. The use of this technique should be restricted only to patients already intubated and artificially ventilated. This has now been included in the IRC guidelines and recommended as the quickest, safest way to decompress a tension pneumothorax in the field.

C. Circulation

Treating or preventing secondary injury has been an underlying principle throughout this chapter. The same emphasis that was placed on preventing hypoxemia must now be applied to the prevention of hypoperfusion.

Although aggressive fluid administration in major trauma patients has been widely recommended for many years, this practice has recently been questioned. The first concern was raised by Kaweski et al. [45], who analyzed data from 6,855 trauma patients and concluded that the mortality was not influenced by prehospital fluid administration. A

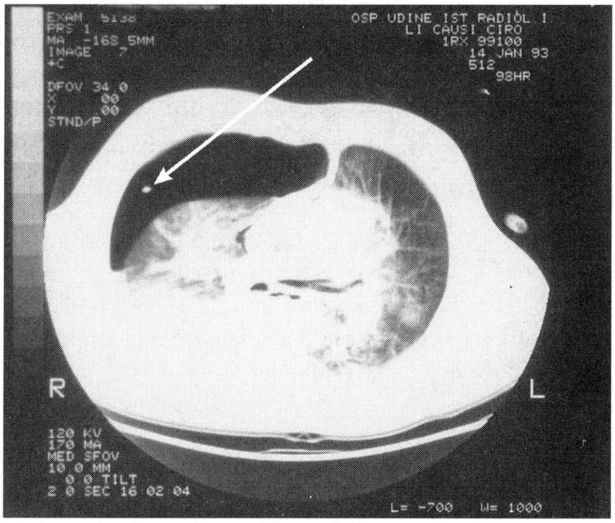

Figure 4 Prehospital decompression of a tension pneumothorax with a small (2.2-mm diameter) chest tube. A CT scan on admission to the emergency room shows the drain (arrow) within a persisting pneumothorax of large size.

more recent paper from Bickell and colleagues [46] went further, demonstrating a better outcome in patients with penetrating trunk trauma if they did not receive any prehospital infusion. Before these reports, trauma patients had often been regarded as a homogeneous group in terms of initial fluid resuscitation. Following Bickell's paper, the importance of immediate access to surgery following penetrating trauma and the hemostatic effect of hypotension was better recognized.

A debate has ensued as to whether fluid restriction should be applied to blunt trauma. Few data are as yet available. It is important to recognize that in penetrating trauma the anatomical damage is generally confined to the track of the penetrating object, whereas in blunt trauma, especially in road accidents, the whole body has been subject to acceleration or deceleration forces, and third space fluid loss may be much greater. The likelihood of worsening bleeding by administering fluids is different in blunt trauma, as discussed below. Equally important, 70% of major blunt trauma cases are associated with a severe head injury. In such cases, the deleterious effect of hypotension has been unequivocally demonstrated; a good outcome is often critically dependent on administering fluids to correct hypovolemia and maintain a normal or high blood pressure. Brain injured patients who are hypotensive in the prehospital phase have a 15 times higher risk of poor outcome [47]. The administration of crystalloids to correct hypovolemia does not increase intracranial pressure in these patients [48]. Updated therapeutic strategies incorporating these findings have been established for the prehospital care of head trauma patients with and without multiple injuries [39].

The need to keep blood pressure high enough to assure brain perfusion despite the loss of autoregulation has been emphasized in the Brain Trauma Foundation guidelines for the management of severe head injury [49]. A systolic pressure over 120 mmHg or a mean arterial pressure of more than 90 mmHg are considered to be appropriate target pressures in the prehospital setting, as they are in the hospital. Similar recommendations have been adopted in Europe, although a lower systolic pressure (110 mmHg) has been accepted as an adequate target.

The results of studies on penetrating trauma cannot be extrapolated to multiple blunt trauma patients, with or without head injury. Many of the lesions responsible for hemorrhage, such as bone fractures, are often self-tamponading; restoring blood volume and blood pressure does not necessarily lead to an increase in blood loss. In the case of hemorrhagic injuries involving the body cavities (i.e., hemoperitoneum or hemothorax), a compromise must be sought between the need to perfuse vital organs and the theoretical risk of aggravating bleeding. The judgment of how much fluid to give depends on the pattern of injuries identified in the individual patient, as well as taking into account any delays associated with extrication or diagnostic procedures. Experimental data from blunt trauma studies in animals demonstrate a higher mortality rate in animals that received no fluid therapy. The best survival rate was achieved when the volume of crystalloid equalled twice the blood loss [50].

It seems reasonable to tailor the approach to a hypotensive trauma patient according to the type of trauma. Head-injured blunt trauma patients require a higher blood pressure than blunt trauma victims with no injury to the brain, and they are likely to benefit from more aggressive fluid resuscitation. Patients with penetrating injuries to the torso or the abdomen, on the other hand, should receive limited infusion volumes. Guidelines for prehospital fluid therapy in the trauma patient have been developed (Table 7) based on the principles described, and have been approved by the IRC [39].

The pressure targets in the guidelines should be regarded as theoretical. It remains essential to incorporate sound clinical judgment into critical decisions. While the guidelines are useful as an aid to limiting fluids infusions, they may need to be overridden. Sometimes it is necessary for fluid administration to keep up with blood loss, and this may require high volumes.

In studies of fluids given by paramedics or basic life support (BLS) crews, the volume administered has often been so small as to be ineffective [45]. The volume expected

Table 7 A Suggested Differential Approach to Prehospital Fluid Therapy in Multiple Trauma

Type of trauma	Fluids	Pathophysiologic rationale
Multitraumatized (blunt) *with* head trauma	The minimum amount with the maximum speed to keep systolic blood pressure >110 mmHg; Mean blood pressure >90 mmHg	Perfusing the brain despite the loss of autoregulation
Multitraumatized (blunt) *without* head trauma	The minimum amount with the maximum speed to keep systolic blood pressure >90 mmHg	Perfusing the vital organs without enhancing ongoing bleeding and minimizing delay to diagnostic facilities and surgery
Penetrating trauma	The minimum amount with the maximum speed to keep systolic blood pressure >70 mmHg	Perfusing at least the brain without increasing blood loss and minimizing delay to surgery

to balance loss can be inferred from the classic classification of shock. In order to achieve maximal infusion rates in the prehospital setting, flexible bags (rather than glass bottles) and pressurizers are essential, as is the case in the hospital (Fig. 5). The time-honored recommendation of two large-bore (14G.) intravenous cannulae cannot be overemphasized. When this is not feasible, alternative routes should be considered (e.g., central venous or intraosseous). The choice depends on the skills of the rescue teams and the equipment available, as discussed elsewhere.

Once the fluid infusions have been established, pressure targets are considered simultaneously with other field maneuvers. In following this approach, blood pressure and tissue perfusion can be restored without delaying the time to definitive care and with beneficial effects on outcome.

Even more controversy exists about the types of fluids to use. This is dealt with in greater depth in another section of the book. For the polytraumatized patient, it can be said that even if the various solutions are of equal efficacy, the ''low-volume'' fluids (i.e., colloids, hypertonic solutions) have potential advantages in the prehospital environment. Logistic problems such as weight and space occupied in a prehospital backpack, together with the tendency to cause hypothermia, are reduced if fluids with the lowest volume for a given circulatory effect are used. Hypertonic solutions also have the theoretical advantage of reducing intracranial pressure, and indeed have reduced mortality in hypotensive, brain-injured patients [51]. Nevertheless, the evidence in the literature is insufficient to permit a definitive preference to be declared.

Hypothermia in the multiple trauma patient is a well-recognized problem and is exacerbated by aggressive fluid resuscitation. Body temperature decreases by 0.3°C for each liter of infusion at 20°C and by much more if the infusions are colder. Whichever solutions are used, every effort must be made to keep them warm before and during infusion.

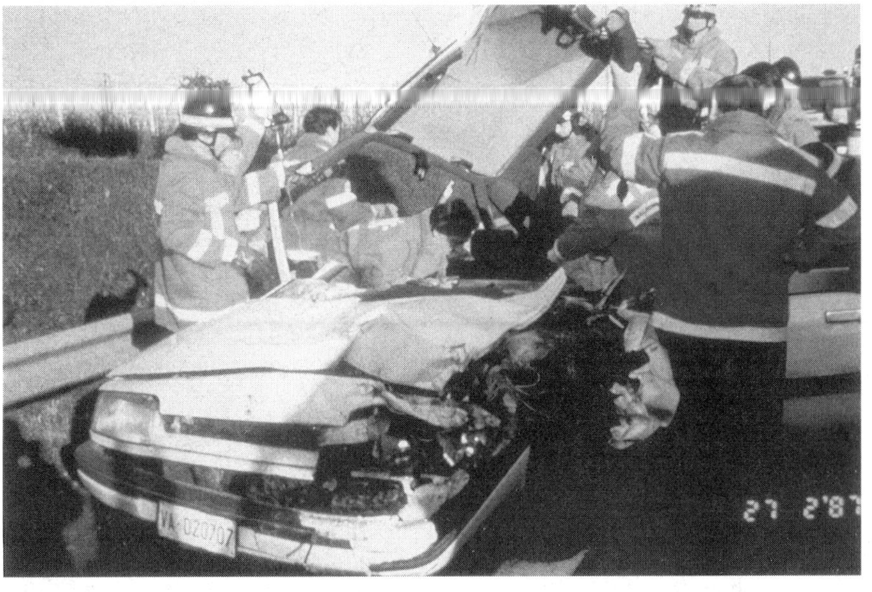

Figure 5 High-volume fluid infusions with pressure bags.

III. HOW AGGRESSIVE IS AGGRESSIVE ENOUGH?

Trauma is an extremely time-sensitive condition. Every procedure performed in the prehospital setting must be measured against time. The goals of prehospital trauma care are to avoid the development of hypovolemia, hypoxia, hypercarbia, and acidosis, and at the same time to ensure rapid transport to a definitive care center and to facilitate early surgery when needed. Patients involved in accidents in urban areas usually reach a well-equipped hospital quickly, reducing the need for prehospital stabilization. On the other hand, patients from rural areas more frequently need resuscitation and stabilization, both at the scene and during transport to the hospital.

In an attempt to improve the quality of prehospital care, physicians, nurses, and paramedics have been trained to provide ALS, including procedures such as tracheal intubation, decompression of a tension pneumothorax, and placement of intravenous cannulae. Therapeutic procedures on the scene are expected to reduce mortality and morbidity. Surprisingly, few studies have addressed the effectiveness of ALS interventions, and their results have often been controversial. Most U.S. studies [52] have been unable to demonstrate any benefit of ALS at the scene in terms of survival or reduction in hospital stay. In Europe, where there is widespread support for prehospital care delivered by physicians, the results of an admittedly small number of studies are more encouraging, suggesting clear benefits from ALS [14,53,54].

Several reasons help to explain the discrepancies in the apparent effectiveness of prehospital interventions. First, many of the authors investigating the differences between ALS and BLS failed to differentiate between blunt and penetrating trauma. As clearly demonstrated by Lerer and Knottenbelt [55], the key to improving survival from penetrating injuries lies in rapid transportation to the hospital by the quickest means available (including private cars!). Attempted prehospital stabilization of shocked patients with major injuries to the heart or large intrathoracic vessels is rarely worthwhile, although in a very small number of well-documented cases of witnessed traumatic cardiac arrest, immediate thoracotomy was lifesaving. In general, ALS rarely provides any extra benefit in this type of injury.

On the other hand, many blunt trauma patients require prolonged extrication from a vehicle [24]. Increased prehospital time with inadequate resuscitation is likely to increase the risk of secondary injuries. There is more scope for prehospital stabilization to make a difference in blunt trauma.

To minimize study bias and to allow valid conclusions to be drawn, blunt and penetrating injuries must undergo separate analysis. Moreover, many of the investigations were conducted in urban areas, which appropriate facilities can be reached in a reasonably short time. The results therefore cannot be easily extrapolated to extraurban areas, where the transport time to a trauma center is often prolonged. Without appropriate field ALS, the victims of a major trauma in a remote rural area have a seven times higher risk of death than in an urban area [56].

A second (and more contentious) explanation for the discrepancies between the reported effectiveness of prehospital ALS in different parts of the world has been put forward. Although the same term advanced life support is used throughout the world, the procedures undertaken and the training of the personnel who carry them out are often very different. To expect ALS maneuvers to reduce mortality and morbidity, they must be performed with a high level of proficiency. Unfortunately, this is often not the case.

In the Winchell and Hoyt study [31], almost 50% of trauma patients with a GCS <9 failed to undergo intubation when cared for by ALS paramedics. Although the nonintubated patients had a much higher mortality, all the patients were considered to have received ALS because they were cared for by an ALS team.

While there is little information on the frequency of prehospital chest decompression in the field, some discrepancies are evident in the extent to which tension pneumothorax is suspected and treated. Schmidt et al. [41] reported a decompression rate of 0.5% in a series of severely injured patients rescued by ALS paramedics, but a rate 20-fold higher in patients with comparable injuries when treated in the field by surgeons. A decompression rate of about 10% has been reported by other ALS teams staffed by skilled physicians [14,43,44].

As already mentioned, several studies have concluded that prehospital fluid administration is ineffective in reducing mortality. The average amounts of fluids given were so small as to make any benefit unlikely, however, and there were delays in the field to insert cannulae. This can be interpreted as inefficient implementation of field ALS procedures rather than as a limitation of the advanced techniques themselves.

In the debate about the efficacy of field ALS following trauma, there is indeed a problem of definition. What constitutes an ALS team is open to different interpretations, and even when the interpretations are similar the implementation often falls short of the declared aims.

In a regional audit [14] of severe trauma in a population of 1.2 million, a highly significant reduction in mortality was observed in those treated by fully qualified anesthesiologists working in the HEMS compared with those treated by BLS ambulance staff. In the ALS group, all head trauma patients with a GCS <9 were intubated at roadside; 14% of the severe trauma cases underwent prehospital chest decompression, and patients who were hypotensive at the scene received over 2 liters of fluid (colloids and crystalloids) before arriving at the hospital. In a more recent review of more than 900 comatose trauma patients, the same HEMS team intubated 97% of those with a GCS <9 and 67% of those with a GCS between 9 and 12. Prehospital mortality in patients with major trauma found alive at the scene was as low as 1.5%.

In order to compare ALS practices in different systems, clearer definitions and better quality control are required. These need to address organizational aspects as well as the skills and training of prehospital personnel, and cannot be achieved without reliable data collection.

A. Multiple Organ System Failure

Multiple organ system failure (MOSF) is a major cause of hospital death in patients with multiple trauma. Its reported incidence varies widely, ranging from 14–42% of ICU trauma patients who survive more than 48 hr [57]. Postinjury MOSF has a bimodal temporal distribution, with an early peak around day 3 and a delayed peak one week after injury. Both early and late MOSF are characterized by a high incidence of respiratory failure. Patients with early MOSF have more cardiac dysfunction, while late MOF is characterized by a higher incidence of infections and hepatic failure.

Several factors are associated with the development of MOSF: a high ISS, hypotension on admission to the ER, the need for more than six units of blood within the first 12 hr, acidosis, and an increased lactate level. Patients over age 55 have an independent risk factor for late MOSF, but not for early MOSF. Patients with injuries involving the chest and the abdomen are at greater risk of developing MOSF than patients with severe trauma to the head.

There appears to be a correlation between the frequency of MOSF and the level of care in the prehospital setting. The improvement of rescue systems and on-scene therapy has led to a significant reduction in both early and delayed complications. Shackford et al. [58] reported a lower incidence of sepsis and MOSF after establishing the trauma system in San Diego County. Regel et al. [59] showed that prehospital intubation was associated with a reduction in MOSF.

IV. CONCLUSIONS

Clear definitions are essential to allow data to be compared. Epidemiological studies must include data from the prehospital phase. Prehospital mortality and prehospital preventable deaths should be considered separately from their in-hospital equivalents.

Penetrating and blunt trauma need different approaches and separate prehospital strategies.

The majority of major traumas associated with MVAs or occurring at work or in sports affects multiple body regions. Head injury is the most frequent finding.

Aggressive prehospital advanced trauma life support can improve mortality and morbidity, but the personnel involved must be skilled enough to carry out strategies that have shown to be effective.

Advanced life support for prehospital trauma care of multiple trauma patients should include

- Tracheal intubation for patients with a compromised airway, hypoxia, or a GCS <9 (and perhaps those with a GCS between 9 and 12).
- Field chest decompression in trauma patients suspected of having a pneumothorax. (Initial confirmation by needle thoracentesis is recommended.)
- Aggressive fluid resuscitation in hypotensive, head-injured patients. Differential blood pressure targets for blunt trauma patients with a serious head injury (SBP 110–120 mmHg), blunt trauma patients without a head injury (SBP 90 mmHg), and penetrating injuries (the least amount of fluid to maintain cerebral perfusion).

Careful quality control of the performance of prehospital ALS is needed, paying particular attention to delays in the field and to the effectiveness of the procedures undertaken.

REFERENCES

1. C Murray, A Lopez. The Global Burden of Disease: A Comprehensive Assessment of Mortality and Disability from Disease, Injuries and Risk Factors in 1990 and Projected to 2020. Cambridge, MA: Harvard University Press, 1996.
2. WF Dick, PJF Baskett, C Grande, et al. Recommendations for uniform reporting of data following major trauma—the Utstein style. Eur J Emerg Med 6:369–387, 1999.
3. G Nardi, L Lattuada, F Scian, S Di Bartolomeo, et al., Epidemiological study on high grade trauma. Min Anesth 65:348–352, 1999.
4. CW Schwab, DR Kauder. Trauma surgeons on violence prevention: Ready, willing and able? J Trauma 40:671–672, 1996.

5. G Trinca. Reducing Traffic Injury: A Global Challenge. Melbourne, Australia: AH Massina, 1988.
6. XCN Mock, GJ Jurkovich, D nii-Amon-Kotei, et al., Trauma mortality patterns in three nations at different economic levels: Implications for global trauma system development. J Trauma 44:804–812, 1998.
7. N Stocchetti, G Pagliarini, M Gennari, et al. Trauma care in Italy: Evidence of in-hospital preventable deaths. J Trauma 36:401–405, 1996.
8. JD Cooper, FT McDermott, SM Cordner. Quality assessment of management of road traffic fatalities at a Level 1 Trauma Center compared with other hospitals in Victoria, Australia. J Trauma 45:772–779, 1998.
9. LM Hussain, AD Redmond. Are pre-hospital deaths from accidental injury preventable? Br Med J 308:1077–1082, 1994.
10. IN Papadopoulos, D Bukis, E Karalas, et al., Preventable prehospital trauma deaths in a Hellenic Urban Health Region: An audit of prehospital trauma care. J Trauma 41:864–869, 1996.
11. HR Champion, WS Copes, WJ Sacco, et al. The major trauma outcome study: Establishing national norms for trauma care. J Trauma 30:1356, 1990.
12. PL Lane, G Doing, A Mikrogianakis, et al. An evaluation of Ontario trauma outcomes and the development of regional norms for trauma and injury severity score (TRISS) analysis. J Trauma 41:4, 731–734, 1996.
13. DF Gorman, DN Teanby, MP Sinha, et al., The epidemiology of major injuries in Mersey region and North Wales. Injury 26:51–54, 1995.
14. G Nardi, D Massarutti, R Muzzi, et al. Impact of emergency medical helicopter service on mortality for trauma in North-East Italy: A regional prospective audit. Eur J Emerg Med 69–77, 1994.
15. DW Spaite, DJ Tse, TD Valenzuela, et al., The impact of injury severity and prehospital procedures on scene time in victims of major trauma. Ann Emerg Med 20:1299–1305, 1991.
16. D Demetriades, H Belzberg, J Asensio, et al. The impact of a dedicated trauma program on outcome in severely injured patients. Arch Surg 130:216–220, 1995.
17. FT McDermott, SM Cordner, AB Tremayne, et al. Evaluation of the medical management and preventability death in 137 road traffic fatalities in Victoria, Australia: An overview. J Trauma 40:520–532, 1996.
18. CK Van der Sluis, HJ ten Duis, JHB Geertzen. Multiple injuries: An overview of outcome. J Trauma 38:681–686, 1995.
19. DD Blackbourne. Injury-vehicle correlations in the investigation of motor vehicle accidents. In: CH Wecht, ed. Legal Medicine 1980. Philadelphia: Saunders, 1980, p. 1.
20. RH Daffner, ZL Deeb, AR Lupetin, WE Rothfus. Patterns of high-speed impact injuries in motor vehicle occupants. J Trauma 28:498–502, 1988.
21. SJ Mucci, LD Eriksen, KA Crist, LA Bernath, PK Chaudhuri. The pattern of injury to rear seat passengers involved in automobile collisions. J Trauma 31:1329–1331, 1991.
22. BJ Simon, P Legere, T Emhoff, VM Fiallo, J Garb, Vehicular trauma triage by mechanism: Avoidance of the unproductive evaluation. J Trauma 37:645–649, 1994.
23. BA McLennan, SB Rizzoli, FD Brenneman, BR Boulanger, PW Sharkey, JP Szalai. Injury pattern and severity in lateral motor vehicle collisions: A Canadian experience. J Trauma 41: 708–713, 1991.
24. G Sanson, S Di Bartolomeo, G Nardi, et al. Road traffic accidents with vehicular entrapment: Incidence of major injuries and need for advanced life support. Eur J Emerg Med 6:285–291, 1999.
25. DB Reath, J Kirby, M Linch, et al., Injury and cost comparison of restrained and unrestrained motor vehicle crash victims. J Trauma 29:806–811, 1989.
26. GT Loo, JH Siegel, PC Dischinger, et al. Airbag protection versus compartment intrusion effect determines the pattern of injuries in multiple trauma motor vehicle crashes. J Trauma 41:935–951, 1996.

27. D Doyle, M Muir, B Chinn. Motorcycle accidents in Strathclyde Region, Scotland during 1992: A study of the injuries sustained. Health Bull (Edinb) 53:383–394, 1995.
28. R Orsborn, K Haley, S Hammond, RE Falcone. Pediatric pedestrian versus motor vehicle patterns of injury: Debunking the myth. Air Med J 18:107–110, 1999.
29. EG Pfenninger, KH Lindner. Arterial blood gases in patients with acute head injury at the accident site and upon hospital admission. Acta Anaesth Scand 35:148–152, 1991.
30. PE Pepe. Resuscitation of the patient with major trauma. Curr Opin Crit Care 1:479–486, 1995.
31. R Winchell, DB Hoyt. Endotracheal intubation in the field improves survival in patients with severe head injury. Arch Surg 132:592–597, 1997.
32. JL Oswalt, JR Hedges, BE Soifer. Analysis of trauma intubations. Am J Emerg Med 10:6, 511–514, 1992.
33. G Nardi. Helicopters in emergency medicine. In: European Society of Anaesthesiologists, eds. London: ESA Refresher Courses, 1996.
34. E Soreide, C Deakin, D Baker. Prehospital trauma management for the anesthesiologist. Anesth Clin of North Am 17:33–44, 1999.
35. GM Vilke, DB Hoyt, M Epperson, et al. Intubation techniques in the helicopter. J Emerg Med 12:217–224, 1994.
36. H Frankel, G Rozycki, H Champion, JD Harviel, R Bass. The use of TRISS methodology to validate prehospital intubation by urban EMS providers. Am J Emerg Med 15:630–632, 1997.
37. JC Criswell, MJA Parr. Emergency airway management in patients with cervical spine injuries. Anaesthesia 49:900–903, 1994.
38. F Adnet, F Lapostolle, S Boiron, B Hennequin, G Leclercq, M Fleury. Optimization of glottic exposure during intubation of a patient lying supine on the ground. Am J Emerg Med 15:1–3, 1997.
39. Italian Resuscitation Council, Trauma Committe. Prehospital Trauma Care. IRC ed Compositori Bologna, 1998.
40. S Di Bartolomeo, GF Sanson, G Nardi, et al. A population based study on pneumothorax in severely traumatized patients. J Trauma (in press).
41. U Schmidt, SB Frame, ML Nerlich, et al. On-scene helicopter transport of patients with multiple injuries—Comparison of a German and an American system. J Trauma 33:548–553, 1992.
42. MM Baldt, AA Bankier, PS Germann, et al. Complications after emergency thoracotomy: Assessment with CT. Radiology 195:539–543, 1995.
43. U Schmidt, M Stalp, T Gerich, et al. Chest tube decompression of blunt chest injuries by physicians in the field: Effectiveness and complications. J Trauma 44:98–101, 1998.
44. CD Deakin, G Davies, A Wilson. Simple thoracostomy avoids chest drain insertion in prehospital trauma. J Trauma 39:373–374, 1995.
45. SM Kaweski, MJ Sise, RW Virgilio. The effect of prehospital fluids on survival in trauma patients. J Trauma 30:1215–1218, 1990.
46. WH Bickell, MJ Wall, PE Pepe. Immediate versus delayed fluid resuscitation for hypotensive patients with penetrating torso injuries. New Eng J Med 331:1105–1109, 1994.
47. RM Chestnut, LF Marshall, MR Klauber. The role of secondary brain injury in determining outcome from severe head injury. J Trauma 34:216–222, 1992.
48. MH Zornow, DS Prough. Fluid management in patient with traumatic brain injury. New Hor 3:488–493, 1995.
49. R Bullock, R Chestnut, G Clifton. Guidelines for the Management of Severe Head Injury. New York: Brain Trauma Foundation, 1996.
50. L Riddez, L Johnson, RG Hahn. Central and regional hemodynamics during crystalloid fluid therapy after uncontrolled intra-abdominal bleeding. J Trauma 44:433–439, 1998.
51. CE Wade, JJ Grady, GC Kramer, RN Younes, et al. Individual patient cohort analysis of the efficacy of hypertonic saline/dextran in patients with traumatic brain injury and hypotension. J Trauma 42:S61–S65, 1997.

52. JS Sampalis, A Lavoie, JI Williams, et al. Impact of on-site care, prehospital time and level of in-hospital care on survival in severely injured patients. J Trauma 34:256–261, 1993.
53. C Kirk. The first 1000 patients admitted to the Royal London Hospital. In: R Earlam, ed. Trauma Care—Helicopter Emergency Medical Services. London: 1996.
54. J Schuttler, B Schmitz, AC Bartsch. The efficiency of emergency therapy in patients with head-brain, multiple injury: Quality assurance in emergency medicine. Anaesthesist 44:850–858, 1995.
55. LB Lerer, JD Knottenbelt. Preventable mortality following sharp penetrating chest trauma. J Trauma 37:6–12, 1994.
56. DC Grossman, A Kim, CS Macdonald, et al. Urban–rural differences in prehospital care of major trauma. J Trauma 42:723–729, 1997.
57. FA Moore, A Sauaia, E Moore, et al. Postinjury multiple organ failure: A bimodal phenomenon. J Trauma 40:501–509, 1996.
58. SR Shakford, RC Mac Kersie, TL Holbrook, et al. The epidemiology of traumatic death. Arch Surg 128:571–577, 1993.
59. G Regel, M Stalp, U Lehman, A Seekamp. Prehospital care: Importance of early intervention on outcome. Acta Anaesth Scand 110 (suppl.):71–76, 1997.

23

The Patient With Penetrating Injuries

KIMBALL I. MAULL

The Trauma Center at Carraway and Carraway Methodist Medical Center, Birmingham, Alabama

PAUL E. PEPE

University of Texas Southwestern Medical School and Parkland Memorial Health System, Dallas, Texas

I. INTRODUCTION

Penetrating injuries may be arbitrarily divided into wounds caused by sharp instruments, wounds caused by firearms, and impalements. Worldwide, stab wounds cause the greatest number of penetrating trauma casualties. In certain parts of the world, including the United States, the majority of penetrating wounds are caused by firearms [1]. Regardless of their etiology, most penetrating wounds result from interpersonal violence or violence that is self-inflicted. This fact has profound significance to prehospital rescue personnel, who usually have little initial insight into the circumstances surrounding the incident and who may be at considerable risk if the perpetrator(s) remain in the immediate vicinity. Coordination of rescue efforts between and among rescue personnel, law enforcement officials, and others in the community may be required to enable rescue efforts to safely proceed. While *Do no harm* may be the time-honored rule of trauma care, *Protect thyself* is always the first rule for the prehospital rescuers, who cannot do their job if they, too, fall victim to violence.

Once the security of the incident scene is assured, the most important priority for rescue personnel is to determine how best to get the penetrating trauma victim to the appropriate medical facility alive [2]. Loss of vital signs is rapidly followed by loss of cardiac electrical activity. With rare exception, ''trauma arrest'' in the prehospital phase is uniformly fatal [3]. Although there are documented instances of successful emergency department thoracotomies for patients who arrive with no vital signs, virtually all such survivors have penetrating cardiac wounds with tamponade [4]. In the elderly, one must consider the possibility of nontraumatic cardiac arrest followed by injury. Death generally awaits patients with other injury mechanisms, including the penetrating trauma associated with exsanguination. This concept opens the ongoing debate concerning how much treatment in the field is appropriate. While there is certainly room for individualizing cases and considering transport times in the decision paradigm, except for taking the time needed to establish an airway, delay in transport must be avoided. With certain types of traumas—and penetrating trauma in particular—circumstances may exist in which immediate evacuation is unsafe for either the victim or the rescuer (or both). Under such conditions, rescue personnel may perform interventions that under other circumstances would be undertaken only in transit or upon arrival in the emergency department (ED). It is axiomatic that trauma is a time-sensitive disease, that it is important to minimize scene and transport times, and that local protocols should reflect these critical priorities. Nonetheless, experienced prehospital rescue personnel can often reliably estimate whether the patient's outcome is dependent on rapid transport to the closest hospital for lifesaving procedures that cannot be done in the field (e.g., hypotension with impending arrest from a gunshot wound to the abdomen), or if it is indicated to transport the patient an additional distance to a verified trauma center for definitive trauma care. These types of decisions are still difficult and require an organized approach to the care of the injured (i.e., a trauma care system) [5].

II. TYPES OF PENETRATING AGENTS

A. Knife Wounds

Wounds caused by sharp instruments, such as stabbings or slashings, may cause major injury, shock, and death, but in general, are not as serious as those caused by gunshot or shotgun wounds. Stabbings are common, however. The knife, or any variety thereof, is ubiquitous in our society, and while most knives are used for legitimate purposes, the knife is an effective wounding agent.

There appears to be a gender-specific difference in wounding mechanisms (Fig. 1). Women appear to attack with a knife held with the handle up, striking in a downward arc so that the penetration of the wound extends inferiorly, assuming that the victim is in the upright position at the time of the attack. Men hold the knife with the handle down and penetrate more directly or with a slight upward arc. Although these generalizations do not always hold, obtaining a history of the circumstances of the trauma incident may assist the clinician in establishing the anatomy of the injury, and guide local wound exploration if this option is selected by the examining physician.

B. Impalements

Impalements may be caused intentionally by leaving a sharp object imbedded in the body, or may be incurred unintentionally by impacting a sharp structure in a fall, deceleration incident, or explosion. Occasionally the victim may be impaled on an immovable object, challenging the ingenuity and resources of the rescue service and requiring close coordination with hospital-based emergency medical or surgical staff. As a general rule, impaled objects should not be removed in the field. Such removal should be an exception to this rule and made only after possible dangers of removal have been considered. The reason for leaving impaled objects in place relates to their tamponade effect and the risk of hemor-

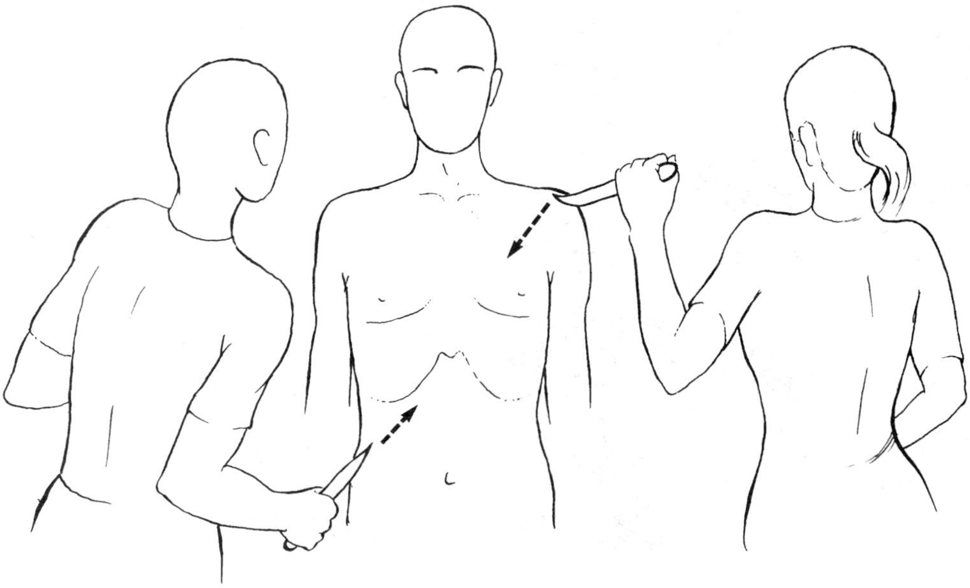

Figure 1 Artist's depiction of the differences in stabbing techniques typically employed by women and men.

rhage upon their removal. In most instances of impalement, the object should be removed only in the operating room (Figs. 2a,b). At times it may be more prudent to remove an impaled object prior to transport. Such circumstances occur when the impaled object cannot be stabilized, exceeds the dimensions of the transport vehicle, or in the opinion of field personnel is likely to cause further damage during transport.

C. Gunshot Wounds

In most countries, gunshot wounds are not commonly encountered outside of wartime. There are important exceptions, however. In the United States, firearm violence is the second leading cause of trauma deaths and constitutes a major portion of urban trauma center operative experience [1]. In South America, Colombia's annual firearm deaths approach 30,000, the highest per capita peacetime rate in the world–101 per 100,000 population. Other sites where gunshot wounds are likely to be encountered include Russia, South Africa, and the Middle East.

Firearm deaths fall into three categories: *homicide, suicide, and unintentional injuries.* The latter make up a small (3.8%) but important subgroup of casualties, because unintentional firearm injuries are overrepresented among the pediatric population.

Ballistics is the study of a missile in flight. Wound ballistics refers to the study of a missile within tissue, and by implication, the wounding potential of various missile types. Several factors determine the tissue damage from firearms, but the most important is the velocity of the missile. The kinetic energy KE imparted to the tissue is related to the mass m of the missile and its velocity v and is defined by the following equation:

$$Ke = m/2 \times v2$$

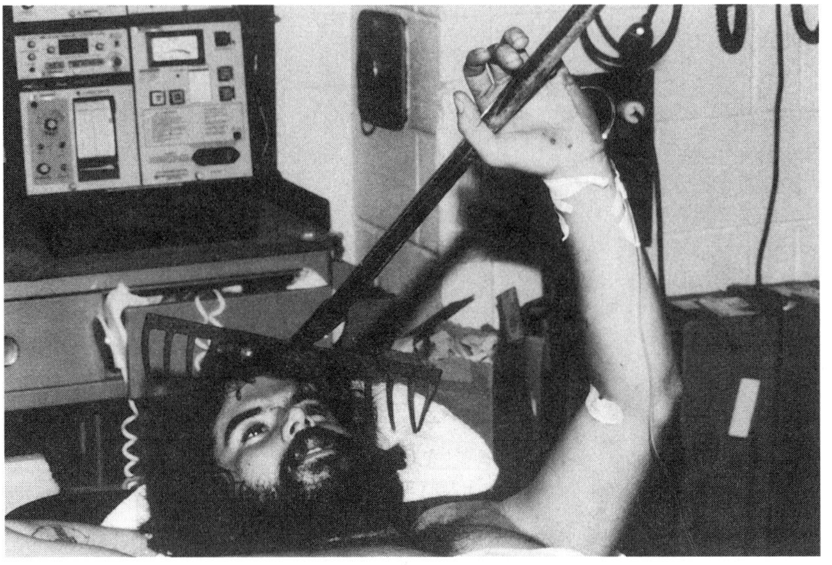

(a)

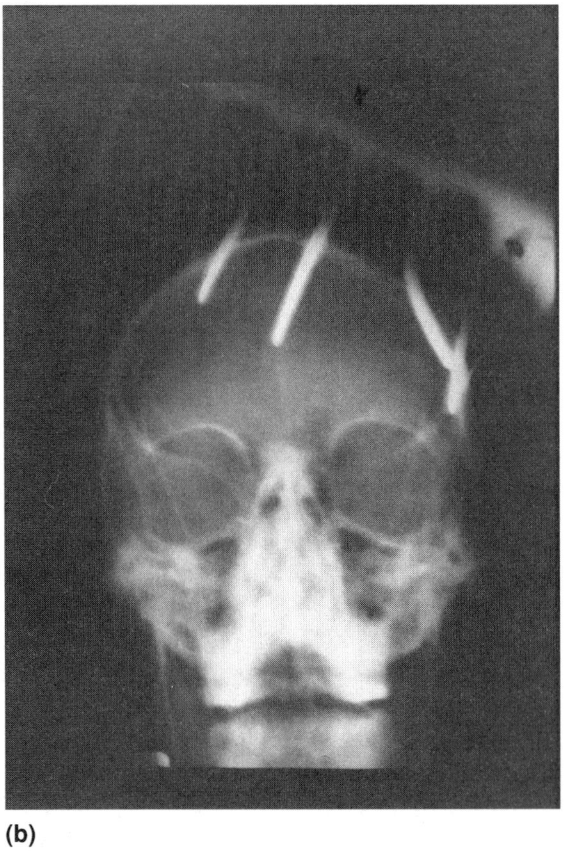

(b)

Figure 2 (a) ED photo of man impaled with garden rake during altercation. Note patient is awake and ''stabilizing'' the impaled object. (b) Skull films showing teeth of rake imbedded in frontoparietal portion of cranial vault. Rake was removed in the operating room at time of craniotomy.

If the mass is doubled, the KE is doubled; doubling the velocity quadruples the KE. It is therefore evident that as the velocity of the missile increases, the KE rises exponentially.

Firearms can be defined as low-velocity (<1000 ft/sec), midvelocity(1000–2000 ft/sec), or high-velocity(>2000 ft/sec). Most handguns are low-velocity weapons, although magnum loads can push the missile velocity to exceed 1000 ft/sec. Although firearms are defined by their muzzle velocity (i.e., the speed at which the missile leaves the barrel), it is the velocity at which the missile strikes the body (impact velocity) minus the velocity at which the missile exits the body (residual velocity) that determines the total KE absorbed by the body. As the missile passes through the body, it creates "cavitation." The "permanent cavity" is the actual tract that the missile takes through the body. The "temporary cavity" refers to the field of destruction extending out from the missile tract as the KE is dissipated to the tissue. This temporary cavity is directly related to the velocity of the missile as it passes through the body, and inversely proportional to the elasticity of the wounded tissue. Low-velocity bullets create only a small temporary cavity, so tissue damage is confined to the missile tract. High-velocity gunshot wounds cause extensive damage to tissues beyond those struck by the missile itself. Positive and negative pressures alternate as the missile exits, sucking foreign material in at both the entry and exit sites.

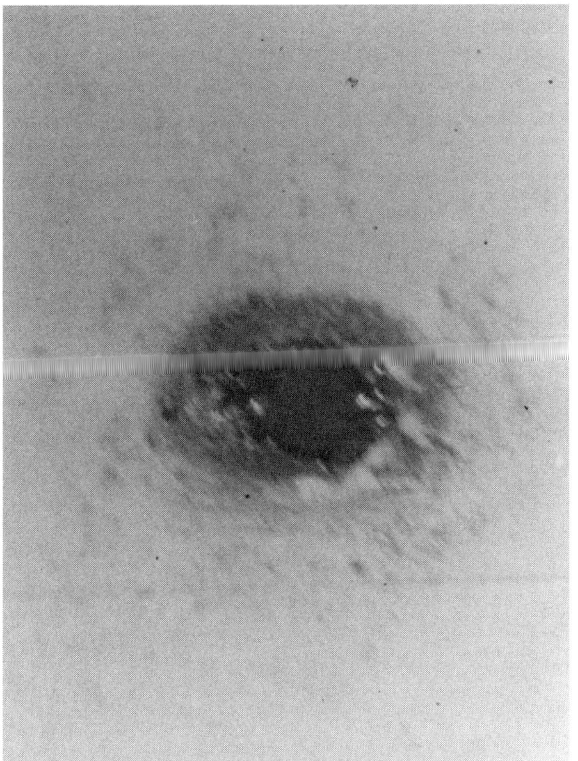

Figure 3 Entrance wound from self-inflicted abdominal gunshot. Note well-rounded margins and peripheral stippling. Internal injuries included perforation of the stomach, pancreas, and aorta.

Damage to bone is greatest because bone is virtually free of elastic tissue. Damage to lung is least because of its high elastic tissue content.

There are several other aspects of wound ballistics that relate to the extent of tissue damage. Missile mass, shape, and deformability are important. Large bullets are more injurious than small bullets, given the same impact velocity. Bullets that strike the body with a large, flat surface from excessive yaw or ''wobble'' or are easily deformed to ''pancake'' upon impact, are certain to dissipate more energy to the tissues than bullets that retain their aerodynamic shape, and strike the body straight on. Certain types of ammunition are designed to deform on contact (e.g., soft point and hollow point rounds), and are often retained in the body, thereby creating maximum tissue damage. Other missiles may tumble within tissue, creating a similar effect. Other factors that affect the severity of wounds include the part of the body struck and the distance between the barrel and the victim. Missiles that have poor aerodynamic form (e.g., spheres), will lose their velocity over shorter distances than missiles that have good aerodynamic form. As a rule, metal jacketed bullets, especially those shot at high velocity, retain their aerodynamic form, and the impact velocity may approximate the muzzle velocity even at great distances (''high-powered rifles'').

Of concern in today's environment is the tendency toward the use of multiclip rapid-fire weapons that cause multiple wounds, often in close proximity to each other. The tissue destruction can be extensive. Forensic concerns dictate that evidence be preserved, including all clothing and any bullets that are lodged superficially or lying about the patient. It is often helpful to attempt to confirm entrance and exit wounds. Entrance wounds typically have round or oval margins with smooth, sometimes slightly stippled margins (Fig. 3). Powder burns around the wound suggest that the barrel of the weapon was close

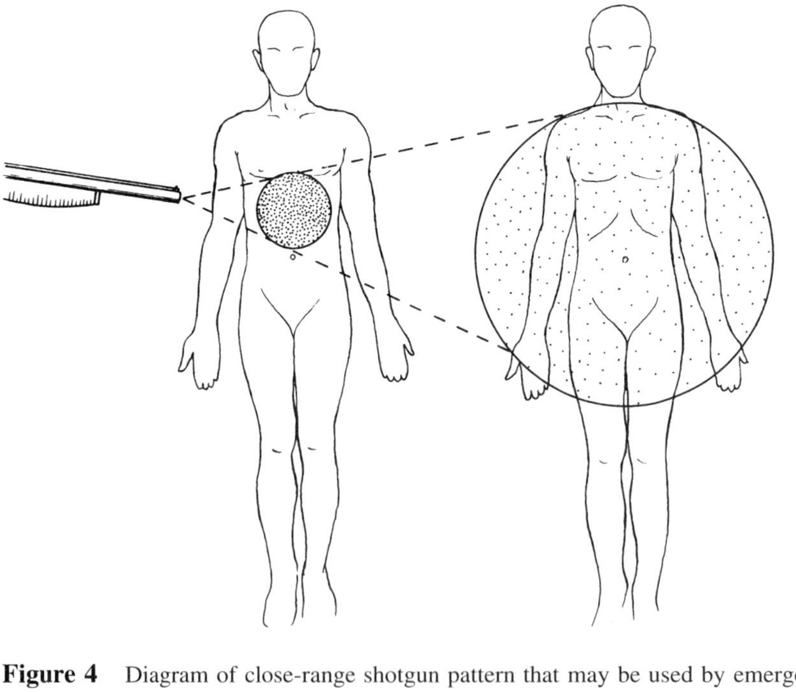

Figure 4 Diagram of close-range shotgun pattern that may be used by emergency personnel to estimate distance between gun and victim.

to or applied to the skin [6]. The exit wound will have none of these characteristics. Exit wounds may be the same size and shape as the entrance wounds or they may be larger, depending on missile deformity within the tissue. Regardless of the size or configuration of the wound(s), extensive internal damage may be done with little external evidence to alert the rescuer. The absence of an exit wound provides little clue to the nature of the internal injuries.

D. Shotgun Wounds

Injuries caused by shotguns can be highly lethal but are dependent on the distance between the victim and the barrel. At ranges over 15 yards (5 meters), the injury potential of shotguns begins to fall off rapidly. At close range (<4 ft or 1–1.5 meters) shotgun wounds can be devastating, creating extensive tissue loss, contamination, and early death. Pellets contained within shotgun shells show poor aerodynamics, but collectively have a large mass. If the distance between the perpetrator and the victim is not known, one can predict the wounding potential by measuring the spread of the shot pattern (Fig. 4). If the pattern of shot is confined within a small area, rescue personnel may assume a close-range wound and triage accordingly.

III. PATHOPHYSIOLOGY OF PENETRATING TRAUMA

Severe injury to vital organs usually results in death at the scene. Patients with penetrating wounds to the head, neck, heart, or pulmonary hilum, and great vessels in the thorax or abdomen may reach the hospital alive but require immediate operative intervention if they are deemed salvageable. In a review of scene deaths in Arizona, Meislin et al. noted that 60% were caused by firearms [7]. Death was immediate in most cases, emphasizing the important role of prevention in any strategy to decrease firearm deaths. The greatest immediate risk to the patient is exsanguination, which may be external or internal or exist in combination. If bleeding is strictly external (e.g., from a penetrating extremity wound), field personnel can readily estimate the severity of the hemorrhage, implement appropriate measures to control further blood loss, and begin volume replenishment. If bleeding is internal and ongoing, the patient will develop a dilutional anemia that reflects the physiologic response of shunting extracellular fluid into the intravascular space. Intracellular fluid passively moves out of the cells into the extracellular space and the cells build up an oxygen debt. This must be replaced within a certain period or the cells die [8]. While the trend toward a dilutional anemia begins immediately, in rapid response systems this phenomenon is more theoretical than real. Clinically, this preterminal period is recognized by a falling hematocrit and a rising base deficit. If the acidosis persists or worsens despite volume replenishment, the patient will likely die. In patients with bleeding that can effectively be controlled in the field, volume replenishment should begin as soon as possible without extending the prehospital phase of care. In these circumstances it is not unreasonable to initiate an intravenous infusion on the scene provided that intravenous access is achieved promptly. Delaying transport for multiple attempts at venous access is potentially harmful, especially since Lewis has shown that volumes of fluid infused en route to the hospital are inconsequential in systems with average transport times [9]. Despite difficulties with motion and restricted contact with the patient, intravenous lines should be started in the ambulance, and infusions of Ringer's lactate solution initiated. In general, hospital emergency personnel appreciate the advantage of having large-bore intravenous access arrive with the patient.

The role of prehospital volume infusions has been studied in victims of penetrating trauma with ongoing internal hemorrhage not amenable to prehospital control. The initial work by one of the authors (P.E.P.) has led to a growing body of knowledge based upon the assumption that hypotension may be a protective mechanism by curtailing further blood loss, limiting hemodilution, and promoting spontaneous clotting until definitive surgical control of bleeding can be accomplished in the operating room. Supporting this hypothesis is the recent finding that among hypotensive patients with penetrating torso wounds, those whose blood pressure was allowed to remain low by fluid restriction until the bleeding could be operatively controlled had better outcomes than a like group treated by traditional resuscitation [10].

In this context, the principles of prehospital care must be to preserve red cells (either at the scene by direct control of hemorrhage or by rapid evacuation to a trauma center for definitive operative control), saturate those red cells with oxygen, and circulate the saturated red cells to vital organs [11]. Patients fare far better with their own red blood cells than with massive transfusions. There thus appear to be two clear messages from these studies: hemostasis at the earliest possible moment is critical, and aggressive blood pressure elevation prior to the control of internal bleeding is detrimental [12].

A. Maximizing Oxygen Delivery: Preemptive Endotracheal Intubation

The importance of oxygenating the red blood cells is reflected in a study from Seattle in which 131 patients with prehospital cardiopulmonary arrest from trauma were studied [13]. Almost all the survivors were young, intubated, and had penetrating trauma. Almost all (90%) of the blunt victims died. The remarkable survival of 70% of the patients with penetrating wounds correlated with endotracheal intubation and the brevity of time to the trauma center. The penetrating wound in the survivors was typically a knife-induced injury, amenable to rapid hemorrhage control. In a similar study from Los Angeles, prehospital blunt and penetrating pulseless, unconscious patients were compared [14]. Survival was low in both groups: five out of 382 in the blunt group and four out of 497 in the penetrating group. All blunt survivors had poor neurologic outcomes. Three of the four penetrating survivors had stab wounds, all had electrical activity in the field, and neurologic outcomes were favorable.

Early intubation makes a difference because those who are apneic or in deep shock underinflate their lungs, leading to intrapulmonary shunting and critical hypoxemia and hemoglobin desaturation [15]. It is speculated that by providing high concentrations of oxygen through endotracheal intubation, the decreased volume of red cells is sufficiently oxygenated to provide the additional margin of cellular support needed to survive until definitive surgery can be carried out. Without endotracheal intubation, it is rare for any trauma victim to survive more than 5 min in an apneic, pulseless state, even with cardiopulmonary resuscitation.

IV. PENETRATING WOUNDS BY SITE

Like the disease cancer, the term trauma represents a number of different entities linked by a common response. Both trauma and cancer can be viewed as distinct entities with their own clinical findings. For trauma, these findings include injury mechanism, physiologic response, and site of injury. In considering penetrating trauma as the injury mechanism, it has already been demonstrated that there are significant differences between injuries caused by stabbing and those caused by other forms of penetrating trauma, especially gunshot wounds. It is also clear that the anatomic location of the penetration determines to a great extent both the survivability of the wound and whether or not long-term impairment is likely in those who do survive.

A. Head/Craniofacial

Scalp lacerations typically occur in the setting of blunt trauma, but can occur from knife slashings or cutting with glass bottles. The scalp is a highly vascular structure, and victims can quickly bleed to the point of hypotension. Control of scalp bleeding in the field is usually ineffective unless pressure is directly applied to the scalp at pressure points just beyond the laceration. The use of Raney clips is a simple, effective technique that should be available in every emergency facility [16] (Fig. 5). Their use in the field is as yet unreported in the literature.

Stab wounds about the head may gain entry into the cranium when they pass through the nose or orbits. The anterior fossa is particularly at risk, which may incur vascular injuries and neurologic deficits. Gunshot wounds to the head are particularly sensitive to missile velocity because of the inherent lack of elasticity of brain tissue and the volume expansion limitations imposed by the cranial vault. Further, bullets passing through the skull often carry bone fragments with them, which become secondary missiles. Sudden, exaggerated elevations in intracranial pressure (ICP) follow high-velocity impacts and may directly affect brain stem function [17]. Those who survive the initial insult commonly develop elevated ICP, which leads to their demise. Current thinking holds that any bullet wound that crosses the midline is incompatible with survival. Unless the bullet exits the skull, rescue personnel are unable to determine the immediate extent of intracranial involvement. Since the brain is highly sensitive to impaired perfusion and hypoxemia, the principle responsibility of prehospital rescue personnel is to prevent the secondary injuries from hypotension and/or hypoxia therefore, the field approach should be to vigorously resuscitate and support the patient in transit to the trauma center. If the wound proves

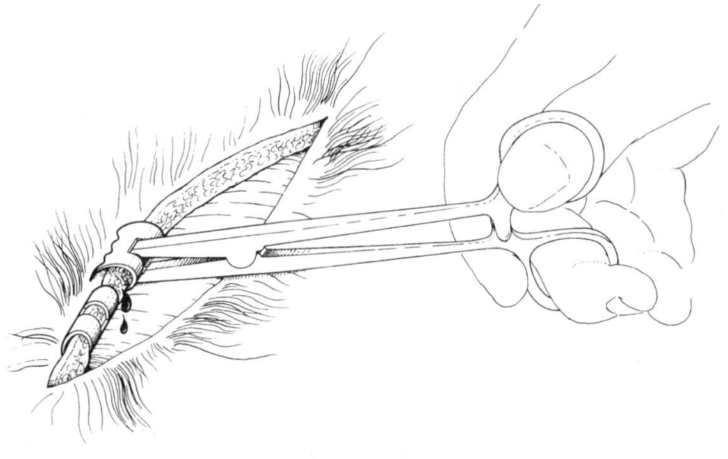

Figure 5 Depiction of means of applying Raney clips to hemorrhaging scalp laceration. (From Ref. 16, with permission.)

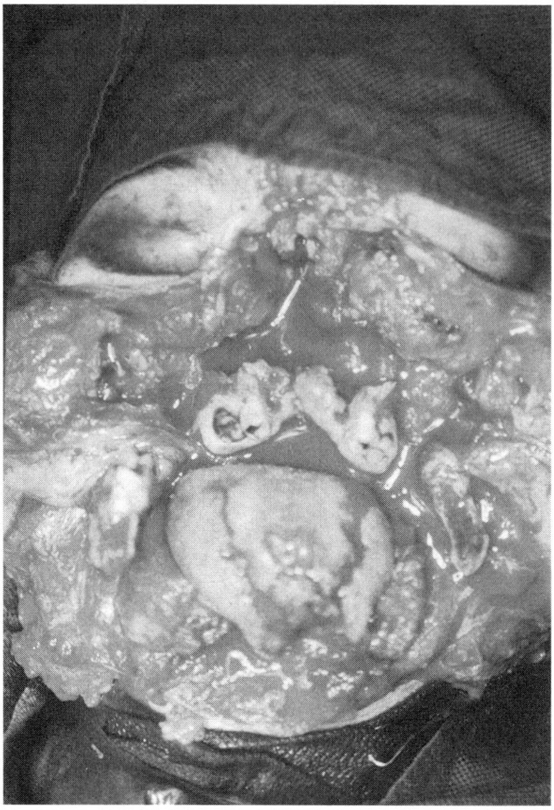

Figure 6 Facial wound showing extensive soft tissue destruction. (Courtesy of David B. Reath, M.D., Knoxville, TN.)

fatal, early efforts at resuscitation may reap benefits should the patient qualify as an organ donor. Wounds to the face may also impact bone or teeth, causing secondary missiles and increasing the soft tissue injury. Exsanguinating hemorrhage is a much greater risk with penetrating wounds of the face than with primary wounds to the cranium or brain. Penetrating injuries superior to the angle of the mandible may cause injury to the internal carotid artery just below the base of the skull and present an immediate threat to life from exsanguination. Self-inflicted gunshot or shotgun wounds to the face are often incurred when the individual places the barrel of the gun beneath the chin (Fig. 6). If the brain is spared, airway obstruction, massive hemorrhage, and soft tissue loss present the principal challenges [18].

B. Neck

Penetrating wounds to the neck often present challenging management problems in the field.

The *airway* may be directly injured or may be compromised by early and progressive neck swelling. The trachea is usually deviated to the side opposite the accumulating hematoma, leading to difficulty in intubation. There may be bleeding directly into the airway. Acute airway compromise may progress rapidly and impair ventilation.

Bleeding externally is also a potential problem. In addition to blood spreading through the soft tissues, the partial laceration of the carotid artery produces sustained pulsatile bleeding, causing hypovolemic shock. The *cervical spinal cord* may be injured, and if this injury is complete and above the third cervical vertebra, respiratory paralysis ensues. Cervical cord damage below the third cervical vertebra may spare portions of the phrenic nerves and allow some diaphragmatic excursion. Most of these patients will require assisted ventilations. Penetrating wounds to the *upper esophagus* or *hypopharynx* may produce significant intraoral accumulation of blood, especially if the patient's level of consciousness is impaired. If the patient cannot protect his or her airway, this must be recognized immediately and a definitive airway placed.

C. Thorax

Penetrating chest wounds range from the trivial, requiring no treatment, to the acutely life-threatening, in which airway placement and rapid transport to a trauma center offer the only potential of survival [19]. Significant thoracic injuries are accompanied by chest pain, respiratory distress, or both. Shock may rapidly follow. Possible injuries may involve the lungs, heart, or great vessels. There are three principle injuries that may be life-threatening and are of concern to prehospital rescue personnel: tension pneumothorax, pericardial tamponade, and massive hemothorax. Table 1 demonstrates that these entities are not always easy to distinguish. Simple (closed) pneumothorax or an open pneumothorax converted to a closed pneumothorax by the application of a dressing are not life-threatening and will not be further considered. While definitive management must await the patient's arrival at the hospital, placement of an airway is always indicated if the patient is having difficulty breathing. In most patients, this will enhance the chances of survival.

In patients with *tension pneumothorax*, however, endotracheal intubation and positive pressure ventilation may hasten the patient's demise. In this condition, air passes through a lung wound and overlying defect in the visceral pleura to fill the pleural space. The effects are not immediate and the intrapleural air must collect over time. With positive pressure ventilation, the process is accelerated. The lung on the affected side collapses but still allows air to escape into the pleural space. The opposite lung is compressed, leading to hypoxemia. More important, the elevation in intrapleural pressure interferes with venous return. With mediastinal shift, kinking of the great veins may occur, further compromising cardiac filling. The patient becomes hypotensive from low cardiac output, and in combination with hypoxemia, the patient may sustain a cardiopulmonary arrest.

Table 1 Comparison of Clinical Findings of Tension Pneumothorax and Pericardial Tamponade

Finding	Tension pneumothorax	Pericardial tamponade	Hemothorax
"In distress"	Yes	Yes	Yes
Hypotension	Yes	Yes	Yes
Potential for cardiac arrest	Yes	Yes	Yes
Distended neck veins	Yes	Yes	No
May occur with precordial wound	Yes	Yes	Yes
May occur with peripheral torso wound	Yes	Yes	Yes
Absent or diminished breath sounds	Yes	No	Yes
Tracheal deviation	Yes	No	No

Clinical tip-offs to the diagnosis include absent breath sounds on the affected side, distended neck veins, tracheal deviation to the side opposite the developing tension, and shock without other apparent cause. Unfortunately many of these patients have other potential causes of shock, especially if multiply wounded. Hypovolemic patients may not demonstrate distended neck veins, and in thick-necked individuals the trachea may not be palpable. Tension pneumothorax must be considered in any patient with a penetrating thoracoabdominal wound.

Treatment is by needle thoracostomy, which relieves the tension and allows equilibration between the intrapleural pressure and ambient pressure, a condition tolerated by most patients for the duration of prehospital transport. Eckstein and Suyehara studied field needle thoracostomy in Los Angeles [20]. In their series, 108 patients had thoracic needles placed in the field. Of this number, 96 were victims of penetrating trauma. Improvement was noted in 12 (12%), with objective improvement in vital signs in five patients. They concluded that needle thoracostomy improves outcome in a subset of patients with chest injuries. Schmidt et al. reported on the benefits of chest tube insertion by physicians in the field [21]. This German study, largely of blunt trauma, nonetheless confirmed the therapeutic effectiveness of prompt chest decompression for pneumothorax.

Pericardial tamponade may occur following any thoracoabdominal wound, depending on trajectory. When the wound is precordial, the possibility of tamponade is heightened. The pericardium is normally separated from the myocardium by a potential space that contains a small amount of serous fluid. If the heart is penetrated, blood will escape from the affected cardiac chamber and begin to fill the pericardial sac. The deleterious effect on hemodynamics is not immediate. There is a finite volume that the pericardial sac can accommodate before tamponade critically compromises the cardiac filling. As this threshold is reached, an additional small volume of pericardial blood significantly affects the amount of blood pumped by the heart and the patient develops profound hypotension and is at risk of dying. *Pericardiocentesis* has been used with mixed success, but in recent years has been discouraged. Problems with the technique relate to the difficulty in confirming needle or catheter placement, the clotting of pericardial blood and failure to aspirate, and the risk of injuring the heart, including the potential for coronary artery laceration.

Classically the diagnosis is made by inspecting the wound site and appreciating that the patient is at risk. Neck vein distention is the most reliable sign. Muffled heart sounds occur, but their significance is difficult to appreciate in the prehospital setting. At this time the best management is rapid transport to a facility staffed and equipped to intervene surgically since virtually all paitients with pericardial tamponade from penetrating wounds require operative management.

Massive hemothorax may arise from penetrating injury to any major vascular structure in the chest, including the heart, great vessels, lung, or internal mammary or intercostal vessels (Fig. 7). Clinical manifestations may be scant except for hypotension. If the hemithorax is filling with blood, the breath sounds may not be transmitted as well on the affected side, raising the suspicions of prehospital rescue personnel. It is important to recognize that massive hemothorax is a form of hypovolemic shock that cannot be effectively treated in the field. In this context, treatment measures described elsewhere in this chapter pertain, including oxygen enrichment, ''hypotensive resuscitation,'' and rapid transport. The prehospital placement of a tube thoracostomy is not indicated since it may release the limited form of tamponade, leading to exsanguination. Intravenous lines for volume infusion must be in place prior to evacuation of the hemothorax, which is best done at the hospital or in the operating room.

16. B Turnage, KI Maull. Scalp laceration: An obvious ''occult'' cause of shock. South Med J 93:265–266, 2000.
17. HA Crockard, FD Brown, LM Johns, S Mullan. An experimental cerebral missile injury in primates. J Neurosurg 46:776–783, 1977.
18. RB Fratianne, CS Cocanour. Exsanguinating craniofacial trauma. Adv Trauma Crit Care 7: 159–173, 1992.
19. AS Gervin, RP Fischer. The importance of prompt transport in salvage of patients with penetrating heart wounds. J Trauma 22:443–448, 1982.
20. M Eckstein, D Suyehara. Needle thoracostomy in the prehospital setting. Prehosp Emerg Care 2:132–135, 1998.
21. U Schmidt, M Stalp, T Gerich, M Blauth, KI Maull, H Tscherne. Chest tube decompression of blunt chest injuries by physicians in the field: Effectiveness and complications. J Trauma 44:98–101, 1998.
22. KI Maull, JW Snoddy, BW Haynes. Penetrating wounds of the buttock. Surg Gyn Ob 149: 855–877, 1979.
23. KL Mattox, WH Bickell, PE Pepe, J Burch, D Feliciano. Prospective MAST study in 911 patients. J Trauma 29:1104–1112, 1989.
24. KI Maull. Role of military antishock trousers. In: RR Ivatury, CG Cayten, eds. Textbook of Penetrating Trauma. Baltimore: Williams and Wilkins, 1996, pp. 170–175.
25. M Eckstein, K Alo. Effect of a quality improvement program on paramedic on-scene times for patients with penetrating trauma. Acad Emerg Med 6:191–195, 1999.
26. SI Koury, L Moorer, CK Stone, JS Stapczynski, SH Thomas. Air vs. ground transport and outcome in trauma patients requiring urgent operative interventions. Prehosp Emerg Care 2: 289–292, 1998.
27. KI Maull, TJ Esposito. Trauma system design. In: KL Mattox, DV Feliciano, EE Moore, eds. Trauma. New York: McGraw-Hill, 2000, pp. 57–68.

24

Prehospital Trauma Management of the Pediatric Patient

ALEKSANDRA J. MAZUREK

Children's Memorial Hospital and Northwestern University Medical School, Chicago, Illinois

PHILIPPE-GABRIEL MEYER

Hôpital-Necker Enfants Malades, Paris, France

GAIL E. RASMUSSEN

The Meridian Anesthesiology Group, Meridian, Mississippi

I. PEDIATRIC TRAUMA

A. Pediatric Injury Patterns

For children and teens injury is often part of the experience of growing up. Parents may sometimes wonder if indeed it is possible that children will survive to reach adulthood. Statistics worldwide show accidental injury to be the number one cause of death from the age of 1 to 25 years. It is also a major source of long-lasting disabilities. In many instances, children who sustain a severe traumatic injury will never regain social and developmental capabilities and will require extensive rehabilitation resources for the rest of their lives. Since as many as 50% of trauma deaths occur immediately at the scene, only the prevention of accidents can effectively decrease trauma morbidity and mortality. In Europe, as in North America, home is most often the setting for the accidents of childhood, but with the exception of burns, such accidents represent a small proportion of severe trauma. Although the home is the site of a majority of traumatic events for children and adults, the residential street is the most lethal environment [1].

In *urban* settings, falls from heights and accidents involving pedestrians struck by cars are the most frequent sources of severe trauma. Falls from heights account for 35% of accidents and occur mainly during the spring and summer among preschool children [2]. Thirty to 40% of accidents involve pedestrians who are struck by cars. These accidents occur primarily at the end of the school day among children older than 6 years of age. After 6 years of age, the severely injured child is most likely to be either a pedestrian hit by a car or an unrestrained passenger. Pediatric-aged passengers are less often injured severely in urban areas. The mandatory use of specific restraints and speed restrictions have decreased the incidence of severe head trauma. In *rural areas*, high-speed collisions are responsible for 15–20% of severe pediatric injuries. Most of the time they involve nonrestrained children who are thrown out of a vehicle or children who are improperly restrained with seat belts unsuitable for their size. Subsequent spinal cord injuries and head injuries are frequent and result in a high incidence of severe neurological disabilities [2,3]. Because farming and forest work in rural areas require the use of heavy machinery, there is always the potential for severe mutilating injuries, usually to the limbs.

Among other perils for toddlers is the possibility of death by *drowning*, most often in the family swimming pool, or by *choking* incidents. Choking is common at the age of 18 to 24 months when curiosity about the world is great and the easiest way to explore is by putting enticing objects in the mouth. The absence of molars and the immature coordination of swallowing and breathing leads to choking and aspiration of a foreign object into the airway. Current U.S. statistics, however, indicate a downward trend in the death rate from choking since the 1980s, perhaps because of effective educational campaigns conducted by physicians, the food industry, and toy manufacturers. A similar downward trend has been noted in the drowning rate [4].

Among preteens and teens, *bicycle* injuries are more prevalent in boys (10:1) than in girls aged 10 to 13 years. In the absence of uniform bicycle helmet laws in the United States, when head injuries occur, they are serious. Australians have decreased the frequency and severity of head injuries from bicycle accidents by 80% by instituting mandatory helmet laws. Inventions such as in-line skates or all-terrain vehicles add new patterns of injuries, most often involving males. It has been suggested that the competitive and daring natures of adolescent boys as well as raging hormonal storms may be factors [5,6].

A striking difference exists between the United States and Western Europe in the area of intentional injuries to children. *Gunshot and stab wounds* are anecdotal in the pediatric population in Europe, and except for sporadic cases, are accidental. Blunt trauma accounts for more than 98% of the cases of injury to children. The uniquely American phenomenon—gunshot injuries in children—is worth separate mention. Practically unlimited access to all kinds of weapons in the United States fosters criminal activity, accidents, and suicides. Gunshot-related deaths are the domain of 15 to 18 year olds. The latest available statistics indicate that there were 34,040 firearm deaths in the United States in 1996. Of those who died, 9,459 were 24 years old or younger (Table 1). Although rural settings are not free of guns, the incidence of gun-related deaths there is much lower than in cities.

The clinical entity of *child abuse* was first acknowledged in the United States in the 1960s; it is still to be acknowledged in many other corners of the world. The growing bank of information on the subject places the burden on the physicians and other health care workers and teachers to recognize child abuse and deal with the consequences of making the diagnosis [7]. Physical violence in any form leaves psychological wounds as well as physical marks in children of all ages. To treat only the body is not enough. Equal

Table 1 Deaths from Firearms in the United States (1996)

Age (years)	Number of deaths
<1	11
1–4	77
5–14	605
15–24	8,766

Source: Adapted from National Vital Stat. Rep. 47(9), 1998.

effort should be directed to healing the psychological scars of injured children. In spite of the proven need for such treatment, contemporary society is not always prepared to finance support for healing the after effects of violence, which are intangible and not easily measured. It is up to us to learn more through research and to educate the public and the government about this need.

B. Children Versus Adult Trauma Victims

1. Pathophysiology

Children have anatomic features that put them at risk for specific injuries [8]. The volume of a child's head is disproportionately large for the rest of the body, and the cervical muscles are weak. Protective reflexes such as putting the arms forward during a fall are absent in small children. For these reasons, the head is the most frequently injured region of the body in children with trauma. Head trauma can be present in more than 80% of those severely injured. In children, the skull is thinner and cerebral myelin, which is an efficient protective layer for long neural fibers, is less developed, leading to more frequent diffuse axonal injuries. The rise of intracranial pressure is more frequent and rapid. In severe trauma, a child's brain is more prone than an adult's to impaired cerebral vasoreactivity, which leads to diffuse vasodilatation and brain swelling in the early phase following trauma [9].

The weakness of the *respiratory muscles* in children decreases the ability to adapt ventilation to increased respiratory demand. Respiratory distress in severely traumatized children may be present before resuscitation in as many as 45%. Apart from its direct life-threatening consequences, when respiratory distress is not recognized and properly treated it may cause secondary brain injury [10].

Direct *abdominal trauma* results mainly in spleen and liver injuries, which are generally amenable to conservative treatment. The adipose tissue of the abdominal wall, efficient for the dissipation of kinetic energy, is thin and does not protect the abdominal organs against a direct impact. Pelvic and thoracic bone structure is not sufficiently developed in children to act effectively as a natural bumper. Indirect lesions resulting from deceleration forces are less frequent and more difficult to assess. A blunt intestinal injury is found in less than 10% of children with abdominal trauma, but the incidence may exceed 50% in improperly restrained occupants of a vehicle involved in a high-speed collision.

Although children are also susceptible to thoracic injuries, rib fractures are infrequent. The energy that is not absorbed at the level of the chest wall will dissipate easily in the parenchymal structures and may result in severe pulmonary and cardiac contusions in more than 30% of severely injured children, even without evidence of rib fractures. Finally, hemothorax may result in rapid mediastinal compression that must be relieved quickly [2].

Orthopedic injuries are most frequently associated with severe trauma. Except for complex pelvic ring dislocations, which are very unusual, bone injuries do not usually result in significant blood loss or endanger the life of a traumatized child.

II. RESUSCITATION AND THE INITIAL MANAGEMENT OF TRAUMA

Pediatric cardiac arrest, unlike that of an adult, is rarely a primary event and rarely originates in the heart. More commonly a respiratory event leads to hypoxic cardiac arrest. Airway obstruction, possible at various levels, is responsible for the final critical event. The initiation of cardiopulmonary resuscitation (CPR) in injured children is no different from that in adults and follows the advanced trauma life support (ATLS) algorithm from A to E. The notable exception is the relative ease for developing hypothermia that increases with diminishing patient size. In the prehospital environment heat loss should be a priority; since active heating cannot be undertaken until the patient is in a controlled environment, preventive measures must begin on the scene of injury.

The management of a child's airway presents a challenge, even to a highly skilled health provider, when those skills have been applied primarily to treating adults. A lack of familiarity with the various pieces of equipment required for the airway management of children and the small size of the patient are sources of stress for the caregiver and may cause life-threatening complications. A toddler's neck is short, the tongue is large and posteriorly positioned, the larynx is situated high in the neck, and the head is large in proportion to the rest of the body, making laryngoscopy more difficult. Upper airway obstruction is more frequent in children than in adults when the level of consciousness is depressed [11]. In infants and young children an airway may be obstructed by the collapse of abundant soft tissue in the upper airway (pharyngeal collapse) and/or the presence of enlarged tonsils and adenoids. Obstruction may occur after fluctuation in the level of consciousness or swelling of soft tissues. The airway is usually opened by positioning the head chin up, performing a jaw thrust, and most important, applying positive pressure ventilation. Application of 5 to 7 cm H_2O of positive pressure can open a child's airway. To perform this maneuver effectively, one must be trained and maintain the skill. It is recommended that emergency medical service (EMS) personnel undergo continuous refresher training in pediatric resuscitation to sustain their skills and confidence. This laudable goal, however, is rarely attained [12]. In the United States, emergency medical technicians (EMTs) and paramedics attend to children in only 10% of their cases; therefore they have fewer opportunities to practice their professional skills on children than on adults.

Fewer attempts at prehospital emergency tracheal intubation (ETI) are made in children than in adults, even in children with no vital signs. When pediatric intubation is performed in the field by paramedics, only 25% of children with trauma who require ETI are successfully intubated. Intubation is delayed until arrival at the hospital in 50–75% of cases, and the success rate ranges from 7–42% [13–16]. Life-threatening complications that result directly from ETI attempts in the field have been reported in as many as 25% of all cases. In one study in Pennsylvania, only 9% of children intubated at the scene or in a local hospital received adequate drugs before intubation [15]. Attempts at ETI without first administering drugs may explain the high incidence of unsuccessful ETI reported in the literature. Indications for ETI in the field include head trauma with a score on the Glasgow coma scale of (GCS) ≤ 8, or in a combative and restless patient with a rapidly deteriorating level of consciousness. Additional indications, determined on an individual basis, are severe associated facial or chest trauma and airway obstruction.

The role of airway adjuncts is limited in securing oxygenation in children. The Combitube and the esophageal obturator or similar devices have no application in children because they are made only in adult sizes. The laryngeal mask airway (LMA), on the other hand, comes in a variety of sizes to fit any child. This device is rapidly gaining a reputation as a rescue method in establishing a clear airway and is included in American Society of Anesthesiologists' difficult airway algorithm. Its use in the field has not yet been approved in the United States.

According to advanced cardiac life support (ACLS) principles, the trachea is intubated in the field when necessary. Once it has been determined that tracheal intubation is indicated, proper sedation/analgesia is mandatory. In our experience, the risks of regurgitation, aspiration of gastric contents, laryngospasm, increased intracranial pressure during laryngoscopy, and airway trauma must be ever-present concerns for those treating pediatric trauma patients, all of whom are considered to have "a full stomach." A protocol used at Children's Memorial Hospital in Chicago includes a hypnotic (thiopental 1–5 mg/kg or only lidocaine 1–2 mg/kg); midazolam for anxiolysis; ketamine 1 to 2 mg/kg for hypovolemic patients; a short-acting, nondepolarizing muscle relaxant: rocuronium 1.2 mg/kg or suxamethonium 2 mg/kg; and a short-acting opioid (fentanyl 1–2 μg/kg) [17]. At Necker Hospital in Paris, the protocol for drug administration for ETI includes flunitrazepam 0.025 to 0.05 mg/kg or midazolam 0.1 to 0.25 mg/kg, fentanyl citrate 0.001 to 0.005 mg/kg or sufentanil 0.0003 mg/kg, and vecuronium 0.2 mg/kg. Ketamine may be used as an induction agent (1–2 mg/kg) when there is no head injury. These techniques must be only used by trained personnel who are capable of rapidly controlling the child's airway and who are knowledgeable of the drug pharmacology. The need for *analgesia or sedation* continues during transportation of mechanically ventilated children. Physicians with expertise in pediatric anesthesiology and resuscitation, certified nurse anesthesist (CRNA) and PICU nurses, and to a lesser extent paramedics with clinical experience of pediatric resuscitation under direct supervision of a physician, are qualified in this area.

The frequency of attempted and failed awake intubation in the field may also reflect difficulty in obtaining IV access in children. Gaining emergency venous access is often very difficult or not possible for untrained personnel. The best success rate for pediatric IV access reported in the field in the United States is 68%; this number declines to 49% in children younger than 6 years of age [18]. Intraosseous (IO) infusion has been proposed as the first-line alternative for the administration of drugs and emergency fluid loading [19,20]. This method for vascular access is suitable primarily for small children.

Tracheal intubation should be as atraumatic and as rapid as possible. *In-line stabilization* of the cervical spine must be maintained constantly during intubation, and flexion or rotation movements must be avoided. The oral route is preferred until a basal skull fracture has been ruled out and the airway has been secured. After careful preoxygenation, external cricoid pressure is maintained until the endotracheal tube has been successfully placed in the trachea. Controlled ventilation is then employed and adjusted during transport according to feedback from pulse oximetry and capnography monitors. The goal is to secure normoxia and normocarbia ($PaCO_2$) between 32 to 35 mmHg (4.2–4.6 kPa). To assure effective ventilation of a child's lungs, continuous IV sedation is needed. Gastric decompression by means of an orogastric tube is always used. Tension pneumothorax has to be ruled out promptly, especially in children whose lungs are being mechanically ventilated. If a pneumothorax is present, needle evacuation or an emergency thoracostomy should be performed by the field physician prior to transport of the child, especially when air transport is required. Among 188 consecutive head-injured children admitted to Necker Hospital in Paris over 2 years, as many as 78% of the severely traumatized children were intubated in the field. This number increased to 98% in children with the most serious injuries and reflected the liberal indications for prehospital ETI. Although junior physicians did experience difficulties with intubation in the field, failed attempts or life-threatening complications from field intubation were rare. An endobronchial intubation was the most frequent complication, occurring in approximately 18% of cases. The main problem with field intubation was the underuse of drugs to facilitate it; 12% of children were emergently intubated without prior administration of drugs, and 67% of them experienced immediate reactions to laryngoscopy (e.g., coughing, hypertension, tachycardia). Inadequate administration of drugs was more likely to happen in the hands of less experienced physicians [21]. A similar experience was reported from medical teams from the Helsinki area [22].

In the United States pediatric field intubations by paramedics were associated with a high failure/morbidity rate. In several studies the combined field, referring hospital, and children's hospital emergency department intubations had a 31% complication rate [5,23]. With growing awareness of the difficulty of the task and increasing frequency of the use of IV drugs to facilitate intubation, recent results are more optimistic [12,13,24].

A. Triage and Field Decisions: Scoop-and-Run or Stay-and-Stabilize

Based on the Korean and Vietnam War experiences, the North American triage philosophy calls for swift patient transfer to the most competent medical facility (a level 1 trauma center) rather than time-consuming resuscitation and stabilization before transport. The time between the accident and arrival at the emergency room, at which critical care can be initiated, is the first variable used for predicting the quality of the outcome [25]. One current opinion is that "any hospital is a better hospital than an ambulance." Management at the scene delays the time to definitive care, may increase blood loss from a penetrating injury, and may be deleterious instead of beneficial to the patient [26]. Only lifesaving maneuvers are performed in the field by emergency personnel in the United States tracheal intubation, IV access, and CPR (ACLS)—a triage philosophy often referred to as "scoop-and-run." Scoop-and-run is particularly applicable to pediatric patients, who as a rule make prehospital caregivers (emergency medical technicians [EMTs], paramedics) uneasy. For instance, in one urban area, for each 20 adult intubations there was only one pediatric intubation [27]. Children come in various sizes, and so does the equipment suitable for them, which may be unfamiliar to many paramedics. In some cases, because of the low frequency of pediatric trauma, the proper equipment for treating children may be missing from the ambulance. The literature examining the management of comatose children by *prehospital medical teams* demonstrates that the principles for prehospital advanced life support (ALS) should not be *routinely* applied. Instead, minimal basic life support (BLS) management is employed at the scene and the patient is rapidly transported to the first hospital at which ALS can be initiated [28–30].

In the European approach, the rule is to bring the critical care capabilities of the hospital and the expertise of a physician to the scene of the accident. In this philosophy, mobile intensive care unit (MICU) crew members must be professionals with special training and expertise. Because of the high cost and limited availability of trained teams, decisions to send MICUs to the scene of accidents are under tight medical control.

One difference between the application of ALS principles in North America and in Europe is that gaining venous access is considered a priority of management *in the field*. Although gaining venous access is more difficult in children than in adults, in our experience (Paris) a team consisting of a physician and a qualified nurse makes it feasible in most cases. All severely injured children brought to our trauma center had established venous access. A similar experience has been reported in other European countries [2,22]. In the hands of field physicians, a more unconventional external jugular vein catheterization or central venous access through the femoral or internal jugular veins is more often successfully employed and carries less morbidity [31]. By contrast, in the United States, in children less than 18 months of age IV access is gained in only 30% and not attempted in 70%. Intraosseous infusion has become an excellent and accepted alternative and is already improving the rate of successful IV infusions [18,32]. The prevention of hypoventilation is the major goal for the initial management of severe head trauma. Chest injury can be present in as many as 30% of children who have sustained a high-energy impact. The combined deleterious effects of hypoventilation from depressed consciousness and of lung injuries or oxygenation contribute to the development of secondary brain injury, which are especially associated with hypotension. The risk in normotensive and normoxic children is approximately 22% [10]; hypotension and/or hypoxia upon admission quadruples the risk of mortality in children. The correlation between initial hypoxemia and the severity of disabilities or survival has been noted, but because of the vast differences among the protocols used and the small number of patients included in studies of pediatric trauma, an analysis of the direct influence of prehospital treatment on morbidity and mortality is difficult. Sophisticated at-the-scene management is mainly beneficial for children who are less severely injured and in whom mortality is prevented by such prompt management. Of children intubated in the field, 90% reach the hospital with normoxia and normo- or slight hypocarbia. Mechanical ventilation should be initiated early and closely monitored [33].

In the scoop-and-run philosophy, triage principles are derived from those of the battlefield. Children are managed minimally at the scene, promptly removed from the field, and transported to the first hospital for aggressive care. Secondary interhospital transportation is then arranged if further specialized management is required. The "stay-and-stabilize" philosophy has been derived from the experience of civilian trauma, in which blunt trauma is predominant. In these situations, the need for prompt transportation to the operating room for emergency surgical hemostasis of bleeding lesions is infrequent because wounds are not caused by gunshot or stabbing. Critical care management is initiated at the scene before direct transportation to a tertiary care center. When the anticipated transport time for an unstable child is long, a stop at the nearest hospital for stabilization and minimal exploration may be preferred [34]. Whatever the philosophy of transport is, common triage guidelines can be drawn for definitive care. A brief example of these guidelines is found in Table 2, along with the elements to be considered in rating the severity of pediatric trauma.

Table 2 Medical Triage Scheme for Pediatric Trauma

- Elements of severity
  - Accident-related
    - Mechanism of the accident
      - High-speed pedestrian/motor vehicle accident (>40 km/hr)
      - Fall from height (>3 meters)
      - Unrestrained victims of high-speed motor vehicle accident
      - Penetrating or crush injuries
    - Associated factors
      - Prolonged extrication (15 min or more)
      - Ejection from motor vehicle or projection
      - High-energy impact with other severely injured victims
  - Patient-related
    - Primary lesions
      - Severe head injury or spinal injury plus neurological deficit
      - Multiple injuries or extensive explorations required
      - Age less than 5 years
- Estimated severity
  - Glasgow coma scale equal to or less than 8, pediatric trauma score less than 7
- Medical dispatching principles
  - If stable after scene management, direct transport to trauma center
  - If unstable, direct prompt transport to trauma center whenever possible
  - Scoop-and-run for rapid evaluation at the next available hospital; plan secondary interhospital transfer

There is no proven evidence in the literature that either type of management increases the survival and improves the functional outcome. For obvious ethical reasons randomized studies cannot be designed in this area.

B. Analgesia for Trauma

Trauma is a major source of pain, which is aggravated by fear and anxiety. Treating children with pain is often neglected in many prehospital situations. Extrication maneuvers, manipulations, and transport add painful stimuli in children who may already be suffering from bone fractures and other injuries. Analgesia and/or sedation are frequently indicated during trauma scene management before transport. Minor analgesics, such as paracetamol, have limited effects and application in this setting. The equipment to administer anesthetic gases is cumbersome, and nitrous oxide is contraindicated in the presence of a child's potentially expanding pneumothorax.

Regional anesthesia can be an attractive alternative to the use of opioids. A femoral nerve block using 1% lidocaine (maximum dose 5 mg/kg) can be performed safely and rapidly, requires only minimal training, and provides good analgesia for femoral shaft fractures. Brachial plexus nerve block by the axillary approach and many other peripheral nerve blocks can be used in the field by *qualified individuals*, particularly in case of limb entrapment or prolonged extrication.

Patients with multiple trauma suffer from stressful, painful stimuli which, apart from creating unacceptable pain, can aggravate life-threatening lesions. Some indications for the need to administer general anesthesia in the field are prevention of an acute rise in intracranial pressure in patients with severe head trauma who require endotracheal intubation and controlled ventilation, severe pain from extensive or multiple fractures or crush injuries, and predictable prolonged extrication from a crash site. At the scene, various degrees of sedation may be provided with hypnotics such as benzodiazepines or etomidate. Low doses of fentanyl (1–3 μg/kg) or sufentanil (0.3 μg/kg) offer efficient analgesia with minimal cardiovascular adverse effects. Benzodiazepines such as midazolam (0.1–0.3 mg/kg) or flunitrazepam (0.015–0.03 mg/kg) may be used in combination with analgesics. Because of dose-dependent ventilatory depression and the risk of thoracic rigidity (especially in young children), the use of these drugs must be restricted to personnel who can intubate a child immediately and provide adequate monitoring and precise drug titration. Physicians with training in anesthesiology, certified nurse anesthetists, and to a lesser extent, medical technicians with specific training in pediatric resuscitation who are directly supervised by an experienced physician are qualified for these techniques. The undesirable cardiovascular effects associated with benzodiazepines are frequently mild in children, and these drugs effectively prevent early posttraumatic seizures after head trauma.

III. SHOCK AND RESUSCITATION IN PEDIATRIC TRAUMA

A. Recognition of Shock

One of the major difficulties in pediatric resuscitation is the recognition of shock in the trauma patient. Once identified, shock requires timely intervention to enhance successful management. Pediatric trauma patients differ from their adult counterparts in their ability to maintain an adequate heart rate and blood pressure in spite of a large intravascular volume deficit. Heart rate and blood pressure in traumatized children are thus relatively insensitive measures of shock. A blood-volume deficit may continue untreated up until the point of circulatory collapse and cardiopulmonary arrest. Signs that herald hypotension and bradycardia in adult patients may not be observed in children until 40–50% of circulating blood volume has been lost. Once this point has been reached, effective resuscitative efforts may be difficult. Resuscitation may be hindered not only by a failure to recognize the severity of shock, but also by the inability to gain adequate access to circulation in patients with intense peripheral vasoconstriction [35].

Especially in the prehospital setting, the primary and secondary evaluation of a pediatric patient must integrate a constellation of clinical findings to lead to timely recognition of shock and hasten its treatment. The nature and extent of the traumatic insult must be considered with respect to the clinical status of the child. To recognize shock and abnormal vital signs, the provider must first be familiar with the normal range of pediatric vital signs for a patient's age group (Table 3). Because a child can maintain blood pressure in the face of substantial blood-volume loss, one must be able to identify tachycardia as one of the first signs of hemorrhagic shock. To treat it effectively and recognize this situation promptly and immediately, several clinical variables (Tables 4 and 5) must be integrated on initial assessment in the field.

B. Venous Access

Venous access is a major challenge in pediatric trauma patients. The most likely sites for rapid cannulation in a pediatric patient are the antecubital veins or the saphenous veins. The site selection is determined by the location of the traumatic injury. If peripheral access fails, which is common because a child may be intensely vasoconstricted after injury, then

Table 3 Normal Range of Vital Signs for Pediatric Patients

Age	Weight (kg)	Systolic blood pressure (mmHg)	Heart rate (beats/min)
Newborn	3	60	170–180
6 months	5–6	70	160–170
1 year	10	80	150
4 years	15	80	120
6 years	20–30	80–100	100
10 years	30–35	80–120	90

Source: Ref. 46.

Table 4 Blood-Volume Loss and Clinical Signs of Shock

Blood-volume loss	Clinical signs of shock
Up to 20%	CV: slightly elevated HR, weak, thready pulses CNS: irritable and combative Renal: decreased urine output Integument: cool to touch, capillary refill 2–3 sec
Approximately 25%	CV: tachycardia, thready, distal pulses CNS: confusion, lethargy Renal: decreased urine output to minimal Integument: cold extremities, mottled, cyanotic
Up to 40%	CV: hypotension, tachycardia can degenerate to bradycardia and asystole CNS: comatose, posturing Renal: no urine output Integument: cold, cyanotic, pale

Table 5 Clinical Variables in the Assessment of Shock

Primary
- Adequacy of oxygenation and ventilation
- Heart rate
- Blood pressure
- Capillary refill: normal less than 2 sec
- Differential pulses: central versus peripheral
- Level of consciousness
- Hypothermia

Secondary
- Urinary output: desired 0.5–1 ml/kg/hr
- Oxygen saturation
- Acid-base status
- Central venous pressure measurements

other approaches should be attempted. In a prehospital setting (in the United States) central venous access may not be attempted as it would be in a hospital or emergency room setting or in Europe, but catheterization of deep veins such as the femoral or jugular with short over-the-needle catheters could be a valuable alternative for qualified individuals. The external jugular vein, though, remains the favorite for many prehospital practitioners. The next quickest alternative is the IO route (Figs. 1 and 2). The Pediatric Advanced Life Support curriculum recommends that "during CPR in children 6 years old or younger, intraosseous access should be established if reliable venous access cannot be achieved within three attempts or 90 seconds, whichever comes first" [20,36,37]. This technique is performed by using a short needle with a cannulated tip to enter the vascular marrow cavity of bone. The most common site chosen is the anterior tibial surface just below the tibial tuberosity (Fig. 1). One then angles the needle away from or distal to the epiphyseal growth plate at the knee. Aspiration of bone marrow confirms proper needle placement, as does easy infusion of a test dose of fluids. Any IV agent that is used in resuscitation can be given via a properly placed IO line. The learning curve to place an IO line is relatively short. The IO route may be used under the extreme circumstances usually found at an accident scene; however, an IO line should not remain in place for more than 6 hr. It is a temporary measure to access the circulation and begin resuscitation until a more permanent route can be established. It should be noted that insertion of the IO needle can be very painful in a conscious child. Among the few contraindications to this technique the most crucial is that an IO line is not placed in a fractured extremity in which the marrow space may have been disrupted or in patients with osteogenesis imperfecta whose bones may crack and fracture easily. In these patients the standard IV route is the only alternative.

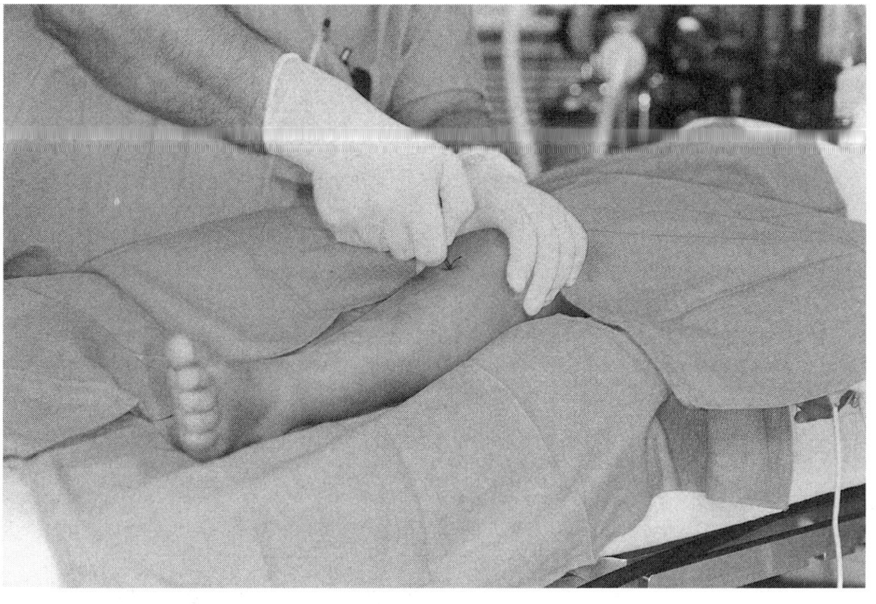

Figure 1 Insertion of intraosseous needle.

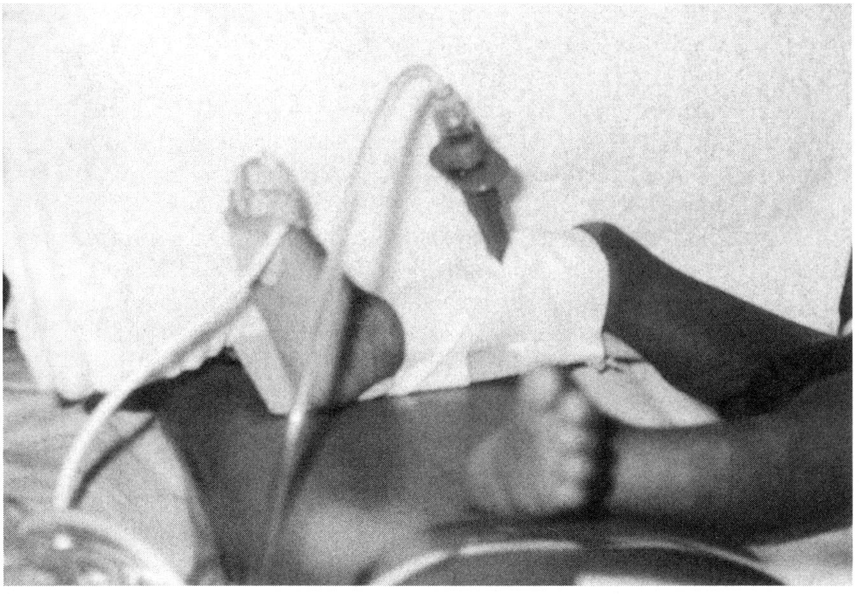

Figure 2 Intraosseous needle in situ.

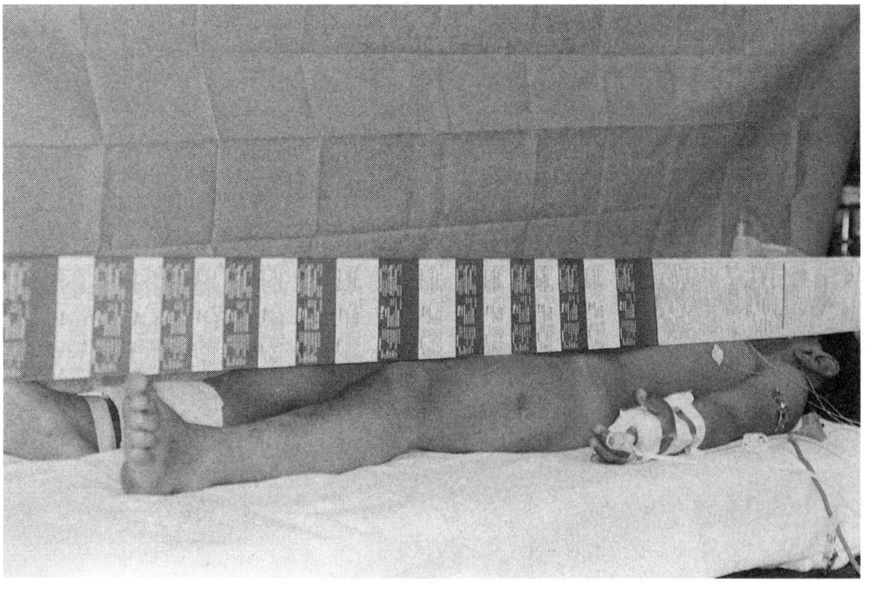

Figure 3 BROSELOW™ pediatric emergency tape.

C. Fluid Management

Appropriate therapy in treating a pediatric patient in shock is to begin with a bolus of 20 ml/kg of crystalloid solution such as lactated Ringer's, plasmalyte, or normal saline. This volume may be given as a bolus up to three times, with reassessment of the status of heart rate or blood pressure between each bolus. In patients who sustain burn injuries, a greater volume of fluid resuscitation may be required. Depending on the percentage of body surface area burned, the initial volume needed may be 30 to 40 ml/kg infused as fast as possible.

In the prehospital setting, crystalloids are used and are universally available. Colloids are reserved for large-volume resuscitations—for burn patients, for example—or as a second-line fluid for resuscitation. There has been recent interest in the use of hypertonic saline solutions (3–7.5%) for use in initial low-volume resuscitation. Approximately 4 ml/kg of a hypertonic solution can increase circulating blood volume equivalent to an increase after 30 ml/kg of standard crystalloid solutions. The advantage of hypertonic saline solutions in pediatric patients may become more pronounced because the lack of adequate venous access hinders the ability to conduct large-volume resuscitation. The need for a much smaller resuscitation volume with hypertonic solutions to adequately affect circulating blood volume is potentially advantageous in the pediatric trauma population [38] (see Sec. IV.E). Hypertonic resuscitation should only be used by individuals trained in its use.

One other difficult aspect of managing pediatric trauma is the need to estimate the age or weight of a child before resuscitation. An advance in this area are length-based measuring tapes (Fig. 3), which estimate the patient's weight, drug doses, and size of emergency equipment (e.g., endotracheal tubes). One simply measures the child from head to foot and the tape estimates a weight based on the length. Some tapes have calculations for resuscitative drugs and endotracheal tube size based on estimated weight, while others are color coded to correspond to resuscitation kits for various weights. This type of tape has taken some of the guesswork out of initial resuscitation and eliminates the delays caused by estimating the size or weight of a child [39].

IV. HEAD INJURY IN CHILDREN

A. Incidence and Severity

Children with head injury represent almost 80% of severely injured children. They are particularly at risk for pathophysiological changes during the initial phase of management. Of the immediate threats to life after trauma, secondary brain injury is the first. It is impossible to reverse the primary damage from direct application of mechanical forces at the time of the initial impact, but an injured brain is highly susceptible to additional insults such as hypoxemia and hypoperfusion during the first minutes and hours following trauma. Every systemic adverse event, including hypotension, hypoxia, induced osmotic edema, and hypercarbia, may contribute to secondary lesions and adversely affect outcome. Because the quality of care rendered during initial management has the most impact on outcome there is a rational basis for aggressive care of head trauma victims [10,40]. The goals of early medical management are twofold.

To rapidly evaluate the severity of the head injury and the potential for further deterioration

To initiate critical care as soon as possible to avoid secondary brain insults, such as hypoxemia and hypotension

In an analysis of deaths in traumatized children transferred to a referral center, it was found that 30% of deaths might have been avoided by prompt evaluation and management of brain, abdominal, or chest injuries to prevent acute cardiac decompensation. Severe physiological change, if untreated, may lead to secondary insults on the vital organs. These changes are more likely to occur in the early phase following trauma and during transportation, particularly in patients who were unstable before transport. A significant relationship between the incidence of physiologic deterioration and increased severity of illness during interhospital transport has been reported. Secondary brain insults caused by hypoxemia, cerebral hypoperfusion or expanding mass lesion, shock related to unrecognized or inadequately treated hemorrhage, and acute respiratory failure caused by undiagnosed airway obstruction were the main causes of potentially preventable deaths and a major source of long-term disabilities [28,41]. The influence of early management on the prevention of secondary insults has been illustrated. As many as 53 of 100 children who died from trauma could have been saved with an optimally functioning emergency medical system. Errors in the management of children who could have been saved occurred at the scene in 36%, during transport in 23%, and during definitive care in 17%. The medical rescue of a traumatized child in the field often depends on the emergency system in the city or rural area in which the trauma has taken place [42]. The key to adequate management is early intervention and aggressive care.

Diffuse lesions occur twice as often in children as in adults. They are frequent in victims of high-energy impact. Brain swelling, which results from acute increased cerebral blood flow secondary to cerebral vasodilation, is a common first response of a child's brain to severe insult. In many series, the mortality rate is more than 50%, or three times that for children with other lesions [9]. Although the most frequent cause of rapidly increasing intracranial pressure is brain swelling or diffuse cerebral edema in children older than 6 years, an acute intracranial hematoma requiring emergent surgical evacuation must be ruled out whatever a child's age.

B. Cervical Spine Injury

Vertebral and spinal cord injuries are rare in children who survive severe trauma. Pediatric cases represent 7–15% of spinal cord injuries [43]. In toddlers and small children, the large volume of the head and the weakness of the cervical muscles put the upper cervical spine at particular risk for severe lesions. A classical source of error in the overdiagnosis of upper cervical lesions is the observation of a ''false'' cervical dislocation at the level of $C_{2\text{-}3}$ and C_7-T_1 that is physiological in children younger than 3 years of age. Spinal lesions, which are frequently associated with head injuries, carry a high risk of mortality or severe neurological disability in those who survive. A protocol for evaluation of the cervical spine appears in Table 6. It should be emphasized that complaint of *neck pain is a hallmark of cervical injury*. In children older than 3 years of age involved in high-speed motor vehicle collisions, burst fractures of thoracic vertebra (Chance fracture) can be associated with severe spine injuries and intestinal tears resulting from deceleration forces. Burst fractures must be systematically ruled out. Whatever the age of the child, spinal cord injury without radiological evidence (SCIWORA) of lesions is difficult to diagnose and frequently results in severe neurological deficits. Spinal cord injury is particularly difficult to recognize in the presence of coma. A high degree of suspicion of such

Table 6 Protocol for Evaluation of the Cervical Spine

1. Any child who comes in having suffered trauma and who has a Glasgow coma score of 8 or less or evidence of a severe force of trauma either by history or examination, needs to have the cervical spine cleared at some stage.
2. Children over the age of 13 years are biomechanically adults from a cervical spine point of view and can be considered to have a cleared C spine if C_1 to C_7 is intact on lateral C-spine X-ray.
3. Under the age of 13 years, an intact lateral C spine is not considered sufficient. Because of the danger of ligamentous injury without bony injury, a child must either (1) be awake and verbalize that he or she has no neck pain or (2) have adequate flexion-extension neck X-rays performed with a neurosurgical house officer present. The X-rays must be read by an attending radiologist or attending neurosurgeon prior to being ''cleared.''
4. Children who are intubated and cannot be moved for flexion-extension pictures, or who are too sick to be moved for flexion-extension pictures because they complain of neck pain or are not able to do so, will have their hard collars changed to fitted cervical collars within 24 hr.
5. Every effort will be made to evaluate the status of the neck of a child who is going to the operating room. It may well happen that children are ''not cleared'' before surgery, but that will be only because it was not possible to clear them with certainty, not because efforts were not made to do so.

Source: Committee on Trauma, Children's Memorial Hospital, Chicago, 1999.

an injury should prompt an emergency evaluation with magnetic resonance imaging. Although spinal cord injuries are infrequent in children surviving trauma, an extracranial neurological injury must be suspected, and the patient should be immobilized on a spine board. Children are immobilized in a hard neck collar or with the head taped to the board between sandbags or IV fluid bags. Spinal shock is rare in the acute phase of trauma in children; however, it can result in hemodynamic instability with hypotension and bradycardia. This condition can be confounded with vascular collapse from an associated hemorrhagic lesion.

C. Evaluation of Neurological Distress

The first minutes spent at a trauma scene must be devoted to the evaluation of life-threatening lesions. Neurological examination includes evaluation guided by the GCS, which can be adapted for use in children younger than 2 years of age (Table 7). A score on GCS ≤ 8 clearly defines coma in a patient with no verbal response or eye opening, whatever the motor response. In comatose patients, the motor component indicates the level of the rostrocaudal lesion. It is of major importance to evaluate the level of consciousness at the scene before sedating the child. In as much as 10% of initially comatose children, the first early CT-scan evaluation will be normal. The main reason for this paradox is that a CT scan performed within the first 2 hr after head injury is not sensitive enough to detect small petechial contusions, which will be frequently depicted at a later examination. The GCS score determined before resuscitation, and especially its motor component, is well correlated with outcome [2,9,44]. In children younger than 2 years of age, a rapidly expanding intracranial hematoma can be responsible for significant blood loss relative to total blood volume. It is important to recognize the hemodynamic signs of a hematoma before intracranial hypertension develops and leads to errors of diagnosis. An extensive

Table 7 Glasgow Coma Scale

Eye-opening response	
Spontaneous	4
To speech	3
To pain	2
None	1
Verbal response[a]	
Oriented	5
Confused conversation	4
Inappropriate words	3
Incomprehensible sounds	2
None	1
Best upper limb motor response	
Obeys commands	6
Vocalizes	5
Withdraws	4
Abnormal flexion	3
Extensor response	2
None	1

[a] Children less than 2 years of age should receive full verbal score for crying after stimulation.
Source: Ref. 47.

scalp laceration also may cause heavy blood loss. In such instances, the child requires immediate hemostasis and volume replacement. A neurological evaluation is then completed by an examination of pupil size and reactivity. Unilateral mydriasis can be noted immediately after severe head trauma, but must be interpreted cautiously if it is associated with facial trauma. Mydriasis may be caused by local trauma or may be a sign of an *acute compression of the ipsilateral* hemisphere with resulting third nerve palsy. Although an acute extraparenchymal hematoma can cause brain compression and requires *prompt surgical evacuation*, it represents less than 10% of the lesions in comatose children after a head trauma [2,9]. Unilateral mydriasis is at times the result of diffuse axonal injury and is not related to a focal brain lesion requiring surgical treatment. A focal neurological deficit can be noted soon after head trauma. Like mydriasis, this localizing neurological sign should be interpreted cautiously in the multiple trauma patient because a focal neurological deficit can result from diffuse axonal injuries or from an associated orthopedic injury. With the exception of the fronto-orbicular and oculocardiac reflexes, brain stem reflexes should not be evaluated until an associated spinal cord injury has been ruled out.

D. Ventilation and the Brain

The relationship between cerebral blood flow (CBF) and arterial CO_2 partial pressure ($PaCO_2$) has been recognized for many years. Under physiological conditions, every 1 mmHg variation of $PaCO_2$ induces a 2 ml/100 g/min variation in CBF. This relationship is modified when hypoxia and/or hypotension are present. In children with severe head trauma, cerebral hemodynamics and reactivity to CO_2 are modified. The initial phase of brain ischemia immediately following trauma seems to be brief. A rapidly succeeding phase of relative hyperemia frequently results from acute cerebral arterial vasodilatation. The cerebral hemodynamic condition cannot be assumed in the prehospital phase, but hypercarbia, and to a lesser degree hypoxia, are known as major ventilatory factors contributing to early intracranial hypertension. Both occur in more than 50% of comatose patients at the scene of accidents. Controlling the airway and initiating controlled ventilation is one of the most useful emergency interventions in severe head trauma. Prompt intubation and airway control at the scene of the accident have been found effective in previous studies and are correlated with increased survival and functional outcome [2]. Indications for emergent intubation are liberal in patients with a GCS score of 9 or less.

Preservation of cerebral perfusion pressure is the main goal of the management of head-injured patients. Many associated factors may contribute to hypotension in prehospital settings. Severe head injury by itself can be the first cause of hypotension. The precise mechanism is not known, but a possible explanation is the exhaustion of endogenous catecholamines after a massive release in the first minutes following trauma. Associated hemorrhagic lesions may cause hypotension, especially in small children with low total blood volume. Finally, in rare cases, neurogenic shock may cause hemodynamic instability. Whatever the precise etiology of hypotension, there is no time for complex pathophysiological discussion in prehospital settings. After hemostasis of evident sources of hemorrhage, hemodynamic stabilization is vital. A mean arterial pressure within the range of normal values for the age is mandatory. The fear of potentially increasing cerebral edema with extensive vascular fluid loading must be balanced against the always-present risk of rapid development of secondary brain injury when cerebral perfusion is critically decreased. The first step for hemodynamic stabilization is to rapidly establish at least one large-bore venous access for fluid and drug administration. The best fluid to use is still controversial. Because isotonic fluids will not increase cerebral edema, isotonic saline and colloids solutions may be used liberally when needed to restore cerebral perfusion pressure. Small-volume fluid resuscitation with hypertonic saline solutions is an efficient way to stabilize hemodynamics. This modality of treatment is more common in Europe. It has the associated advantage of decreasing intracranial pressure and could be used in prehospital settings, particularly in the presence of hypotension and intracranial hypertension. There is still uncertainty regarding dramatic changes in plasma osmolality in children. It may be the principal means of decreasing moderate intracranial hypertension when continuous small-volume infusions are used, however. When fluid resuscitation is not sufficient to rapidly restore hemodynamics, vasopressive drugs could be added. Continuous infusion of dopamine (2–20 μg/kg/min) or epinephrine (0.1–1 μg/kg min) are the most efficient to improve mean arterial pressure.

E. Fluid and Electrolyte Balance and the Brain

There are two major threats to already traumatized brain cells: glucose and hypotonic fluid. In the first hours following trauma, insulin resistance and impaired cerebral intake of free glucose are common. Hyperglycemia is associated with impaired outcome in severely head-injured children [45]. The prevention of hyperglycemia is an argument for exclusive use of glucose-free isotonic solutions for basic fluid maintenance in the first hours following a severe head trauma. Variations in plasma oncotic pressure influence peripheral edema but not cerebral edema; decreased plasma osmolality increases directly both peripheral and cerebral water content and edema. The main goal of basic fluid maintenance is to preserve or to slightly increase plasma osmolality. Fluid and electrolyte maintenance is different from fluid loading for hemodynamic stabilization and compensation for blood loss. Fluid loading is necessary to maintain adequate cerebral perfusion pressure to compensate for blood loss. *Hypotonic* solutions, such as lactated Ringer's, increase both peripheral and cerebral water content. The best solution to be used to compensate for water and electrolyte losses is normal saline.

Mannitol has long been used to decrease cerebral edema, especially in the presence of high intracranial pressure; 25% mannitol is a crystallized solution that must be warmed before IV infusion, however. Moreover, it can—at least theoretically—increase intracranial extraparenchymal bleeding. Mannitol is used only after examination with a CT scan has eliminated the possibility of acute epidural hematoma. For these reasons its use in prehospital settings is difficult. The only indication for use of mannitol in such a setting may be evidence of immediate life-threatening brain herniation persisting after adequate hemodynamic and ventilatory resuscitation.

Plasma osmolality and cerebral free water outflow can be increased by hypertonic solutions. Hypertonic saline solutions are valuable alternatives to mannitol. They can be infused without special preparation, and they have a similar effect on increased intracranial pressure. As a continuous infusion, they increase plasma osmolality and cerebral perfusion pressure without adverse effects and have beneficial effects on mean arterial pressure. They may be ideal in the future for prehospital basic fluid management of children with severe head injuries. Until further data become available, their use must be restricted to health care providers experienced in using this method of volume resuscitation.

V. CONCLUSIONS

Traumatic injuries remain the number one killer of the pediatric population worldwide, and no preventive measures can be too great.

Unlike the situation in adults, in pediatric multiple trauma, 80% of cases include head trauma. Prehospital management should be focused on timely and aggressive prevention of secondary CNS injury. Expert skills in pediatric airway management are the prerequisites.

Training and retraining of prehospital providers has to be synchronized with the advances and changes in clinical practice, such as use of the IO route for emergency drug management and fluid resuscitation and new measuring tapes to estimate the size of pediatric patient for rapidly estimating drug doses.

Physical trauma is accompanied by psychological devastation of the young that should be addressed in the course of treatment.

The role of hypertonic solutions in pediatric trauma resuscitation warrants further investigation.

REFERENCES

1. A Mazurek. Pediatric injury patterns. Internet Anesth Clin 32:11–25, 1994.
2. GA Orliaguet, PG Meyer, S Blanot, MM Jarreau, B Charron, C Buisson, PA Carli. Predictive factors of outcome in severely traumatized children. Anesth Analg 87:537–542, 1998.
3. JG Avery, RH Jackson. Children and Their Accidents. London: Edward Arnold, 1993.
4. Accident Facts. National safety council. Itasca, IL: 1997.
5. DK Nakayama, KB Pasieka, MJ Gardner. How bicycle-related injuries change bicycling practices in children. Am J Dis Child 144:928–929, 1990.

6. T Wood, P Milne. Head injuries to pedal cyclists and the promotion of helmet use in Victoria, Australia. Accid Anal Prev 20:177–185, 1988.
7. MF Altieri. Child abuse: When to be suspicious and what to do then. Postgrad Med 87:153–156, 1990.
8. D Jaffe, D Wesson. Emergency management of blunt trauma in children. New Eng J Med 324:1477–1482, 1991.
9. EF Aldrich, HM Eisenberg, C Saydjari, TG Luerssen, MA Foulkes, JA Jane, LF Marshall, A Marmarou, HF Young. Diffuse brain swelling in severely head-injured children: A report from the NIH Traumatic Coma Data Bank. J Neurosurg 76:450–454, 1992.
10. FA Pigula, SL Wald, SR Shackford, DW Vane. The effect of hypotension and hypoxia on children with severe head injuries. J Pediat Surg 28:310–314, 1993.
11. WG Elliott. Airway management in the injured child. Internat Anesth Clin 32:27–46, 1994.
12. MA Wayne, CM Slovis, RG Pirrallo. Management of difficult airways in the field. Prehosp Emerg Care 3:290–296, 1999.
13. D Brownstein, R Shugerman, P Cummings, F Rivara, M Copass. Prehospital endotracheal intubation of children by paramedics. Ann Emerg Med 28:34–39, 1996.
14. DK Nakayama, WS Copes, W Sacco. Differences in trauma care among pediatric and pediatric trauma centers. J Pediatr Surg 27:428–431, 1992.
15. DK Nakayama, T Waggoner, ST Venkataraman, M Gardner, JM Lynch, RA Orr. The use of drugs in emergency airway management in pediatric trauma. Ann Surg 216:205–211, 1992.
16. WC Boswell, N McElveen, N Sharp, CR Boyd, CI Franz. Analysis of prehospital pediatric and adult intubation. Air Med J 14:125–128, 1995.
17. AJ Mazurek, B Rae, S Hann, JI Kim, B Castro, CJ Coté. Rocuronium versus succinylcholine: Are they equally effective during rapid-sequence induction of anesthesia? Anesth Analg 87: 1259–1262, 1998.
18. KA Lillis, DM Jaffe. Prehospital intravenous access in children. Ann Emerg Med 21:1430–1434, 1992.
19. RS Seigler, FW Tecklenburg, R Shealy. Prehospital intraosseous infusion by emergency medical services personnel: A prospective study. Pediatrics 84:173–177, 1989.
20. DH Fiser. Intraosseous infusion. New Engl J Med 322:1579–1581, 1990.
21. PG Meyer, GA Orliaguet, MM Jarreau, B Charron, R de Sauverzac, PA Carli. Complications of emergency tracheal intubation in severely head-injured children. Paediat Anaesth 10:253–260, 2000.
22. P Suominen, C Baillia, A Kivioja, R Korpela, R Rintala, T Silfvast, K Olkkola. Prehospital care and survival of pediatric patients with blunt trauma. J Pediat Surg 33:1388–1392, 1998.
23. DK Nakayama, MJ Gardner, MI Rowe. Emergency endotracheal intubation in pediatric trauma. Ann Surg 211:218–223, 1990.
24. TR Paul, M Marias, PT Pons, KA Pons, EE Moore. Adult versus pediatric prehospital trauma care: Is there a difference? J Trauma 47:455–459, 1999.
25. N Kissoon, JJ Tepas, III, RJ Peterson, P Pieper, MO Gayle. The evaluation of pediatric trauma care using audit filters. Pediat Emerg Care 12:272–276, 1996.
26. MM Krausz, M Bar-Ziv, R Rabinovici, D Gross. ''Scoop and run'' or stabilize hemorrhagic shock with normal saline or small-volume hypertonic saline? J Trauma 33:6–10, 1992.
27. SJ Stratton, LA Underwood, SM Whalen, CS Gunter. Prehospital pediatric endotracheal intubation: A survey of the United States. Prehosp Disas Med 8:323–326, 1993.
28. ML Ramenofsky, A Luterman, E Quindlen, L Riddick, W Curreri. Maximum survival in pediatric trauma: The ideal system. J Trauma 24:818–823, 1984.
29. Textbook of Trauma Anesthesia and Critical Care. St.Louis: Mosby-Year Book, 1993.
30. JS Seidel, D Parkman-Henderson, P Ward, BW Wayland, B Ness. Pediatric prehospital care in urban and rural areas. Pediatrics 88:681–690, 1991.
31. PG Meyer. Pediatric trauma and resuscitation. Curr Opin Anaesth 11:285–288, 1998.

32. I Claudet, C Alberge, MC Bloom, F Fries, MC Lelong-Tissier. Intraosseous infusion in children. [in French]. Ann Fr Anesth Rean 18:313–318, 1999.
33. LJ Michaud, FP Rivara, MS Grady, DT Reay. Predictors of survival and severity of disability after severe brain injury in children. Neurosurgery 31:254–264, 1992.
34. DL Johnson, S Krishnamurthy. Send severely head-injured children to a pediatric trauma center. Pediat Neurosurg 25:309–314, 1996.
35. JD Tobias. Shock in children: The first 60 minutes. Pediat Ann 25:330–338, 1996.
36. American Heart Association. Pediatric Advanced Life Support. Elk Grove Village, IL: American Academy of Pediatrics, 1994.
37. RJ Smith, DP Keseg, LK Manley, T Standeford. Intraosseous infusions by prehospital personnel in critically ill pediatric patients. Ann Emerg Med 17:491–495, 1988.
38. SJ Teach, RE Antosia, DP Lund, GR Fleisher. Prehospital fluid therapy in pediatric trauma patients. Pediatr Emerg Care 11:5–8, 1995.
39. G Hughes, H Spoudeas, IZ Kovar, HT Millington. Tape measure to aid prescription in paediatric resuscitation. Arch Emerg Med 7:21–27, 1990.
40. M Gausche, RJ Lewis, SJ Strattom, BE Haynes, CS Gunter, SM Goodrich, PD Poore, MD McCollough, DP Henderson, FD Pratt, JS Seidel. Effect of out-of-hospital pediatric endotracheal intubation on survival and neutological outcome: A controlled clinical trial. JAMA 283: 783–790, 2000.
41. DK Nakayama, ML Ramenofsky, MI Rowe. Chest injuries in childhood. Ann Surg 210:770–774, 1989.
42. ML Ramenofsky, TS Morse. Standards of care for the critically injured pediatric patient. J Trauma 22:921–933, 1982.
43. WH Lam, A Mackersie. Paediatric head injury: Incidence, aetiology and management. Paediat Anaesth 9:377–385, 1999.
44. PG Meyer. Critical care management of severe paediatric trauma: A challenge for anaesthesiologists. Paediat Anaesth 9:373–376, 1999.
45. LJ Michaud, FP Rivara, WT Longstreth Jr, MS Grady. Elevated initial blood glucose levels and poor outcome following severe brain injuries in children. J Trauma 31:1356–1362, 1991.
46. American College of Surgeons. Advanced Trauma Life Support. Instructors' manual. 5th ed. Chicago: Committee on Trauma, American College of Surgeons, 1994.
47. GJB Teasdale. Assessment of coma and impaired consciousness: A practical scale. Lancet 2: 81–84, 1974.

25

Trauma in the Elderly

ERAN TAL-OR and MOSHE MICHAELSON

Rambam Medical Center, Technion Institute, Haifa, Israel

I. INTRODUCTION

A. Demographics of Trauma in the Elderly

Trauma in the elderly is a growing problem due to the increase in life span. During the twentieth century, the number of people in the United States under the age of 65 tripled. At the same time, the number of people 65 and over jumped *by a factor of 11* [1]! *The Census Bureau predicts that the elderly population will more than double between now and the year 2050, to a total of 80 million.* The rate of death from trauma in the elderly group is high. Although the death rate from unintentional injury per 100,000 persons is 35.4 for all ages combined, it rises to *90.3 for persons older than 65 years of age* [2].

Not only do people live longer, but the quality of life is greater, so *more elderly people are involved in driving, working outside the home, and participating in other activities, including sports and dangerous pastimes, which add to the risk of getting injured.*

Another factor that contributes to injury is the environment we have created. For example, housing is geared toward younger people, who are more agile, and little consideration is given to the needs of the elderly, particularly in terms of safety.

Old people are more prone to injury for several reasons. They are slow to notice upcoming hazards due to hearing and vision problems. They are also slow in responding to danger because of their slow reaction times. Other problems are daytime sedation caused by medications and alcohol and medical conditions such as seizures, fainting, vertigo, and gait disorders. Furthermore, the elderly with the same injury as younger people experience greater morbidity and mortality [3], *and the rate of mortality increases with multisystem trauma* [4].

Table 1 Three Leading Causes of Death in the Elderly in the United States (1998)

Cause	Number	Percentage
Falls	13,500	41
Motor vehicle crashes	8100	25
Burns	1250	4

Note: From all elderly deaths (>65 years).
Source: From the National Safety Council, Chicago, 1998.

B. Mechanisms of Injury

The three leading causes of accidental death in the elderly are falls, motor vehicle crashes, and burns (Tables 1, 2).

1. Falls

The U.S. Department of Health and Human Services reported to Congress in 1989 that falls represent the second greatest source of economic loss due to injuries in the United States. *In Australia, falls of the elderly constitute 80% of all deaths* caused by falls in all age groups [5]. Falling is one of the most common causes of trauma among the elderly [6]. Falling is the cause of death in 12% of cases for all age groups combined; however, it is the cause of death in 41% of trauma cases involving persons aged 75 and over.

The elderly are more prone to injuring themselves while falling. (The incidence of hip fractures in the elderly is fourfold that among younger age groups [7]. Falls frequently result from environmental hazards, such as poor lighting, slick floors, hazardous furniture, low beds, and toilets. The list is endless. The major causes of falls in the elderly are summarized in Table 3.

2. Motor Vehicle Crashes

In 1996, a total of 43,449 people of all ages died from motor vehicle crashes in the United States. Of these, 7,539 (17.35%) were elderly, and this number will increase [2]. In Australia, 284 elderly people died from motor vehicle crashes [5] in 1997, which was more than in previous years. The reason for the increase is that there are more elderly people on the road—as drivers and as pedestrians. The explanations offered for the difficulties the elderly have on the roads include age-related declines in sensory (e.g., vision or hearing) and cognitive functions and physical impairments due to medical conditions, all of which

Table 2 Three Leading Causes of Death in the Elderly in Australia (1997)

Cause	Number	Percentage
Falls	997	63
Motor vehicle crashes	294	19
Burns	39	2.5

Note: From all elderly injury-related deaths (>65 years).
Source: From Ref. 5.

Table 3 Causes of Falls Among the Elderly

Change in age and environmental hazards
Cardiac dysrhythmias
Orthostatic hypertension
Dizziness/vertigo
Syncope
Vertebral-basilar insufficiency
Drugs

may affect some older persons' driving ability [8,9]. Added to this is the timidity that increases in the elderly, which can be dangerous on the roads.

Furthermore, the mortality of elderly pedestrians is the highest of all age groups. It was found that at the same injury severity score (ISS), the mortality rate in the elderly is much higher than in others [10]. The death rate per 100,000 is higher for people 70 years of age or older than for people in any other group except those younger than 25 [11].

3. Burns

Burns are the third leading cause of death from trauma in the elderly. The most common reasons for the high death rate are scalding from hot tap water, spilled liquids in the kitchen, and ignition of fabrics by faulty heaters or cigarettes [12]. The rate gets much higher among people who live alone. In the United States, more and more people are living alone in their elderly years: 32% of people aged 65 to 74 and 57% of those over age 85 [1]. Elderly people with burns are more prone to morbidity and mortality than younger people with the same burn injury [12].

II. PHYSIOLOGICAL CHANGES IN THE ELDERLY

The human body is built with a large functional reserve, which is supposed to last a lifetime. It is a well-established fact that because of this a young person can have a kidney or lung removed without any limitation in activity. As the body ages, however, this vast reserve is used up, and by the time a person reaches old age, he or she is left with little or no reserve at all. The loss of this functional reserve is caused by aging and disease [13]. The human body begins aging during the individual's twenties, and this process continues over the years. Until now there has been no way to stop this natural process, although there are ways to slow it.

A. Nervous System

Brain mass is diminished in old age, partly due to a loss of neurons and partly from a reduction of blood flow to the brain. All these changes cause memory problems, dementia, and deterioration in cognitive function. Silent strokes add to the problem.

In the peripheral nerves, large nerve fibers are lost and there is hypertrophy of glial cells. This causes a reduction in nerve conduction velocity and an increase in reaction time up to 30%, which leads to impairment of all the cutaneous senses, including pain.

Most old people suffer from hearing loss and impairment of eyesight, partly due to changes in the cornea, lens, and retina.

B. Lungs

Disease and normal aging processes destroy alveoli, which reduces the ability to deliver oxygen. The dead space grows and functional residual capacity (FRC) and expiratory reserve volume decrease. Closing volume may exceed the FRC, causing part of the lungs to be unventilated and leading to atelectasis, a ventilation–perfusion mismatch.

The compliance of the chest wall and lung decreases. The respiratory muscles age and become weaker, reducing the forced expiratory volume (FEV_1). All these changes interfere in the ability of the body to supply oxygen in larger amounts when demanded in stress.

C. Cardiovascular

As the years go by, the contractility and elasticity of the heart decrease. Cardiac output decreases by 1% per year and stroke volume by 0.7% per year, starting at the age of 20. After 40 years of age, peripheral resistance increases by 1% each year. These changes decrease perfusion, especially in the kidneys and the splanchnic and cutaneous vessels. The arteries lose their elasticity, and deposits of calcium and cholesterol narrow their lumen. The veins become torturous and also lose their elasticity.

D. Kidneys

By the age of 80, renal perfusion is reduced by half and the kidneys lose 30% of their mass. This is caused by a reduction in the number of nephrones. The ability to concentrate urine is diminished.

E. Liver

In aging, there is a decrease of 35% of the liver due to loss of hepatocytes. Blood flow is reduced by 35%.

F. Skeletal

Bone cell mass and muscle strength are also reduced, along with the ability of the bone marrow to function.

III. INITIAL ASSESSMENT AND MANAGEMENT

In the elderly trauma patient, and in other adults and in children, initial assessment and management are performed *according to the guidelines of advanced trauma life support* (ATLS) [14]. The next paragraph will highlight only the points that are different in the elderly and need special consideration, understanding that the overall protocol is the same as that discussed in earlier chapters.

In assessing the elderly trauma patient, the patients medical history is extremely important. Knowledge of pre-existing deficits and infirmities and of medication being taken helps in the interpretation of findings and identification of acute changes that are a result of the trauma. For example, a patient who is taking beta-blockers might not present with tachycardia, even in a state of shock. Blood pressure of 120/80 would be considered normal in a young adult; in an elderly person, a blood pressure of 160/90 might be low and suggestive of occult bleeding.

A. Airway and C-Spine Control

Securing the airway in an elderly patient is especially challenging. Pre-existing conditions may make it more difficult. Many elderly people have loose, inconveniently placed, or very carious teeth, along with lax cheek muscles (Fig. 1) and resorption of the mandible. Arthritis of the temporomandibular joint may limit mouth opening and cause additional problems. Chin lift and jaw thrust may not open the airway, in which case an oral or nasal airway must be used. Trauma to the mouth area may cause loose teeth or a dental prosthesis to block the airway.

When the patient must be ventilated, the mouth space must be cleared of foreign bodies and false teeth. Bag ventilation must be carried out with an oral airway in place. It might be possible to ventilate the patient with a dental prosthesis in place for protection of the mouth space. (The authors' preference is to remove any prostheses and insert an oral airway).

The best way to supply oxygenation and adequate ventilation is *intubation and controlled ventilation*. During intubation, extra consideration must be given to the soft tissues, as injuries in the elderly tend to bleed easily, especially in the nose.

A patient in a borderline conscious state or with a compromised airway requires a definitive airway since elderly patients deteriorate faster than young adults.

Extra care is also warranted when controlling the cervical spine. Rheumatoid arthritis, which is common in the elderly, weakens the cervical ligaments [15]. Abrupt movements may injure the ligaments and cause dislocations of the dense (C_2). Any movement of the cervical spine must be made very carefully, *even if the mechanism of the injury dose not suggest spinal damage*.

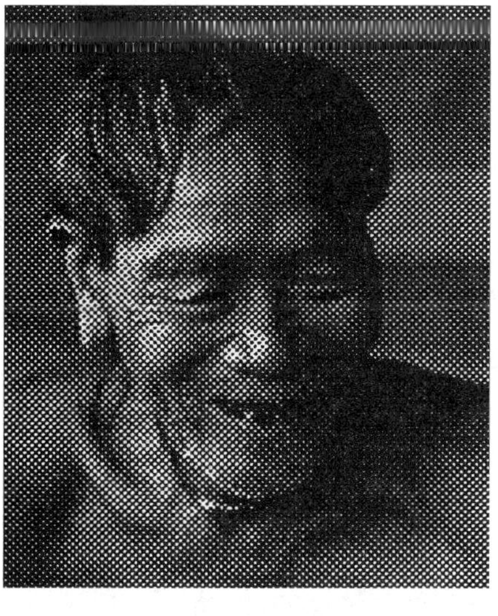

Figure 1 Old man's face with lax tissue and loose teeth.

B. Breathing

In the elderly, support of ventilation must be more aggressive than in younger patients because of the reduction in lung capacity and the decrease in respiratory reserves. In patients with dyspnea and in whom chest injury is suspected, the decision to intubate and ventilate must be made in the early stages (of initial assessment). This includes those suspected of having flail chest, pulmonary contusion, and tension or simple pneumothorax (open and closed) *after decompression* of the chest.

Bag-mask ventilation should not be used for the reasons noted earlier. It is *preferable to intubate and ventilate*.

The elderly suffer from rib rigidity, which makes them prone to *sustain rib fractures, even in seemingly mild incidents*. Fractures can lead to tension pneumothorax or delayed hemothorax, which have significant morbidity [16]. The patient must be reassessed carefully before and after ventilation looking for tachycardia, subcutaneous emphysema, saturation falls, and/or diminished breath sounds in one or both lungs.

Jugular vein distention may not be seen, because of hypovolemia. Chest decompression should be carried out early, when necessary, with needle application and chest drain. During ventilation, the patient must be kept on high saturation and *normocapnia*; the use of a pulse oximeter and capnograph will help. It is important to monitor the airway pressure by the feeling of the bag in the hand or by monitoring the pressure in the ventilator.

Elderly people will not tolerate a chest injury as well as younger people can. Since they may have compromised breathing and a lower tidal volume, an injury to the chest may lead to a reduction in oxygenation and ventilation. Intubation and ventilation may be needed in cases that would not call for intubation in young adults. Ventilation of the elderly must be performed carefully; a chest drain must be placed as soon as possible. Since the patient might have lung adhesions, ''needle application'' will not help. The elderly trauma patient might have lung diseases that interfere with breathing and make oxygenation and ventilation difficult to achieve. Chronic obstructive pulmonary disease (COPD) and emphysematous lungs may cause extra injury or complications if the wrong ventilation parameters are used.

All this points out that obtaining as much as is possible of the patient's medical history is essential. *A pulse oximeter is a must* in the elderly for monitoring their oxygenation status. It also might be problem in patients with PVD.

C. Circulation

The elderly are more susceptible to shock. Their cardiovascular reserve is lower, which means they have a reduced capability for cardiovascular compensation, thus their *blood pressure will fall when a smaller* amount of volume is lost.

Tachycardia will start later because of the heart's inability to increase its pace as a result of disease or medications (beta-blockers), *therefore tachycardia is not a reliable sign of shock in the elderly*. Low blood pressure is not tolerated well by the elderly, and shock should be fought *vigorously with fluids to decrease the time of hypoperfusion*. Fear of overhydration and pulmonary edema should not cause a delay in administering the correct amount of fluid. There is no place for vasoconstrictive medication in the treatment of hypovolemic shock in the elderly.

In some elderly patients, *a blood pressure of 120/80 may mean hypotension*, as they suffer from hypertension and their normal blood pressure is much higher. Check mental status (sign of low perfusion).

Treatment consists of placement of a minimum of two large-bore intravenous lines. Central vein pressure (CVP) must be considered; also it is a debate whether or not an overload of fluid can cause ARDS [17,18] Central vein pressure will help to monitor the fluid status, and will be done only on long rides to the hospital (*if the transport time is more than 20 min*).

Intravenous fluid therapy starts with a balanced salt solution (such as Ringer's lactate). If the patient is not hemodynamically stable and does not respond after a bolus of 2 liters, a bolus of *colloid solution* may be useful in the prehospital phase since there is no blood in this time. Blood pressure should be measured at this time. In the elderly more than in the young, most of the time it is more valuable monitoring, since their ability to compensate blood loss is limited and changes in their blood volume will be reflect earlier.

D. Disability

When attempting to assess the neurologic status of the elderly trauma patient, a few points must be taken into account. First, some elderly may be in a confused state prior to the injury. Second, a previous cardiovascular accident may have left the patient with neurologic deficits not related to this trauma. Third, eye disease, such as cataracts or status after cataract removal, may alter pupil reaction (glass eye!). All of these possibilities should be taken into consideration when assessing the patient's neurologic status.

E. Exposure and Hypothermia

Exposure is an important part of the first survey to ensure that no injury is missed. *Elderly people are prone to hypothermia* due to malfunctioning of temperature control and peripheral vascular disease. It may be present on arrival at the scene or may develop quickly from uncovering the patient and from the field temperature of administered fluid. Extra consideration must be taken to minimize heat loss, therefore undressing the patient should be postponed until arrival at the hospital. All fluids must be warmed by any means that can work in the prehospital phase. In addition, *the ambulance or helicopter should be warmed.*

F. Adjuncts to Primary Survey and Resuscitation

Electrocardiographic (ECG) monitoring (with a 12-lead ECG) is required in trauma patients, and all the more so in the elderly, who are vulnerable to cardiac arrhythmias (for instance VF in a driver crashing his car), cardiac hypoperfusion, and myocardial infarctions and who suffer from coexisting cardiac diseases. These conditions must be added to the differential diagnosis in the elderly.

1. Gastric Catheter

As in younger patients, a gastric catheter is indicated as a *diagnostic and therapeutic process*. It reduces stomach dilatation, decreases the risk of aspiration (but does not prevent it entirely), and allows assessment of oropharyngeal bleeding (swallowing blood) or actual injury to the upper digestive tract.

2. Urinary Catheter

Urinary output is a sensitive monitor for hemodynamic state and volume status, *although it takes more than an hour to obtain any result* (evaluation of urine output).

There is therefore no place for a urinary catheter in urban areas when the prehospital transport time is less than an hour. If the hospital is more than an hour away and there are no contraindications, a urinary catheter *could* be inserted. *This can be a big pitfall in elderly men*, however, some of whom suffer from benign prostate hyperplasia. It is very difficult, if not impossible, to insert a catheter in these patients. In this case, *no additional attempt should be made*.

IV. CONCLUSION

The elderly represent the fastest-growing segment of the population [1]. Prehospital assessment and management of the elderly must include a variety of special considerations due to the pathophysiologic changes caused by aging. Elderly trauma patients sustain distinct patterns of injuries, have a unique response to stress, and are more likely to suffer serious consequences from trauma compared with younger patients [17]. When possible, early assessment of the elderly needs to include knowledge of the patient's medical history, pre-existing diseases, and any medication taken. This information will be valuable for understanding the physical findings and not missing injuries that may be masked by pre-existing diseases or medication (e.g., not detecting tachycardia in a patient who takes a beta-blocker). Since the elderly have a lack of reserve, they cannot tolerate hypotension, hypoventilation, or hypothermia as well as younger patients. Management must be rapid and aggressive, and the elderly patient must be kept oxygenated, well perfused, and warm, which means high oxygen saturation, good blood pressure, and covered with a warm blanket in a warm area.

Prehospital care providers' assumptions about an elderly trauma patient should include the following:

1. The injuries are probably more severe than they look based on the first assessment and findings.
2. There are underlying medical problems and diseases that will worsen the outcome.
3. The elderly patient has greater instability and lack of reserve.
4. The injuries will have a more overwhelming affect on an elderly patient than on a younger patient.
5. Assessment and management must be rapid and aggressive.

REFERENCES

1. Economics and Statistics Administration. Bureau of the Census. May 1995.
2. The Centers for Disease Control and Prevention (CDC). Death and Death Rates for 10 Leading Causes of Death in Specified Age Groups. 1996.
3. T Osler, K Haels, B Baack, et al. Trauma in the elderly. Amer J Surg 156:537–543, 1988.
4. SP Zietlow, PJ Capizzi, MP Bannon, MB Farnell. Multisystem geriatric trauma. J Trauma 37(6):985–988, 1994.
5. Australia National Injury Surveillance Unit, 1997.
6. A Ciccone, JR Allegra, DG Cochhrane, et al. Age-related differences in diagnoses within the elderly population. Amer J Emer Med 16(1):43–48, 1998.
7. P Kannus, J Parkkari, H Sievanen, et al. Epidemiology of hip fructures. Bone 18(1 suppl): 57s–63s, 1996.

8. JA Gresset, FM Meyer. Risk of accidents among elderly car drivers with visual acuity equal to 6/12 or 6/15 and lack of binocular vision. Ophthal Physiol Opt 14(1):33–37, 1994.
9. MK Janke. Age-Related Disabilities That May Impair Driving and Their Assessment: Literature Review. Sacramento, CA:California Department of Motor Vehicles, report no. RSS-94, 1994.
10. PW Perdue, DD Watts, CR Kaufmann, AL Trask. Differences in mortality between elderly and younger adult trauma patients:Geriatric status increases risk of delayed death. J Trauma 45(4):805–810, 1998.
11. Insurance Institute for Highway Safety (IIHS). Facts, 1996 Fatalities: Elderly. Arlington, VA: IIHS, 1997.
12. A Manktelow, AA Meyer, SR Herzog, HD Peterson. Analysis of life expectancy and living status of elderly patients surviving a burn injury. J Trauma 29(2):203–207, 1989.
13. DD Trunkey, FR Lewis. Current Therapy of Trauma. 4th ed. St. Louis: Mosby, 1999, pp. 92–94.
14. American College of Surgeons, Committee on Trauma Advanced Trauma Life Support. 6th ed. Chicago: American College of Surgeons, 1997.
15. BJ Simon, Q Chu, TA Emhoff. Delayed hemothorax after blunt thoracic trauma: An uncommon entity with significant morbidity. J Trauma 45(4): 1998.
16. RD Miller. Anesthesia. 3rd ed. New York: Churchill Livingstone, 1990, p. 2014.
17. CA Stamatos. Geriatric trauma patients: Initial assessment and management of shock; STNS. J Trauma Nurs 1(2):45–54, 1994. e 45, Number 4, October 1998 Volume 45, Number 4, October 1998

26

The Pregnant Trauma Patient

SUSAN KAPLAN

MCP Hahnemann University, Philadelphia, Pennsylvania

HANS-R. PASCHEN

Amalie Sieveking-Krankenhaus, Hamburg, Germany

Trauma is the leading cause of death in women of child-bearing age under 35 and occurs in 6–7% of all pregnancies [1]. Motor vehicle accidents and falls are the two major causes of injury, while other less common causes include gunshot and stab wounds, domestic abuse, suicide, electrocution, and burns.

The incidence of trauma increases with each trimester of pregnancy (see Fig. 1). Approximately 8% of traumatic injuries occur in the first trimester, 40% in the second trimester, and 52% in the third trimester [2]. The higher incidence of third trimester injuries is aggravated by gait disturbances, shift of the center of gravity, and the anatomic protuberance of the pregnant abdomen.

Mechanism of injury is either by blunt or penetrating forces. Mild blunt trauma due to falls is common during pregnancy and generally has no sequelae. With more significant blunt trauma, the uterus absorbs the major impact, and the most common complications (see Table 1) include: placental abruption, uterine irritability, premature labor, premature rupture of membranes, abdominal pain, cramping, tenderness, infection, and leakage of amniotic fluid. More serious injuries include: amniotic fluid embolism, pelvic venous embolism, and uterine rupture.

Gunshot and stab wounds are the most common forms of penetrating injuries. The gravid uterus, especially in the third trimester, is the organ most commonly affected. Fetal outcome is poor, with morbidity and mortality reported from 41–71% [3].

Maternal mortality in both blunt and penetrating trauma is due primarily to exsanguination, although abdominal organ injury, retroperitoneal hemorrhage, and uteroplacental

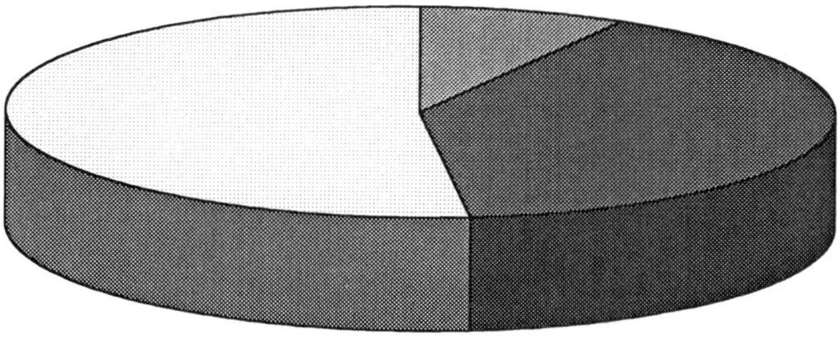

Figure 1 Incidence of trauma during pregnancy.

injury are also common causes of maternal death. Fetal morbidity and mortality is largely dependent upon maternal outcome.

Traumatic placental abruption is the leading cause of maternal and fetal complications following trauma [4]. Occult uterine bleeding may be massive and may result in fatal exsanguination or irreversible disseminated intravascular coagulation (DIC) if not treated early. The protuberant abdomen makes the uterus especially vulnerable in vehicular accidents, although the use of three-point automobile restraints has reduced this incidence dramatically. The gravid uterus cushions injury to other abdominal organs, often protecting the stomach, pancreas, diaphragm, and mesentery at the point of impact. Bleeding from enlarged uterine, pelvic, and retroperitoneal vessels may not be protected, however, and pelvic hemorrhage from sheared vessels can be massive.

Fetal insult is significant in both blunt and penetrating trauma. Intrauterine fetal demise is common. Hypoxia, asphyxia, and hypovolemia may not necessarily cause fetal death, but significant neurological and other developmental abnormalities may result. Fetal skull fracture and intracranial hemorrhage are two common sequelae from trauma during gestation. If maternal injuries are not recognized and treated quickly and aggressively, seemingly mild injuries may result in significant morbidity and death for mother and child.

Table 1 Complications of Trauma in Pregnancy

Placental abruption
Uterine irritability
Premature labor
Premature rupture of membranes
Abdominal pain
Cramping
Uterine tenderness
Leakage of amniotic fluid
Infection
Amniotic fluid embolism
Pelvic venous embolism
Uterine rupture
Fetal hemorrhage and death
Maternal hemorrhage and death

Because the physiologic state is so different during pregnancy and because two lives are at stake, it is important to understand the differences between trauma occurring during pregnancy and that occurring in the nonpregnant individual. This chapter summarizes normal maternal physiology and its impact on trauma management in emergent prehospital care, specific injuries and modifications of treatment in pregnancy, on-site analgesia and anesthesia, fetal assessment, problems upon arrival at the hospital, and perimortem delivery.

I. NORMAL MATERNAL PHYSIOLOGY AND ITS IMPACT ON TRAUMA MANAGEMENT

Initial resuscitation of the pregnant trauma victim differs only minimally from that of the nonpregnant trauma victim. The airway, breathing, and circulation (ABCs) of resuscitation are always priorities. Advanced trauma life support (ATLS) guidelines [5] regarding airway management, ventilation, and maintenance of cardiovascular stability for the pregnant trauma victim are identical to those guidelines for the nonpregnant population. Normal anatomical and physiological changes of pregnancy mandate some modifications in the care of the pregnant patient, however.

A. Airway

Capillary engorgement of the respiratory vessels during pregnancy causes mucosal edema of the oronasopharynx, larynx, and trachea. Hormonal effects of increased estrogen and progesterone production result in friability and easy bleeding of mucosal surfaces. Soft tissue swelling of the face and neck often distorts an otherwise normal airway.

Airway obstruction, hypoxemia, and moderate to severe hemorrhage with minimal manipulation occur rapidly in a *normal* pregnancy. These physiological changes limit the safety margins of airway protection. When there has been associated trauma, these safety margins are narrowed even further. Hypoxia occurs quickly, and endotracheal intubation may be difficult if not impossible. Only small endotracheal tubes (ETT) may pass through engorged and edematous arytenoids and vocal cords. Endotracheal tube size should not exceed 7.0 to 7.5 mm outer diameter, and often a 6.0 or 6.5 mm ETT may be necessary.

Intubation with cricoid pressure and rapid sequence induction with cricoid pressure are the preferred techniques for airway access in the majority of pregnant trauma victims. When difficult intubation is encountered and the airway cannot be easily controlled, alternative methods of airway access should be used earlier rather than later. The laryngeal mask airway (LMA) and Combitube are two alternative airway devices. The LMA, although relatively easy to insert, does not protect against aspiration of gastric contents [6,7]. The Combitube may be a better alternative. It should be emphasized, however, that *either* device can and should be used when airway access is necessary and cannot be achieved quickly with endotracheal intubation. If these techniques fail, a surgical airway should be obtained.

B. Respiration and Oxygenation

Respiratory alterations are significant during pregnancy (see Table 2). Dyspnea is common in the majority of healthy pregnant patients at term, especially in the supine position. This is due to physiological reduction in expiratory reserve volume, residual volume, and functional residual capacity (FRC) during pregnancy (see Fig. 2), closure of airways, and

Table 2 Respiratory Changes in Pregnancy

Total lung capacity	Decreased/unchanged	−5–0%
Expiratory reserve volume	Decreased	−20%
Residual volume	Decreased	−20%
Functional residual capacity (FRC)	Decreased	−20%
P_aCO_2	Decreased	−10 torr
Closing volume	Unchanged	—
Minute ventilation	Increased	+45–50%
Respiratory rate	Increased/unchanged	+15–0%
Oxygen consumption	Increased	+20%
Tidal volume	Increased	+45%

increased oxygen consumption. Should painful contractions begin, oxygen consumption increases even more, approximately 60% above baseline. Exogenous oxygen via nasal cannula or mask should always be provided in the spontaneously breathing pregnant victim, or via ETT in the obtunded patient.

Tilting of the patient to the left reduces dyspnea in the majority of pregnant patients (see Sec. II.), and healthy patients will often do this spontaneously. In a severely trauma-

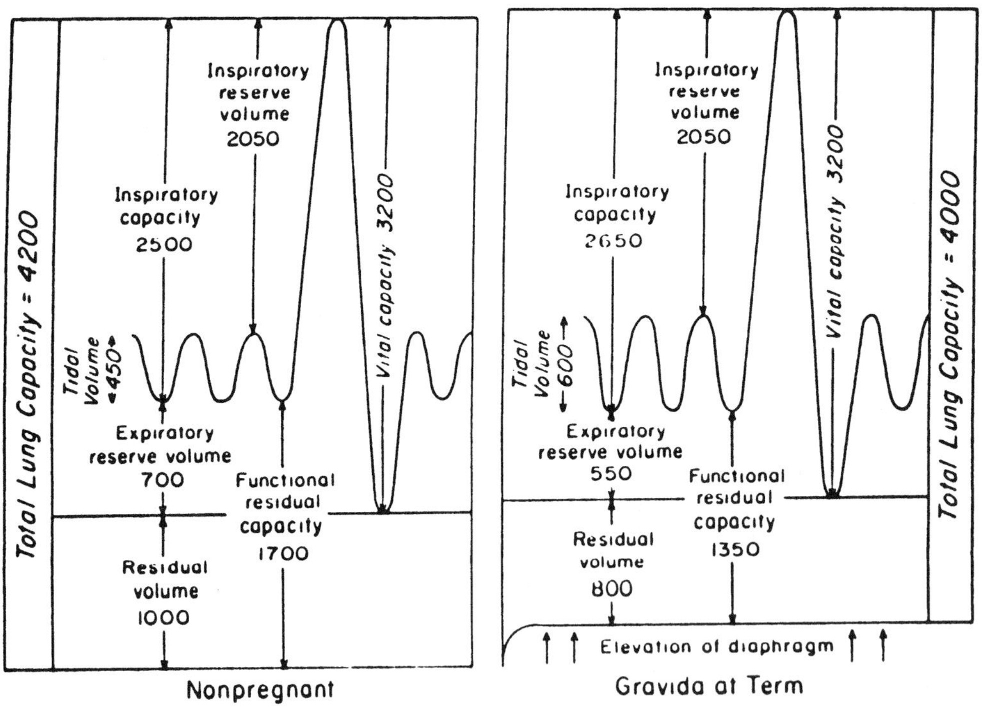

Figure 2 Pulmonary volumes and capacities during pregnancy, labor, and postpartum period. (From Ref. 7a.)

tized patient or in a patient with severe pain from injury or contractions, self-tilting does not often take place. It is therefore imperative that the trauma team be aware of positioning throughout care. The pregnant female should *always* be positioned in a 10° to 20° left-sided tilt (exception: the right side may be used if there is objective clinical evidence, such as fetal heart rate monitoring or fetal ultrasound, that the fetus tolerates the right side better than the left).

C. Cardiovascular System

Total blood volume, plasma volume, and red cell volume increase throughout pregnancy (see Table 3, Fig. 3). The maximum increase in circulating blood volume occurs by 30 to 32 weeks gestation, and by the late third trimester, blood volume has expanded by 1000 to 1500 ml above the nonpregnant volume. The increase in plasma volume exceeds red cell volume, resulting in a relative anemia, the so-called physiologic anemia of pregnancy. Although this physiologic anemia is normal, hemoglobin and hematocrit levels of less than 11 grams/dl or 33%, respectively, are considered abnormal.

Cardiac output (CO) increases progressively throughout pregnancy and reaches a maximum of 50% above the nonpregnant state by the twenty-eighth week of gestation. The increase in CO is due to an increase in both heart rate and stroke volume. Blood pressure generally remains unchanged, secondary to a decrease in both systemic and pulmonary vascular resistance.

Changes in the electrocardiogram are common. Left axis deviation due to the horizontal displacement of the heart within the chest from diaphragmatic elevation is normal, as is sinus tachycardia. Depressed ST-T segments and nonspecific ST-T changes are often observed, but these do not necessarily represent pathological events [8].

It is important to maintain maternal hemodynamics as close to normal as possible throughout pregnancy, as both mother and baby are affected by hypotension. Uterine blood flow (UBF) is a pressure-driven system (see Fig. 4) and is directly proportional to maternal blood pressure [9]. No autoregulatory mechanism exists for UBF, and perfusion of the uterus and placenta (and therefore oxygenation of the fetus) is determined solely by the mother's hemodynamic status. In the prehospital setting, aggressive volume resuscitation, left uterine tilt, and exogenous oxygen therapy are imperative for maternal and fetal well-being.

Table 3 Cardiovascular Changes in Pregnancy

Blood volume	Increased	+35–40%
Plasma volume	Increased	+45–50%
Red blood cell volume	Increased	+20%
Cardiac output	Increased	+40–50%
Stroke volume	Increased	+30%
Heart rate	Increased	+15%
Total peripheral resistance	Decreased	−15%
Systemic vascular resistance	Decreased	−20%
Mean arterial pressure	Decreased/unchanged	−15–0%
Central venous pressure	Unchanged	—
Blood pressure	Unchanged	—

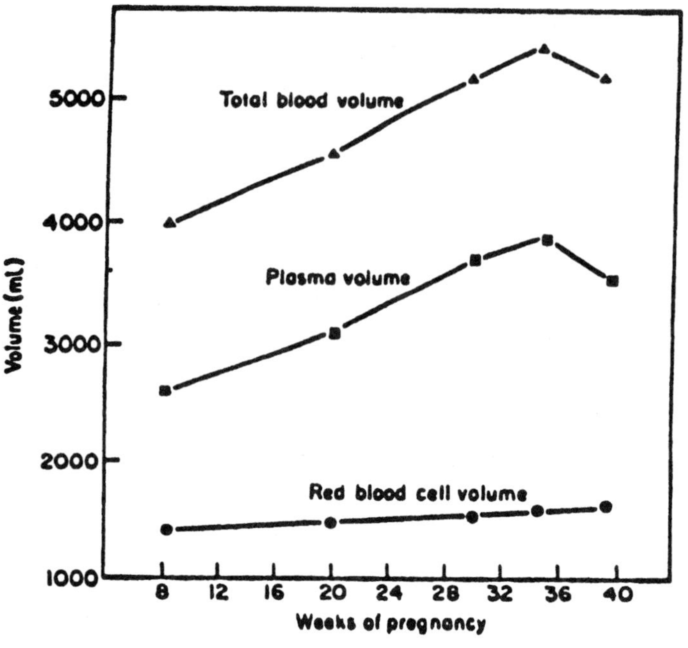

Figure 3 Changes in total blood volume, plasma volume, and red blood cell volume in normal pregnancy. Note the continued increase in red blood cell volume and plasma volume late in the third trimester. (From Ref. 10a.)

D. Gastrointestinal System

Mendelson [10] originally described the syndrome of pulmonary aspiration and chemical pneumonitis in pregnancy in 1946. Roberts and Shirley [11] demonstrated in the early 1970s that approximately 25% of normal women at term were at risk of aspiration because of gastric volumes in excess of 25 ml and gastric pH of less than 2.5.

The stomach is anatomically rotated upward into a horizontal lie, which interferes with normal lower esophageal sphincter tone. Incompetency of the lower gastroesophageal junction results in significant reflux in the majority of pregnant women. Effects of excessive estrogen and progesterone production, as well as the horizontal lie, reduce gastric emptying time. Gastric pH is reduced (i.e., more acidic), and gastric volume is increased.

These anatomic and physiologic changes of pregnancy place the normal pregnant female at increased risk of pulmonary aspiration. Although early airway protection is

$$\text{Uterine Blood Flow (UBF)} = \frac{\text{Uterine Arterial Pressure (UAP)} - \text{Uterine Venous Pressure (UVP)}}{\text{Uterine Vascular Resistance (UVR)}}$$

$$\text{UBF} = \frac{\text{UAP} - \text{UVP}}{\text{UVP}}$$

Figure 4 Uterine blood flow.

imperative in any trauma victim, it is especially important in the pregnant trauma victim. Cricoid pressure is essential during intubation attempts or mask ventilation.

E. Hematologic System, Vascular Access, and Volume Resuscitation

Pregnancy is considered a hypercoagulable state. Red cell volume is increased, as is total blood volume. There is mild thrombocytopenia, although platelet function generally remains unchanged. Circulating levels of clotting factors VII, VIII, and X and fibrinogen increase. Plasma fibrinogen levels generally exceed 400 mg/dl in normal pregnancy and fibrin–fibrinogen complexes also increase slightly.

Prolonged maternal bleeding will invariably lead to coagulopathy in both nontraumatic and traumatic situations (see Table 4). When trauma and pregnancy are combined, there is a very high risk of dilutional thrombocytopenia, DIC, and exsanguination from both nonobstetrical and obstetrical injuries. Hemorrhage can and will be massive.

Normal uterine blood flow is approximately 700 ml/min. Enlarged spiral arteries, venous lakes, and increased myometrial blood volume will cause rapid and fatal exsanguination if traumatic placental abruption remains undiagnosed and untreated. Occult blood up to 5 liters (essentially the blood volume of the average female) can be sequestered behind a large placental abruption (see Figs. 5 and 6). Occult uteroplacental hemorrhage as well as bleeding from caval tears, aortic dissection, or retroperitoneal hemorrhage can produce a rapid consumptive coagulopathy that will progress to irreversible DIC and death.

Controversy currently exists regarding on-site volume resuscitation vs. ''scoop-and-run'' in prehospital management of the trauma victim. Recommendations for the pregnant trauma victim are essentially nonexistent. Obviously, clinical decisions must be tailored to each victim, but these are the authors' recommendations for prehospital care of the pregnant trauma patient.

The age, health, and normally expanded blood volume of the pregnant female will often mask signs and symptoms of hypovolemic shock. Maintenance of normal maternal blood pressure will help prevent hypoxic insults to both mother and fetus. A primary goal of prehospital care of the pregnant trauma victim should be early restoration and maintenance of normal maternal hemodynamics via rapid and aggressive volume resuscitation. Even if vital signs are within the normal range, if the mechanism of injury suggests hemorrhage, a high index of suspicion should be maintained and volume resuscitation should be continued prophylactically.

One or two large-bore intravenous lines (16-gauge or larger are ideal) should be started, and non-dextrose-containing crystalloid solutions should be administered rapidly.

Table 4 Causes of Coagulopathy in Pregnancy

Rapid activation of clotting cascade
Consumption of clotting factors
Release of placental hormones causing uterine atony
Dilutional thrombocytopenia
Occult uterine bleeding
Hypothermia
Hypovolemia
Massive blood transfusions

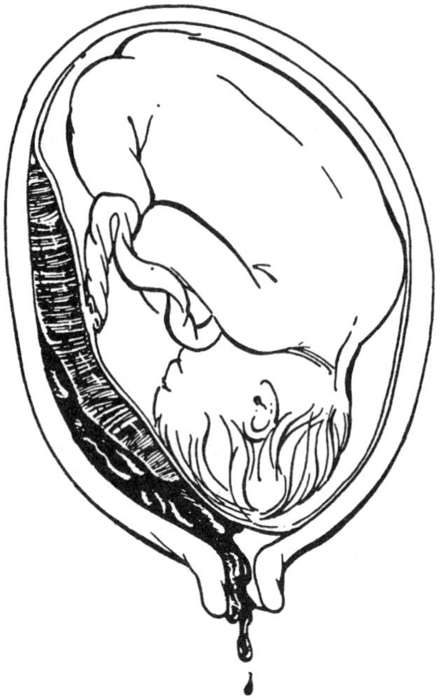

Figure 5 Abruptio placenta with visible vaginal bleeding. (From Ref. 11a.)

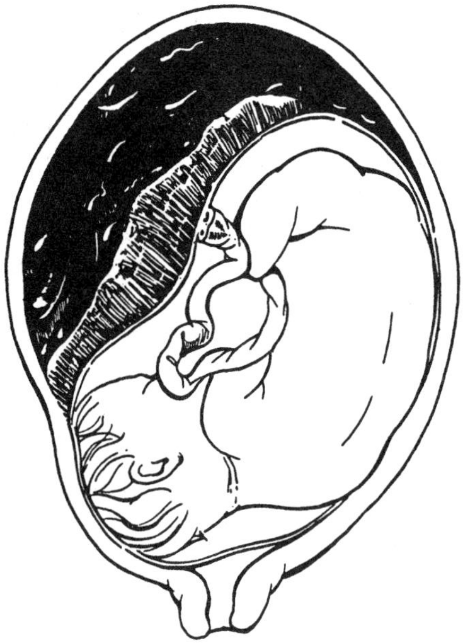

Figure 6 Abruptio placenta with concealed vaginal bleeding. (From Ref. 11a.)

Dextrose-containing fluids may cause fetal insulin surge, resulting in potentially severe fetal hypoglycemia at delivery. For each liter of suspected or real blood loss, three liters of crystalloid should be infused. If blood pressure cannot be stabilized with crystalloid, colloid should be added. Vasopressors can be used, but those with both alpha and beta properties (e.g., ephedrine) are preferred over pure alpha agents (e.g., phenylephrine). In desperate situations, military antishock trousers (MAST) trousers can be used as long as the abdominal compartment is not inflated.

II. AORTOCAVAL COMPRESSION SYNDROME

Venous return is altered significantly during pregnancy, especially during the second and third trimesters. The enlarging uterus impairs blood return from the inferior vena cava (IVC) at its bifurcation, causing a decrease in venous return to the heart. To compensate, collateral vessels enlarge and drainage of the lower extremities to the heart is enhanced via engorged azygous and epidural veins [12]. The gravid uterus also causes obstruction of the abdominal aorta, resulting in reduced cardiac outflow. Although the aortic outflow obstruction has minimal maternal effect, uteroplacental flow may be significantly impaired, especially in the supine position. Maternal baroreceptor reflexes normally result

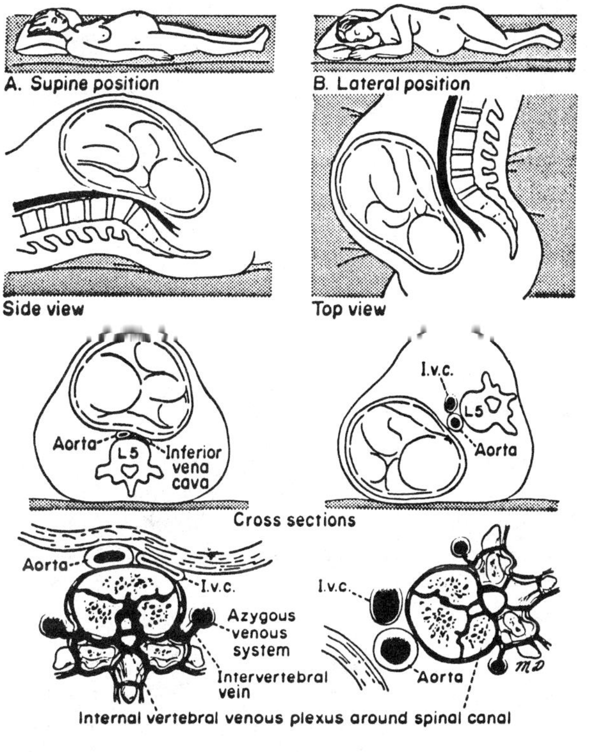

Figure 7 The effects of the pregnant uterus on the inferior vena cava and the aorta in the supine position (A) and the lateral position (B). The marked aortocaval compression in the supine position causes venous blood to be diverted to and through vertebral venous plexus, which becomes very engorged, thus reducing the size of the epidural and subarachnoid spaces. (From Ref. 12a.)

Table 5 Signs and Symptoms of Aortocaval Compression

Hypotension
Tachycardia
Palor
Shortness of breath
Lightheadedness, dizziness
Nausea, vomiting

in sinus tachycardia and peripheral vasoconstriction in response to any reduction in blood pressure. If the baroreceptor reflexes are inhibited for any reason, significant hypotension may result.

Howard et al. [13] noted that dyspnea was common in up to 25% of normal pregnant women in the third trimester when they assumed a recumbent position. In 1953, the hypotension and symptoms accompanying it were described, and the term *supine hypotension syndrome* of pregnancy was coined. In 1964, Kerr and colleagues [14] radiographically demonstrated complete obstruction of the IVC by the gravid uterus in the supine position. Later, Bienarz and co-workers [15] confirmed partial aortic occlusion in the same recumbent position. Current standard obstetrical practice includes positioning of the pregnant mother in a left uterine displacement (LUD) position to prevent the syndrome now called *aortocaval compression syndrome* (see Fig. 7, Table 5).

Avoidance of aortocaval compression is essential in the care of the pregnant trauma victim. Although there is partial compensation of reduced venous return to the heart via enhanced flow through the azygos and epidural veins, displacement of the uterus off the IVC and aorta will prevent physiologic hypotension and will minimize uteroplacental insufficiency. The clinician may then be able to differentiate physiologic hypotension from that caused by maternal hemorrhage or acute spinal shock. In both the prehospital setting and throughout care until delivery, every pregnant woman in the late second trimester or beyond should be positioned with left uterine displacement, or if spine injury is suspected, stabilized on a long backboard in a left 10° to 20° tilt.

III. SPECIFIC INJURIES OF THE PREGNANT TRAUMA VICTIM

Trauma during pregnancy threatens two individuals. By virtue of its inherent physiologic changes, pregnancy may cause a significant modification of a woman's response to catastrophic insult. Care and treatment must be modified to accommodate this altered physiologic state and to protect the viability of the developing child.

A. Head Injuries

The most common cause of traumatic head injury in Europe and the United States is vehicular trauma and is *the leading cause* of maternal morbidity and mortality. The goal in treatment of the head-injured victim is to prevent hypoxia and hypoxemia and is identical to that of the nonpregnant trauma victim.

Mechanical ventilation to maintain normocarbia (recall that in the pregnant female, *normal* $PaCO_2$ is 28 to 32 mmHg by 12 weeks gestation and remains slightly decreased until term), head elevation of 30° to 45°, hyperosmotic diuresis (mannitol 0.25–1.0 gm/kg, furosemide 1 mg/kg), corticosteroids, and barbiturates are routine clinical measures to reduce elevated intracranial pressure (ICP). Hyperventilation should be avoided, as it may compromise uteroplacental blood flow by decreasing maternal cardiac output and blood pressure. Incremental adjustments in maternal ventilation will often allow a reduction in ICP without compromise to the fetus. During labor, skeletal muscle contractions, not uterine contractions, cause increased ICP, and efforts should be made to prevent or reduce skeletal muscle movement.

B. Cervical Spine Injuries

Patients with suspected cervical spine injury must be immobilized until complete clinical neurological evaluation (including radiographic evaluation) has excluded pathology. The pregnant trauma victim, just as the nonpregnant victim, should be immobilized with a cervical collar. If no collar is available, manual in-line axial stabilization should be maintained. Rigid collars reduce flexion and extension to 30% of normal, and rotation and lateral movement is reduced to 50% of normal. The combination of rigid cervical collar, backboard, and taping of the head reduces movement to 5% of the normal range. Examination and transport of the pregnant patient should be modified by tilting the stretcher 10° to 20° to the left. This maneuver assures correct vertebral immobilization while simultaneously preventing aortocaval compression syndrome.

C. Thoracic Injuries

Management and occurrence of chest injuries are essentially the same in pregnant and nonpregnant patients. Pulmonary contusions, pneumothorax, pneumohemothorax, hemothorax, rib fractures, flail chest, and myocardial contusion are the most common injuries. Early airway control and oxygenation are critical, and aggressive treatment of pulmonary injuries is important due to the increased risk of maternal and fetal hypoxia. Placement of thoracostomy tubes for pneumothoraces should be one or two interspaces above normal because of the elevation of the diaphragm from the gravid uterus [3].

D. Abdominopelvic Injuries

Today women continue their active daily lives throughout gestation. Vehicular accidents and falls are the major causes of traumatic injuries in pregnancy. In early pregnancy, the young fetus is protected by the maternal bony pelvis, strong maternal abdominal muscles, and cushioning by amniotic fluid. The elastic fixation of the uterus optimizes protection in the first trimester [17]. Beyond the twelfth week of gestation the uterus is no longer protected by the bony pelvis, and abdominal trauma may cause direct injury to the fetus (see Fig. 8).

The widespread use of seatbelts has reduced the number of deaths and injuries in road traffic accidents [18]. Nevertheless, restraining devices may themselves increase fetal morbidity and mortality via placental abruption and may increase the incidence of fetal fractures by deceleration forces (see Figs. 9 and 10). Discrete evidence of bruising across the thorax under the site of the shoulder harness or of the lower abdomen should raise the suspicion of occult hemorrhage and injury.

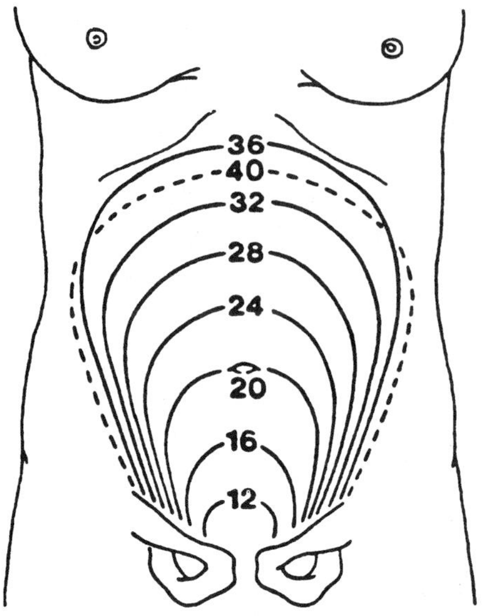

Figure 8 Increasing fundal height according to week of gestation. At term, the fundus approaches the xiphoid process, which can obscure normal physical signs associated with intra-abdominal disease. (From Ref. 16.)

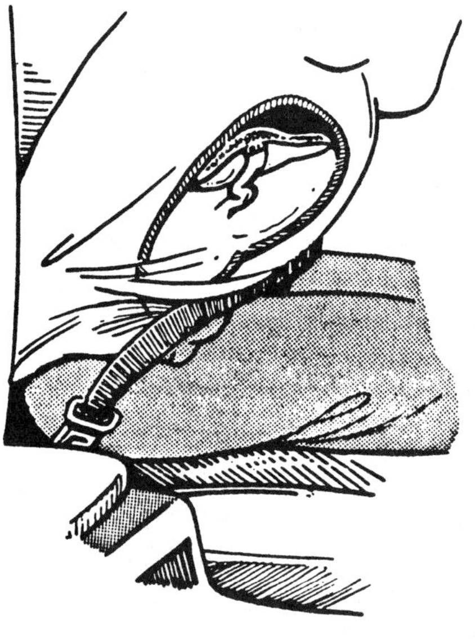

Figure 9 Seatbelt use without shoulder belt. (From Ref. 3.)

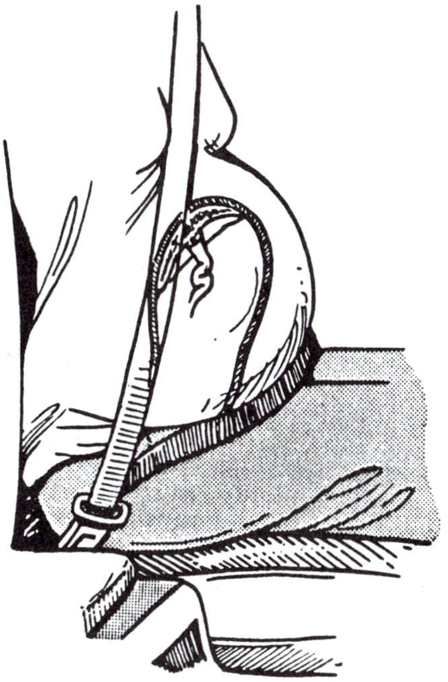

Figure 10 Shoulder and lap belt. (From Ref. 3.)

IV. CARBON MONOXIDE POISONING

Patients suffering from carbon monoxide poisoning present a confusing and often misleading clinical picture. Maternal symptoms are nonspecific, and serum carboxyhemoglobin levels may not correlate with clinical findings. Carbon monoxide readily crosses the placental barrier and has a higher affinity for binding with fetal hemoglobin (Hgb) than with adult Hgb. This displacement of oxygen by carbon monoxide will cause early fetal death [19]. Airway control and oxygenation are of paramount importance to minimize maternofetal morbidity and mortality. Hyperbaric oxygen therapy is the treatment of choice.

Hyperbaric oxygenation is not contraindicated during pregnancy [20]. The European Concensus Conference on Hyperbaric Medicine [21] has shown that hyperbaric oxygen treatment during pregnancy does not elevate the incidence of congenital malformation or premature delivery. Every parturient with proven CO inhalation should be transferred to a center with a hyperbaric chamber for immediate treatment.

V. ON-SITE ANALGESIA AND ANESTHESIA

Pregnancy should not limit or restrict the use of any pharmacological or resuscitative treatment routinely indicated after trauma. This is especially true for pain relief for on-site analgesia or surgical intervention. At the trauma scene, intravenous narcotics and sedatives should not be withheld from the mother because of concern regarding potential depression of the fetus. Pain causes release of vasoconstrictive stress hormones, and these hormones will reduce fetal perfusion via impaired uterine blood flow. Opioids and seda-

Table 6 Induction Agents for General Anesthesia in the Pregnant Trauma Victim

Thiopental: 1.0 to 3.0 mg/kg
Etomidate: 0.1 to 0.2 mg/kg
Propofol: 0.5 to 1.0 mg/kg
Ketamine: 0.25 to 0.5 mg/kg

tives can be used safely in pregnancy as long as they are administered carefully and the patient's vital signs are monitored continuously.

If surgical intervention is necessary at the trauma scene, regional anesthesia is preferred over general anesthesia whenever possible. There is minimal effect of local anesthetics upon the fetus from regional techniques, and further depression of the baby from general anesthetic drugs is avoided. If hemodynamic stability is a concern or if regional anesthesia is contraindicated, however, general anesthesia with preoxygenation, cricoid pressure, and rapid sequence induction is the anesthetic of choice. Induction agents include thiopental, etomidate, propofol, and ketamine in significantly reduced doses in the presence of suspected or known hypovolemia (see Table 6). Muscle relaxation is best provided with succinylcholine, although high-dose, nondepolarizing muscle relaxants can be used when succinylcholine is contraindicated (see Table 7).

VI. FETAL ASSESSMENT IN THE PREHOSPITAL SETTING

Fortunately, the pregnant trauma victim is a rare event. Although all precautions should be taken to protect the fetus, priorities in resuscitation should be centered on the mother. Immediate resuscitation of the mother is the best antidote for survival of the fetus (see Table 8). Continuous LUD positioning and 100% mask oxygenation at the scene and throughout care and transport is imperative for improved fetal outcome.

Table 7 Muscle Relaxants for Rapid Tracheal Intubation in the Pregnant Trauma Victim

Depolarizing agent	
Succinylcholine	1 to 1.5 mg/kg
Nondepolarizing Agents[a]	
Vecuronium	0.3 to 0.4 mg/kg
Rocuronium	0.6 to 1.0 mg/kg
Rapacuronium	1.5 to 2.0 mg/kg
Mivacurium	0.25 to 0.3 mg/kg[b]
Cisatracurium	0.25 to 0.4 mg/kg[b]

[a] Patient ready for intubation approximately 60 to 90 sec after injection.
[b] Use with caution. Give priming doses (0.02 mg and 0.01 mg, respectively) 2 to 4 min prior to intubating doses. Both drugs may cause histamine release and hypotension, especially when given rapidly.

Table 8 Primary Causes of Traumatic Fetal Morbidity and Mortality

Maternal death
Maternal hemorrhagic shock
Placental abruption
Uterine rupture
Direct fetal injury

In the field, diagnostic equipment is generally unavailable for fetal assessment, and the emergency physician must rely on indirect fetal signs. Although evaluation of the fetal heart rate (FHR) is the most reliable parameter of fetal viability, in the prehospital setting auscultation may be difficult if not impossible due to environmental noise. Fetal movement at the trauma scene is the most trustworthy sign of fetal viability.

Complaints by the patient of abdominal pain and palpation of a rigid uterus may be indicative of placental abruption. The patient will often report vaginal bleeding, although a large volume of blood may be concealed behind the fetus or a closed cervix. Should labor begin at the trauma scene, tocolytic therapy is *not* recommended, as uterine contractions may prevent severe uterine hemorrhage. Immediate transport to an obstetrical facility for possible cesarean section is mandatory.

VII. PROBLEMS AND PITFALLS UPON ARRIVAL AT THE HOSPITAL

Evaluation of the pregnant trauma victim should be the same as that of a nonpregnant victim with several modifications. Maximum oxygen therapy is essential for both mother and baby because of reduced FRC and should be administered throughout care. The gravid uterus must be displaced to prevent aortocaval compression syndrome. The fetus should be monitored continuously and the obstetrical care team should be involved from the onset. Although every effort should be made to protect the fetus, priorities in resuscitation revolve around the mother. To reiterate, the best outcome for the fetus is a good outcome of the mother.

A. Diagnostic Imaging

The most common mistake in the workup of the pregnant trauma victim is avoidance of essential radiographic studies for fear of teratogenicity to the fetus. Although unnecessary radiation should be avoided, the use of diagnostic imaging studies should be based on *maternal* injuries and not on theoretical risk to the fetus. The greatest vulnerability occurs during rapid organogenesis (2 to 12 weeks gestation). Beyond this period, exposure of less than 5 to 10 rads is unlikely to significantly increase radiation risks, and the diagnostic benefits of the study will usually prevail. Lead shielding of the abdomen is required when other organ systems are evaluated.

Ultrasonography is an essential diagnostic tool in the workup of the pregnant trauma victim. Its portability allows bedside evaluation of both mother and fetus in the emergency unit simultaneous with resuscitative care. Real-time ultrasonography is used routinely to assess fetal movement, cardiac activity (as early as 6 weeks with an abdominal probe and 4 weeks with a vaginal probe), gestational age, and placental integrity. The fetal biophysi-

Table 9 Biophysical Profile (BPP) Scoring

Fetal variable	Normal findings	Abnormal findings	Scoring
Fetal breathing (FB)	At least one episode, 30-sec duration, in 30-min interval	Absent FB or FB <30 sec duration in 30-min interval	0–2
Gross fetal movement	Three or more body/limb movements in 30-min interval	Two or less body/limb movements in 30-min interval	0–2
Fetal tone	One episode or more active extension and flexion of limb or body	Absent fetal movement or slow extension and flexion of limb or body	0–2
Amniotic fluid volume (AFV)	At least one pocket amniotic fluid 2 cm in vertical length	Pocket amniotic fluid <2 cm in vertical length	0–2
Fetal heart rate (FHR)	Two or more episodes FHR acceleration > 15 beats/min (bpm), 15-sec duration, associated with fetal movement in 20-min interval	Fewer than two episodes FHR acceleration or acceleration >15 bpm in 20-min interval	0–2

cal profile (BPP; see Table 9), amniotic fluid index (AFI), and color Doppler flow studies are additional studies used to determine fetal well-being.

B. Fetal Assessment

Upon arrival at the hospital, electronic FHR monitoring should begin immediately, although fetal monitoring should never interfere with maternal resuscitation. During defibrillation, fetal monitors must be removed from the mother. Fetal heart rate monitoring may reveal fetal tachycardia, bradycardia, or variable or late decelerations. Should nonobstetrical surgery be necessary, electronic FHR monitoring should be maintained preoperatively, intraoperatively, and postoperatively. Most clinicians now monitor FHR for up to 24 hr after traumatic injury. Fetal well-being can be further assessed with ultrasonography (e.g., BPP, AFI, and Doppler flow studies). Uterine contractions should also be monitored whenever possible so that premature labor can be determined early and appropriate tocolytic therapy initiated.

C. Diagnostic Peritoneal Lavage

Diagnostic peritoneal lavage (DPL) is routinely performed in suspected abdominal injuries in both pregnant and nonpregnant trauma victims. Beyond the first trimester of pregnancy, open DPL via a small periumbilical incision is preferred, as closed DPL via needle paracentesis may be less accurate and more dangerous (uterine perforation, direct fetal injury). Surgical intervention is based on positive DPL findings [22]: erythrocyte count greater than 100 cells/mm^3 lavage fluid, leukocyte count greater than five cells/mm^3, elevated amylase, and the presence of bile, fecal matter, or bacteria.

D. Surgical Delivery of the Fetus

When hemorrhage cannot be controlled and the survival of the mother is in doubt, surgical delivery of the fetus based on gestational age and potential viability may be the only option for fetal salvage. Cesarean delivery becomes necessary (1) when there is uterine rupture; (2) when fetal distress outweighs the risk of premature delivery; (3) if nonobstetrical surgery cannot be performed because of impaired exposure; and (4) if maternal death appears imminent.

VIII. CARDIOPULMONARY RESUSCITATION AND PERIMORTEM CESAREAN DELIVERY

A. Cardiopulmonary Resuscitation

The risk of cardiac arrest during pregnancy is fortunately rare, estimated to be approximately 1:30,000 pregnancies [23]. Prior to the advent of modern high-risk maternal medical care, the leading causes of morbidity and mortality during pregnancy were eclampsia, sepsis, and cardiovascular disease. Over the last four decades, the leading cause of maternal mortality has been trauma [24].

Should cardiac arrest occur at the trauma scene, maternal and fetal outcome is generally grave despite aggressive heroic interventions. Nevertheless, cardiopulmonary resuscitation (CPR) should begin immediately, and prompt tracheal intubation is imperative. Statistics are limited as to the successful outcome of CPR in pregnancy, but data from nonpregnant patients indicates that external chest compression improves cardiac output by approximately 30% above normal [25]. Successful outcome is dependent upon the efficacy of the external compressions.

Optimally, CPR is performed with the patient placed supine on a hard, flat surface. During pregnancy, however, this supine position exacerbates reduced cardiac output, and LUD positioning is necessary. In the field this is generally accomplished by placing the patient in a left lateral position on a backboard, but this position makes external cardiac chest compressions virtually impossible. An effective compromise is to rotate the pelvis at least 30° by manual displacement or by insertion of a wedge (pillow, blanket, shirt, IV bag, anything available) under the right hip.

Defibrillation and drug application guidelines per Advanced Cardiac Life Support [26] are applicable in both nonpregnant and pregnant trauma. Hesitation in the use of resuscitative drugs because of concern for the fetus can hinder effective care of the mother. Although the fetus may be adversely affected by the application of resuscitative drugs, the needs of the mother come first and all appropriate drugs should be given.

B. Perimortem Cesarean Delivery

Timing of perimortem cesarean delivery in these extremely grave circumstances remains controversial, and recommendations are vague. Whether to institute CPR before, during, or after cesarean delivery is also controversial.

Postmortem cesarean section has been described since antiquity. Although fetal outcome is dismal, current recommendations are as follows. When imminent death of the mother is anticipated, prompt delivery should be attempted if there is any possibility of fetal salvage (see Table 10). Factors influencing the decision for or against surgical deliv-

Table 10 Perimortem Cesarean Delivery

Risk of cardiac arrest during pregnancy: 1 in 30,000 pregnancies
Most common cause of maternal death: Maternal trauma
Most common cause of fetal death: Maternal death
Best fetal outcome: Delivery within 5 min of maternal cardiac arrest; gestational age >26 weeks
Optimized maternal CPR: Postdelivery

ery include: cause of maternal arrest, time interval from arrest to delivery, gestational age, probability of neonatal survival, and availability of appropriate personnel to care for mother and neonate. Johnson and associates [27] describe a modified protocol for perimortem delivery, identifying two treatment groups based on uterine size. If the uterus is less than 20-week size (level of the umbilicus), surgical delivery is unlikely to be beneficial to either mother or fetus. If the uterus is at the 20-week size or greater, emergency delivery should begin within 4 min of maternal arrest.

The ''4-minute rule'' is based on the findings of Katz and associates [28], who reviewed 61 cases of postmortem cesarean section. The best fetal outcome occurred when cesarean section was initiated within 4 min of maternal cardiac arrest and delivery of the fetus within 5 min. Any further delays in surgical delivery resulted in a rapid decline in fetal survival. If cardiac arrest occurs in the prehospital setting, cesarean delivery is still advised even if there is a prolonged time interval between arrest and delivery. Obstetrical input is helpful in the decision-making process.

Perimortem cesarean delivery has been performed for the primary purpose of fetal rescue. Maternal benefits of delivery may be significant as well, however. The gravid uterus, even with LUD positioning, causes a significant reduction in cardiac output and impedes effective aortic outflow. After delivery, abdominal vessels are relieved of their occlusion, maternal oxygen requirements are diminished significantly, and production of carbon dioxide and hydrogen ions by the uteroplacental unit are decreased. In addition, uterine contraction normally returns a volume of blood immediately after delivery such that cardiac output increases by 60–80% [29]. Cardiopulmonary resuscitation at this point may provide adequate cardiac output and improve successful outcome. DePace and colleagues [30] and O'Connor and Sevarino [31] report restoration of spontaneous maternal circulation after cesarean delivery despite failure of predelivery CPR.

A particularly difficult ethical issue arises when there is documented evidence of maternal brain death yet there is still the possibility of a viable birth. If a decision is made to maintain life support of the mother, specific guidelines should be followed. Prentice-Berkseth and co-workers [32] have outlined a management plan for postmortem delivery based on successful outcomes reported in the literature. Guidelines include minimum gestational age for delivery; ongoing fetal assessment using BPP, electronic FHR monitoring, and amniocentesis to determine lung maturity; administration of steroids to enhance fetal lung maturation; maternal cardiopulmonary and nutritional support; and treatment of specific maternal abnormalities such as diabetes, hyperthermia, and hypotension.

IX. CONCLUSION

Trauma during pregnancy is a double tragedy. Fortunately it is a rare event. To ensure successful outcome of mother and child, knowledge of maternofetal physiology is important and modifications of resuscitative techniques are essential. Any woman of child-bearing age (from early teens to midforties) should be considered gravid until determined otherwise. If a protuberant abdomen does not give a visual clue or if the patient and her family cannot provide appropriate information, pregnancy should be assumed until a serum or urine pregnancy test can be performed.

Aortocaval compression syndrome and increased metabolic and oxygen demands put the pregnant victim at greater risk of hypoxia, occult hemorrhage, and hemodynamic instability. Although the health care team should focus attention on survival of the infant, resuscitative efforts should be directed toward the mother. Care should be swift and organized, and transfer to an obstetrical center should be prompt after initial on-site stabilization. Cardiopulmonary resuscitation should be initiated early in the event of cardiopulmonary arrest. In dire circumstances, perimortem cesarean section should be performed. Fetal outcome is best when surgery is within 4 min of maternal arrest and delivery is within 5 min.

Fetal outcome is dependent upon maternal outcome.
Left uterine displacement is essential throughout care to avoid physiologic hypotension (aortocaval compression syndrome).
Oxygen therapy is essential throughout care due to increased maternal metabolic requirements and reduced FRC.
Occult uterine hemorrhage should *always* be suspected.
On-site stabilization vs. "scoop-and-run": Aggressive on-site volume resuscitation with non-dextrose-containing solutions is recommended over scoop-and-run.
Liberal use of narcotics and sedatives is recommended when indicated.
The obstetrical team should be involved as early as possible.
If there is cardiopulmonary arrest, CPR should be initiated at the scene.
If there is doubt of maternal survival, but *any* hope of fetal salvage, perimortem cesarean section should be performed.

REFERENCES

1. D Baker. Trauma in the pregnant patient. Surg Clin North Am 62:275, 1982.
2. HJ Buchsbaum. Penetrating injury of the abdomen. In: HUJ Buchsbaum, ed. Trauma in Pregnancy. Philadelphia: WB Saunders, 1979, pp. 82–100.
3. L Doan-Wiggins. Trauma in pregnancy. In: GI Benrubi, ed. Obstetric and Gynecologic Emergencies. Philadelphia: Lippincott, 1994, pp. 64, 65, 71, 72.
4. TM Goodwin, MT Breen. Pregnancy outcome and fetomaternal hemorrhage after noncatastrophic trauma. Am J Ob Gyn 162:665–671, 1990.
5. American College of Surgeons. Advanced Trauma Life Support. Chicago: American College of Surgeons, 1997.
6. S McClune, M Regan, J Moore. Laryngeal mask airway for Caesarean section. Anaesthesia 45:227, 1990.
7. PS Gataure, JA Hughes. The laryngeal mask airway in obstetrical anaesthesia. Can J Anaesth 42:130, 1995.

7a. JJ Bonica, ed. Principles and Practice of Obstetric Analgesia and Anesthesia. Philadelphia: Davis, 1967.

8. CM Palmer, MC Norris, MC Giudici, et al. Incidence of electrocardiographic changes during cesarean delivery under regional anesthesia. Anesth Analg 70:36–43, 1990.
9. B Glosten. Anesthesia for obstetrics. In: R Miller, ed. Anesthesia. 5th ed. Philadelphia: Churchill-Livingstone, 2000, p. 2030.

10. CL Mendelson. The aspiration of stomach contents into the lungs during obstetric anesthesia. Amer J Ob Gyn 52:191–205, 1946.
10a. DD Moir, MJ Carty. Obstetric Anesthesia and Analgesia. Baltimore: Williams and Wilkins, 1997.
11. RB Roberts, MB Shirley. Reducing the risk of acid aspiration during cesarean section. Anesth Analg 53:859–868, 1974.
11a. D Willis. Bleeding in pregnancy. In: GI Benrubi, ed. Obstetric and Gynecologic Emergencies. Philadelphia: Lippincott, 1994, pp. 136, 137.
12. AP Harris, CR Barton, CR Baker. The pregnant trauma patient. In: JK Stene, CM Grande, eds. Trauma Anesthesia. Baltimore: Williams & Wilkins, 1991, p. 303.
12a. JJ Bonica. Obstetric Analgesia and Anesthesia. Amsterdam: World Federation of Societies of Anesthesiologists, 1980.
13. BK Howard, JH Goodson, WF Mengert. Supine hypotension syndrome in late pregnancy. Am J Ob Gyn 1:371–377, 1953.
14. MG Kerr, DB Scott, E Samuel. Studies of the inferior vena cava in late pregnancy. Brit Med J 1:532–533, 1964.
15. I Bienarz, JJ Crottogini, E Curachet. Aortocaval compression by the uterus in late human pregnancy. Am J Ob Gyn 100:203–217, 1968.
16. R Depp. Cesarean delivery and other surgical procesures. In: SG Gabbe, JR Niebyl, JL Simpson, eds. Obstetrics: Normal and Problem Pregnancies. New York: Churchill-Livingstone, 1991, p. 685.
17. G Schuessling, W Senst. Traumatologie und Schwangerschaft. Z aerztl Fortbild 84:159, 1990.
18. Department of Health. Why Mothers Die: Report on Confidential Enquiries into Maternal Deaths in the United Kingdom 1994–1996. UK: Crown Copyright, 1998, pp. 169–171.
19. D Mathieu, F Wattel, R Neviere, et al. Carbon monoxide poisoning: Mechanics, clinical presentation and management. In: G Oriani, A Marroni, F Wattel, eds. Handbook on Hyperbaric Medicine. Heidelberg, Germany: Springer, 1996.
20. DB Brown, GL Mueller, FC Golich. Hyperbaric oxygen treatment for carbon monoxide poisoning in pregnancy: A case report. Aviat Space Environ Med 63:1011–1014, 1992.
21. European Consensus Conference on Hyperbaric Medicine. Lille: 1994.
22. JW Bryant, AS Wheeler. The traumatized obstetric patient. In: FM James III, AS Wheeler, DM Dewan, eds. Obstetric Anesthesia: The Complicated Patient. 2d ed. Philadelphia: Davis, 1988, p. 495.
23. G Rees, BA Willis. Resuscitation in late pregnancy. Anesthesia 43:347, 1988.
24. R Lanoix, V Akkapeddi, B Goldfeder. Perimortem cesarean section: Case reports and recommendations. Acad Emerg Med 2:1063, 1995.
25. BW Baker. Trauma. In: D Chestnut, ed. Obstetric Anesthesia: Principles and Practice. St. Louis: Mosby-Year Book, 1994, p. 1002.
26. American Heart Association. Textbook of Advanced Cardiac Life Support. Dallas: AHA, 1994.
27. MD Johnson, CJ Luppi, DC Over. Cardiopulmonary resuscitation. In: DR Gambling, MJ Douglas, eds. Obstetric Anesthesia and Uncommon Disorders. Philadelphia: Saunders, 1998, p. 59.
28. VL Katz, DJ Dotters, W Droegemueller. Perimortem cesarean delivery. Ob Gyn 68:571, 1986.
29. K Ueland, JM Hansen. Maternal cardiovascular hemodynamics. III: Labor and delivery under local and caudal analgesia. Am J Ob Gyn 103:8, 1969.
30. NL DePace, JS Betesh, MN Kotler. Postmortem cesarean section with recovery of both mother and offspring. JAMA 248:971, 1982.
31. RL O'Connor, FB Sevarino. Cardiopulmonary arrest in the pregnant patient: A report of a successful resuscitation. J Clin Anesth 6:60, 1994.
32. RL Prentice-Berkseth, RM Weinberg, S Ramanathan. Anesthesia for obstetric trauma patients. In: CM Grande, ed. Textbook of Trauma Anesthesia and Critical Care. St. Louis: Mosby-Year Book, 1993, pp. 641–643.

27

The Entrapped Patient

ANDERS ERSSON

Malmo University Hospital, Malmo, Sweden

DARIO GONZALEZ

*Fire Department of the City of New York/
Emergency Medical Services, New York, New York*

FRANS RUTTEN

HEMS Program Netherlands South–West/Rotterdam, Oosterhout, The Netherlands

I. INTRODUCTION

An entrapment situation represents a wide spectrum of different problems to the rescuer. Immediate access to the patient may not be available, and difficult, urgent medical interventions sometimes have to be done in confined spaces under much less than optimal conditions. Time, or rather time to definitive care, is a crucial factor that influences survival and the risk for development of sequel and multiple organ dysfunction [1–3]. Death from trauma follows a trimodial fashion [4,5] (Fig. 1) in which the majority occurs within the prehospital period. Immediate deaths are mainly due to exsanguinations and severe CNS trauma, and are inevitable and unavoidable. The second peak, however, occurs within the following hours and is mainly due to prolonged exsanguinations and respiratory impairment [4,6]. More than half of the patients have an impaired airway, and as much as nearly 70% of the trauma victims have been reported to require intubation in the prehospital phase [7].

To date very few standards for the care and rescue of entrapped trauma patients are based on proven scientific evidence, and implementing incorrect standards may lead to inappropriate conclusions. The prehospital phase is especially difficult to evaluate, as ‘‘medical scene time’’ has been reported to count for only 25% of the total scene time [8] (Fig. 2).

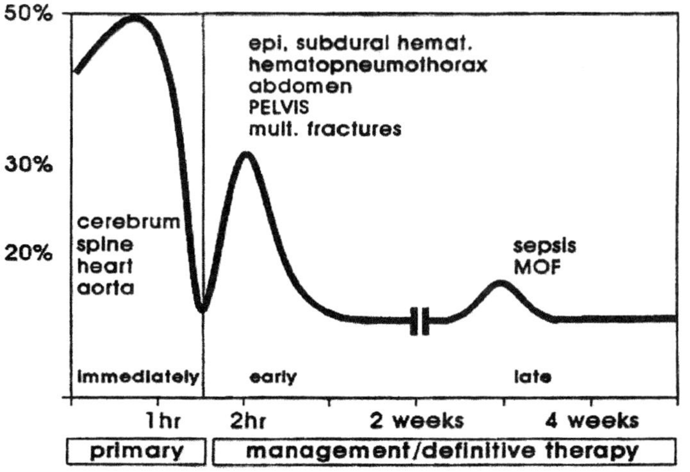

Figure 1 Time correlation and causes of trauma deaths. (From Ref. 4.)

Almost 50% of early trauma deaths have been shown to be potentially preventable by early recognition of impaired vital signs and proper advanced life support (ALS) interventions [3,6,9,2]. Failure to correctly assess the patient and intervene in the early phase in the care of the trauma victim leads to inappropriate and time-consuming actions at the accident site or in the trauma room. This further delays departure and transfer to definitive care and thus increases mortality and the risk for complications.

The overall outcome after prehospital trauma resuscitation has been shown to benefit from increased personnel competence and skill [9], and the needs for defined training standards as well as competence requirements have been highlighted by several authors [10,11,8].

Chain of survival

	Historical definition	Reality
1		Trauma recognition (10 min)
2	Response (10 min)	Response (10 min); arrival to patient
3		contact (5 min)
4	Scene time (20 min)	Scene time (20 min)
5	Scene to hospital (10 min)	Scene to hospital (10 min)
1–5	40 min	55 min

Figure 2 Prehospital scene time consumption. (From Ref. 8.)

In order to minimize time loss and the risk for improper patient handling and to increase coordination, a high degree of bilateral exchange of know-how between the medical and rescue services is needed, and medical training for technical rescue personnel has to be enhanced.

The high incidence of avoidable deaths and morbidity in the prehospital environment and the lack of scientific standards for care and training contrasts sharply to the well-developed in-hospital trauma systems.

Much of the in-hospital rescue effort would be futile and inappropriate if the same principles for the care of trauma patients were not applied in the prehospital environment. This calls for medical command executed by dedicated physicians who recognize the special problems and possess the skills needed to perform in this unique environment.

The role of the physician in the U.S. system is primarily limited to the hospital setting. The prehospital physician role is limited to a relatively small number of emergency medical service (EMS) connected doctors. Most systems within the United States rely on physician volunteers when field responses are necessary. The normal day-to-day functioning of the system relies heavily on physician direction via the use of established assessment, triage, and treatment protocols. This can lead to difficulties when in-hospital physicians respond to a prehospital disaster setting. The typical U.S. hospital-based physician attempts to modify his or her normal day-to-day activities in an unfamiliar and often hostile environment. In order to avoid this dilemma there are two potential options: (1) a limited incident-specific physician role and (2) a ''specialty'' trained physician.

In the limited incident-specific circumstances the role of the physician is one of a limited and defined scope of practice. An example of such a limited role would be the case of an orthopedic surgeon for the amputation of a limb or a cardiologist to manage a complicated cardiovascular emergency. The need for these physicians is limited to nonexistent in the setting of a specialty trained prehospital emergency medicine physician. These physicians must be trained in extensive airway management and immobilization principles and procedures. They must also have training in trauma assessment and management, including the issues related to field anesthesia and extremity amputation.

In the United States this model is established within the urban search and rescue (USAR) medical community. These physicians are specially trained to perform rescues within the collapse environment. Initial development of this specialty was for earthquake response. In the medical response to collapsed building rescues urban paramedics and EMS physicians utilize the same USAR principals. Additionally, this same methodology is utilized for industrial accidents (overturned crane, victims pinned by steel beams, etc.) and rail/subway accidents. These physicians not only require specialty didactic training but also knowledge in the use of specialty equipment for the collapse environment. These medical specialists' primary role is to maintain and sustain patients during the extrication process. These physicians must also be able to initiate preventive management strategies for specific care and incident circumstances. Many of these necessary strategies will be discussed in the chapter.

II. DIFFERENT FORMS OF ENTRAPMENT

A. Motor Vehicle Accidents (MVAs)

Each year an increasing number of people become victims of motor vehicle accidents (MVAs). The yearly deaths rates are appalling, with about 150,000 [1] in the United States 2300 in the United Kingdom [11], and 600 MVAs in Sweden (as a representative for the

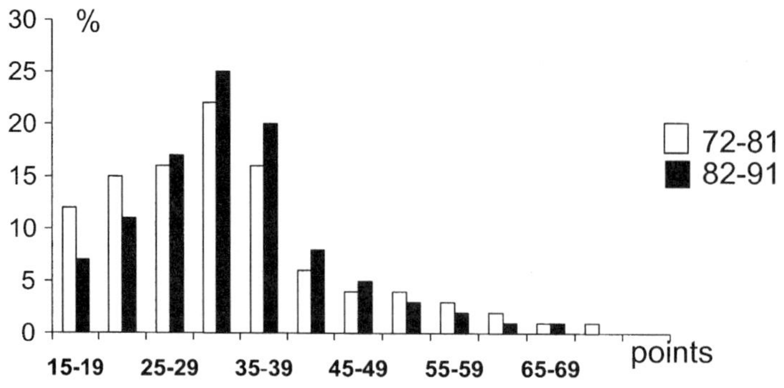

Figure 3 Patient trauma score profiles between 1972 to 1981 and 1982 to 1991 at a level 1 German trauma center. (Adapted from Ref. 3.)

Nordic countries) [12]. The number of seriously injured also is considerable, and a majority of these patient presents with high trauma scores [3]. (Fig. 3).

For the last two decades MVAs have been the dominant cause of blunt trauma in Europe [3] (Fig. 4,5). Of these, crashes involving small cars give rise to most of the entrapment situations [13,7] (Fig. 6).

An entrapment situation indicates a high-energy impact and a high risk for extensive and often concealed injuries [14]. In spite of the increasing use of restraints and cars fitted with sophisticated impact protection systems, injuries to the head, thorax, and extremities are common and have increased during recent decades [3,7] (Fig. 7).

Uncontrolled bleeding and hypoxia are the main causes of early mortality in trauma, and failure to recognize and intervene in these situations account for a high degree of preventable prehospital trauma deaths. In these patients, the state of hypoperfusion and hypoxia is further aggravated by the high incidence of non-season-related hypothermia, which attenuates cardiovascular and pulmonary compensation mechanisms.

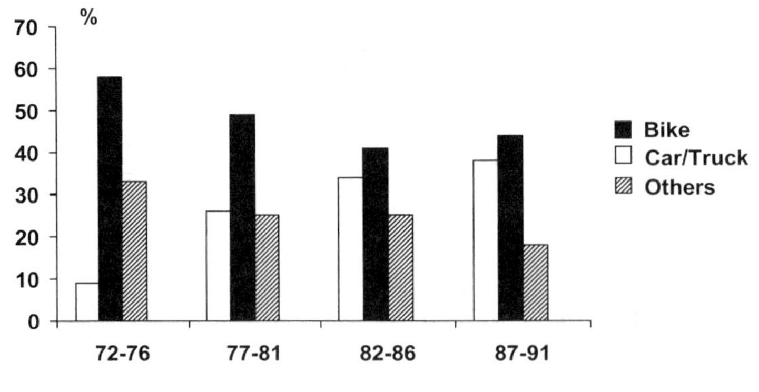

Figure 4 Causes of trauma between 1972 to 1981 and 1982 to 1991 at a level 1 German trauma center. (Adapted from Ref. 3.)

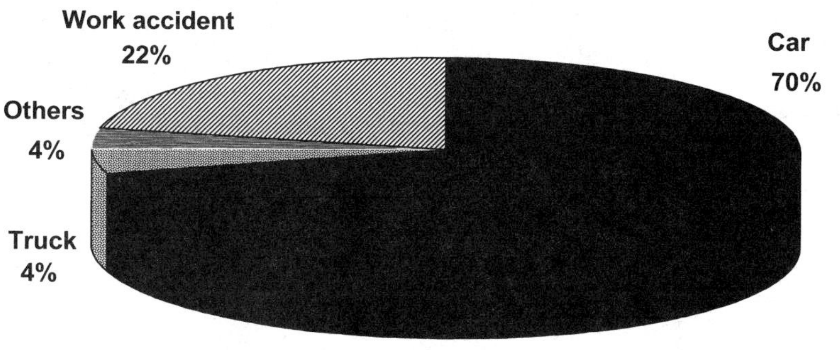

Figure 5 Entrapped patients (type of accident). (Adapted from Ref. 7.)

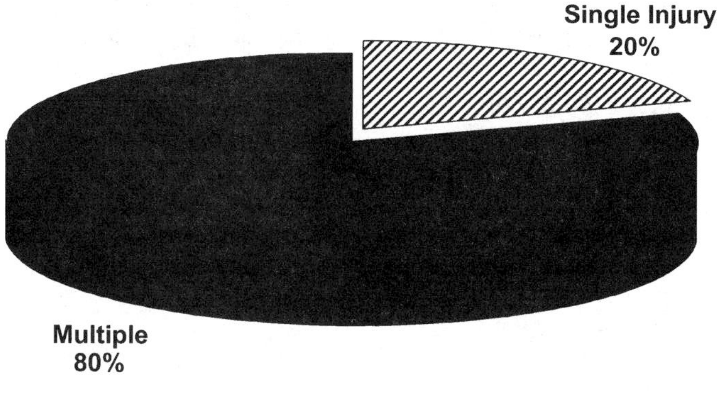

Figure 6 Entrapped patients (multiple vs. single injuries). (Adapted from Ref. 7.)

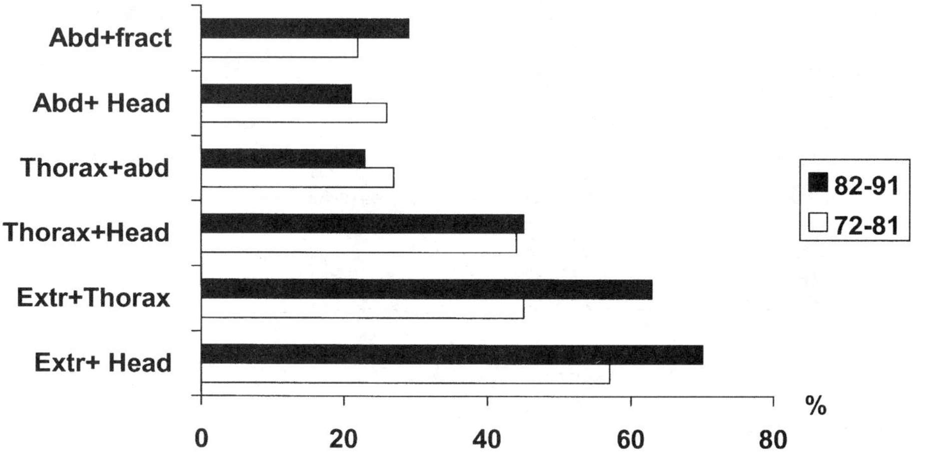

Figure 7 Frequent injury combinations. (Adapted from Ref. 3.)

The immediate care of the entrapped patient thus has to be expedient and appropriate in order to get rapid control over vital functions [13,2,1,15]. Although there has been recent debate about the need for prehospital volume replacement in the case of penetrating torso injury, the need for appropriate on-scene ALS interventions has been well established in numerous studies [13,9,11,16].

During the efforts of extrication and transport, however, improper handling and care of the patient has been reported to significantly increase the risk for neurological disability in patients with spinal trauma [17]. The need for adequate triage and estimation of suspected injuries as well as good standards for prehospital management and extrication are thus vital to improve patient outcome in an entrapment situation.

The overall outcome after prehospital trauma resuscitation has also been shown to benefit from increased personnel competence and skill [9,11], and the need for both defined training standards as well as competence requirements has been strongly emphasized.

All actions performed at the scene of an accident in order to extricate the patient are bound to consume time, which is precious to the patient. An entrapment situation can significantly prolong both the on-scene and rescue time by as much as almost 50% [18]. Previous reports also estimate the time spent to extricate the patient to be 40 to 60 min (Fig. 8).

The overall time spent at the scene has also been reported to be approximately 1 h [3,10], and the scene time has remained about 1 h over the last three decades [3]. This fact and the high number of seriously injured people have led to the call for more developed EMS activities and in Europe have led to the increased involvement of physicians in prehospital trauma care, which has proven to be of benefit in terms of patient outcome [9,17,6].

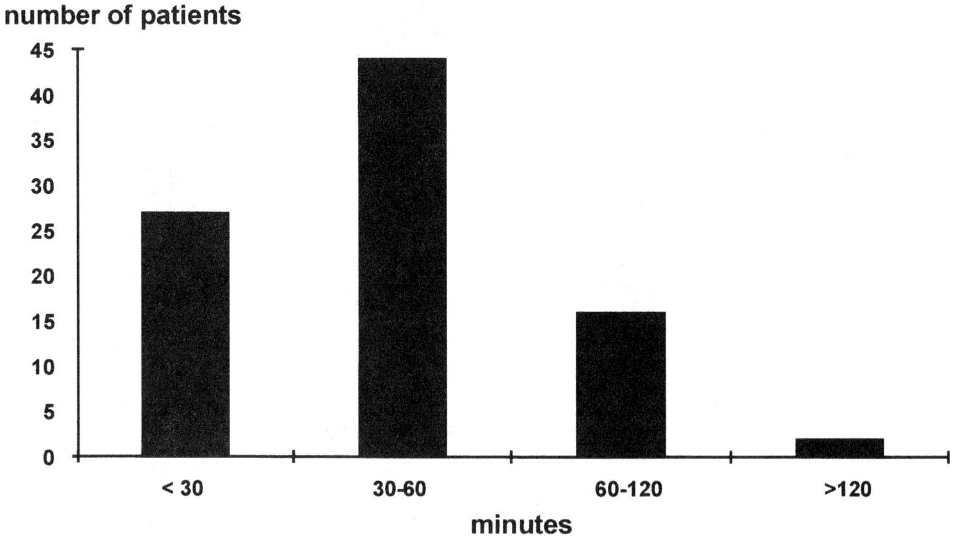

Figure 8 Entrapment times and number of patients per category. (From Ref. 11, with permission from Elsevier Science.)

1. "Scoop-and-Run" vs. "Stay-and-Play"

Prehospital treatment should always focus on not spending unnecessary time at the scene. In the entrapment situation, however, the patient is not immediately accessible and thus needs to be stabilized during the process of extrication.

The involvement of physicians in EMS has been reported to increase the time spent at the scene [16] and can seem to interfere with the initial ''golden hour'' concept in which rapid transport is advocated. Considering the fact that the entrapped patients, in a majority of the cases have sustained multiple injuries and are hypothermic, however, the need for advanced life support in an entrapment situation is high [7,18]. In a recent review of two decades of trauma in Europe, a majority of the victims were shown to have needed invasive actions to secure vital functions in the prehospital phase [3] (Fig. 9).

Within a minimum of the golden hour the patient has to be extricated and vital functions secured. This must be done in an environment in which different interests may conflict.

Vital medical care can thus be unnecessarily held back because of inappropriate extrication procedures, and technical interventions to create access to the patient can in the same way be delayed by insufficient liaison among the different rescue teams. Improvement of rescue strategies and training of the rescue crew have recently proved to reduce scene time, which could be beneficial in the effort to provide appropriate and expedient immediate care [19].

B. Alpine Environment—Avalanche

The victim of an alpine accident (Fig. 9) outside the prepared posts of a ski resort area or in mountain terrain usually is younger and fitter than the average urban trauma population. The greater physiological reserves of such people can be advantageous in a rescue situation, but the behavior of these persons also means that the injury profile is more oriented against trauma and environmental exposure than medical emergencies. The recent growing interest in outdoor sports and especially in ''extreme'' sports have, however, increased the trauma caseload [20–22]. Although people are more concerned about outdoor safety and about being appropriately trained and equipped before taking up de

Volume Substitution	During Extrication	After Extrication	Total
Crystalloid (ml)	530	420	950
Colloid (ml)	600	850	1450
Endotracheal Intubation	31%	38%	69%
MAST			17%
Inotropes			3%

Figure 9 Therapeutic actions. (Adapted from Ref. 7.)

manding outdoor activities. Many accidents still result from inadequate planning and insufficient personal ability to function in a suddenly hostile environment.

Alpine entrapment situations result from the following situations:

- Falls into confined spaces, such as ravines and glacier clefts
- Climbing accidents, in which the victim is stuck on the mountainside
- Suspension injuries
- Disabling accidents in which the victim has to be transported out by means other than by foot
- Avalanche accidents

Apart from the traumatic injuries sustained during the accident itself, hypothermia and altitude-related medical conditions could substantially complicate the rescue operation and deteriorate vital functions (Table 1).

1. Injury Mechanism

Injuries from falls and sports activities in the alpine environment are mostly traumatic, and as such are related to the energy absorption caused by the fall or impact. An aggravated or fatal outcome is apart from the initial trauma due to such external factors as exposure and coexisting medical conditions.

An initial stable situation in good weather with a relatively minor injury such as a broken ankle can, however, very rapidly deteriorate because of limited physical reserves. This can be due to progressive hypothermia, fluid loss, and hypoglycemia as mentioned above, or to time of day, with declining temperatures and sudden weather deterioration at night. In the victim buried by an avalanche, time is even more crucial, and in connection with the presence or absence of an air pocket directly correlated to survival [23]. A fatal

Table 1 Associated Medical Conditions in Alpine Trauma Victims

Event	Medical condition	Consequences for the patient
Inhalation of cold, dry air	Dehydration, asthma	Fatigue, respiratory impairment during exercise, reduced physical capacity, increased susceptibility for hypothermia
Inappropriate clothing that does not divert body moisture from skin surface	Heat loss by convection, hypothermia	Fatigue, lack of initiative, frostbite, immersion injuries (trenchfoot), impaired ability to cooperate in rescue operations, impaired vital functions
Unprepared strenuous exercise (e.g., unexpected weather change)	Hypoglycemia, increased metabolic demands	Fatigue, fear, lack of initiative, impaired decision making, increased susceptibility for hypothermia and injuries
Fall, resulting in suspension in free air attached to climbing rope	Progressives loss of postural vasocontrol, hypothermia.	Hypotension, circulatory collapse, impaired venous drainage and raised ICP if upside down
High altitude	Tachycardia, tachypnoe, epitaxis, cerebral and pulmonary edema	Decreased physical capacity, bleeding, non-trauma-related seizures, respiratory impairment

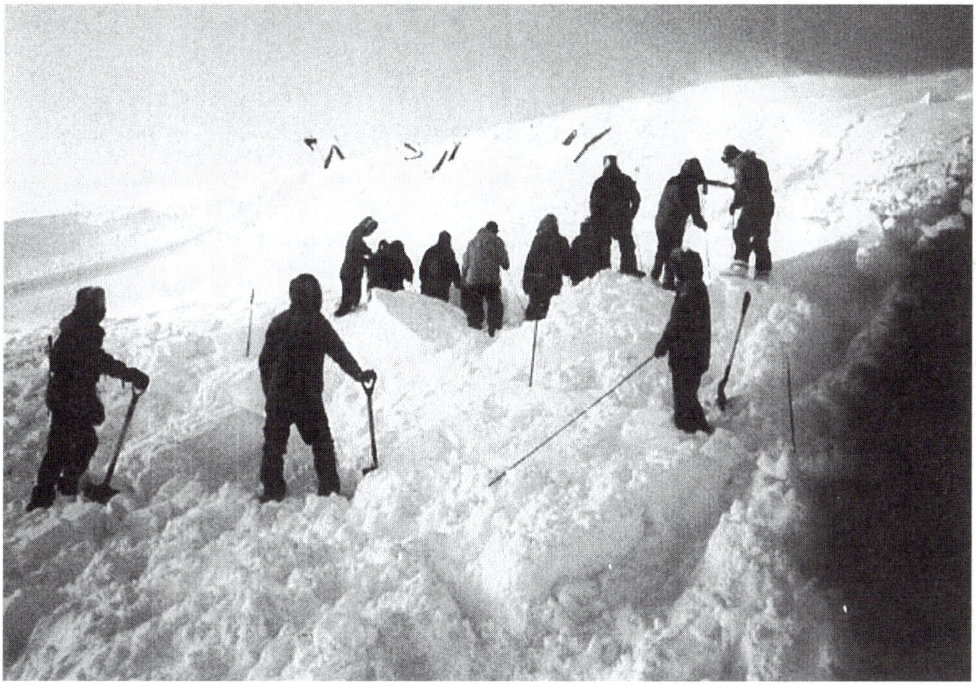

Figure 10 Avalanche search and rescue team. (Courtesy of B. Carlsen, Norwegian Air Ambulance.)

outcome in an avalanche victim is due to hypoxia and subsequent asystole rather than to hypothermia [23,24].

Rapid interventions by rescue teams are thus paramount. Even more important is immediate help from the remaining survivors, as the buried survivors usually lie close to the surface. Fifteen minutes postavalanche there is a dramatic fall in the chance of surviving.

In conducting the search it is also of the outmost importance that the rescue team (Fig. 10) can get information on:

The point at which the victims were caught by the avalanche
The point at which they were last seen
The point of found material
The use of transceivers by the victims

C. Submerged Objects

This is usually a fatal accident, in which the compartments containing people have been flooded (Fig. 11). In rare cases people manage to bail out, but usually restraints, obstructive objects, panic, and jammed hatches and doors prevent escape. Apart from injuries sustained from the impact itself, the submerged position poses exclusive problems to the rescuer.

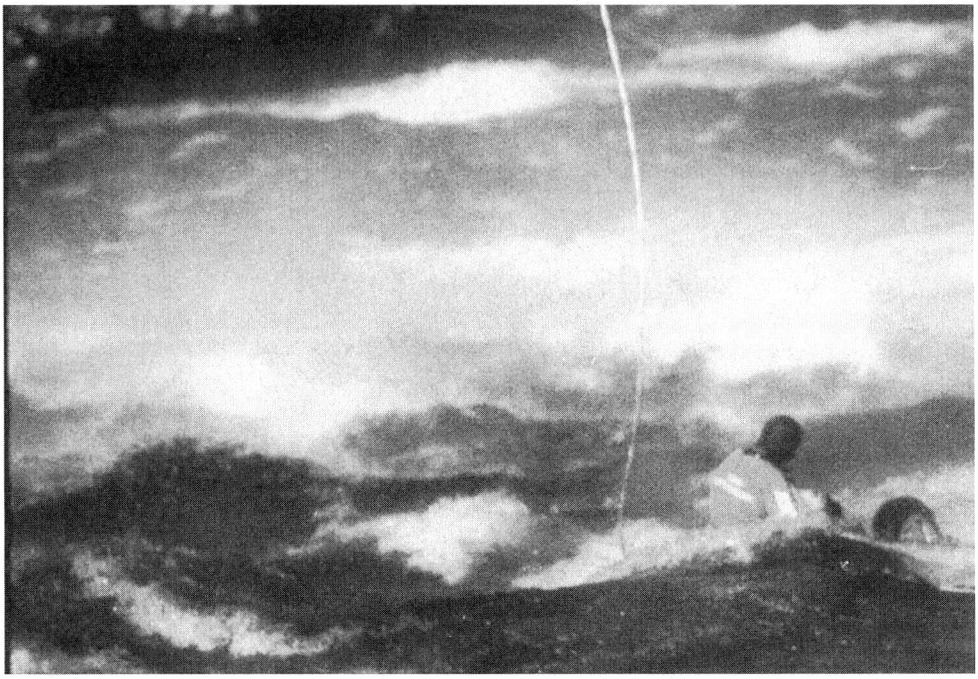

Figure 11 Submerged car after driving off a river bank. (Courtesy of B. Carlsen, Norwegian Air Ambulance.)

These accidents can be divided into the following two major subgroups:

1. *Objects located in or immediately below the surface with a partially flooded personnel compartment or an air pocket.* In cases in which the object is standing on the bottom, it may be accessible from a safe footing, and if so, there might be time to try to winch it to more shallow waters before making entry to an air pocket or opening a closed compartment. If the vehicle is secured in position and time allows, a brief survey of the vehicle and the patients' positions would be helpful in deciding the rescue strategy.

   When access is made the risk of flooding the personnel compartment is imminent, and measures to immediately extricate the patients should be undertaken. Usually reliable estimations of the victims' positions and injuries are almost impossible in the submerged position. An uncontrolled attempt to move the object can endanger the entrapped victims and cause additional injuries because of the increased deformation of the compartment and the loss of the air pocket.

   Access ''on site'' is thus usually preferred, with diver-assisted entry to the compartment. Objects floating on the surface must be carefully handled and secured to prevent the loss of the air pocket.
2. *Completely submerged objects containing an air pocket.* In such cases time is even more crucial since the entrapped victim is breathing a small volume of compressed air. The depth and time of exposure is usually not sufficient to endanger the victim for decompression sickness during the ascent, but the small

amount of compressed air is progressively diluted by exhaled gas, and thus the pO_2 declines with time. When the victim is brought to the surface the rapidly decreasing ambient pressure results in a subsequent fall in pO_2, leading to hypoxia, loss of consciousness, and possible risk of asphyxiation (shallow water blackout) [25]. Because of the pressure drop, the intrapulmonary gas expands during the ascent. If not exhaled it can result in pulmonary barotrauma and air embolization

Apart from hypothermia and traumatic injuries, the victims have been immersed for a period of time. The increased venous return caused by the water pressure would have induced an increased diuresis due to stimulation of stretch receptors in the right atrium and thus a reduction in plasma volume. When lifted out of the water, the sudden decrease in venous return, isolated or in conjunction with hypovolemia from exsanguinations, can result in cardiovascular collapse. Immersed victims should thus always be recovered supine.

D. Buildings, Subways, Caves, and Underground and Confined Spaces

There are many different forms of entrapment that vary in location and in needed rescue skills. These different forms of entrapment include buildings, subways, and underground and confined spaces.

Entrapment within buildings may be due to entombment within closed spaces. These are commonly referred to as void spaces. In this situation the victim may or may not have associated injuries, but egress from the location is restricted. The space exit may be blocked by debris, or the exit may lead out into open air (Brooklyn collapse). The exit may therefore be so dangerous that the victim must remain in the void space. Additionally, the rescue personnel must consider the potential of a secondary building collapse, a stairwell collapse, or even an elevator collapse.

Underground entrapment may be within a collapsed structure or secondary to a trench collapse. The victim who is entrapped in a trench may die of immediate traumatic injuries or die secondary to airway compromise. Suffocation within a trench is due to restricted chest movement. Lung expansion is a passive process, and the inability of the chest wall to expand results in failure to generate necessary negative pressures. This is similar to what is seen in restricted lung disease or stiff-chest-like syndrome secondary to thermal thoracic burns. The entrapment may also affect oxygen transfer due to the aspiration of soil and the resultant occluded airway. The entrenchment situation may also result in significant traumatic injuries. These can be blunt and or penetrating chest, abdomen, or extremity injuries.

This type of entrapment may also lead to significant spinal trauma. This mandates cautious rescue of entrapped victims and the ability to appropriately immobilize these individuals. It is critical that existing injuries not be exacerbated and rescue injuries not be created. This consideration must be tempered with the possibility of secondary collapse and subsequent rescuer injuries or death. The fear of exacerbating (or creating) a spinal injury while a patient remains hypoxic or becomes anoxic is a misplaced field triage decision. An additional consideration is the development of crush syndrome (a.k.a. traumatic rhabdomyolysis). If a patient escapes crush syndrome the assessment should exclude the possibility of compartment syndrome. This can lead to severe nerve injury or in the case of the latter acute renal failure (see Appendix I).

Subway incidents are similar to train or rail incidents, but their confined underground location makes them unique in the rail rescue environment. Train entrapment is essentially broken down into two rescue environments. The first is the disentanglement of victims from within the subway car. This is a medical rescue situation that needs to focus on penetrating and blunt trauma rather than issues related to crush syndrome. These may extend from hemorrhage control or partial or complete amputations to closed thoracic or abdominal trauma. The second issue of subway rescue is the situation referred to as the "man-under" situation, which occurs when individuals fall under trains. The medical management of the victims must be integrated with the extrication process. Medical assessment is critical to determine the victim's survivability to provide *only* lifesaving medical intervention. This should not extensively delay extrication procedures. It may be necessary to make an amputation decision at this time.

Extrication and medical survival must be balanced with respect to time. Traumatic injuries are often fatal, and the primary process is often a body retrieval.

The medical rescue process is one that occurs in a potentially volatile environment. This is the case in a subway crash or derailment event. The potential of secondary collapse of the subway tunnel can be directly related to destabilization of the tunnel structure. The increased collapse potential is often precipitated by the removal of debris from part of the remaining support structure. The debris removal may undermine hidden dangers from within the tunnel environment. These may include secondary street collapse and the undermining of adjacent buildings. The clearing process may also create a subway hazmat incident. The clearing of debris can and has disrupted fuel tanks or heating boiler units. Another hidden danger is from the electrified track system. Under all circumstances the power cutoff should be accomplished prior to the initiation of patient care. Personal safety is of the utmost and primary concern. Unfortunately power systems sometimes get activated inadvertently. There should be a local on-site system to warn all rescue personnel of the status of the electrical system. (Often a high-wattage light across the track system provides a rapid visual warning system.) Another rescuer danger is from smoke and/or dust. This may be from the rescue zone or carried to the rescue work site from distant locations. It is surprising how well smoke and dust are carried through the tunnel system by moving trains. They can effectively function like a large system fan. A fact of life in subway rescue is the limitation of normal communication systems. This type of rescue relies heavily on point-to-point and face-to-face communications. This must be taken into account, and the key to success is prior planning. Needless to say, this goes hand and hand with a support system that anticipates the medical rescue needs.

1. Cave Rescues

Cave rescue scenarios are situations that can have catastrophic results for the rescuer as well as the victim. This type of rescue begins with an individual who is by definition unable to extricate himself. This may be further compounded by associated physical injuries.

The rescuer may unknowingly be entering a location with a potentially toxic environment. The issue of unsafe air quality may be due to constituent cave gases. These may actually be present or there may be a potential for their release or accumulation. This issue mandates the need for constant environmental monitoring. Under extreme circumstances this may require the rescuers to don a self-contained breathing apparatus (SCBA) or other external sources of air (i.e., self-contained underwater breathing apparatus–

SCUBA). The cave rescue also has the potential to be conducted in extreme darkness with poor communications. A site hazard survey conducted prior to the commencement of any rescue attempt is a necessity. This should include the location of pits, holes, trip hazards, waterfalls, and siphons. The potential for an initial or secondary collapse (e.g., mining or water tunnel incident) must be part of this rescue assessment. The potential for hypothermia to the victim and/or the rescuer should be assessed.

A mine rescue is not one that is conducted in a static environment. There is the potential for flooding (changing tides or flowing underground rivers) from existing water sources. There is also the potential for flooding due to ''outside'' weather conditions.

One should not forget that caves (and tunnels) become natural drains in rainstorms. The potential of infectious disease is often overlooked. A potential source may be from resident cave animals.

One disease of concern is rabies, which may be the consequence of a bat bite or secondary to breathing aerosolized rabies-infected urine. Locating victims may only be the beginning of a protracted rescue process. Victims pinned into small crevices may require prolonged extrication. This increases the potential for crush syndrome (secondary to limited or restricted range of motion with resultant muscle compression), compartment syndrome, hemorrhage, or long bone cervical spine injury (fracture or contusion). The combination of confined spaces with low crawls and squeeze points makes the use of traditional extrication transport equipment difficult if not impossible. All of these points add to the potential medical decompensation of the patient. The victims also may need to be transported to extended distances or time (due to terrain obstacles), which may further add to the need for in-field extended medical management. Medical care will at best be only acceptable for the circumstances, since it will be provided in a cold, wet, dark, muddy environment.

Rescue for entrapped victims in cave incidents should only be undertaken by experienced splancners and personnel experienced in trench rescue practices. These personnel should have, at a minimum basic cave skills, experienced rock-climbing skills, rope skills, and experience in rescue and the provision of medical care in the out-of-hospital environment.

III. CARE OF THE ENTRAPPED PATIENT

The entrapped patient is a unique clinical enigma. These patients are some of the most difficult to triage, treat, and assess. Their clinical picture will change at almost a moment's notice. They have stressed their physiological and psychological body systems. They work in conjunction and sometimes at odds to present a complicated clinical picture. They present with a combination of mixed medical and trauma conditions. Often the extent of their true injuries remains hidden until they become life-threatening conditions.

A. Injury Potential: Medical vs. Traumatic

The entrapped patient is one who has the potential for a combination of medical and traumatic injuries. It is extremely important that both aspects be pursued in the assessment of the entrapped patient. Listed in Table 2 are categories of injury potential that should be included in the differential diagnosis of any entrapped victim.

Table 2 Medical and Traumatic Conditions to Consider in the Entrapped Patient

Medical	Pathophysiology	Clinical syndrome
Crush syndrome (a.k.a. traumatic rhabdomyolysis)	Myoglobin from compressed muscle; increased K^+ and acidosis	Acute renal failure Cardiac arrest
Asphyxia	Low O^2 delivery to cells	Hypoxia
Toxic gases	Displace O^2; interfere with O^2 functioning	Hypoxia
Concrete dust	Interfere with normal airway functioning; resultant bronchospasm	Hypoxia
"Lack of oxygen"	Decreased O^2 content	Hypoxia
Bronchospasm	Reactive airway secondary to underlying disease or environmental irritant	Hypoxia; respiratory distress
Hydration/nutrition states	Starvation ketosis; dehydration	Nutritional starvation; dehydration or hypovolemia
Decreased environmental temperature	Alteration in body temperature; alteration in body functions	Hypothermia
Increased environmental temperature	Alteration in body temperature; alteration in body functions	Hyperthermia Heat illness Heat cramps Heat stroke
Traumatic		
Blunt		
Head, neck, and body	Bony injuries; cervical spine and long bone trauma; internal bleeding	Fractures; contusions; sprains; hypovolemia
Airway	Interferes with oxygen exchange	Traumatic asphyxia; flail chest; rib fractures
Penetrating		
Airway	Interferes with oxygen exchange	Pneumothorax; hemothorax; tension pneumothorax
Exsanguination	Internal or external hemorrhage	Hypovolemia

B. Crush Syndrome

The field experience with crush syndrome was extensively studied and documented during the Tangshan earthquake. On July 28, 1976, a magnitude 7.8 earthquake struck the city of Tangshan in China. This single event resulted in the injury of 350,300, with 242,769 deaths. Approximately 20% of the victims suffered from crush syndrome.

Modern-day crush syndrome does not exist in a vacuum. It exists as part of a spectrum of soft tissue injuries. These consist of: crush injury, "pin job," compartment syndrome, traumatic asphyxia, traumatic rhabdomyolysis, and crush syndrome.

Crush syndrome has a long-standing history but has gone unaddressed, undertreated, and undiagnosed. German literature of the 1800s described a clinical syndrome known as Meyer Betz disease. This syndrome was characterized by muscle pain, weakness, and dark urine. This syndrome fell into obscurity, only to be revised during the London blitz of 1941. Trapped and entombed bombing victims would suffer muscle injury associated with kidney failure. This clinical syndrome remained an enigma until modern disasters rediscovered this old disease. This became quite clear with the documented review of the Tangshan earthquake.

Crush syndrome runs a predictable course. Patients survive for days in the entrapped environment (in the ''hole''), then unexplainably and unexpectedly die shortly after rescue. Similar patients that survive are those who are treated early and aggressively ''in the rubble!''

Interrelationships between the different forms of soft tissue (muscle) injury are described below. Crush injury is a local limited and direct muscle injury. Mechanism may be any means of transmitting force directly to muscle tissue. Compartment syndrome is a local limited muscle injury that results in blood flow impairment. This impairment is secondary to the generation of excessive intracompartmental pressures that result in the net reduction in vascular flow. A severe compression of the thorax and retrograde flow of blood cause traumatic asphyxia from the right heart into the head and neck. Crush syndrome is a ''local'' muscle injury that manifests itself in systemic signs and symptoms. The primary insulting substance associated with crush syndrome is the muscle protein myoglobin. Extended compression of muscle tissue also results in the release of toxic substances into the circulation. These result in renal and cardiac complications. The production of released myoglobin is a function of time and compressed muscle mass.

Crush injury is limited, and only involves local tissue (muscle) injury. This is the result of direct muscle trauma. In the incidence of an MVA victims may become trapped for limited periods of time. Such an accident is referred to as a pin job. This direct muscle trauma precedes the development of crush syndrome. The effects of crush syndrome are *local only* until tissue is released and reperfused. Adverse affects begin immediately upon tissue release (transport phase). Patients survive entrapment despite severe crush injury. Muscle tissue in compression is the primary culprit. Muscle is exquisitely vulnerable to sustained compression. Compression may come from either debris or body weight. The inability to move and relieve pressure can have devastating effects. The time frames for developing crush syndrome can range from 1 to 6 hr. The overall clinical effect is a function of muscle mass and time.

Compartment syndrome is the result of increased pressure within closed soft tissue ''compartments'' secondary to muscle injury. This clinical entity is usually the result of buttock, forearm, and leg compression. The net result of compartment syndrome is compromised vascular flow resulting in ischemic necrosis. This in itself is the first stage of crush syndrome.

Crush syndrome is the net result of muscle tissue compression that leads to muscle breakdown and the release of myoglobin and cellular breakdown products into the general circulation. The sequelae of muscle breakdown are increased CPK levels with associated renal failure and acidosis with potassium shifts. The clinical dysfunction is the net result of cells functioning without oxygen due to disrupted local blood supply. Cell membrane disruption will affect the normal structure and function of cellular systems. Local capillary membrane leaks and ''reoxidation'' injury begin as micro injuries that result in macro physiological complications. These can be reflected in the increase of potassium levels (hyperkalemia), acid production (acidosis), myoglobin release (myoglobinuria), capillary leak, and muscle enzyme and ''toxin'' release. One devastating effect of releasing compressed tissue is secondary to associated capillary leak. Hypovolemia with associated hypotension can lead to irreversible shock. A subsequent effect of shock is the development of severe acidosis and its accompanying complications. Shifts in cellular functions move in the oxyhemaglobin dissociation curve, affecting the efficiency of cellular oxygenation.

Myoglobin remains the primary culprit that results in renal shutdown followed by multisystemic organ failure. The association of acidosis and myoglobin within the renal tubular collection system may have devastating results. The precipitation point of myoglobin is directly affected by the acidotic environment. The lower the pH (acidosis) the earlier the myoglobin precipitates, resulting in acute renal failure. Cardiovascular compromise may ultimately result in ventricular fibrillation or other potentially fatal arrhythmias. Pulmonary (disseminated intravascular coagulation, acute respiratory distress syndrome, and noncardiogenic pulmonary edema), hepatic, and vascular injury are additional insults that can have devastating cumulative consequences. All of these are the resultant effects of releasing compressed muscle tissue.

Prerelease of entrapment, clinical findings may range from the painless crushed extremity to a hypersensitive extremity. The limb may have palpable or absent pulses. Postrelease clinical findings may consist of agitation, hyperestesia, or anesthesia. The patient may demonstrate severe pain with or without progressive swelling of the extremity. Patients may demonstrate systemic problems at any time during the rescue despite their initial clinical presentation. These may result in death from the following causes: relative hypovolemia, cardiac arrest, kidney failure, shock (distributive, cardiogenic), shock lung adult respiratory distress syndrome (ARDS), multiple organ failure/death, and diffuse bleeding disseminated intravascular coagulation (DIC).

Diagnosis is critical and is primarily based on three factors: a high index of suspicion, identification of a potential crush mechanism, and detection of early subtle signs and symptoms of crush syndrome.

Medical management is very focused yet limited in its scope and nature. ECG abnormalities should make the clinician suspect alterations in potassium levels or acidosis or electrolyte changes, all of which will respond rapidly to effective early intervention. Potassium and acid management responds well to a variety of strategies, including sodium bicarbonate, insulin and glucose combination, B_2 agonist, calcium administration, and diuretics with continuous cardiac monitoring. The minimization of kidney injury is based on the principal of maximal perfusion and diuresis. Prerelease management is directed at the prevention of kidney shutdown and its associated acidosis.

Management in the rubble is directed at basic time-proven strategies. These include attention to the ABCs (airway, breathing, and circulation) of resuscitation. Early and when necessary aggressive fluid management via intravenous (IV, saline lock or even oral route) infusion is critical. The issue of oxygen utilization versus air is one that is often neglected. There is strong evidence to counter the view that a little oxygen never hurts. The generation of systemic free radicals and their deleterious effect is championed in the sports medicine literature. The injudicious use of oxygen plays havoc with the rescue environment. The iatrogenic creation of oxygen pockets and its potential interaction with high-temperature cutting tools (torches) are not usually addressed by the on-scene medical personnel. Often the only real issue is airway protection from dust and debris. The better alternative would be the use of ''breathable'' air. Psychological support is critical to prevent victim panic and also to provide an easy tool to victim status.

Changes in mentation, speech pattern, respiratory rate, and level of activity are all part of the ongoing medical monitoring and assessment. The issue of management in the rubble requires deliberate assessment of the incident crush potential and the likelihood that this diagnosis should or should not be entertained. The medical personnel on the scene should also consider the incident specifics as to the best way of integrating medical care into overall rescue efforts. This requires at least basic knowledge of collapse potential and structure support strategies. The patient's pre-existing physiologic health is another critical factor that can introduce a positive or negative survival factor. Delayed or protracted rescues on debilitated patients may require a customization in the rescue and medical management strategies. An already impaired patient will have unexpected physical responses. It is critical that the on-scene medical personnel have the ability to predict potential rescue victim decompensation. Environmental (temperature) factors are often ones that no one involved in the rescue effort is able to control, but often simple environmental mitigation efforts can result in increased survivability and decreased morbidity. Immobility and entrapment are protective and are effectively dismantled during the rescue phase and become clinically apparent during the transport phase of a rescue. Critical to the rescue effort is the directive Look and observe.

C. Crush Syndrome Complications: Interrelationships

1. Airway

Field management of the entrapped patient is often directed at the prevention of any future injury or exacerbation of an existing problem. The underlying principal is most critical when addressing airway issues.

Protection of an adequate airway can be accomplished by the use of a nonrebreather mask that prevents or limits the entry of dust or other irritants into the upper and lower airways. In this situation the primary objective is airway protection and not the delivery of oxygen. Definitive airway management may be necessary based on clinical assessment. Possible procedures may include the use of endotracheal or nasotracheal intubation techniques. Both methods will gain airway control but are of limited practicality in the collapse environment. In the event of an inability to intubate the patient, a cricothyroidotomy (surgical airway) should be performed. In either situation the ventilation of the patient may be via bag-valve mask (BVM) or via a portable high-frequency ventilator. These methods may serve to secure the airway but have limited usefulness in the confined space environment. They become difficult methods of ventilation when the patient requires transport out of an entrapment area. Patients often need to be carried in various positions through areas in which space is limited in height and depth. Under these circumstances the ability to continuously provide positive pressure for ventilation may become easily compromised.

The issue of resuscitation gas may not be as obvious as it appears. In the prehospital setting it is the usual practice to administer oxygen freely and liberally. Oxygen toxicity is limited to the patient with high (100%) prolonged administration or patients with chronic obstructed lung disease (COPD; emphysema). In the collapse or entrapped environment the role of oxygen is a controversial one. The unnecessary use of oxygen can result in the production of *oxydases*. In the rescue environment the indiscriminant use of oxygen can result in dangerous flammable gas collections (i.e., concentrations) in the enclosed space. For these reasons there should be a very clear and compelling reason for the use of oxygen. Under most circumstances the use of ''breathable'' air (not *medical* air) is more than sufficient. The source of air from the other rescue workers can be from the self-contained breathing apparatus (SCBA).

In a situation in which there is an unstable or unmanageable airway, joint team assessment is critical. The use of definitive airway adjuncts must be factored in with the practicality of extraction. By discussing these issues other nonmedical rescue personnel can often contribute significantly to the information pool. These discussions may accentuate the urgency of the patient's situation and affect the rescue approach. The key to airway maintenance begins with control of the environment and strict adherence to the rule that no entry shall be permitted until the structural situation is declared to be relatively "stable."

2. Concrete Dust

Concrete dust is an issue of special concern in the entrapped environment and its immediate airway injury. The access of concrete dust into the patient's airway can have fatal consequences. The mixture of concrete dust in the airway with moisture can result in the development of airway concretions. In the worst case scenario these concretions can form space-occupying molds of the patients airway. Additionally, the mixture of concrete dust and moisture can result in varying degrees of airway chemical burns (with associated irritation, inflammation, and soft tissue swelling). These burns are the result of concrete additives, especially lime, placed in combination with moisture.

Intermediate injury can be the result of the disruption of ventilation system integrity. This exposure can present itself as an upper respiratory infection (URI) or in some cases as pneumonia. The offending organism may result in mycoplasma pneumonia or Legionnaires' disease.

Long-term injury can result from asbestos exposure, especially in the case of long-term smokers. The rule of thumb should be that there *is* asbestos until proven otherwise.

3. Bronchospasm

Bronchospasm can be the result of various atmospheric irritants. In this situation the best solution is to limit the total time of exposure or remove the victim or the rescuer from the environment as soon as is possible or most practical. The airway should be protected with some form of a mask (nonrebreather or even a dust mask). The medical management for these patients is the frequent and liberal use of bronchodilators and controlled irritant exposure. These patients must be monitored closely (respiratory status) for decompensation. The use of steroids should be considered early and administered intravenously.

4. Environment

Temperature as it relates to the rescue environment is another critical factor that must be added to the mix of rescue concerns. Environment extremes can be a danger to rescuers as well as victims. Under the prolonged effects of the environment rescuers may exhibit impaired judgment and fatigue. Where professionalism and basic safety procedures would normally dictate actions, risk taking and shortcuts may be the end result. The environment of concern may not be as austere or friendly as the external outside world. Assessment of the immediate entrapment area is a necessary early area of evaluation.

Hyperthermia is defined as failure of the normal thermoregulatory system of the body. A factor that must be considered is the temperature humidity index (THI) or the wet bulb globe temperature (WBGT). This will allow for better assessment of the true relative temperature variation within the rescue space. This can be seen as a factor in such cases as an underground subway rescue, where the work temperature may be as high as 105° to 110°F with outside temperatures in the low 90s. The correction may be limited to or as simple as providing forced air circulation. The basic pathophysiology of hyperthermia is the ultimate collapse of the central nervous system, hypovolemia, cardiovascular collapse, hepatic failure, and renal decompensation.

The other extreme of elevated temperature is the issue of hypothermia. Accidental hypothermia is the drop of the body core temperature below 35°C (95°F). This may be secondary to environmental conditions such as cold, cool, moist, wind seasonal factors, or an intrastructural environment that is secondary to the collapse conditions. The medical rescue team should monitor the reported wind chill factor (WCF) to appreciate the effective victim temperature exposure. These can be related to moisture/water from broken water pipes or secondary to fire-suppression efforts. The basic pathophysiology of hypothermia is multifaceted in its systemic repercussions. Hypothermia affects the cardiovascular system (collapse and failure), respiratory system (hypoventilation), central nervous system (disorientation and confusion), and renal (cold diuresis with resultant hypovolemia). Environmental hypothermia must be corrected where possible before (or to limit the development of patient clinical hypothermia) the victim's physiologic condition deteriorates.

5. The Heat Sink

A heat sink is a substance that aggressively absorbs heat from its surroundings, usually in an attempt to reach thermal equilibrium with its immediate environment. In the rescue environment the main culprit to address is *concrete*. Other heat sinks that may affect patient conditions (and therefore viability) are such things as water, snow, ice, stone, ground, and metal. If these factors are not addressed they may result in a drop of body temperature that is actually independent of moderately favorable surrounding environmental conditions.

Management is directed at one common goal: to remove the patient from contact with an heat absorber or to limit the total contact surface area. This may simply require the utilization of a nonconductive (insulating or inefficient) interface (e.g., blanket, dry cloths). It is extremely important that the efforts not be made to correct patient hypothermia but rather to prevent a further deterioration in the clinical status. Failure to correct any environmental extreme is directly correlate to victim survivability.

6. Hydration/Nutrition States

Dehydration is a factor that will impair or have a negative overall effect on survivability as well as the morbidity and mortality rate. The maintenance of fluid and hydration status may not simply be an issue of replacing the patient's insensible losses. It is critical that the rescue efforts not fall into a negative hydration status. Maintain daily hydration needs (insensible losses) and adjust for the rescue space environment with augmentation losses secondary to entrapment. Other clinical conditions must also be part of the general assessment, such as third spacing due to crush injury, crush syndrome, compartment syndrome, and gastrointestinal ileus. Other volume losses that must be considered are such things as internal or external bleeding, vomiting, and diarrhea. Management is directed toward the monitoring of existing medical conditions and preventing further clinical deterioration. The medical management of fluid resuscitation should be conducted judiciously to avoid iatrogenic overhydration. The most optimal route of fluid resuscitation when possible is via the oral hydration route. If this is not possible or practical then IV 0.9% normal saline should be administered. Rescue personnel should make every effort to keep fluid status at a slightly negative balance. Insensible losses and acute loss replacement are the optimal goal. Judiciously hydrate the patient to avoid iatrogenic acute pulmonary edema. The medical team may choose to monitor urine output as a measure of hydration status. Where the resources exist, monitoring the electrolyte status may be possible. For those with electrolyte-monitoring capabilities the water deficit in liters = total body water (TBW) = [0.6 × weight in kg] minus (desired [Na^+]/measured [Na^+]). The clinician should use limited or controlled pain management for a patient who requires continual monitoring of his or her mental status.

7. Nutritional Concerns

Nutritional support (supplementation) is not required in most cases. The use of unnecessary food supplements may subject the trapped victim to the potential for aspiration. Should the victim require nutritional support the use of IV glucose bolus's should be considered. A portable glucometer for measuring blood glucose levels should be part of the medical rescue tools. Protracted rescues such as in Kobe, Japan, the Philippines, and Mexico City all had live rescues extending from 10 days to 2 weeks. In such cases the medical rescue will need to provide supplemental nutrition. This should *not* include such things as diuretic-inducing substances. Items such as coffee may induce or exacerbate volume-depletion status. This also includes smoking, which will result in peripheral vasoconstriction with resultant heat loss and environmental contamination. Another restricted item includes alcohol, which will result in heat loss due to peripheral vasodilatation and alteration in the victim's mental status.

8. Medications

The overall goal is to maintain medical stability for ''most'' chronic conditions. Not all medications should be omitted or excluded, but rather should be dealt with on a case-by-case basis. Cardiac and seizure medications should be administered. Medications that are diuretic in nature should not be administered unless increased failure is noted. The use of antibiotics in the rescue setting is unnecessary and should be discontinued. Special caution should be used when the patient is on chronic oral hypoglycemic agents. The rescue team should monitor blood sugar levels and treat only with short-acting IV hypoglycemic agents. Oral hypoglycemic medications should *not* be used because of their long-acting properties. Immediate active intervention should not be automatically instituted but become a function of the patient's clinical status. Vasodilator drugs should be avoided and only used on a case-by-case basis.

9. Trauma

Penetrating Trauma

The basic tenants of trauma remain in place. Monitor and stabilize the airway and ensure the patency and adequacy of ventilations. Stabilize the cervical spine as is situationaly feasible. Monitor vital signs to establish baseline parameters. This will enable the medical team to establish a trending pattern. Hemorrhage control and necessary resuscitation should be addressed early. Evaluate for evidence of a pneumothorax (caution not to convert an open pneumothorax into a tension pneumothorax), tension pneumothorax, or flail chest. The presence of any protruding objects should remain and stabilize in place. Intravenous access should only be instituted if medically indicated. Incident specifics require review for established injury patterns. Such is the case with explosion specifics (with and without the collapse scenario): propane, incendiary devices, flammable fluids, or gases.

Blunt Trauma

Blunt trauma injuries are common to victims of collapse, especially in cases of earthquakes. This was an all too frequent scenario in the case of the Tangshan and Kobe earthquakes, with a significant percentage of patients demonstrating long bone and cervical spine injuries. Collapses will also cause a significant number of head injuries from falling debris. The management of potential cervical and long bone fractures should be undertaken (immobilization) as soon as possible and practical in the collapse environment. Instruments such as the long boards may not be universally acceptable. Their use is limited by angles of victim removal, and the rescuer must consider his or her inflexible diameter with respect to the exit (removal) path.

The use of plastic skeds (semi-rigid plastic sheaths) may be the best option. They are limited by decreased stability and decreased immobilization capability but with the advantage of conforming to the contours of the entrapped space (increased ability to remove from confined space).

Chest Trauma

Chest trauma offers a unique clinical dilemma. The net result of this type of injury may be impaired mechanical excursion of the chest wall, resulting in decreased oxygen and carbon dioxide exchange. This impaired exchange may result in clinical hypoxia or hypercarbia. This type of injury (or impairment) resembles the effects of restrictive lung disease in which stiff inefficient respiratory muscles exist. Traumatic asphyxia is a situation in which the patient's traumatic lung injury is usually limited. Even with limited injury his or her ability to passively expand his or her lungs secondary to mechanical excursion of the outer chest wall is severely impaired. These patients will survive quite well (despite their morbid appearance) if rescue efforts are rapid in the sense of relieving the mechanical restriction. These patients must also be evaluated for pneumothorax, tension pneumothorax, flail chest, or simply for broken ribs.

D. General Airway Procedures

General airway procedures do not change with respect to the basics of evaluation and resuscitation. Under normal conditions the use of oxygen by clinicians is an automatic action. Unless a contraindication can be demonstrated, the oxygen flow begins (almost universally) with patient contact. In the collapse environment this can result in changes in ambient oxygen concentration.

This can significantly affect the speed and safety of an entrapped victim rescue operation. Even if oxygen concentrations remain well within safe environmental parameters, there is always the issue of gas pockets and increased gasmonitoring frequency. The need for administrating supplemental oxygen to these patients can be questioned in most cases. The medical effort would be better served if it would concentrate on maintaining a clear and unobstructed airway. Under these circumstances the use of breathable air is quite acceptable (to the victim as well as to the rescue personnel). Within the United States the common source of such air is found on all rescue vehicles. This is the self-contained breathing apparatus SCBA, which is used by all firefighters for entry into dangerous environments. This source of breathable air with free flow into face mask will (under most rescue circumstances) keep most dust from entering the victim's airway. Definitive airway maintenance and final procedures are a function of incident logistics. In general order of preference they are: nonrebreather mask without oxygen, nonrebreather mask with oxygen, endotractacheal tube, nasotracheal tube, and cricothyroidotomy. There is no one answer or approach; each situation must be assessed on its own merits and resolved accordingly.

E. Amputation

Field amputation is a radical procedure and should not be undertaken without due consideration of the patient's short- and long-term outcome. The consideration and mental intellectual evaluation may be undertaken early, but this option is only implemented when normal extrication procedures have *failed*. This option must not be viewed as a heroic procedure but rather one in which the only choice was that of life over limb.

The general indications for field amputation are the following:

1. The patient *will* die if removal is not rapidly achieved.
2. All methods of extrication (with respect to time) have failed.
3. The limb is severely shredded, with only minimal tissue connecting the extremity (clearly an unsalvageable extremity).
4. For the purpose of victim (corpse) identification when extrication is not feasible (i.e., fingerprints).

Only a physician who is trained in entrapped patient rescue and environment should perform the ultimate procedure. In order to make the appropriate decision, information material as to the structure and technical rescue logistics must be obtained from nonmedical rescue personnel. This is very different from the surgeon in the operating suite, and requires a physician who has previously interacted with such personnel.

Ultimately the final decision to cut is made by a physician, with joint decision input from all of the following rescue team members:

1. Building/team engineer: establishes building stability (how long the structure will remain upright in its present state)
2. Rescue personnel: establish the true time parameters for the actual rescue/removal from entrapment
3. On-scene medical: establishes victim (probability) survivability on a best-guess basis to survive the extrication process under the restraints of the projected rescue and extrication time

Once the on-scene physician has made the decision that limb removal is the only viable option, the following issues must be addressed for medical logistical planning. These general principles must be considered as the medical team proceeds with its necessary actions. The first general principle is the acknowledgment that

1. Field amputations should be considered primary, not definitive procedures:
2. All field amputations will require in-hospital debridement and revision:
3. Field amputations should never violate a joint space.
4. *Above all maximize length* (for revision and rehabilitation considerations).

The issue of field anesthesia is a critical one, since within the U.S. prehospital system there are no field anesthesiologists. The prehospital emergency physician must therefore be knowledgeable in the use of anesthetic agents. This last requirement is not a simple, straightforward issue. Even under the best of circumstances the appropriate selection and use of anesthetic agents is extremely difficult. Some may champion the role of the noncollapse physician, but only in extreme emergencies (nonavailability of a field physician) should another physician be permitted into the collapse environment. You are asking someone to work totally out of his or her environment, and simply stated this is no place for on-the-job training. The field physician should be trained and have access to IV anesthetic and possibly paralytic medications. Only under the most extreme conditions should anesthetic agents be omitted. (This should be immediately followed by a benzodiazepine in an attempt to induce retrograde amnesia to the immediate event.) This method should only be imployed under the threat of imminent collapse. The choice of anesthetic, sedative, and or paralytic agent should be a function of (1) physician comfort and experience, (2) training, and (3) availability.

The recommended field general procedure is one that has been advocated by the NATO field amputation guide; it is an excellent resource for use under austere field conditions. These procedures may be modified by physician training, and in the end be totally at the discretion of the physician. These amputation procedures follow the general rule of speed with bleeding control. Remember that the patient will need to be removed to a tenuous environment immediately after the procedure, therefore use of tissue flap and pressure dressing is critical to patient survivability. The choice of field amputation devices are limited and dictated by entrapment circumstances and physician training.

One such item can be the traditional rigid orthopedic handsaw. It is simple to use and allows for fairly good control of the cutting area. Another device that can be utilized in the collapse setting is the Gigley saw. This is a diamond-impregnated stainless steel wire. Control is quite easy and can cut through long bones very quickly. The use of the Gigley saw is also very useful in awkward environments in which finding a working space is a concern. The final and last choice for amputation equipment is the cordless reciprocating saw with a 6-in. cutting blade. This tool has the absolute worst cut with respect to neatness. The spray of bone and blood is significant, and body fluid contamination is unavoidable. The advantage to this tool is speed. In the situation in which building stability and rescuer safety is most critical, we can sever a femur in 20 to 30 sec. Every one of these items mandates immediate surgical debridement and a secondary final procedure. The issue of bleeding control is critical for the patient undergoing a field amputation. The managing physician should apply a tourniquet proximal to the amputation site until the procedure is completed.

On *stable* patients (within ''relatively'' stable structures) a scalpel skin incision with attempted isolation and tie-off of the major vessels should be attempted. On the *unstable* patient tying off the major vessels may not be possible due to time constraints. Under these circumstances speed and not technique becomes the critical factor. A skin flap should be used as compression dressing in addition to extensive pressure dressing. The physician may also use purse-string sutures to aid in bleeding control. Ultimately rapid procedure within the confines of the collapse environment and rapid (as is possible) transport to a definitive care facility will dictate patient survivability.

F. Analgesia and Anesthesia During Motor Vehicle Entrapment

It should be stressed that analgesia is an important factor in the quality of medical assistance during motor vehicle extrication. Excessive pain in trauma patients may result in a worse outcome because of many factors.

1. Negative Effects of Excessive Pain in Trauma

Hypertension
Increased blood loss

Increased oxygen consumption
Increased intracranial pressure (ICP) in head injury
Lesser diagnostic feedback
Negative psychological effects
Negative effect on therapeutical measures
Negative effect on rescue measures
More chance of chronic pain

For these reasons adequate analgesia is important, even in difficult situations, such as motor vehicle entrapment.

In Europe, many emergency medical systems involve physicians. Especially when anesthetists are involved who are also specially trained in the prehospital environment, high-quality anesthetic care can be delivered.

Because of the special circumstances during extrication of an entrapped victim, only highly experienced physicians can find the right balance between adequate analgesia and the risks of possible side effects. When an analgesic causes a respiratory depression, for example, airway management and ventilation support should be given. In the case of entrapment and minimal space around the head of the patient this can be difficult. Another side effect that shouldn't be neglected is the risk of hypotension. In a sitting, hypovolemic patient, such as is found in a motor vehicle entrapment, the blood pressure can decrease tremendously when the patent given a sedative or a narcotic. Titration therefore should be performed carefully.

It is essential that physicians or paramedics are trained in special techniques for airway and ventilation management under these circumstances when giving analgesia or sedation. These special airway maneuvers are principally the same as in the hospital. The difference, however, is the difficult access to the patient. A patient with an obstructed airway needs an open airway immediately. Immediate release is in most cases too late to prevent choking or at least hypoxic brain damage. Airway maneuvers should be performed even when there is difficult access to the patient. With proper training this has been shown to be possible. The same can be said about endotracheal intubation. In most situations it is not possible to intubate the patient from the top of the head while he or she is lying on a table or stretcher. For that reason it is necessary to train people to intubate from different positions around the patient, like ''face-to-face'' intubation, sitting at the right side of the patient's head, or lying on the ground at the head side of the patient with the elbows on the floor. Only when these techniques are trained in simulations, can performance in reality be safe.

The general rule in these situations is: when the patient needs an open airway, he or she will get it immediately. Only in exceptional situations is immediate release necessary for reasons of airway obstruction or ventilation impairment.

The choice for the right analgesic technique depends on the following:

The condition of the patient
The intensity of the pain
The situation of the entrapment
The skills and experience of the physician or paramedic
The medical equipment and medications available
The possible side effects of the drug

All analgesics should be administered intravenously. The only exception could be ketamine, the only agent that could be given safely and effectively intramuscularly when needed. Titration doses are dependant on the condition of the patient, the age of the patient, and the intensity of the pain. In general the endpoint of analgesic therapy is a situation in which the patient can tell the pain is still present but the intensity is acceptable. Side effects will occur more often when the pain disappears totally. Giving the drug slowly intravenously in small boluses and avoiding high-peak plasma levels, can diminish the occurrence of side effects of narcotics.

2. Side Effects of Intravenously Administered Narcotics

Respiratory depression
Circulatory depression
Vomiting
Uncooperative motions
Muscle rigidity (opioids)
Disappearance of clinical symptoms

Ketamine is a drug with a special place in anesthesia/analgesia in the field. It is able to induce amnesia, analgesia, and a state of unconsciousness or sleep without relevantly reducing reflexes or muscle tone. Ketamine still is the most suitable single drug anesthetic in the field or in wartime. If possible ketamine should be combined with a benzodiazepine, like midazolam, in a dose of 2.5 to 5 mg when giving more then 0.3 mg/kg BW. In a low dose (<0.3 mg/kg BW) ketamine mainly has an analgesic effect where psychological side effects are minimal. When administering higher doses, a benzodizepine should be given in combination with ketamine, which avoids psychological side effects in most cases. Ketamine in doses of 1 to 1.5 mg/kg BW are sufficient for pain-free extrication in most cases and has a duration of 10 to 15 min. Although pharyngeal reflexes are believed to be intact after induction with ketamine, they may not be sufficiently protective against pulmonary aspiration of gastric contents.

Regional anesthesia in the field can be very useful in some cases. One of the most important blocks that can be used in the case of a femoral fracture is a femoral nerve block. In particular, fractures of the distal two-thirds of the femur can be treated sufficiently by a femoral nerve block. In a proximal femoral fracture, pain relief will be only partial in most cases.

In general pain relief is an important task for health care providers dealing with motor vehicle entrapment. Hospital personnel, however, have to be trained to get experience in special techniques related with the more difficult environment. Too often it is said that things would be impossible while experienced people can show that a lot is possible in a safe and effective way.

IV. EXTRICATION TECHNIQUES AND RESCUE OPERATIONS

A. General Aspects

Entrapped trauma victims have a high risk for extensive injuries and often have severe impairment of vital functions [3,9]. Such a patient is not immediately accessible and because of that is exposed to further injuries. Delayed and insufficient airway control, uncontrolled exsanguinations, and hypothermia are major threats to the patient, and must be dealt with expediently. The extrication efforts in themselves may also be deleterious if not undertaken with proper knowledge of the underlying mechanism, suspected injuries, and without coordination and liaison within the rescue team [11,10,2].

According to the prehospital trauma life support (PHTLS) [26] manual, global evaluation of vital functions should be accomplished within 15 sec after gaining access to the victim, followed by a primary survey. No more than 5 to 10 min should be allowed at the scene before the patient is en route to the hospital.

Although the mean time from the occurrence of an accident to the arrival at the EMS facility in most EMS systems is about 8 to 10 min, an entrapment situation significantly increases the time spent at the accident scene [26,16]. The average rescue time is somewhere between 45 to 60 min when the patient is entrapped, and has remained fairly constant during the past two decades [3,11,10]. About an hour is thus spent at the accident scene before the patient can begin to be transported to the hospital.

Most of the golden hour is thus already spent, and in order to prevent profound shock due to ongoing exsanguinations, inadequate oxygenation, and exposure, medical interventions at the accident scene have proven to be advantageous [9,19,27]. Appropriate training of rescue teams and the use of defined protocols and algorithms have been shown to greatly improve performance and to reduce the time spent at the accident scene, however [11,10,19]. The need for close contact and liaison within the team and with the on-scene commander (OSC) is paramount.

B. Motor Vehicle Accidents

1. Strategy, Techniques, and Safety Precautions

Method of Approach

The Scene. All actions at the scene are supervised by the OSC. The fire and EMS vehicles are parked so as to protect the accident site from other traffic and facilitate passage of the rescue vehicles. The crew is organized to previously assigned tasks. The accident scene is divided in two areas with a 5- and 10-meter radius, respectively (Fig. 12). Only the necessary equipment is allowed within the 5-meter radius. All medical equipment used is placed in or on the vehicle to prevent damage from boots and heavy tools. Scrap is continuously brought outside the inner radius. Before entering, the vehicle should be secured and carefully stabilized. The risk of fire should be ruled out and measures for immediate fire extinguishing undertaken. When entering the vehicle all personnel should beware of the dangers of nontriggered air bags and impact-reduction devices and be sure not to position themselves between such a device and the patient. After gaining access to the victim and after the global survey is completed, two different approaches of extrication are available, depending on the situation and the patient's condition.

Immediate extrication because of a life-threatening situation, either from environmental hazards or because of severe deterioration of the patient's vital signs, which cannot be managed inside the vehicle. The rapid extrication procedure, even when carried out properly, may aggravate already existing injuries, thus rapid extrication should be reserved for emergencies only. A rapid extrication procedure should not take longer than 2 to 3 min once the decision is made. A common reason for rapid extrication is a compromised airway. Special training

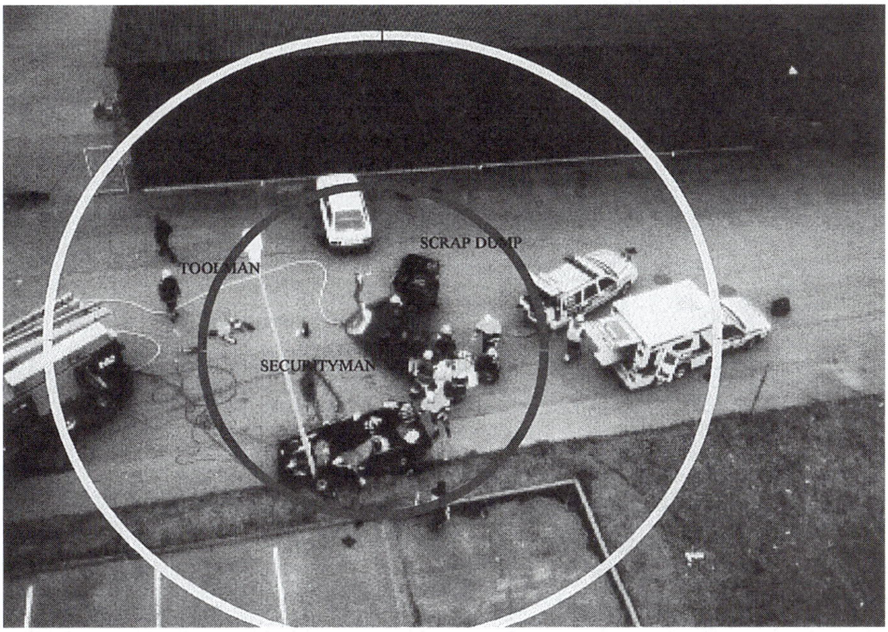

Figure 12 Organization of the accident scene. (From Ref. 19.)

in field airway management can minimize the need for this potentially harmful procedure.

Controlled extrication with maintained control of vital functions after rapid assessment and stabilization of the patient.

Rapid Extrication. Three routes are available. The patient is slid out on a spine board either sideways through one of the doors or through the rear window. This is an uncontrolled emergency maneuver in which only minimal spinal protection and airway control can be provided, and it requires good coordination and trained manpower to be successful. During the extrication the patient's neck should be protected with manual in-line stabilization. The use of a short spine board facilitates extrication, especially when using the route through the rear window (Fig. 13).

Controlled Extrication. The first priority is to gain access to the patient. This can be achieved through a window or by removal of a door. If possible the approach should be made in the patient's field of vision to gain rapid attention, to reassure the patient, and to prevent unnecessary movement of the patient's head. When the windows are removed, blankets or plastic sheets are used to protect the patient from glass debris. When appropriate the patient can be fitted with goggles (Fig. 14). Once access is obtained, manual in-line stabilization is applied to protect the C spine, and a rapid global survey is done.

Personal Protection. All personnel wear helmets, goggles, and protective gloves to protect them from sharp edges and glass debris. Vinyl examination gloves are worn under the protective ones to protect from contamination during medical interventions.

After the wreck is stabilized enough room must be created to allow medical interventions and immobilization of the patient before extrication on a spine board. This is usually

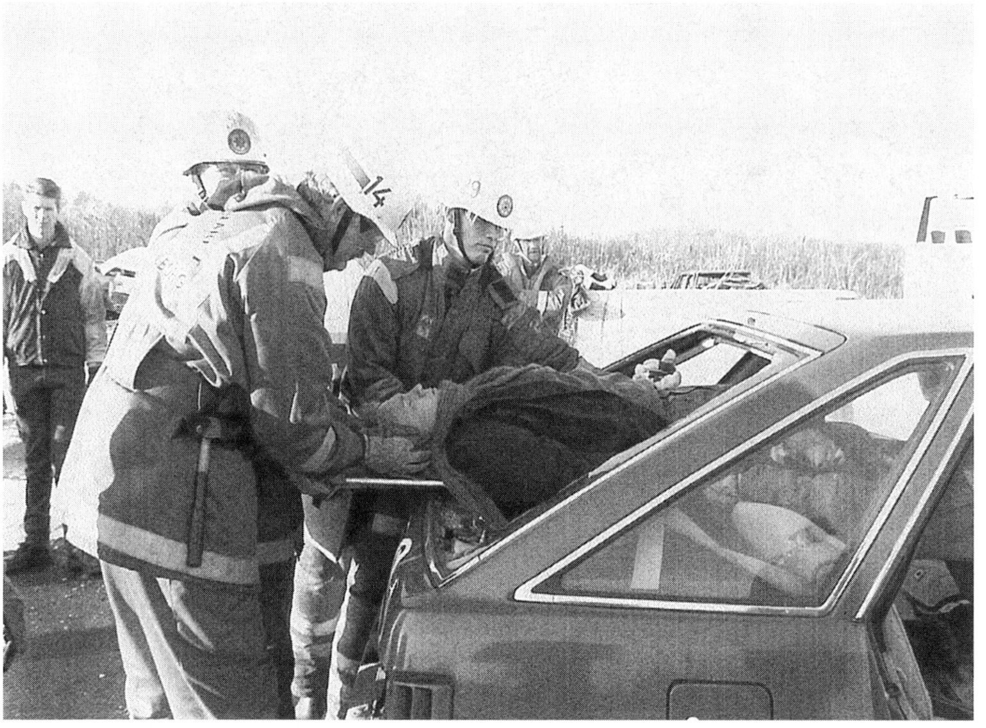

Figure 13 Rapid extrication through a rear window.

most easily achieved by removing the roof. Best access is obtained if the roof is totally removed, since this allows extrication over the rear seat and trunk. This procedure also avoids the risk of the roof falling back on the rescuer attending to the victim. The rear seat and trunk also give a good support for the spine board and allow the team to slide the patient out of the wreck without any sideways or turning maneuvers. When enough room is created a short spine board is slid down behind the patient and the backrest (Fig. 15). The spine board is held firmly during this maneuver. The backrest of the seat is then cut or pulled down and the patient is gently extricated over the rear of the vehicle. The patient should then be fully immobilized with a hard collar and an extrication device (Kendrik extrication device—KED).

Overturned Vehicle. Access is obtained either by cutting the side, which is then folded down, or by the rear section, which is forced open by expanders after cutting the rear supporting posts. The patient is best slid out on a short spine bord, thus allowing acceptable medical control and monitoring. If the patient is strapped in a head-down position, slide the patient out in the prone position on a short spine board. Once outside put a vacuum mattress on the patient's back. Activate the mattress. Gently logroll the patient between the spine board and the mattress to a supine position. Maintain manual in-line stabilization during the procedure.

On the Side. Access is obtained by cutting the upper supporting posts. The roof is folded down and a short spine board is put between the center console and the driver's seat. The passenger seat backrest and the handbrake handle can serve as supports for the

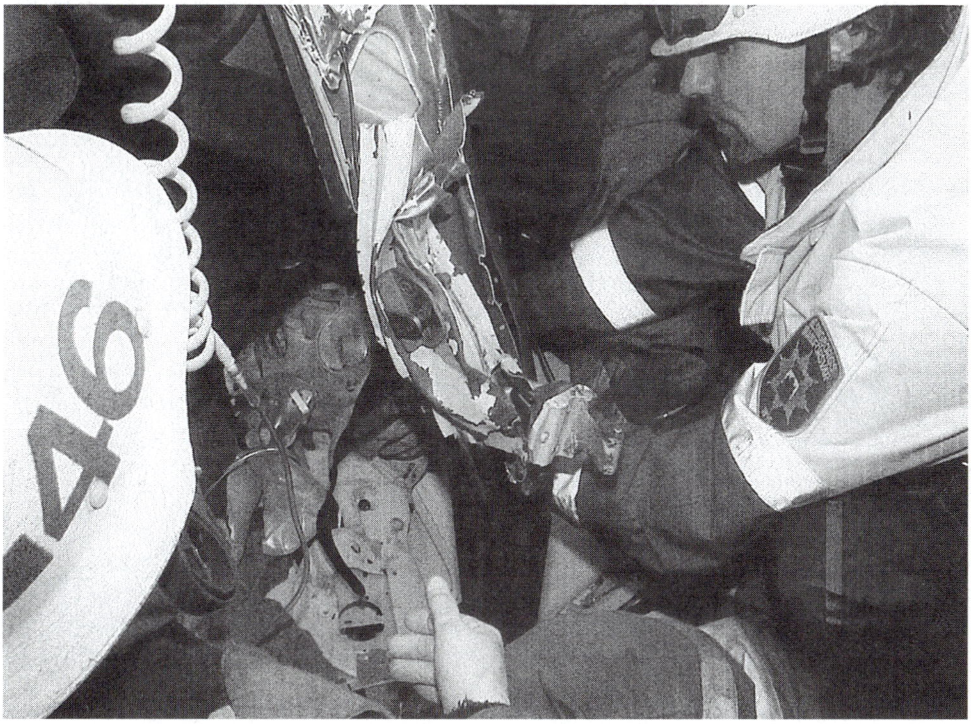

Figure 14 Patient fitted with goggles as protection during extrication.

spine board. The spine board is held securely, and after immobilization and with careful observation of the patient's vital signs and in-line stabilization, the restraints are cut and the patient is gently slid onto the spine board.

This can be done either with the patient on his side or in a supine position. When extricating victims from the "ground side" the spine board is placed on the ground. In every situation in which the vehicle is in any position other than on its wheels the extrication has to be conducted with an appreciation of the victim's position and how the restraints are holding the patient.

The wreck might be unstable, and it might not be possible to create enough room for adequate maneuvers and interventions once the patient starts to deteriorate. The victim also has a higher risk for severe and extensive injuries because of the kinematics of the accident. Because of this, a high readiness to convert to a rapid extrication procedure is mandatory.

Of the total time spent at the accident scene only about 25% is "medical time" [8] (i.e., time when appropriate medical actions are made). The rest of the time can be divided in time spent at various rescue, medical, and technical procedures. As time is very strongly correlated to patient outcome [4], the reduction of the time spent at the scene should be in favor of the patients' outcome. Recently, the use of a team approach has been suggested as a method to save crucial time for the patient [19]. This approach uses a system of defined tasks and a working protocol (Table 3). The crew can be organized as suggested

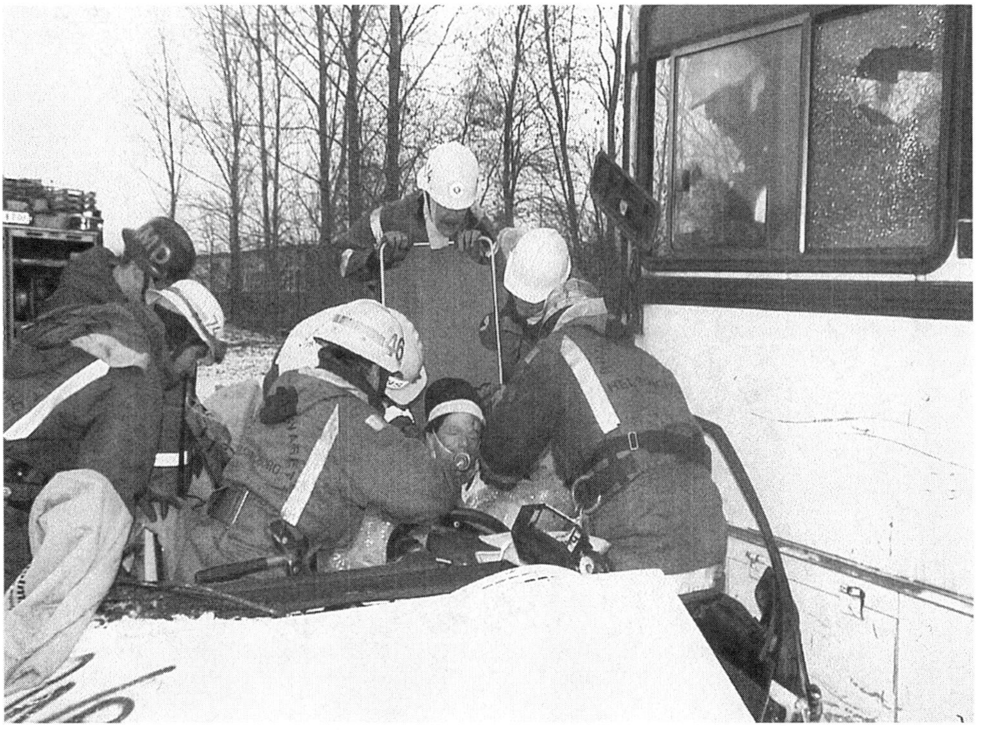

Figure 15 Short spine board placed behind the patient.

Table 3 Extrication Protocol

Safety/access	Stabilize the vehicle. Cut the electrical power. Create rapid access for one person. Establish manual in-line cervical spine stabilization and determine if an immediate life-threatening situation exists. Decide if ''controlled extrication'' has to be abandoned.
Read the accident	Estimate the energy absorption involved and what injuries to suspect. Photo document the scene for the benefit of the emergency room staff. Three pictures are taken (overview, site of impact, patient position).
Triage	Number of patients, priority, and extrication procedure. Frequently reassess.
Primary survey and resuscitation	ALS according to the ABCDE principles of the ATLS and PHTLS concepts. Frequently reassess.
Immobilization and ABC control	Keep the manual in-line stabilization. Apply cervical collar. Apply KED vest if appropriate. After extrication, immobilize the patient in a full body vacuum mattress or on a long spine board. Frequently reassess the patient's condition and the need to abandon the chosen extrication strategy.
Extrication	Extricate on a short or long spine board.

Table 4 Crew Composition

Extrication	Task
Fire captain	On-scene commander (OSC)
Firefighter	Security
Firefighter	Tools
Firefighter	Technician 1
Firefighter	Technician 2
Patient care	
Ambulance paramedic 1	Immediate patient access
Ambulance paramedic 2	Oxygen and airway
EMS paramedic	Photo documentation, communication
EMS Physician/nurse	Medical command and triage, advanced life support

in Tables 4 and 5. Using a preset flow scheme can facilitate the work on the scene. Decisions to abandon the chosen strategy because of deterioration of the patient or environmental hazards are taken by the OSC (Fig. 16, Table 3).

C. Inside Buildings and Confined Spaces

1. Confined Spaces

Confined spaces are in the most general terms areas of limited egress and access. Additionally, these locations have a significant potential for rescuer injury and secondary collapses (if applicable). They can also cause problems in the rapid identification and location of trapped victims.

Critical to this is the unemotional assessment of victim survivability. The question is whether this operation is a victim rescue or body retrieval/recovery. This determination

Table 5 Crew-Assigned Tasks

Function	Person	Task
OSC	Fire captain	Takes command and decides the extrication strategy.
Security	Security man	Checks for fuel leaks or other hazardous material around the wreck, prepares for immediate fire extinguishing, disconnects the power supply, and stabilizes the vehicle with rubber pads and straps. During the extrication process he continuously removes scrap and debris to outside the 5-meter radius, puts covers on sharp metal edges and using plastic shields or blankets protects the patient from glass and debris throughout the process.
Tools	Tool man	Provides the appropriate tool to the two *technicians* who cut the vehicle.
Cutting	Technicians	Operation of mechanical extrication tools.
Patient care	EMS staff	Makes a primary survey, applies manual in-line stabilization of the C spine, and stabilizes vital functions according to PHTLS principles.

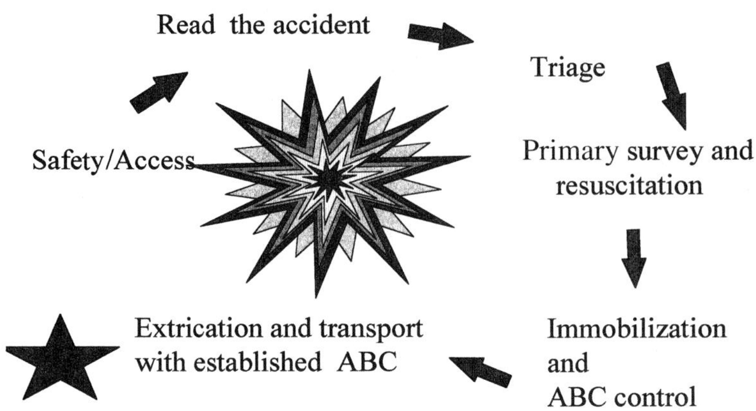

Figure 16 The accident scene. (From Ref. 19.)

will dictate the extent of acceptable risk for the rescue personnel. Rescuer training is a mandatory prerequisite to avoid repeating errors of rescue history. Some of these instances are as follows:

Virginia Beach Fire Department: one worker and one firefighter killed in a rescue within a ship's hold
Binghamton, New York: one worker killed and 14 firefighters injured in an underground sewer pipe rescue
Phoenix, Arizona: one worker and one firefighter killed, with injuries to 14 firefighters from a rescue in an aboveground storage tank
Lancaster, Pennsylvania: one firefighter and two paramedics killed in a rescue attempt from a septic tank

Ultimately the risk–benefit ratio must direct rescue efforts.

Confined space rescue requires a common terminology and minimal knowledge base for both medical and nonmedical personnel. This requires us to set a few of the basic tenants of confined space sciences. A working definition of a confined space is as follows:

Large enough for someone to physically enter and work in
Limited exit and entry
Not a normal space for extended continuous occupancy

All confined spaces should be treated with respect and cautious pessimism.

The confined space should be viewed as a location with a potentially hazardous environment. These environmental dangers may be from disrupted utility systems (i.e., gas, electrical, water, and sewage) within the space. Other dangers may result in victim or rescuer hypothermia, hyperthermia, cold water immersion, and even electrocution. Bites from animals such as arthropods, snakes (envenemation), spiders, ticks, scorpions, and mammals are not uncommon. To the surprise of some rescuers plants and vegetation are things that can result in a severe case of contact dermatitis. The environmental dangers may be physical, and the space contents may engulf or submerge anyone who enters. The site may be structured so that entrapment or asphyxiation by wall contours or sloping floors may occur. The space may also taper to very small (with respect to volume) and inaccessible spaces. Additionally the area may contain many other incident-specific safety or health hazards (collapsing walls, floors, dust, smoke, etc.), all of which the medical personnel should be aware.

All involved rescue personnel in both medical and technical rescues *must* have minimal basic, joint, standardized training certification. All involved personnel must also have their own personal protective equipment (PPE), such as a mask, goggles, multiple flashlights, gloves, and either steel toe-shank shoes or appropriate climbing footwear. Critical to the use of PPE is a general working knowledge of all basic on-scene rescue equipment. Medical personnel (as well as all other involved parties) must have and must conform to specifically assigned tasks, roles, and responsibilities. The rescue should have an established command structure. It should have a designated team leader who probably should *not* be the rescue physician. This general format should follow the recognized incident command structure (ICS) model.

Rescue skill training (including cross-training) should be conducted on an ongoing basis. Medical personnel ideally participate in simulated rescues with all necessary equipment. Ultimately a significant percentage (at least 50%) of the participants should have actual rescue experience.

Training components should include the following:

Use of operational confined space rescue plans
Personal protective equipment
Retrieval systems
Rope rescue
Use of racks, pulley systems, carabiners, descending devices (Fig. 8), and rescue seat harness
Rappelling skills

Confined space training must stress the safety issues in a potentially dangerous environment. This includes a working knowledge of lockout/tag-out procedures. This procedure attempts to isolate machinery. All equipment should be marked and physically locked so as to prevent accidental operation or powering. In this procedure only the person who has placed the lock and tag is permitted to remove the tag-out. This process is intended to avoid the inadvertent repowering (electrical, gas, water, steam, etc.) of on-line machinery.

Proper removal techniques include knowledge of confined space hazards, both physical and environmental. Environmental hazards include both environmental and physical factors. Environmental atmospheric conditions may be some of the most potentially lethal or injurious issues faced by the rescue team. These include such conditions as an oxygen-deficient atmosphere a flammable atmosphere, and a toxic atmosphere. This requires ongoing atmospheric and personnel monitoring. Physical hazards are also items that must be monitored, and their injury potential must be assessed. These physical hazards include such things as temperature extremes, including the associated clinical effects of hypothermia and hyperthermia. Noise decibel monitoring is often not monitored and is often looked at as an unavoidable cost of doing business. Physical engulfment by sand, coal, grain, water, mud, and so on are potential dangers for rescue personnel and victims alike. Fall hazards on wet surfaces or in floor openings are critical scene evaluation components. Falling objects can cause death and injury, especially to those who are not trained in the scene-assessment basics. Sources of released energy or materials (steam, water, electricity, gas, etc.) are additional.

Confined space rescue may not only result in physical injury but may also precipitate acute psychological trauma. Psychological reactions can exacerbate or uncover previously controlled or unknown phobias: dark (black, lightless space), animals, and closed spaces. All of these can result in fear (real and perceived), panic, and uncontrolled anxiety.

2. Inside Buildings

Rescue operations in high-density urban areas offer unique opportunities for true urban search and rescue operations. This requires the ongoing search activities while the city's normal daily activities continue. This is particularly true when one considers the situation of the single structural collapse.

This was the situation in the Oklahoma City bombing (of the Murrow Federal Building) in 1993. A similar situation occurred with a single building propane explosion in Puerto Rico. One was a nine-story federal office building and the latter a combination storefront/apartment building. Another example of a unique circumstance is the incident that occurred in New York City's Times Square in 1998. This situation was due to a construction accident, specifically the partial collapse of an external construction elevator. This was unique in that the search and rescue resources were developed into the building structure to assist in any potential injuries to the fire rescue services that were overseeing the dismantling of the elevator. The dismantling required the closing of Times Square to all traffic (pedestrian and vehicular). The issue that was not appreciated (by the public) was that the potential drop or fall zone was 1.5 times the total height. This 50-story elevator had a potential drop zone of 75 stories in a 360° swing.

Additional safety precautions require cooperation with public safety personnel (i.e., the police) in order to maintain necessary perimeter control. This includes pedestrians, traffic, and even helicopter (news helicopters) activity. Often the obvious areas of perimeter control are addressed, but ''invisible'' and distant dangers may not be addressed. In multiple collapses in New York City the subway service had to be suspended in order to prevent uncontrolled vibrations.

Traffic and proximal rail traffic can result in secondary collapses. Pedestrian traffic control is more of a safety issue. Large crowds can obstruct the flow of emergency equipment or be a potential source of new victims. In all instances there must be a mandatory site evacuation of any attached or proximal buildings.

In almost all incidents mandatory evacuation does not permit the occupants the luxury of removing personal items. These may include important documents, family photos, or even their pets. Animals left behind on an extended stabilization process can become an emotional as well as a public relations item. The question of pet rescue is a sensitive issue that requires an objective risk assessment. The problem is the human rescuer risk vs. the likelihood and benefit of pet retrieval. The decision must take into account the likelihood of the pet owner entering the structure to save his or her pet. The ability of pets to survive even the most difficult and Spartan environments is well documented in multiple earthquakes. Occupants may also make efforts to access the structure to retrieve ''irreplaceable'' documents. One should not assume that people would follow direction and approach such issues in a logical, objective manner.

Rescue operations are a function of multiple factors. Some of these are such general issues as the type, degree, and class of collapse. The type can include high-rise, single family dwelling, or subway tunnel collapse. This may be a single isolated structure or multiple adjacent regional structures. There may be single or multiple victims, all in varied states of health. This requires all medical rescue personnel to gather medical intelligence and gain a working knowledge of the existing normal medical background. The rescue operations must assess the likelihood of survivors vs. the likelihood of secondary deaths.

The class of collapse will also dictate the potential for survivors. This requires the return to the basics of building triage, things such as a pancake collapse vs. a void structure situation. In the urban environment the availability of resources should be explored and exploited. This may include such items as heavy-duty construction equipment, auxiliary power supplies, water, and personnel.

D. Building Triage and Assessment

Nonrescue physicians are often a danger to themselves, to the victims, and to the technical rescue personnel. The physician must be trained in and oriented toward the rules of rescue. The physician should also be aware of the structure signs and symptoms. Just as any astute physician would be aware of the signs of a heart attack or the symptoms of shock, the same can be said about the collapse environment.

Most rescue teams employ a standardized marking system. These markers usually include the following:

1. Entry time and date
2. Up-to-date number of bodies in the location
3. Building safety hazards: fall, slip, hanging, drop
4. Biohazards: body fluids, laboratory samples, sharps
5. Identification of entering group (no single/solo entries)
6. Close-out procedures with exit marking

The on-scene physician should also be aware of basic building assessments. The standardized approach to structure collapse potential includes the engineer's overall collapse potential. There must be identification of potential fall hazards (some of which can weigh into the hundreds of pounds), such as hanging concrete, filling cabinets, and so on. The location of trip hazards and walk hazards where precipitous drops can have fatal consequences must be identified, as well as building microenvironmental hazards. Hazardous materials (hazmat) should be located and clearly marked. These may include various household or industrial chemicals, asbestos potential, or compromised sewage systems.

The microenvironment should also include the discontinuation of building services, such as water, electricity, and gas. The rescue field physician should be aware of structure void space potential and the presumed location of any such spaces, as well as daily weather conditions, including potential changes in climatic conditions. Such physicians should make an assessment as to their probable impact on the patients as well as the rescue team. The information reports should also include precollapse building utilization, such as a hospital, pediatric medical facility, and tuberculosis ward.

Places such as sewage treatment plants and industrial chemical treatment or storage plants all have their own unique dangers. There is no excuse for medical personnel who enter a collapse zone with little or no knowledge of basic safety procedures and equipment. All rescue personnel should have their own redundant personal lighting, such as flashlights and strobes. The rescue personnel should not assume that building lighting is infallible and will always be there. This should be independent of the time of day. The interior of a hole is as dark at noon as it is at midnight. Additionally, it is critical that all medical personnel only perform building entry with a partner or as part of a group entry. Building traffic control and 100% personnel accountability is an absolute must. One should also be aware of the benefits and limitations of supplemental support structures. It does not hurt in the general information and assessment phase to ask about general load-bearing limits.

All personnel should either have or be with someone who has a monitored radio communication device. No medical rescue physician should enter the collapse zone without steel toe-shank safety shoes. Additionally they should have and use respiratory protection and appropriate gloves. Medical personnel must often act as an advocate for the basic infection-control procedures.

Often nonmedical personnel will use various mixtures of cleaning and disinfecting agents in an attempt to deal with body fluids. These more often than not create an unsafe environment for all rescue personnel. Where need be rescue personnel may use Tyvek or other disposable outerwear. Medical rescue personnel should be aware of secondary collapse medical hazards that have long-term medical importance. One major issue is the collapsed ventilation system. This may contain a significant growth fungus or bacterial matter. Additionally, the impact of dust irritation on the victims and rescuers can result in delayed respiratory symptoms, therefore medical monitoring must extend to the postincident recovery phase. This period may extend to as long as 10 days postincident.

The physician must at all times assume responsibility for his or her own safety, and should be aware of not only the common fall hazards but also site-specific collapse consequences such as gothic or Christmas tree patterns. He or she must at all times be aware of established exit and entry points as well as emergency escape routes. The physician or medical rescue personnel must have full knowledge of areas *not* to be accessed or altered and collapse ''safety'' zones.

E. Rescue vs. Recovery

Rescue is the process by which live victims are searched for and removed. This is based on the probability and likelihood of live (and viable) recovery. Recovery is the process by which bodies are removed from a collapse site and it is accepted that live victims are no longer obtainable. The delta (difference) of these two functions is the concept of acceptable vs. unacceptable risk. This risk-benefit ratio is not always an easy one to derive or even follow. The philosophical question begs the following question: What is the price of retrieving a corpse; should a rescuer be asked to pay with his or her life? This may on the surface seem fairly straightforward, but multiple rescue operations have demonstrated the risk that people are willing to assume. Rescue of live victims (as per an Armenian earthquake study) demonstrated the possibility of survivors up to 48 hr postincident. There are various rescue and recovery factors that impact on the issue of survivability. The type of structure and its construction factors are critical to the creation of void spaces. The drop of concrete slabs vs. a reinforced steel structure is an example. The basic mechanism and etiology of collapse will in direct proportional basis affect victim survivability. The incident that is secondary to a propane explosion or bomb will have a greater structure death rate than an earthquake incident. The prevailing environment with its weather conditions (inside and outside the building) is a factor that should provide hope in some instances. The benefits of a warm, temperate environment vs. the cold, harsh winter are factors for consideration when patient survivability is being assessed. Finally, the medical and rescue staff must evaluate the medical status, of the normal population base.

Normal medical background noise is critical information when one attempts to establish basic risk–benefit ratios. It is of the utmost importance that these decisions be made on the available information and not on conjecture or emotion.

V. THE USE OF HELICOPTERS IN RESCUE OPERATIONS

A. General Aspects and Use in Rural Areas

The use of rotor wing EMS for search and rescue of entrapped trauma victims can be of great value in rural areas (Fig. 17). In these areas the helicopter provides a flexible and fast facility to transfer medical expertise to the remotely located patient. The rural setting also means a lack of immediate access to sufficient definitive medical treatment, and this calls for special considerations compared to the urban situation.

1. Time of No Therapy

As a consequence of the rural setting, the victim of a medical emergency often has low access to qualified definitive care and may have long transfer times with conventional ground-based EMS. The time to emergency calls has recently been reported to about 45 min in European ski resort areas, and the time of no therapy to just over 1 hr [28]. This time must be seen as a minimum. It can very easily increase substantially, depending on location and weather conditions. In the remote trauma case the use of helicopter emergency medical service (HEMS) systems can shorten the time of no therapy [16]. This, in combination with qualified medical interventions at the scene and the ability to maintain a high standard of therapy during transport, has been shown to improve outcome in trauma patients [16,17,29]. The use of physician-staffed HEMS systems has also been shown to improve performance and the quality of the given therapy compared to paramedic-staffed HEMS programs [17], and as well as to reduce mortality in trauma [9,30–32].

Providing emergency medical assistance over a widespread rural area means significantly longer mission times than in the urban setting. To keep the response times rea-

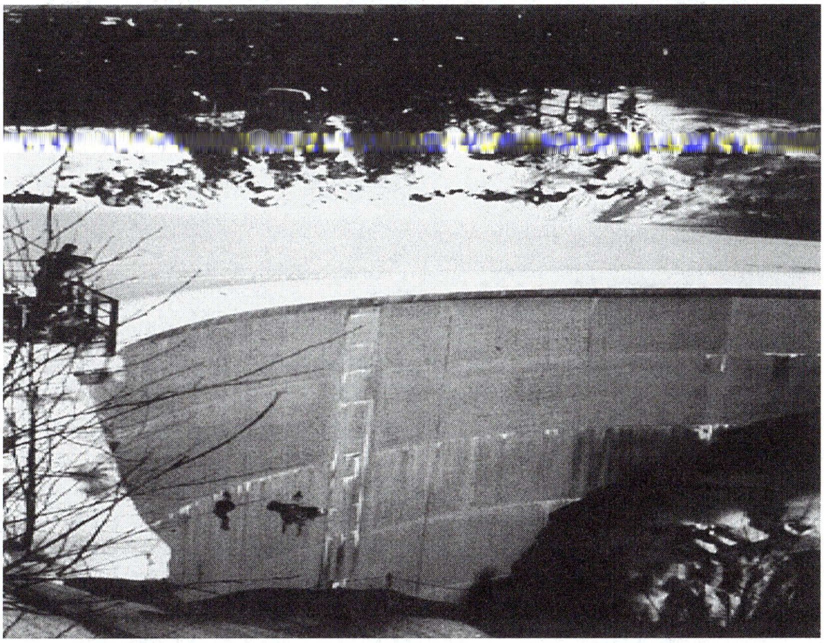

Figure 17 HEMS rescue operation. (Courtesy of B. Carlsen, Norwegian Air Ambulance.)

sonable low, effective triage and dispatch systems are essential for optimum performance of the HEMS system [33,34]. To keep the HEMS facility operational and free to take on new missions, the dispatch center should have medical staff with HEMS expertise available to evaluate all incoming calls.

2. Distance to the Appropriate Receiving Hospital

The fact that the receiving hospital may be distant from the scene increases the needs for qualified medical interventions. ''Swoop-and-scoop'' as practiced in urban areas is seldom applicable in the rural trauma setting, and patients have to be sufficiently prepared for a long transfer before takeoff. This means that in addition to the initial survey, stabilization, and advanced life support, other advanced intensive care procedures must be continued during the transfer. This calls for meticulous planning in terms of equipment and appropriate training of the flight crew. In such a distant setting, the benefit of properly selected and experienced flight physicians is apparent and enhances the versatility of the HEMS system.

Because of longer transit times, remote location, and limited additional resources, the HEMS team has to be self-sufficient and not dependent on hospital control functions. Having the highest level of competence at the patient's side also enables the team to perform advanced medical interventions and on-scene triage to the best suitable medical facility, which might not always be the nearest.

B. Level of Care En Route

The care en route should focus on maintaining vital functions. The general aim to reduce the time spent at the accident scene must be put into the perspective of a substantially extended transfer time before the patient reaches the definite medical facility. In particular, those injuries that are directly related to early death (i.e., intracranial bleeding, and massive hemorrhage from thoracic and intraabdominal lesions, as well as respiratory impairment) have been shown to benefit from on-scene therapy [6].

1. Airway

The indications for intubation and controlled ventilation become more liberalized and interventions are initiated on a much lower threshold of an inadequate airway or respiratory drive. Before takeoff, the airway should be adequately secured. The in-flight situation of a combative and delirious patient is very dangerous, and thus the patient has to be adequately sedated and/or anesthetized, and if needed, out on muscle relaxants. In-flight reintubation of a dislocated orotracheal airway can be very difficult, and therefore the tube should be carefully secured before takeoff. The in-hospital practice of using adhesive tape would not be sufficient in the HEMS setting, and the use of cotton ribbons or commercially available tube holders is strongly recommended. This also better secures the airway during emergency loading maneuvers in which the helicopter is unable to land and shuttle down and instead hovers light on skid (''hot load'') (Fig. 18) and also during transportation in difficult terrain. The use of other aids for establishing an artificial airway, such as the laryngeal mask, may be appropriate for temporary use during an extrication procedure [35], but should preferably be changed to an orotracheal airway before longer transports.

The security of the airway should be evaluated before transportation, and if the airway is to be changed to an orotracheal tube, the decision should be made before takeoff.

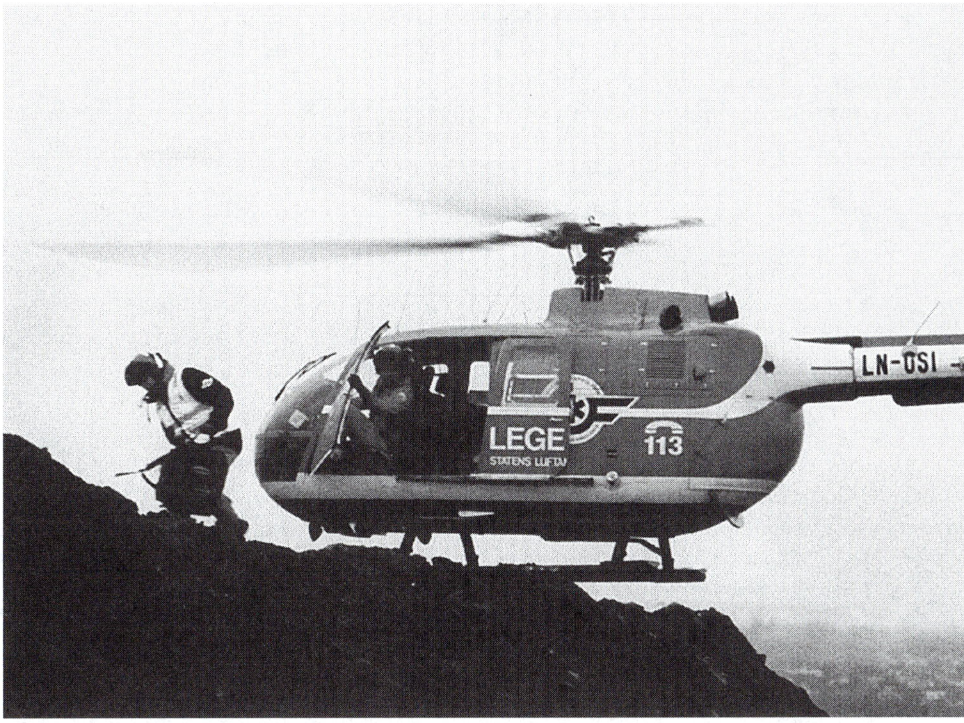

Figure 18 "Hot load." (Courtesy of B. Carlsen, Norwegian Air Ambulance.)

The use of a small pneumatic ventilator facilitates ventilation during patient transport, and can also be used at the accident site and during extrication.

2. Circulation

Controlling ongoing exsanguinations is paramount before takeoff. External compression and fixation of fractures should be applied for that purpose. Vigorous volume replacement has earlier been shown to be of little or no benefit in cases with ongoing and uncontrolled volume losses. Although convincing evidence now exists for withholding prehospital IV fluids in cases with penetrating injuries and short transit times to a definitive surgical facility, extrapolation of this regime to blunt trauma and a longer time span could have a deleterious effect on tissue perfusion [6]. In cases with head injuries, maintaining cerebral perfusion pressure (CPP) is paramount, and thus the use of limited amounts of IV fluids is validated to prevent further cell damage. The aim should not be to resuscitate to restore normal hemodynamics, however, but to maintain hypotensive resuscitation (mean arterial pressure [MAP] 70 to 80 mmHg) [36] to preserve cerebral perfusion and to avoid such consequences of tissue hypoperfusion as impairment of microcirculation, anaerobic metabolism, and profound shock [6].

3. Location of the Patient

The patient can be very remotely located. This means that the medical indication for using the HEMS capability is not solely dependent on the patient's medical condition. Such factors as access to ground EMS, level of training and response times for alternative facilities, patient exposure, and weather conditions also play a significant roll for dispatch and triage. Under these circumstances the HEMS system can be reinforced with mountain rescue groups and avalanche teams with dogs. The HEMS crew operating in such areas should be trained in cooperation with such groups and have customized equipment for working under extreme conditions.

C. Rescue Medical Operations—Difficult Aeromedical Interventions

1. Mountain Rescue Operations

The rescue of patients in remote or inaccessible locations poses a special problem for the rescue organization. Not only must the physician be brought to the patient, he must also be able to deliver treatment to patients with extensive injuries under very difficult situations. A special situation is the rural use of rotor wing EMS in rescue operations in mountain areas with field trauma care and evacuation of often severely injured and hypothermic patients. This situation calls for a multidisciplinary team that is trained and equipped to act in often extreme conditions and that has a high degree of bilateral knowledge in the different disciplines involved, as well as good liaison between the various teams. Trauma in these circumstances is often the result from a fall during climbing, paragliding, base jumps and ski excursions, or other extreme sports. The patient is often more fit than the normal urban trauma population and often below 40 years of age.

2. Technical Aspects

The HEMS team is reinforced with an alpine rescue team, which is responsible for both securing the route and accident site and for accessing the technical aspects during winching and liftoff. About 70% of all patients are accessible by foot, but they might not be able to be evacuated by a ground route. In recent reviews, approximately 20% of all patients requiring air evacuation from the accident site are severely injured. The patients are often located in steep slopes and rock-face terrain and a majority require analgesics and sedative medication before reposition of fractures and evacuation. In about 12% of the cases, the patient has to be intubated and mechanically ventilated on site [28].

Work at the accident scene benefits from using protocols, where defined tasks are carried out within the team. These protocols have to be locally developed but should include some basic functions (Table 6). It is absolutely paramount that the team in the helicopter and on the ground is continuously updated on the progress and plans of the operation. After having vital functions secured, the patient must be prepared for evacuation. This usually means that the patient is recovered in a horizontal position using a horizontal rescue net or a rescue bag (Fig. 19). The use of a rescue loop or harness is often not appropriate since most of the time patients have to be immobilized before transport. If using a net, the spine and fractures must be immobilized the conventional way, using extrication devices, vacuum splints, and cervical collars.

By using a rescue bag the patient can be fully immobilized in a vacuum mattress, which also enables the patient to be lifted without any additional equipment. In locations with limited space the net (Fig. 20) is preferable, as it can be slid under the patient with minimal movement of the patient.

In the process of lifting the patient from the location of the accident, IV lines and airways must be carefully secured and all other equipment fixed well to the stretcher. The orotracheal tube is secured by cotton strings or by using commercially available tube holders, and IV lines are taped to the extremity. Assisted ventilation and CPR must be

Table 6 Suggested Basic Protocol for HEMS Alpine Rescue Teams

Function	Person	Responsibility
Command of operation	OSC	In charge of rescue strategy
Communication	Liaison officer	Responsible for all communication; maintains contact with rescue dispatch centers, HEMS crew, and helicopters as well as with the different team groups; reports status of operation to OSC
Alpine techniques	Alpine security officer	Responsible for securing of patients and personnel; in charge of rope arrangement and securing and descent lines, as well as hoisting and winch operations
Patient access	Climber(s)	Responsible for creating a descent and evacuation route for patients and medical rescue personnel
Medical operations	Leading HEMS physician	In charge of medical triage and operations
Search and rescue (SAR)	Avalanche dog team leader/pilot	Organizing of search patterns in liaison with OSC

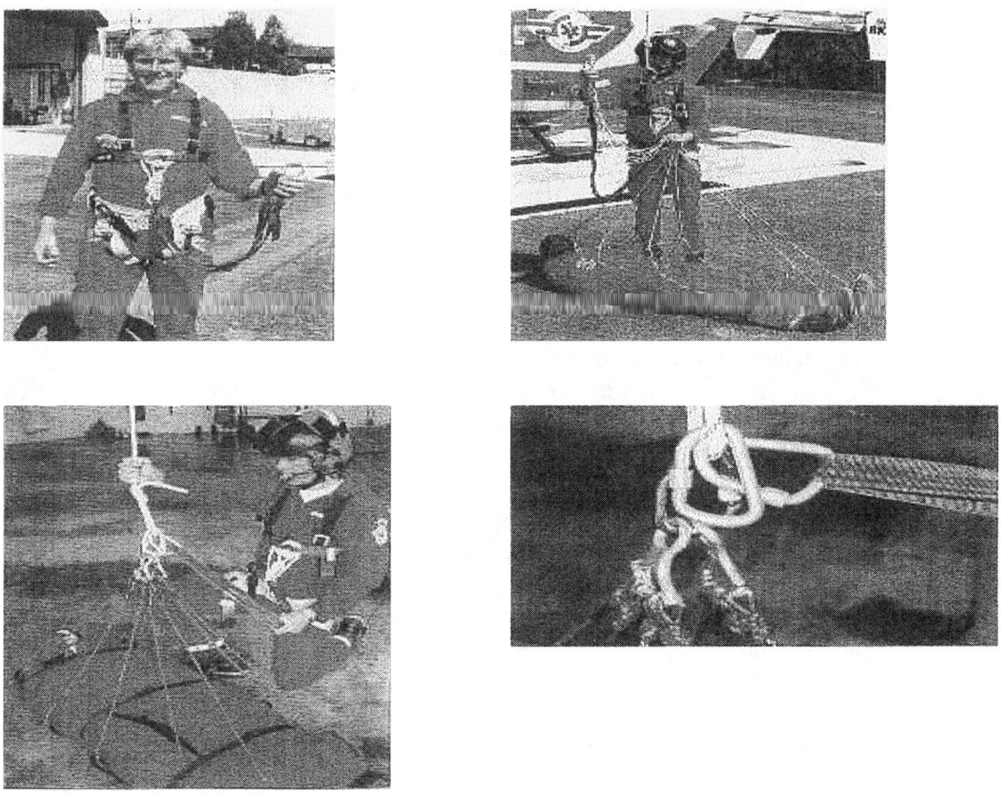

Figure 19 Evacuation net and rescue bag. (Courtesy of Norwegian Air Ambulance.)

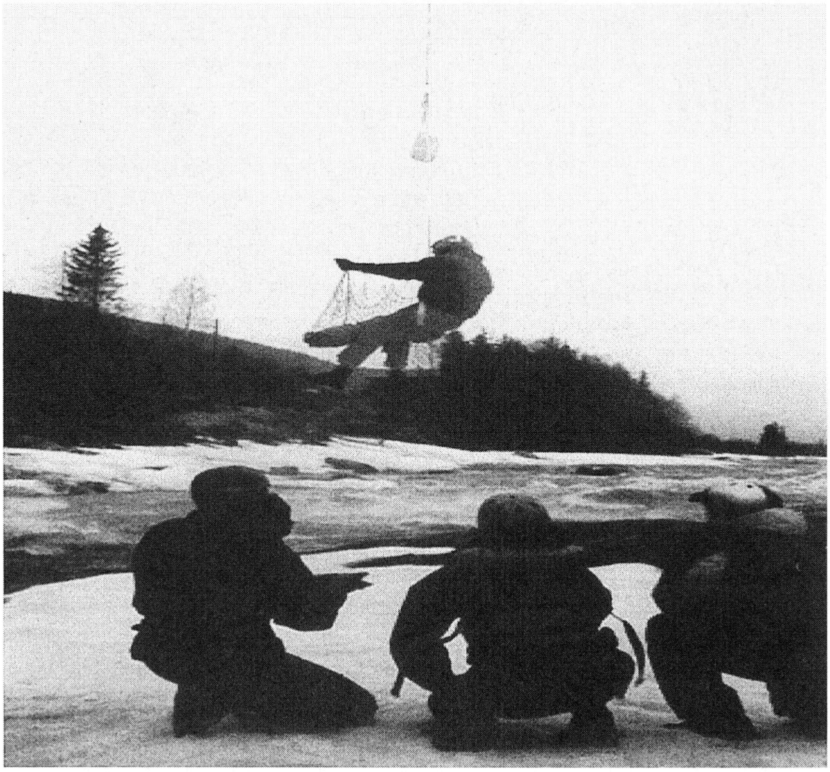

Figure 20 Lift in rescue net. (Courtesy of B. Carlsen, Norwegian Air Ambulance.)

continued during the evacuation. The patient and the physician are attached to the winch cable or rope and lifted to the nearest landing area. During ascent and decent the patient must be protected from hitting the ground or environment, and from debris brought up by the rotor vortex. For that purpose the patient should be fitted with goggles, or else the evacuation stretcher could be fitted with a head cover.

The lift could be conducted either by using a winch or by fixed static ropes fitted to the aircraft. During the lifting procedure communications must be continued between the underslung personnel and the flight crew.

3. Medical Aspects

Because of the position of the patient, a long time may elapse before the patient can get any medical attention and environmental protection. The majority of the patients are also alone on the accident site [28]. Patients are often hypothermic, and in about 10–15% of the cases severely injured with impaired vital functions. Upon arrival, the patient's airway and breathing must be immediately checked and stabilized, and a quick primary survey must be conducted to determine the need for an immediate evacuation.

The patient can be in an uncooperative condition because of injuries, blood and volume losses, and hypothermia. Because of that, a majority of patients require analgesics and sedatives before they can be transported in a controlled fashion.

Besides normal ALS procedures the patient is prevented from further heat loss by protective clothing, and if appropriate should be placed in microfiber-coated waterproof body wrapping. As described above, the patient is best evacuated supine, and hypothermic patients are also better evacuated horizontally because of the risk of impaired vasoregulation and deleterious baroreceptor response in an upright position. To be able to conduct advanced medical treatment, administer analgesics and anesthetics under extreme conditions, and appreciate what is feasible, the flight physician has to be highly trained and experienced. Training programs containing mandatory regularly updated proceedings are highly recommended, as well as outdoor practical training. Treatment at the accident site should focus only on stabilizing conditions for an evacuation to a nearby landing area, at which more advanced ALS can be instituted. Too much medical interference at the accident site can very easily substantially increase the problem of evacuation (e.g., unnecessary intubation), impair patient safety (failure to maintain treatment during evacuation), or increase rescue time. To conduct operations in mountain rescue the different rescue teams have to be trained together on a regular basis. To simplify the work, the use of a specific protocol such as that described earlier is recommended (Table 6).

VI. SPECIAL TOPICS AND SITUATIONS

A. Triage

In the adult patient the primary triage process should follow the well-established procedure of simple triage and rapid treatment (S.T.A.R.T.) (see Appendix II). As a triage algorithm this is a misnomer, but it is an excellent patient-sorting device, allowing for a rapid identification of the dead, nearly dead, and the least injured ambulatory patients. This has been used successfully throughout the United States in the prehospital setting. This allows the identification to occur in less than 30 sec. It was originally developed to identify trauma patients, but has universally also been utilized in the medical scenario. This triage process is used for adults as well as for children. The primary factors of assessment are (1) airway, (2) pulse, and (3) mental status. The on-scene physician should be wary of utilizing standard hospital triage procedures in the out-of-hospital environment. The enemy is time, and the efficient use of this commodity is critical.

B. Public and Media

The media can help you or bury you. The media can often be a hindrance and an annoyance, but only if not used in partnership with rescue activities. The issue of patient confidentiality is critical and should never be violated. This requires an identifiable media source person. This individual should be the conduit for all media communications and is responsible for providing the media with generic real information. This person should hold regular routine meetings, which should be independent of any new incident information. The meetings should continue, even it only to announce that there is no new information. The issuance of rumors is critical, and they should be addressed with factual information and never be dismissed.

Public concerns are often not the concerns of the rescue community, but are real nonetheless. As rescuers we often forget the human impact of an incident and focus on objective clinical matters. The loss of family photos or identification papers can devastate a displaced person. On multiple rescues the ''little'' things provide the most comfort. In the Oklahoma City bombing, the return of a wedding photo or a child's picture from the rubble brought families much comfort. In New York City, the trapped pets of displaced victims brought out a public outcry. This necessitated a pet rescue into a potential collapse zone. The pros and cons of such an act may be debatable, but not to those pet owners. This must be balanced with the risk to human life. Clearly such issues must be addressed before they become a public relations nightmare. It has been our experience that the media is very willing to work with the rescue effort. Treat them with respect and address their concerns.

C. On-Scene Instant Documentation: Photo vs. Run Reports

On-scene documentation is a must for any incident. We recommend the preincident development of incident response and medical management forms. The medical management forms should address the care provided to the victims as well as the rescue personnel (human and canine). The forms should duplicate the normal out-of-hospital forms utilized on a routine basis. These forms should be scanned or the information should be transferred to computer as soon as possible when extended on-scene operations are underway.

Photos are unique information tools. It is paramount that the receiving physician correctly appreciates the energy absorption by the victim in order to correctly triage the patient at his or her arrival in the trauma bay. The use of on-scene photography offers an immediate incident history. Photo information has been shown to be more easily transferred to the trauma bay staff than either verbal information at arrival or written run reports [40]. The information can be faxed and/or modemed to a distant receiving facility for the mechanism of injury information. The use of on-scene digital photography allows the managers to develop and monitor rescue plans in a central command post. This same information can be shared with distant experts for consultation purposes in cases in which they may not be immediately available. Instant photos can also be utilized for hospital information when used in conjunction with the run reports. I recommend that digital and/ or instant photography (still and video) be part of the routine rescue equipment.

D. Environmental Considerations

Environmental issues are critical to the survival of the rescuer as well as the victim. The environmental conditions of concern are micro- and macrometeorological conditions and their affect on the rescue process.

In their most general terms the meteorological concerns are either hyperthermia or hypothermia. Hyperthermia is the detrimental elevation of the surrounding temperature. This can lead to dehydration and various medical heat emergency states. This includes clinical heat cramps, heat exhaustion, or heat stroke. The issue is further complicated by the relative humidity. This is referred to as the temperature humidity index (THI). The combination of heat accumulation and humidity can have devastating affects on victims and rescuers. The resulting dehydration can make trapped victims more susceptible to the renal effects of crush syndrome. Heat and humidity can also increase the rescue stakes by their effects on clinical judgment. Rescue personnel must be monitored for the affects of heat and dehydration on their ability to make competent judgments. This combination can also result in a volume-depletion status that can have multisystem impact. The affects of lowering temperature are very similar to the affects of hyperthermia. Cold significantly impacts the ability of an individual to have sound clinical judgment. Cold diuresis can result in a relative hypovolemic state. Significant drops in body temperature can also result in multisystem organ malfunction. The issue of moisture is a critical operational factor in considering the rescue parameters. The presence of rain or mist results in a drop of relative (if not absolute) temperature.

The other issue of environment is the micrometeorological rescue environment. Rescue in places without heat can drop the relative working temperature. Environmental moisture (broken water pipes or mist) can rapidly deplete the body temperature of both victim and rescuer. Location specifics, such as cave, trench, and subway rescues, can all provide adverse working environments that affect the efficiency of the rescue. The lack of ventilation and/or air conditioning can have a devastating environmental impact. The rescue in the subway environment on a summer day with an ambient temperature of 90°F can result in a tunnel temperature of 120°F. These are conditions that must be continuously monitored and modified where possible.

E. Spinal Injury and Precautions

The incidence and potential of significant injuries are significant issues during earthquakes or building collapses. The increased incidence and frequency of head, neck, and long bone injury has been well documented in multiple earthquakes. It is interesting to note the number of earthquakes that have occurred during the early morning hours. This results in injuries to victims asleep in their homes. This has occurred in Mexico, Turkey, Taiwan, and China, and has resulted in a significant number of spinal, head, and long bone injuries. Daytime earthquakes result in falling debris, and collapsing roadways resulting in musculoskeletal injuries and trapped victims away from the home. The spectrum in this situation decreases the incidence of head trauma since victims are able to remove themselves from danger. Additionally, the daytime event allows people to see the surrounding area and dangerous physical hazards.

This mandates that all medical rescue personnel have a working knowledge of traditional EMS stabilization equipment. This includes the use of neck collars, spine/back boards, and splinting devices. The on-scene medical staff should be capable of maneuvering patients through unusual spaces. This requires, for example, the measuring of space diameters to allow the mobilization device to pass. An average backboard of 36 in. will get through a 32-in. tube. The accepted standard of immobilization is one that often becomes a luxury in the confined space rescue. Victim movement should follow the principle of total patient control with limited and only necessary motion during the extrication process.

Victim extrication may not solely utilize traditional medical skills. The responding medical personnel should have an operational knowledge of rope rescue techniques. It is a fact of life that confined space rescue sometimes requires the use of ropes to access or egress the incident area. The medical personnel may not (probably should not) tie the critical knots, but should have a working knowledge of what is appropriate, acceptable, and safe. Knowledge of anchoring systems (e.g., the bomb anchor) and their application will add to the credibility of the medical staff. Minimal repelling skills and experience should be prerequisites in order to be considered as a senior rescue member. Knowledge of terminology and standard rescue practices should be part of the team's orientation and training. Rescue equipment knowledge—the rack vs. the figure 8 for an elevator rescue—is an additional component in the rope rescue armamentarium. Management and immobilization techniques should be part of the general rescue training and the use of traditional rescue equipment in a nonstandard way. For example the KED extrication device is normally used to immobilize victims of car accidents. In a collapse zone this can roll the patient into a cylinder effectively. Functionally, this serves to decrease the effective victim diameter. Another piece of equipment is the sked extrication device.

This is simply a piece of hard, flexible plastic sheeting. Like the KED, this allows for the ''packaging'' of the patient. Use of the sked allows flexibility in moving patients over debris and through floor holes. This sheet affords protection for the patient from injury by site debris (reinforcement bars, concrete fragments, broken glass, etc.) A combination of extrication equipment and rope rescue procedures will provide for a positive and safe rescue effort.

F. Pediatric Issues

There is a greater incidence of head and cervical spine injury to children in most collapse environments. This is related to three factors: (1) secondary to a greater head to body proportion, (2) the inability of very young children to remove themselves from a dangerous environment, and (3) lax (immature) cervical spinal ligaments as compared to adults. This is especially true in the case of building collapses secondary to an earthquake. The positive aspect of pediatric entrapment is the virtue of young and usually healthy cardiovascular, respiratory, and renal systems. In this case the pediatric patient who has a greater renal, respiratory, and cardiovascular reserve as compared to the adult patient has a decreased likelihood of iatrogenic pulmonary edema with aggressive fluid resuscitation. This is one of the primary early treatments for crush syndrome. The net result is greater survivability from entrapped muscle trauma or crush syndrome, even with an extended entrapment time. A critical issue is the need for pediatric rescue equipment, not modification of adult equipment. This includes not only immobilization and extrication equipment but also pediatric medication administration and dosing schedules.

VII. HYPOTHERMIA IN THE ENTRAPPED PATIENT

A. General Remarks

Motor vehicle accidents represent a major portion of the trauma caseload, and entrapment situations frequently result from accidents involving small cars. Even during winter conditions, people seldom drive a car wearing outdoor clothing, and thus they are more vulnerable to exposure in an accident situation. Hypothermia in trauma is a common problem, and half of all trauma patients have a body temperature below 36°C [18].

Hypothermia in entrapped patients is an underappreciated condition that can heavily influence outcome. Due to long extrication times, extensive injuries, and prolonged exposure, almost all entrapped patients are severely hypothermic (<34 to 36°C). Because of that, an increased risk for developing complications as well as an increase in mortality is seen compared to normothermic trauma victims. Trauma patients with a core temperature ≤34°C have profound impairment of the coagulation cascade and platelet function, leading to both further exsanguinations and the need for massive transfusions. These patients also are more unresponsive to volume and pressor therapy without ongoing volume losses [18,37]. The mortality increases dramatically with decreased core temperature. Below 34°C, mortality increases threefold in patients with the same ISS, and below 32°C the mortality approaches 100%, regardless of injury severity score (ISS).

Exsanguinations, blunt trauma with extensive soft tissue damage, and a low level of consciousness are all frequently found in the entrapped patient. These injuries severely predispose for rapid heat loss and attenuate the normal thermoregulative response (shivering and vasoconstriction) [38]. In addition to this a great deal of these patients are also under the influence of drugs and alcohol. The risk for hypothermia poses a relevant problem in prehospital trauma care and is not limited to a specific season of the year [18]. Early recognition of the risk of hypothermia and early prevention and activation of countermeasures are therefore of great value in the process of prehospital trauma care.

B. Symptoms and Diagnosis

The symptoms of significant hypothermia can be very variable in the prehospital situation and are often misjudged as symptoms of other more obvious injuries in the trauma patient. The patient is less cooperative and may be less responsive than the underlying physical injury might indicate. As a result of this, hypothermia makes the patient more vulnerable to manipulation and should be handled with concern for cardiovascular and neurological instability [38]. Active temperature measurement at the accident scene can easily be achieved by using a tympanic membrane thermometer. Such measurements do not give the accurate core temperature but may give useful information for triage and differential diagnoses [18].

Conclusions drawn from the primary survey depend on the estimated level of hypothermia. Patients with a temperature <34°C should be considered "severely hypothermic," and thus manipulation should be minimal (Table 7).

C. Management

Management of hypothermia in the prehospital phase is mostly a question of preventing further heat loss since active rewarming is neither feasible nor recommendable. The efforts should be focused on minimizing the exposure of the patient and not on diverting more heat and energy away from the patient by medications and cold IV fluids. Due to reduced muscle power the patient may have great difficulties participating or cooperating during a rescue procedure, and the reduced level of consciousness increases the risk for impaired airway or aspiration.

All hypothermic persons are to be considered hypovolemic because of cold-induced diuresis. Keep the patient supine to reduce the risk for ortostatic influence and subsequent triggering of malignant arrhythmia. Keep the patient horizontal during recovery and pickup. The hypothermia is considered deep if <34°C, and leaves the rescuer with a severely compromised patient with limited cardiopulmonary reserves (Table 8).

The management of the hypothermic trauma patient could be divided into the following steps, all of which need special consideration:

Careful primary survey
ABCDE
Isolation from the environment

Table 7 Clinical Implications of Hypothermia

A	Impaired level of consciousness; muscle rigidity; trismus
B	Slow and shallow respiration
C	Weak, slow pulse; cold, pale, skin; distant heartsounds
D	Hyporeflexia hyperreflexia; impaired GSC score
E	Shivering

Table 8 Clinical Management

Alert patient with shivering (temp. >35°C)	Prevent further heat loss. Remove wet clothes and isolate from cold environment. If possible isolate extremities and torso separately. Room temperature; use dry blankets; warm beverages.
No shivering; impaired level of consciousness (temp. 30–35°C)	Always to hospital. Handle like above but nothing oral. Avoid external heating in order to prevent central shunting of cold and acidotic blood, which can further lower core temperature (after drop). Warm IV fluid (1–2 liters) at slow rate to prevent further heat loss. O_2 on face mask. Intubation on strict indications. Avoid unnecessary manipulation.
Deep hypotermia; unconscious patient; impaired circulation (temp. <30°C)	High risk for malignant arrhythmia. Handle with extreme care. No unnecessary manipulation. One IV line. Avoid neck veins. Warm fluid at slow rate. Hypotension and bradycardia IV. atropine only if associated with circulatory impairment. HLR only in case of verified asystoli/v.fib. Poor effect of IV medications. Intubation only if respiratory arrest. Avoid depolarizing muscle relaxants.

Oxygen on face mask
Warm IV fluid if any
Cardiopulmonary monitoring
Transport in normothermic environment

1. Survey and ABCDE

Handling of the patient should be kept minimal, and the femoral artery rather than the carotids should preferably be palpated for pulse to prevent accidental baroreceptor stimulation. The patient should be kept supine because of cold induced hypovolemia and circulatory instability. Shivering and high skin impedance can result in insufficient transmission and artifacts that complicate ECG interpretation and can be misinterpreted as ventricular fibrillation by semiautomatic defibrillators.

2. Isolation from Further Heat Loss

First, the patient should be isolated from the cold environment to prevent further heat loss. In the entrapment situation this usually means covering the patient with blankets and putting on a warm cap. Clothing usually is cut to gain access to the patient. This should be kept to a minimum and done in a fashion that allows the clothing to be put back and cover the patient again after survey and interventions (Fig. 21). The patient should be protected from the environment. This means that all handling of the patient should be done in a sheltered space, protected from rain, snow, or wind. This can often be done by covering the patient or by moving the patient inside an EMS vehicle, but in open terrain shelters of snow- or wind-breaking material can be required. If possible during transport, the torso and the extremities should be isolated separately to prevent central redistribution of cold peripheral blood. The use of electrical heaters and fans has been advocated but does not always apply since they may obstruct the working space, need a power supply, and sometimes cannot be used because of fire hazards.

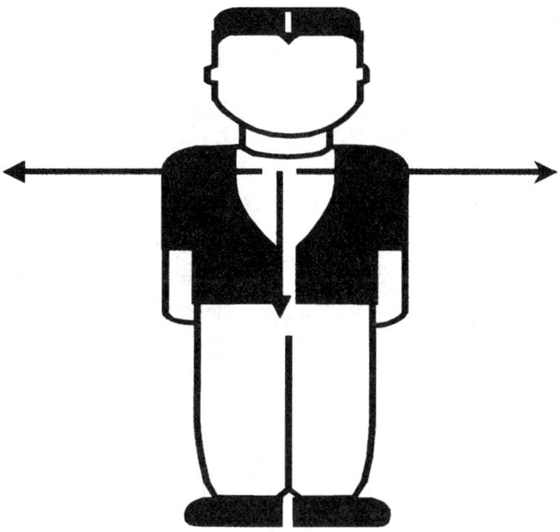

Figure 21 Cutting paths that enable covering of the patient after survey.

Covering the patient is usually more convenient, as the covers can be adapted to fit and do not interfere with operations. Double plastic film containing air cushions (normally used to wrap fragile goods) provides an excellent isolation material and can be cut to fit the patient. Thermal packs can also be used either by themselves or arranged in a vest arrangement that is strapped onto the patient's chest. Once extricated, a microfiber body wrapping with a water-resistant external surface effectively protects the patient from further heat loss.

A novel interesting device (Thermostat™) uses the mechanism of shunting warm blood through the arteriovenous anastomoses in the forearm to the central circulation using negative pressure rewarming. The forearm is fitted through an acrylic mold with an airtight seal around the arm. Negative pressure is applied to override the natural vasoconstriction and a thermal load is applied, which theoretically reaches and warms the core. Initial trials show promising results, and further studies are in progress [39].

3. Resuscitation

Rigid musculature can result in trismus, which complicates intubation and airway mobilization. Application of sedatives and narcotics can increase the heat loss, and vasoactive drugs are less effective in the hypothermic patient. Severe bradycardia can be a sign of deep hypothermia and can progress to therapy-resistant tachyarrythmias if inappropriately managed.

A conservative approach should be taken toward treating arrhythmia other than cardiac arrest. Inotropes are usually of little use in hypothermic and acidotic patients because of generally retarded electrical conduction and impaired myocardial compliance. Cardiopulmonary resuscitation should be continued until active rewarming has been instituted and the core temperature reaches 36°C.

Delivery of IV fluids using uninsulated tubing rapidly and dramatically increases the heat loss even if the fluids have been stored in thermo bags. The IV systems in current use poorly conserve the temperature of the IV fluid over time, thus IV fluids for outdoor use should be warm and delivered in an isolated system. During protracted rescue operations, one should be aware of the dangers of progressing hypothermia, especially in cases with ongoing exsanguinations.

VIII. CUSTOMIZED EQUIPMENT

In extrication situations the rescue crew often has to work in confined spaces and in difficult positions. Because of this, normal equipment used in hospitals can sometimes be troublesome to use. The prehospital situation also calls for customized equipment that has to be modified and developed to master a special situation.

A. Medical Equipment

1. Airway

Securing of the orotracheal tube or the laryngeal mask is paramount. Tape and plasters won't adhere to wet or moist surfaces, but using cotton ribbons or tube holders provides a safer anchorage. Commercially, there are several devices for securing the tube using different kinds of adhesive materials and constrictor fittings. These might do the job, depending on the design and situation, but are costly and not always appropriate. When using the cotton ribbons the cord is double folded and passed behind the tube. The free ends are passed through the loop, and both parts are then tied around the patient's neck.

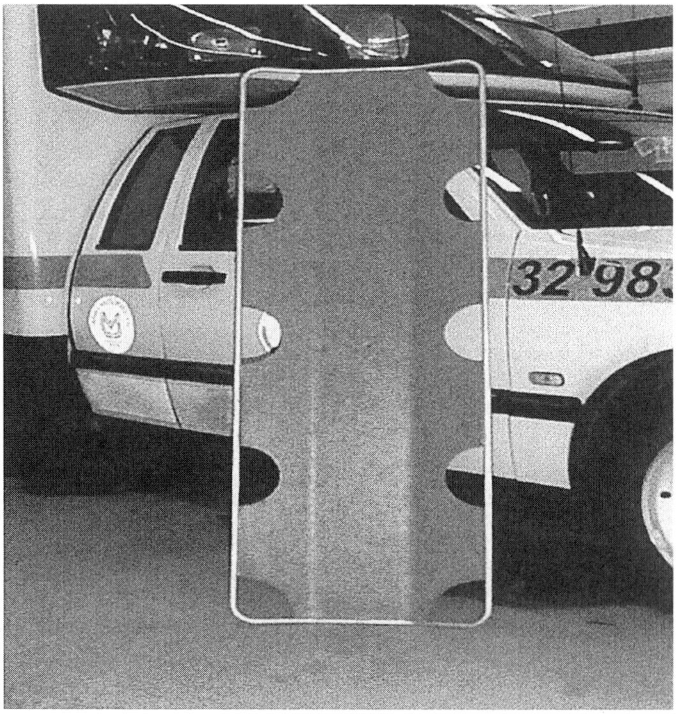

Figure 22 Short spine board.

This provides a good fixation under circumstances in which commercial tube holders sometimes are too bulky to fit (e.g., patients with cervical collars).

2. Spinal Immobilization

During extrication a long spine board will be difficult to handle and maneuver inside an automobile wreck. A shorter spine board enables use in confined spaces and can serve as a support for the victim while cutting restraints and backrests (Fig. 22).

3. IV Lines

A holder for IV infusions that can be attached to even rugged and buckled metal surfaces saves a pair of hands in the rescue work. The holder fits with magnets and is freely adjustable in all directions (Fig. 23).

4. Thermal Protection

Plastic air-containing film provides good insulate capacity (Fig. 24) and can be cut to fit. Using thermo packs stored in a west-like arrangement can also provide thermal energy. Once extricated the patients can be put in whole-body packing with water-resistant rubber outside and a microfleece interior.

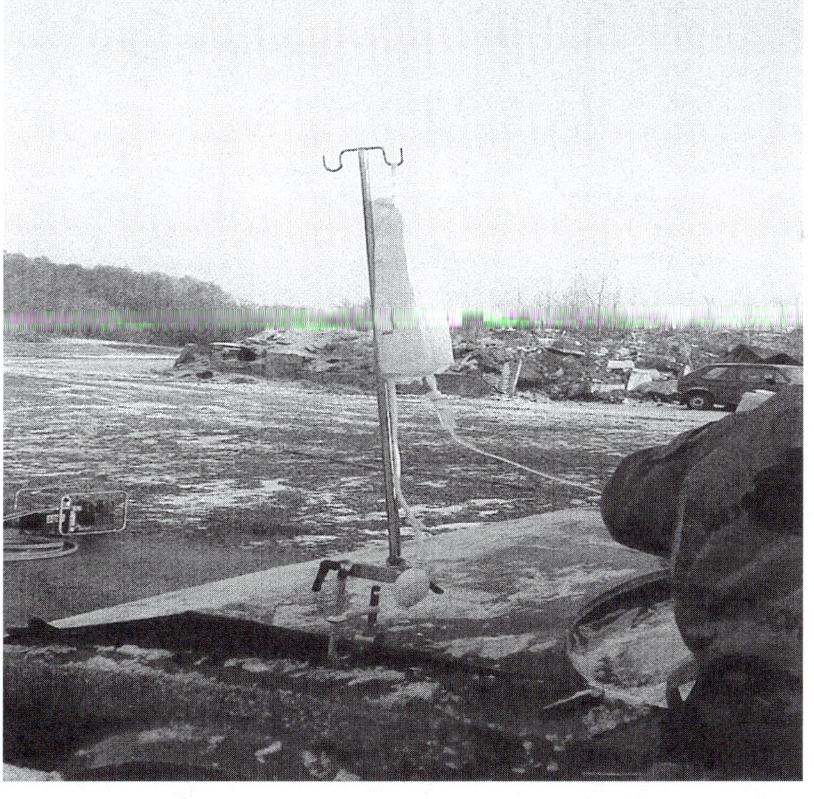

Figure 23 Holder for IV fluids with magnetic or screw fittings.

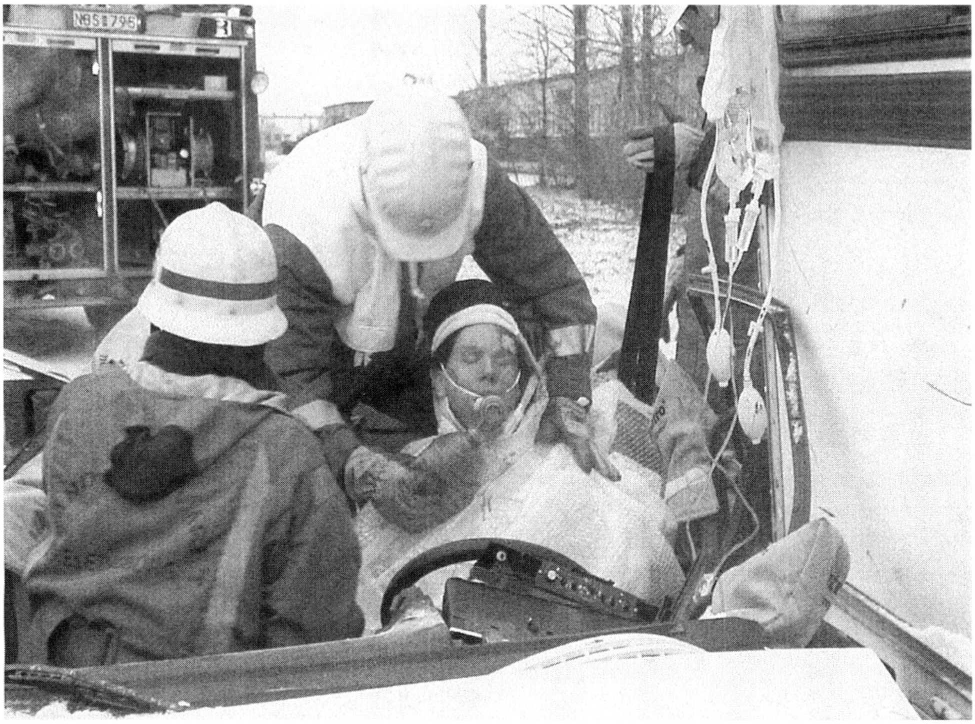

Figure 24 Plastic film with air cushions; used for thermal protection.

B. Technical Equipment

1. Lifting and Immobilization

Helicopter evacuation demands accurate immobilizations and protection from debris and collisions with the environment. This can be done using specially designed stretchers with head covers of full-body vacuum splints with attached horizontal lift straps. A lightweight alternative is a rescue net, which enables horizontal recovery (Figs. 19,20).

2. Tools

Appropriate tools for the assigned tasks are carried along in a holster attached to a belt. Keeping the tools in the holster when not in use minimizes the risk of the tools getting lost in debris and mud at the accident scene (Fig. 25).

3. Glass Protection and Protection from Sharp Edges

When crushing windows the patient is protected from splints by using plastic boards, which are used to push the glass outside the vehicle (Fig. 26). Sharp edges are covered with magnetic fitted Kevlar covers (Fig. 27).

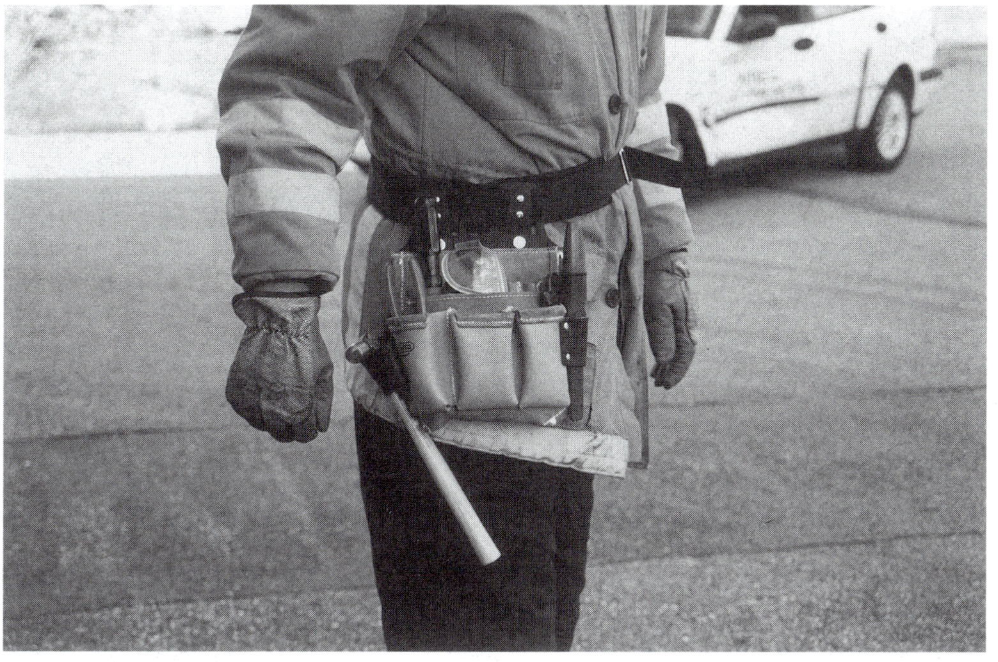

Figure 25 Tool holster.

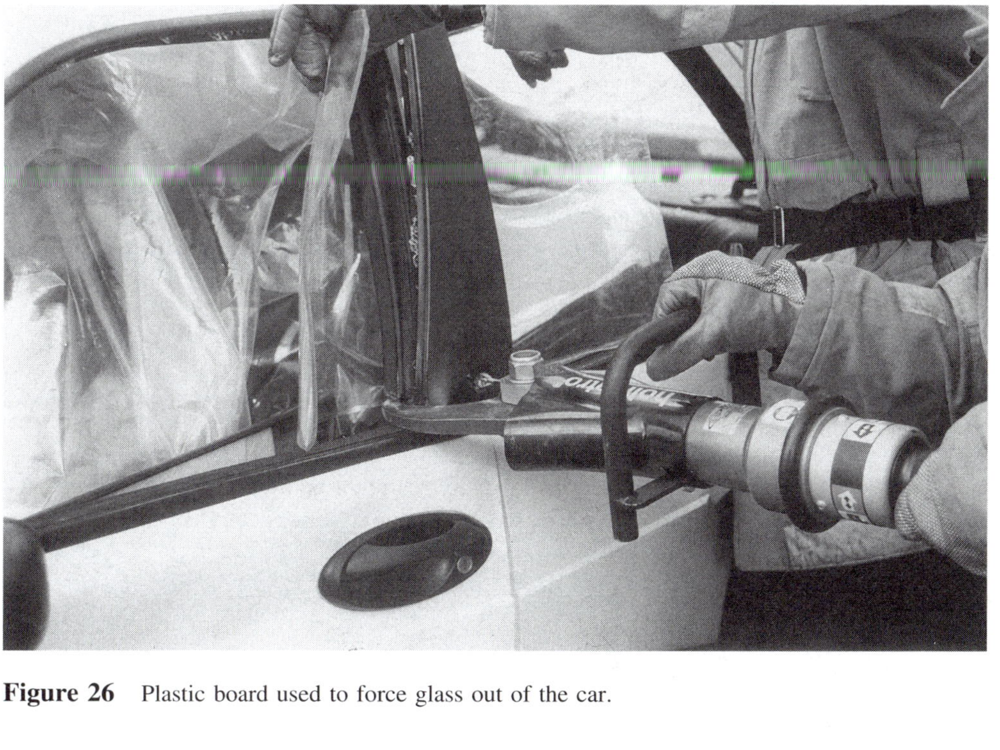

Figure 26 Plastic board used to force glass out of the car.

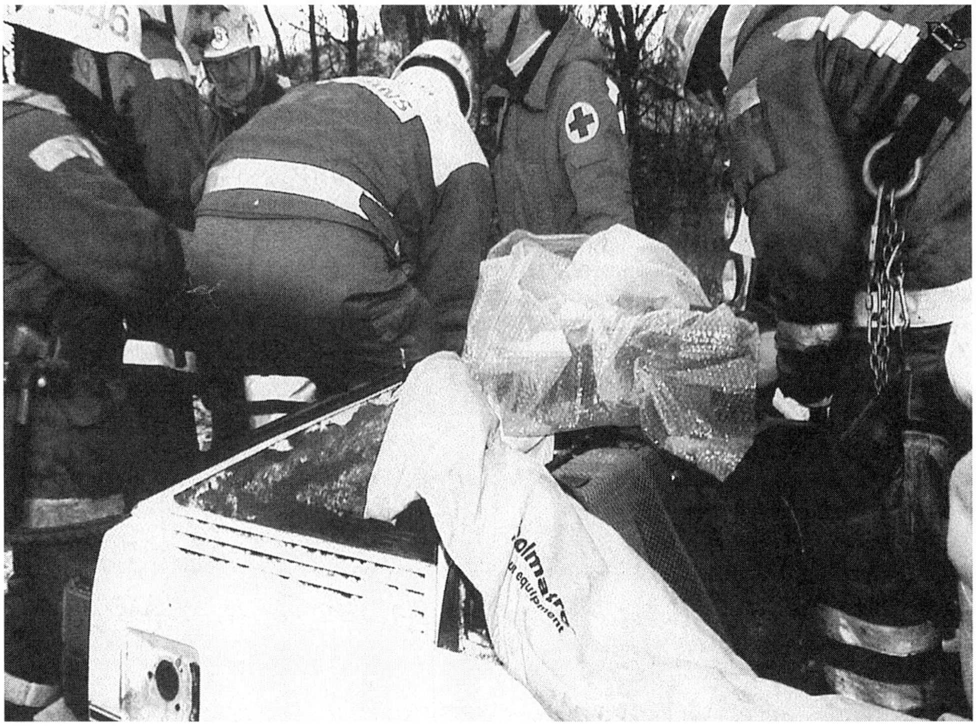

Figure 27 Magnetic fitted covers to protect from sharp edges.

IX. SUMMARY

The entrapped patient poses special problems to the rescue team. Gaining access, providing medical treatment, and performing controlled extrication emphasizes the need for a team approach with organized training to enhance cooperation and liaison within the rescue team. In order to master complex extrication scenarios and not to jeopardize patient and personnel safety, the team must consist of a multidisciplinary staff with broad knowledge in the technical and medical aspects of rescue operations. An entrapment situation is characterized by the following:

High-energy trauma
High incidence of multiple injuries
High incidence of injuries to the head and thorax
High incidence of hypothermia
High incidence of impaired vital functions
High need for on-scene advanced medical treatment and airway maneuvers
Increased risk for worsening of spinal lesions due to improper extrication and transport procedures
Prolonged rescue time due to difficult patient access

REFERENCES

1. TJ Esposito, ND Sanddal, JD Hansen, S Reynolds. Analysis of preventable trauma deaths and inappropriate trauma care in a rural state. J Trauma 39:955–962, 1995.
2. LM Hussain, AD Redmond. Are prehospital deaths from accidental injury preventable? BMJ 308:1077–1080, 1994.
3. G Regel, P Lobenhoffer, M Grotz, HC Pape, U Lehmann, H Tscherne. Treatment results of patients with multiple trauma: An analysis of 3406 cases treated between 1972 and 1991 at a German level I trauma center. J Trauma 38:70–78, 1995.
4. DD Trunkey. Trauma. Sci Am 249:20–27, 1983.
5. A Saudia, F Moore, E Moore, K Moser. Epidemiology of trauma deaths: A reassessment. J Trauma 38:185–193, 1995.
6. G Regel, M Stalp, U Lehmann, A Seekamp. Prehospital care, importance of early intervention on outcome. Acta Anaesth Scand Suppl 110:71–73, 1997.
7. L Lamp, M Helm, JW Wiedringer, KH Bock, Vorschläge zur notärztlichen Strategie bei Einklemmungstrauma. Akt Traumatol 24:163–176, 1994.
8. W Dick. Setting standards and implementing quality improvement in trauma care. Eur J Emerg Med 3:270–273, 1996.
9. J Shüttler, B Schmitz, AC Bartsch, M Fischer. Untersuchungen zur Effzienz der notärztliche Therapie bei Patienten mit Schädel-Hirn-bzw: Polytrauma. Anaesthesist 44:850–858, 1995.
10. PF Mahoney, CJ Carney. Entrapment, extrication and immobilization. Eur J Emerg Med 3: 244–246, 1996.
11. ABM Wilmink, GS Samra, LM Watson, AW Wilson. Vehicle entrapment rescue and prehospital trauma care. Injury 27:21–25, 1996.
12. Swedish Road Traffic Institute. 20, 1998.
13. IS Jones, HR Champion. Trauma triage: Vehicle damage as an estimate of injury severity. J Trauma 29:646–653, 1989.
14. ID Andersson, W Woodford, T Dombal, M Irving. A retrospective study of 1000 deaths from injury in England and Wales. BMJ 296:1305–1308, 1988.
15. KJ Heath. The effect of laryngoscopy of different cervical spine immobilisation techniques. Anaesthesia 49:843–845, 1994.
16. TE Anderson, WD Rose, MJ Leicht. Physician-staffed helicopter scene response from a rural trauma center. Ann Emerg Med 16:58–61, 1987.
17. U Schmidt, SB Frame, ML Nerlich, DW Rowe, BL Enderson, KI Maull, H Tscherne. On-scene helicopter transports of patients with multiple injuries—Comparison of a German and an American system. J Trauma 33:548–555, 1992.
18. M Helm, L Lamp, J Hauke, K Bock. Akzidentelle hypothermie bei traumapatienten. Anaesthesist 44:101–107, 1995.
19. A Ersson, M Lundberg, CO Wramby, H Svensson. Extrication of entrapped victims from motor vehicle accidents: The Crew concept. Eur J Emerg Med 6:341–347, 1999.
20. S Lautenschlager, U Karli, P Matter. Paragliding accidents—A prospective analysis in Swiss mountain regions. Z Unfallchir Versicherungsmed suppl. 1:55–65, 1993.
21. RP Pfeiffer, RL Kronisch. Off-road cycling injuries: An overview. Sports Med 19:311–325, 1995.
22. J Jerosch. Scene and extreme sports varieties: The injury spectrum is changing. Sportverletz Sportschaden 10:VII–VIII, 1996.
23. H Brugger, M Falk, L Adler-Kastner. Avalanche emergency: New aspects of the patophysiology and therapy of buried avalanche victims. Wien Klin Wochenschr 109:145–159, 1997.
24. H Brugger, B Durrer, L Adler-Kastner. On-site triage of avalanche victims with asystole by the emergency doctor. Resuscitation 31:11–16, 1996.

25. PB Bennet, DH Elliott. The physiology and medicine of diving. 3rd ed. London: Ballière Tindall, 1982.
26. PHTLS Manual. 3rd ed. Mosby Lifeline, 1994.
27. G Sanson, S Di Bartolomeo, G Nardi, P Albanese, A Diani, L Raffin, C Fillipetto, A Cattarossi, F Scian, L Rizzi. Road traffic accidents with vehicular entrapment: Incidence of major injuries and need for advanced life support. Eur J Emerg Med 6:285–291, 1999.
28. O Moeschler, S Refondini, C Høfliger, J Freeman. Difficult areomedical rescue situations: Experience of a Swiss pre-Alpine Helicopter base. J Trauma 33:754–759, 1992.
29. JA Moylan. Impact of helicopters on trauma care and clinical results. Ann Surg 208:673–678, 1988.
30. N Demartines, C Meyer, D Scheidegger, F Harder. Helikopter und notarzt an der unfallstelle. Helv Chir Acta 58:223–227, 1991.
31. M Graf, N Demartines, F Harder, D Scheidegger. Polytrauma: Vergleich des spitalverlaufes nach luft (mit notarzt) versus bodentransport (ohne notarzt). Helv Chir Acta 59:649–653, 1992.
32. G Baxt, P Moody. The impact of a phycisian as part of the aeromedical prehospital team in patients with blunt trauma. JAMA 257:3246–3250, 1987.
33. R Northon, E Wortman, L Eastes, D Mohamud. Appropriate helicopter transport of urban trauma patients. J Trauma 41:886–891, 1996.
34. W Schwab, M Peclet, S Zackowski, EM Holmes III, JC Forrester, CN Hensleigh. The impact of an air ambulance system on an established trauma center. J Trauma 25:580–587, 1985.
35. CD Deakin. Prehospital management of the traumatized airway. Eur J Emerg Med 3:233–243, 1996.
36. D Dries. Hypotensive resuscitation. Shock 6:311–316, 1996.
37. A Ferrara, J MacArthur, H Wright, I Modlin, MA McMillen. Hypothermia and acidosis worsen coagulopathy in the patient requiring massive transfusion. Am J Surg 160:515–518, 1990.
38. D Fritsch. Hypothermia in the trauma patient. AACN Clinical Issuses 6:196–211, 1995.
39. E Søreide, DA Grahn, L Rosen. A novel technique for treatment of hypothermia: The combined application of negative pressure and heat to specific surface areas. Proceedings 10th Annual Trauma and Critical Care Symposium, ITAACS, Baltimore, 1997.
40. RC Hunt, RL Brown, KA Cline, JR Krohmer, JB McCabe, TW Whitley. Comparison of motor vehicle damage documentation in emergency medical services run reports compared with photographic documentation. Ann Emerg Med 22:651–656, 1993.

APPENDIX I: Crush Injury

(a) Tissue in compression, consequences

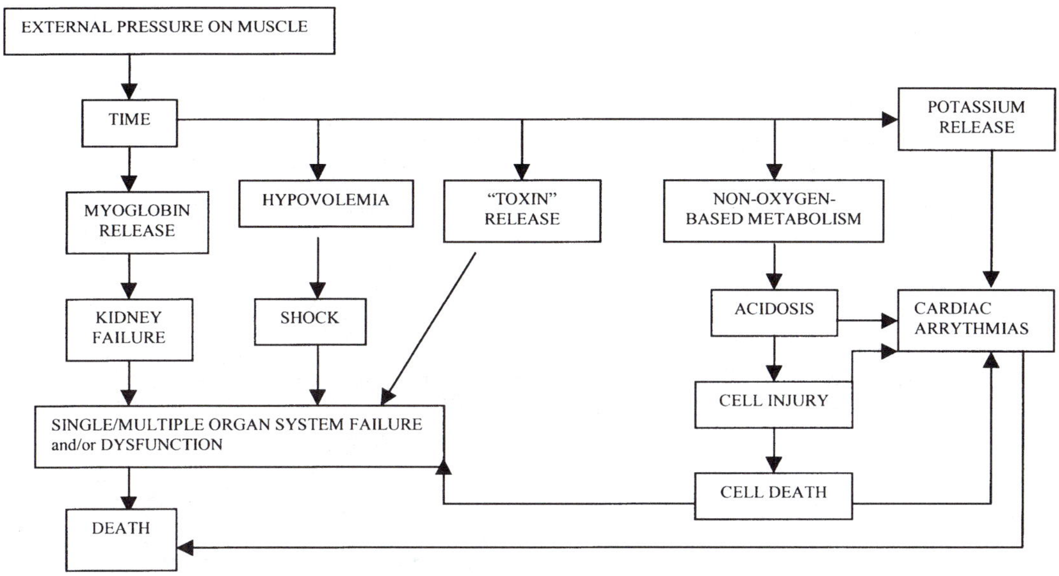

(b) Interrelationships

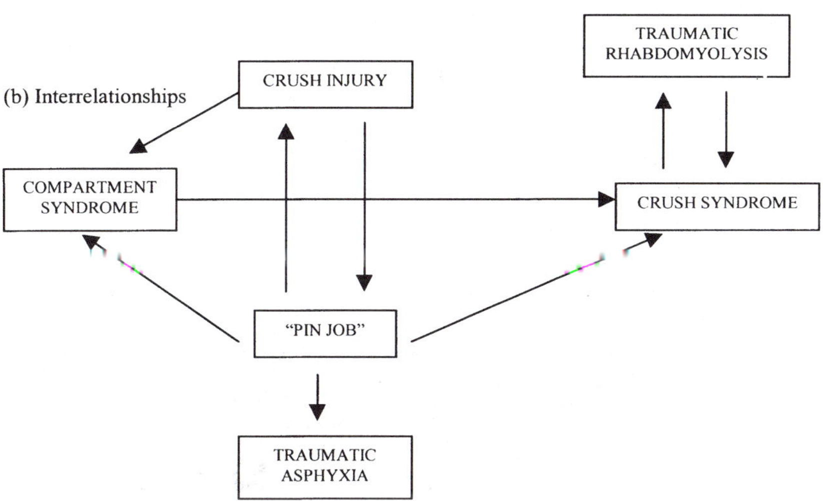

APPENDIX II: Simple Triage and Rapid Treatment (S.T.A.R.T.)

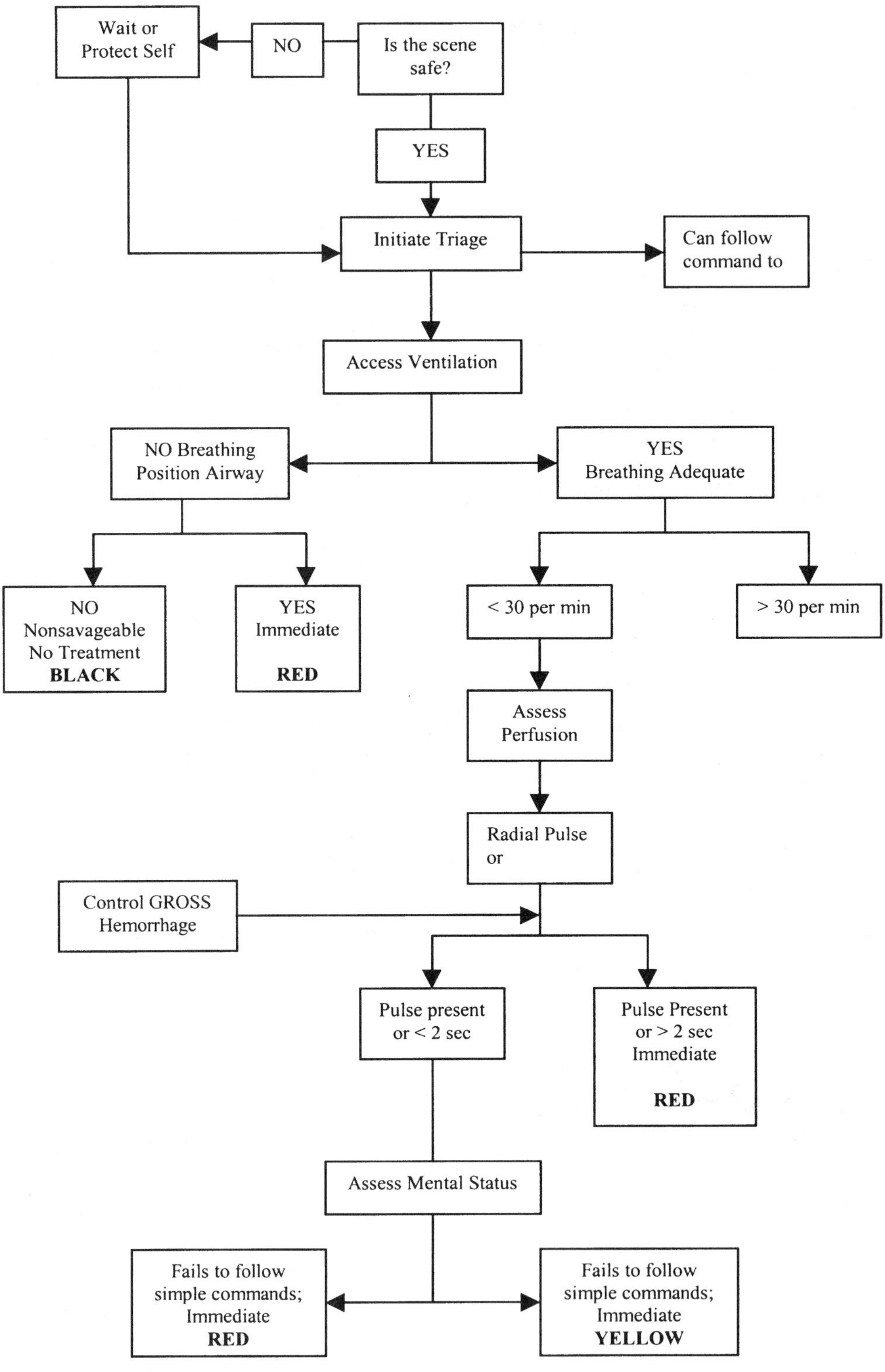

Note: black: nonviable, no treatment indicated, death eminent; red: critical, immediate medical attention, rapid transport; yellow: stable, delayed treatment and transport; green: minor injury, ambulatory.

28

Patients With Orthopedic Injuries

ASGEIR M. KVAM

Ullevaal University Hospital, Oslo, Norway

I. INTRODUCTION

Orthopedic injury is present in 75% of multitraumatized patients [1]. Motor vehicle accidents (MVA) and falls are the causes most likely to be associated with orthopedic trauma [2]. Fractures account for 7.4% of all the injuries sustained by automobile occupants. The incidence of sporting, and especially recreational injuries is increasing. Despite of a lot of preventive and legislative efforts, [occupational accidents] still cause great numbers of orthopedic injuries. Hip fractures in the elderly are responsible for a large burden on the health care system. These patients occupy one-fifth of all orthopedic hospital beds [3].

Preventive efforts have been made to reduce morbidity and mortality. The use of safety belts is one of the most effective means of reducing mortality (around 10%) and morbidity. The combination of air bags and seatbelts offers a further 11% reduction in mortality [2]. Leg fractures in skiing are reduced because of better skiing equipment adapted to the individual. Preventive efforts, with modification of the training systems among Swedish athletes, have caused a decrease in the number of sports-related injuries. The dramatic increase in the number of hip fractures in the elderly is a great challenge in launching preventive efforts. This ranges from attempts at prevention and treatment of osteoporosis to preventing injuries by wearing hip-protecting undergarments [4].

Pelvic and long bone fractures and some amputation injuries may lead to life-threatening hemorrhage. Except for these cases, orthopedic injury in itself is seldom of great urgency (''scoop and run''), and the patient benefits from a well-planned and conducted survey and treatment at the scene. Patients with fractures of larger bones are in danger of developing major physiologic derangements, such as fat embolism, infections, adult respiratory distress syndrome (ARDS), and multiorgan dysfunction (multiorgan failure). In multitrauma patients more ''minor'' orthopedic injuries (e.g., hand injuries) may cause a permanent inability to perform the patient's former occupation. In contrast to injuries to other organ systems, an orthopedic injury may be well stabilized at the scene of an accident, thereby reducing blood loss, pain, risk of infection, and neurological sequela.

This chapter focuses on the general principles of prehospital treatment of orthopedic injury with special emphasis on procedures carried out by anesthesiologists, and a thorough description of equipment and techniques used in the prehospital setting.

A. The Role of Emergency Medical Systems in Epidemiology and Prevention

Detecting the incidence of accidents and injuries, and thereby preventing and stopping the epidemia of trauma is a rather uncommon role of emergency medical systems (EMS). Through documentation and data management it is possible to identify accident locations and perform risk management. Close cooperation with the authorities, for example, may lead to improved sanding of roads after snowfalls or to reduced speed limits on dangerous roads.

II. AIMS AND MEANS OF PREHOSPITAL TREATMENT

Different groups of both professional and volunteer personnel take part in the prehospital care of patients with orthopedic trauma. The working environments and the challenges are different: consider the mountain guide, far away from the civilization versus the paramedic in the city, or the general practitioner at the ski resort, or the specialized anesthesiologist manning the helicopter ambulance.

The general principles of survey and treatment have been simplified and standardized. For each group of personnel the aim is to create an educational system. A quality assurance system must assure that a certain standard of quality of care is achieved. All groups of personnel should, as a minimum, be able to perform the tasks listed in Table 1.

In some countries it is difficult for legal reasons to allow nonphysicians to perform ''advanced'' procedures, such as reducing a tibial fracture with compromised circulation. Every patient is different, and after the primary survey (ATLS; see below) trained personnel should be able to rely on an individual assessment of the situation. In some situations (with entrapped patients, severe pain, and generally unstable patients) prehospital care providers with substantial ''field experience'' may offer the patient more advanced and individual treatment.

Table 1 Desirable Capabilities of All Prehospital Personnel Dealing With Orthopedic Injury

Prevent and intervene against life-threatening conditions
Analyze mechanisms of trauma, perform a simple clinical examination, and recognize the most common kinds of orthopedic injuries
Stabilize injuries with splints and bandages
In cases with danger of secondary damage (e.g., nerve damage, or ischemia) be able to perform a reduction and establish traction on fractured extremities
Administer pain treatment

Table 2 Documentation on Orthopedic Injuries

Mechanism of trauma	Treatment
Time of trauma	Reduction of fractures, time
Trauma energy	Immobilization/splinting
Survey	Pain management
Signs of injury	Fluid therapy
Normal findings (especially neck and spine)	Scoring systems
Free movement of limbs in joints	Glasgow coma score
Distal to injury (examination before and after reduction/splinting)	Revised trauma score
Pulse	
Capillary refill	
Skin color	
Sensibility	
Motor function	
(Reflexes)	

A. Documentation

Every EMS system should have a good system for documentation. The EMS report form should be as simple as possible. The paramedic or physician should concentrate on the patient and not on filling out endless forms. The EMS report form should cover the following subjects:

Documentation of the medical examination and findings
Treatment
Condition of the patient during transport

This is information that is important for further diagnosis and treatment purposes. At the same time it is necessary for legal reasons. The layout of the form should make it easy to obtain important information. For orthopedic injuries, findings concerning sensory/motor and circulatory function should be clearly documented (see Table 2).

The Glasgow coma scale (GCS) [5] and Revised trauma score (RTS) [6] have been shown to correlate well with mortality, and have a good interrater reliability. This allows a longitudinal assessment of the patient to be performed by different observers. These scoring systems are important tools for quality assurance and for comparing different EMS systems. Documentation of problems and complications in treatment are important for quality assurance purposes.

III. MECHANISM OF TRAUMA

An important factor to consider when arriving at the scene of an accident is the mechanism of trauma. This will give important information as far as directing subsequent examination of the patient.

$$\text{Trauma energy } E \approx \text{Kinetic energy} = 1/2\ mv^2$$

The severity of the injuries is often related to the amount of trauma energy. The energy is dependent on the speed before the crash and the rate of deceleration. Patients exposed

Table 3 Factors Often Associated With Life-Threatening Injury

Ejection from vehicle
Death of occupant in same vehicle
Auto crash with significant vehicular body damage
Significant fall
Significant auto rollover, bent steering wheel
Auto pedestrian impact
Significant motorcycle, all terrain vehicle, or bicycle impact
Significant assault or altercation

to high trauma energy will often be subject to severe injury. The events listed in Table 3 are often related to severe injuries [7], and are often associated with multitrauma [8].

IV. MULTITRAUMA AND ORTHOPEDIC INJURIES

Seventy-five percent of multitrauma patients have injuries of the extremities. Fifty percent of patients with open fractures have multiple injuries [9]. Some orthopedic injuries may be life-threatening, mostly because of severe bleeding and development of hypovolemic shock including traumatic amputation, major vascular injury, pelvic fractures with disruption, hemorrhage from open fractures, multiple long bone fractures, and severe crush injury.

The physician and the EMS personnel caring for trauma patients should also pay attention to minor injuries, which often go unnoticed during the initial phase. Permanent sequelae after multitrauma are also influenced by such minor injuries, examplified by a fracture of the navicular bone of the hand or injuries of distal nerves [10]. An early, complete survey of the patient therefore is of great importance.

V. PRIMARY SURVEY OF THE TRAUMA VICTIM WITH ORTHOPEDIC INJURIES

The primary survey is a prioritized series of observations aimed at identifying and treating life-threatening conditions simultaneously. It terms of coordination, by the time this survey is complete, any necessary resuscitation has already been started. When the patient is stable, a thorough secondary survey may be undertaken. It is assumed that the patient is in a safe environment (i.e. no continued danger of fire, traffic accidents, firearm injury, or assault). In general, the patient will not be moved unnecessarily during this survey process.

A. Examination—A-B-C-D-E

The patient is examined where he is initially found. The primary survey follows steps A-B-C-D-E for protocol consistency reasons. Most of the survey is carried out simultaneously with resuscitation efforts and while obtaining the history from the patient. If the patient is unable to report about the accident by himself, detailed accounts of the incident *must* be obtained from bystanders or rescue personnel. Important details are included in Table 4.

Table 4 Medical and Trauma History

Time of accident
Position of patient in vehicle during crash
Speed of vehicle
Direction of falling/ejection from automobile
Wearing of seatbelts (hip and/or shoulder) or helmets
Activation of an airbag?
Consumption of alcohol and/or drugs
Last oral ingestion
Past medical history of relevance

1. A: Airway and Cervical Spine

Is the patient able to maintain a patent airway? Is the airway blocked by the tongue or foreign materials? The initial maneuvers are chin lift or jaw thrust, combined with suctioning or manual removal of foreign debris. *The cervical spine is assumed to be unstable until proven otherwise*, which implies that the head is kept in a neutral position and no movements are allowed before immobilization is applied and enough support personnel are present to maintain the cervical spine in its neutral axis.

2. B: Breathing

A patent airway does not guarantee adequate ventilation. The chest should be exposed for evaluation of breathing. Typical signs of ventilatory impairment are: asymmetrical chest movements, a respiratory rate <10 or >30 breaths per min, abnormal respiratory efforts, and clinical signs of chest injury. Tension pneumothorax, open pneumothorax, and flail chest combined with pulmonary contusion are the major injuries compromising ventilation in trauma patients. The initial management will be bag-valve ventilation with a face mask. (Prehospital endotracheal intubation will be discussed below.) Oxygen should be given to all trauma patients as soon as possible (i.e., upon initial contact).

3. C: Circulation

The loss of erythrocytes and intravascular volume can be disastrous and yet often easily correctable when identified. Hypotension is assumed to be due to hypovolemia until proved otherwise. During the primary survey level of consciousness, skin color and pulse should be evaluated. Pale, white, and cold extremities and especially paleness of the face are signs of hypoperfusion, although a cold outdoor environment also may reduce peripheral circulation. Pulses are palpated at the carotid or femoral artery for rate and quality, with rates above 100 and a ''fine'' thready pulse suggesting a compromised circulation. External bleeding should then be controlled by direct pressure during the initial survey.

4. D: Disability

The initial survey for disability is a brief neurologic assessment, which only involves determining the level of consciousness on a four-level scale (AVPU), along with pupillary size and reactivity. It will already be an integral part of the survey when approaching the patient. The levels of consciousness are listed in Table 5.

Although one at this time may unintentionally observe motor function in the extremities, this is really a part of the secondary survey.

Table 5 AVPU: Level of Consciousness

A—Alert
V—Responds to vocal stimuli
P—Responds to painful stimuli
U—Unresponsive

5. E: Exposure

The fifth part of the initial survey in the advanced trauma life support (ATLS) concept is the total undressing of the patient to facilitate thorough examination. In the prehospital setting this is often unsuitable, as light and temperature do not allow extended examinations. The ''resuscitation phase'' is started at the same time as the initial survey.

VI. PREHOSPITAL INDUCTION OF ANESTHESIA AND AIRWAY MANEUVERS

For simplicity and safety, the prehospital approach to the induction of anesthesia has to be uniform with respect to drugs, equipment, and technique. Performing anesthesia on the scene has many potential hazards, and complication rates are closely related to the qualifications and experience of the prehospital care provider [11]. General anesthesia outside the hospital, as well as in the hospital, should only be performed by anesthesiologists. One must think ''worst case.'' As stated earlier, all patients are considered as having an unstable cervical spine. They should also be assumed to have a full stomach, placing them at risk of gastric aspiration, as well as having raised intracranial pressure. Many of the patients may be hypovolemic. Precautions must be taken because of the lack of diagnostic aids. The anesthetic technique should therefore reduce the risk of cervical movement during intubation, prevent gastric aspiration, prevent increases in intracranial pressure, and maintain cardiovascular stability. In the prehospital phase monitoring during induction of anesthesia reflects these concerns. Monitoring must *at least* include ECG, automatic blood pressure measuring, and pulse oximetry. Capnography is highly desirable. A complete discussion of prehospital monitoring follows.

As in the hospital, an anesthetic plan is made prior to induction. Our ''ideal'' anesthetic technique includes the use of three persons (i.e., an experienced anesthesiologist, a rescue man/paramedic/nurse from the helicopter, and finally an ambulance technician from the local responding unit). The intubation is done in a rapid-sequence procedure with administration of hypnotic and muscular relaxant almost simultaneously. We prefer direct orotracheal intubation, and are reluctant to pass nasogastric tubes before the cranial base has been x-rayed. Confirmation of tube position is done by auscultation with a stethoscope and, if present, by capnography. The patient is ventilated manually (and eventually by the ventilator), and the cervical collar replaced. The endotracheal tube is *secured well*, and the patient is strapped to the backboard again (Fig. 1).

After intubation vital signs are rechecked, bearing in mind that a simple asymptomatic pneumothorax may develop into a tension pneumothorax after positive pressure ventilation, and that circulation may be disturbed by the altered intrathoracic pressures as well as the anesthetic drug effects.

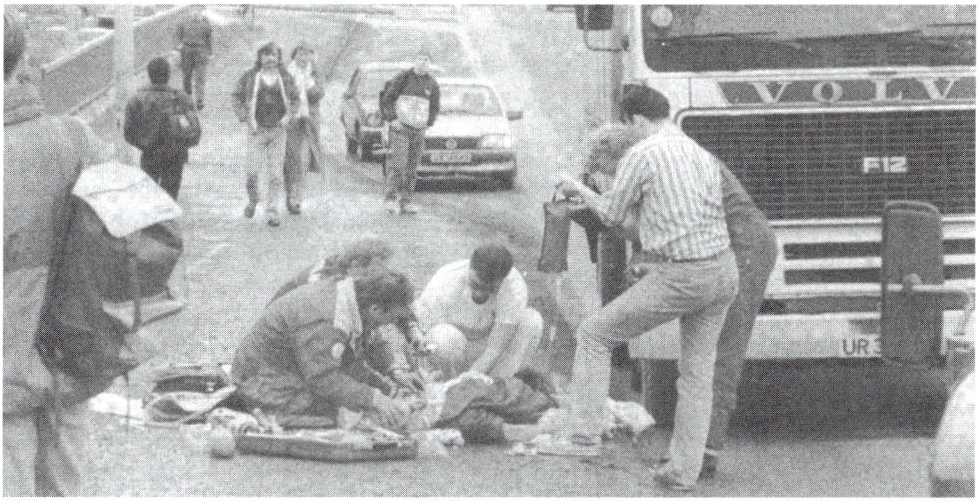

Figure 1 Prehospital anesthesia. A pedestrian has been hit by a truck and is multitraumatized. General anesthesia with endotracheal intubation is performed by the anesthesiologist from Norwegian Air Ambulance, in cooperation with his rescue man and the EMS team. (Photo courtesy of Morten Antonsen, Adresseavisen, Trondheim, Norway.)

VII. HEMORRHAGE AND TREATMENT OF ACUTE HYPOVOLEMIA

Uncontrolled arterial hemorrhage is immediately life-threatening and must be treated at the scene. There are three main ways of controlling such bleeding as shown in Table 6. After an amputation, physiologic regional vasoconstriction and retraction of the vessels, combined with local point pressure, will stop most bleedings. In some cases profuse bleedings may occur. Initially, proximal compression may be needed.

Conversely, a tourniquet may cause ischemic injury. Use for more than 3 hrs may cause an irreversible loss of function [12]. A group of patients arrived at a Norwegian military hospital with applied tourniquets proximal to an amputation injury. Continuous bleeding distal to the tourniquet was frequently observed. Efforts to tighten the tourniquet did not reduce the bleeding [13]. In a review article, Mellesmo and Pillgram-Larsen conclude that tourniquets should not be used in treating bleeding from extremity injuries [14].

Tourniquets should only be used as an exception and only in cases with an entrapped extremity and life-threatening bleeding. On the upper extremity a blood pressure cuff

Table 6 Prehospital Control of External Bleeding

1. Through point control, with localized *pressure* on the bleeding vessel, with a pressure dressing and/or elastic bandage (or rubber bandage) in the vast majority of cases
2. With use of a proximal *tourniquet* (in a few cases, not controlled by direct pressure)
3. Through *ligation* or *clamping* of the bleeding vessels, and only when access to definitive care will be delayed and there is immediate threat to life (very rarely)

Until one of the above methods is established compressing proximal on the arteries may control hemorrhage temporarily should be inflated to a pressure 60 to 70 mmHg above systolic blood pressure. For the lower extremity a broad cuff, with a pressure 80 to 100 mmHg above systolic pressure may be of help. Ligation or clamping is difficult to perform outside the operating room without sufficient equipment and knowledge. It may cause damage to the arteries, and should only be done if other methods fail.

Also, closed fractures may cause severe hemorrhage. The bleeding should be roughly estimated in each patient, as shown in Figure 2. Immobilization and splinting of fractures also contributes to reduce bleeding. According to some authors, extended eleva-

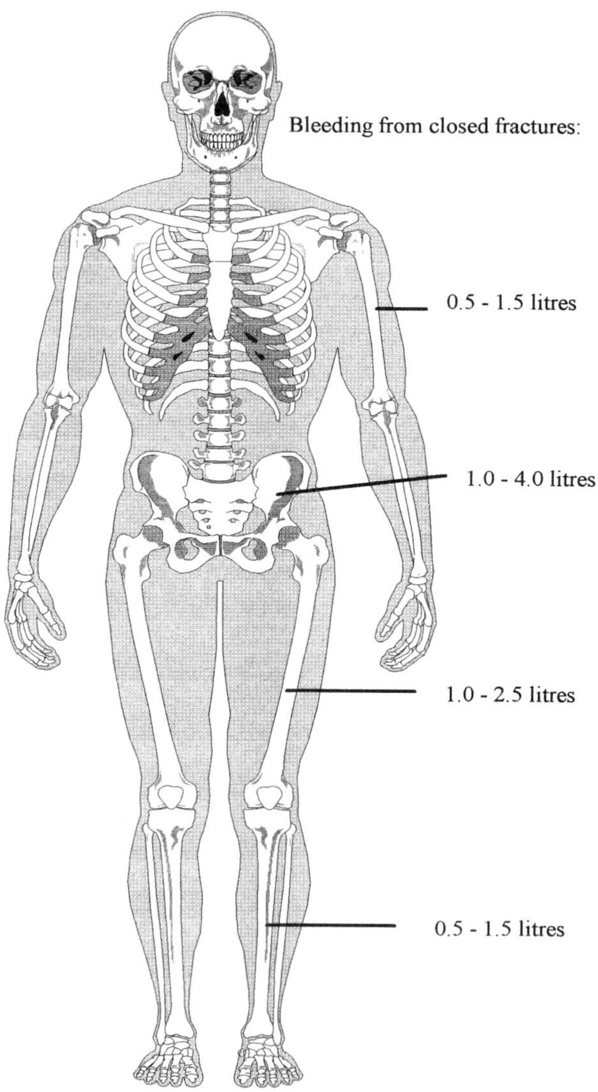

Figure 2 Estimated blood loss from closed fractures. From open fractures the estimated bleeding may be two to three times more.

tion of the bleeding part above the level of the heart increases the risk of developing compartment syndrome (CS) [15].

In conclusion most bleeding may be controlled with localized pressure combined with elevation of the injured part, eventually in combination with compression of proximal arteries. Tourniquets should be avoided if possible and ligation or clamping of vessels should not be performed outside the hospital, unless there are no other alternatives, other methods have been tried, and access to definitive care is going to be prolonged.

A. Fluid Therapy

Studies in animal models indicate that rapid infusions in uncontrolled hemmorrhage may in fact increase the bleeding [16–18]. Pulmonary edema in young, healthy patients after excessive prehospital infusion of crystalloids is reported in two cases in Trondheim, Norway [19]. Further clinical studies will decide whether or not prehospital treatment protocols for fluid therapy have to be changed. When hemorrhage is under control, there is an indication for more liberal fluid therapy. The choice of the ''ideal fluid'' is difficult. A review article by Gould et al. concludes as follows [20]: ''Most clinical studies suggest that there is no advantage to the administration of colloid solution rather than crystalloid in the treatment of hemorrhagic shock. Preliminary studies with hypertonic saline solutions suggest that effective resuscitation can be achieved using relatively small volumes of fluid, but further studies are necessary to verify the safety and efficacy of this therapy.''

B. Prehospital Transfusion: Oxygen Transporting Solutions

In some cases prehospital transfusions may be lifesaving. The authors describe a case with an entrapped patient who was transfused with non-crossmatched homologous blood. Prehospital transfusions are seldom performed in Norway. However, when prehospital transfusions are needed, this is the preferred method. In some countries there are systems for sending blood samples with ambulances for cross matching in the hospital, and then offering the patients transfusions on the scene. There are still no good alternatives to homologous blood. Different synthetic solutions are under development, but clinical studies have neither proved the benefits nor the safety of these products. Prompt transport to the hospital has the highest priority in cases of uncontrolled hemorrhage.

VIII. THE SECONDARY SURVEY OF ORTHOPEDIC INJURIES

A. Clinical Examination: Mechanism of Trauma and Trauma Energy

Before beginning the secondary survey the physician or EMS personnel on the scene should try to understand which mechanisms of trauma and which forces have worked against the victim. The condition of the patient is sometimes so stable that a systematic secondary survey of the patient may be performed before transportation is started. The secondary survey includes not only evaluation of respiration, circulation, and degree of consciousness, but also an examination that includes the skull, spine, shoulders, arms, chest, abdomen, pelvis, hips, and the rest of the lower extremities. A neurological status should also be obtained. Some typical mechanisms causing musculoskeletal injuries are shown in Table 7.

Table 7 Some Typical Mechanisms Causing Musculoskeletal Injury

1. *Direct blow*, in which the injury occurs at the point of impact
2. *Indirect injury*, in which the injury is some distance from the point of impact
3. *Twisting injury*, in which the distal part of the limb is fixed during a twisting movement of the proximal part (skier's injury of the knee)
4. *Overstretch*, due to powerful muscle contractions
5. *Fatigue fractures*, due to long-lasting stress (march fractures)
6. *Pathological fractures*, due to diseases with weakness of the bone (e.g., cancer)

IX. GENERAL PRINCIPLES FOR EXAMINATION AND TREATMENT OF ORTHOPEDIC INJURIES

A. Assessment of the Injured Joint or Limb

The survey should include both history and clinical examination.

1. History

Where is the pain localized?
Which mechanism of trauma?
What was the direction of the force?
Did a swelling occur at once?
Able to put weight through the joint?

2. Examination

An examination of the injured limb should only be performed when it is adequately exposed. In the prehospital setting weather and temperature decide whether or not and how far this is possible. The examination should be performed as described in Table 8. Every

Table 8 Examination of the Injured Limb

Look
- Deformity?
- Discoloration?
- Swelling, localized or general?

Feel
- Is there tenderness, and if there is it in relation to anatomical structures?
- Is there an effusion?

Movement
- Is there a full range of movement in the normal directions?
- Is there pain during movement?
- Is there pain or movement when the joint is stressed in a direction in which movement does not normally occur?

Nerve function and peripheral circulation
- Pulses
- Capillary refill
- Sensation
- Motor function

Table 9 Types of Soft Tissue Injuries

Injury	Mechanism	Findings
Contusion	Direct forces on the joint	Soft tissue edema, hematoma, hemarthrosis; pain, continuously and by palpation
Distortion	Hyperextension of the capsule and the ligaments through indirect forces on the joint	Initially pain solely over the ligament and its anchoring-points to the bone; later, pain and reduced mobility of the joint, caused by hematoma and edema; increasing pain if the injured ligament is extended
Rupture	Same as by distorsion, but with complete rupture of the ligament, or ligament torn out of its anchoring points	Often instability, with subluxation of the joint; edema; often hemarthrosis; pain with reduced mobility, but less or no pain by extension of the ligament compared with distortions

examination of orthopedic injuries must include examination for nerve damage or loss of peripheral circulation distal to the injury.

B. Soft Tissue Injuries of the Joints

The common types of soft tissue injuries are listed with mechanism and findings in Table 9.

C. Other Soft Tissue Injuries

Soft tissue injuries may occur without involving the joints, or resulting in fractures. The mechanism of trauma may be: (1) Direct force (crush injuries) or (2) hyperextension of muscles or tendons (distorsion or rupture). Typical findings are

Pain
Swelling
Hematoma

1. Compartment Syndrome

Compartment syndrome (CS) [25] is characterized by intracompartmental pressures that rise transiently. This may lead to tissue ischemia, depletion of high-energy stores, and cellular acidosis. Hypoperfusion and nerve damage may lead to chronic damage of local tissue and also to the distal part of the limb.

Compartment syndrome may be caused by trauma (crush injuries), overexercise, repetitive motion, and compression. Soft tissue injuries alone or in combination with fractures may in some situations lead to high pressure in muscular compartments of the extremities. This may result in nerve damage and hypoperfusion of tissues distal in the limb.

Due to the serious complications following a fuliminant CS, early diagnosis and the right timing of a fasciotomy is important. The majority of the U.K. trauma and orthopedic surgeons advocate making the diagnosis of CS by a combination of clinical acumen and compartment pressure measurements. The threshold level for surgery is variable among surgeons [21].

In the prehospital situation EMS personnel should be aware of this problem.

Check changes in peripheral pulse and sensation.
Check injury site for increased pressure. (For in-hospital use specially designed manometers are available, but clinical judgment is still important.)
Do not elevate injured limb above level of the heart for a prolonged period.
Do not use pneumatic splints inflated to high pressure.
Epidural blocks should only be established in cooperation with the orthopedic surgeon.

D. Case Study: Avalanche Victims With Soft Tissue Injuries and Hypothermia

The Dovrefjell plateau, a chain of alpine mountains, serve as a barrier against the humid weather fronts coming in from the Atlantic. The weather may change rapidly during wintertime with strong winds and temperatures 20 to 30°C below freezing. At the end of January two groups of climbers have established basecamps in this area. They are both leaving early in the morning for a day ascent on two different mountains. There is only daylight from 9 a.m. to 3 p.m.

The first group of seven men will climb Larstind through a snow- and ice-filled ridge. From basecamp they go 2 hrs on their skis before starting the ascent. After 2 hrs of climbing they have almost reached the top of the mountain when an avalanche is released by the first climber. As they are all tied together in one rope, the whole group is caught. In a few seconds they plummet 400 meters down through the ridge.

As the avalanche stops one man is dead. The others have injuries, some of them serious. They are only partly buried. The temperature is 25°C below freezing and the wind is increasing. They are still situated in rather steep terrain. Two persons have crush injuries in their legs, and are not able to walk. They are moved into a biwak sack, which gives shelter against the wind. After some hours one of them slides out of the sack, and 15 meters down the ridge. The companions have found a poor shelter at a small rock while heading for the basecamp. With only an injured knee the least injured climber reaches the basecamp after a 3 hr walk. The second group, including the author, has partly returned from the climb, and starts a large rescue operation. The attempt to reach the site of the accident failed due to snow and wind.

After a difficult 3-hr drive in five military snow-cats (snowmobiles) the rescue team spots the lights from emergency flares. The four least injured receive first aid inside the snow-cats. They are all suffering from frostbite, moderate hypothermia, and wounds from contact with their ice axes. After a short search in the steep terrain two injured and one dead climber are localized. The two still alive have suffered crush injuries in their legs, serious frostbite in their fingers and teeth, and hypothermia of 30 to 30.5°C. Their skin is partly in contact with snow and wind.

Due to strong pain morphine is injected im (through the clothing). For the person who is still in the biwak-sack it is possible to establish an IV-cannula (causing frostbite on the physician's fingers). The patients and the body are transported on stretchers down the hillside and into the snow-cats. After an hour's ride the helicopters meet us. After a 1 hr flight, the patients reach the hospital in Trondheim (Table 10, Fig. 3).

E. Treatment of Soft Tissue Injuries

The main principles for primary treatment of these injuries are summarized as in Table 11.

Table 10 Summary of Case (Avalanche Victims)

Prehospital treatment
  Monitoring: Core temperature (rectally), ECG, respiration
  Treatment: Analgesics IV/IM; oxygen, passive warming (blankets/removing snow); simple splinting of legs; avoiding movement of limbs (redistribution and decrease in core temperature)
Hospital treatment
  Monitoring: Core temperature, ECG, invasive blood pressure.
  Treatment: Epidural analgesia, fasciotomy of legs, fluid therapy (risk of renal failure due to muscle injury)
Findings, patients 1–7
1. Dead, head injury
2. Head injury, femoral shaft fracture, crush injuries and wounds of arm and leg, frostbite, hypothermia 30.5°C
3. Head injury, femoral shaft fracture, crush injury of leg, frostbite, hypothermia 30°C.
4. Chest trauma, crush injury of underarm, frostbite
5. Abdominal trauma, soft tissue injuries, moderate hypothermia
6. Crush injury, leg
7. Soft tissue injury of femur, wound on elbow from ice axe, moderate hypothermia
Results
  No amputations needed; fasciotomies could be closed without sequela
  Reduced tolerance in fingers/teeth to cold in majority of patients

F. Dislocation of Joints

Typical mechanisms of trauma, findings, and complications are summarized in Tables 12–15. The incidences of different dislocations are shown in Figure 4.

1. Treatment of Dislocations

Normally in the hospital setting dislocations should first be reduced when a fracture is excluded by an x-ray. Under exceptional circumstances in the pre-hospital setting (e.g., if there is very long transportation time to the hospital), dislocations may be reduced on the scene. The indication for prehospital reduction must be weighted between (1) risk of reducing over an unrecognized fracture and (2) risk of obtaining secondary complications due to a long lasting dislocation. This risk varies between different types of luxations. Only trained personnel should perform these procedures.

2. Dislocation of the Shoulder

The mechanism, findings, complications, and treatment of shoulder dislocation is summarized in Table 13.

3. Posterior Dislocation of the Hip

The mechanism, findings, surveys, complications, and treatment of posterior dislocation of the hip is summarized in Table 14.

4. Dislocation of Hip With Prosthesis

The reduction is performed as described in Table 14. After the successful reduction the patient should keep supine with the legs spread. A pillow should be put between the knees to prevent further dislocations.

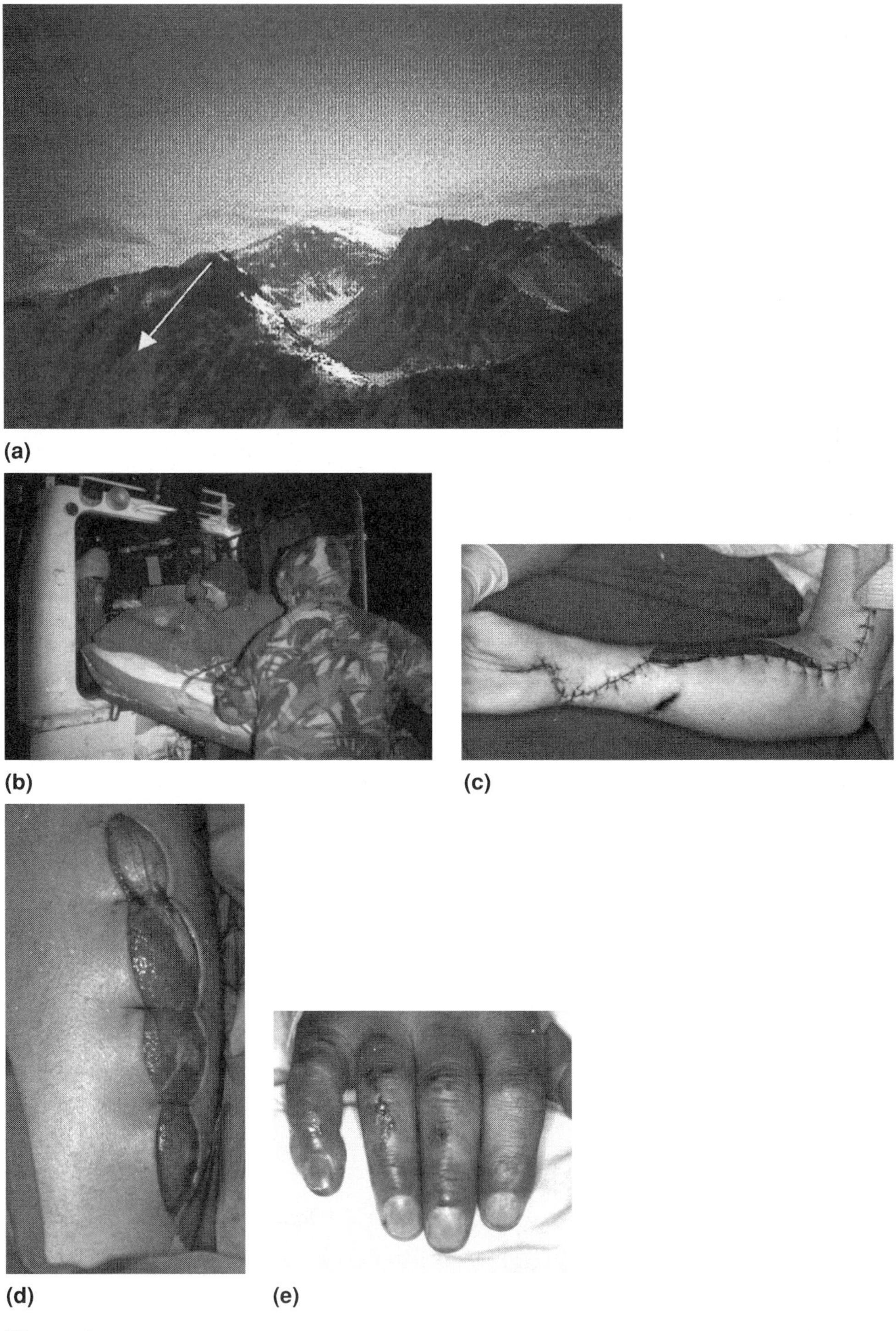

(a) (b) (c) (d) (e)

Figure 3 Avalanche accident. (a) Accident cite, with arrow indicating the direction of the avalanche; (b) rescue; (c) crush injury of arm with fasciotomia; (d) compartment syndrome of the leg/femur; (e) frostbite.

Table 11 Treatment of Soft Tissue Injuries

I-ce	Cool down the injured joint with ice. Ice, or ice bags, should not be put directly on the skin. Avoid frostbite.
C-ompression	The injured joint should be bandaged with an elastic bandage to prevent edema and hematoma. The compression must not compromise the circulation and venous drainage.
E-levation	The injured limb should be elevated to prevent edema and hematoma.
D-rugs	NSAIDs are commonly used. Early start of drug treatment may be useful in soft tissue injuries.
D-octor	Early examination by an experienced and competent physician is important.

Table 12 Dislocations of Joints: Mechanism of Trauma, Findings, Complications

Mechanism	Indirect forces, which pull the bone end out of position. There are traumatic and pathological luxations. Often these lesions are combined with ruptures or distortions of ligaments or the capsule of the joint.
Findings	Pain; deformity of the joint; loss of motion.
Complications	Though ischemia may cause necrosis of the bone, compression nerve damage, and dislocation may be combined with fractures in the joint.

Table 13 Dislocation of the Shoulder: Survey and Treatment

Mechanism	Indirect trauma. In a habitual dislocation, only a small injury/force is necessary.
Findings	The arm is immobilized; displacement of proximal humerus; pain induced by elevating the arm.
Complications	Rupture of the capsule of the joint with or without fractures and lesions of the nerves.
Treatment	If performed within 1 hr after the injury this lesion is easy to reduce, also without analgesics [22]. If a fracture is excluded, the method of *Hippocrates* may be used for reposition of the dislocation. The patient lies on the ground. The physician puts his foot in patient's armpit, traction in caudal direction, with the arm slightly elevated/anteflectated. Use of opioids (morphine) in combination with a benzodiazepine may be necessary.

Table 14 Posterior Dislocation of the Hip: Survey and Treatment

Mechanism	Indirect trauma, force applied to flexed knee (e.g., from a dashboard)
Findings	Pain; internal rotation, adduction and flexion of femur.
Survey	Check distal pulses and function of the sciatic nerve.
Complications	Damage of the sciatic nerve, avascular necrosis of the femoral head.
Treatment	If long transportation time to hospital, qualified personnel should try to reduce the dislocation, as follows [23]: 1. Give analgesics, and explain the procedure to the patient 2. Patient's knee and hip, each flexed 90° 3. An assistant presses the pelvis down on the litter 4. Apply strong upward traction of the femur and rotate back and forth, internally and externally 5. If reduction succeeds and femur head pops back into place, the patient will feel an immediate relief of pain 6. If reduction was successful, the patient may be transported with the leg immobilized in straight position. If not, the leg should be immobilized in 90° of flexion and patient transported promptly to hospital.

Table 15 Dislocation of the Knee: Survey and Treatment

Mechanism	Direct or indirect trauma on the knee
Findings	Severe pain, hyperextension, loss of motion
Survey	Check distal pulses and function of the peroneal nerve
Complications	Ischemia of the leg due to damage of the popleiteal artery; lesions on the peroneal nerve
Treatment	If time to hospital exceeds a few minutes, an attempt to reduce the dislocation should be performed on the scene [23]. 1. Give analgesics and explain the procedure to the patient 2. An assistant applies longitudinal traction to the leg, by hand or by traction splint 3. Keep one hand on the tibia and one on the femur, and use a firm force to guide the joint into position

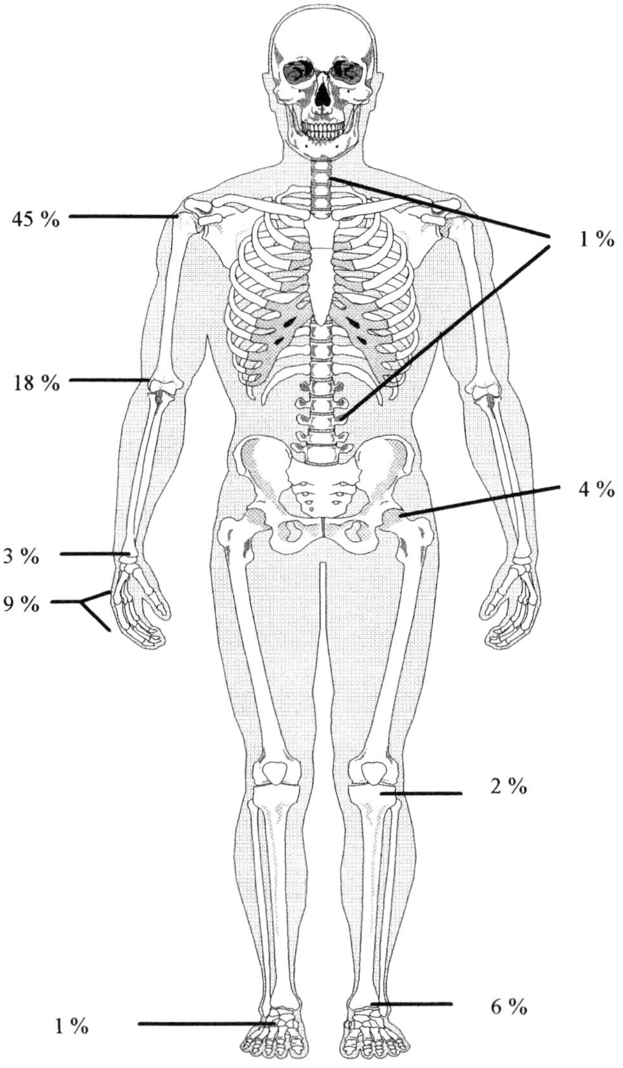

Figure 4 Procentual incidence of dislocations. (Data from Ref. 23a.)

Table 16 Types of Fractures

1. Greenstick; in children, the fracture goes only partly through the bone
2. Transverse, through a direct blow
3. Oblique, through a twisting movement
4. Spiral, through a twisting injury, with a fracture line like a spring
5. Comminuted, where there are more than two fragments, due to powerful direct blow
6. Impacted, through indirect forces, where fragments are jammed together
7. Fractures combined with dislocation of a joint

5. Dislocation in the Knee

The mechanism, findings, survey, complications, and treatment of dislocation of the knee is summarized in Table 15.

X. FRACTURES

A fracture is a complete break in the continuity of the bone. The fracture may be closed, with intact skin, or it may be open, with a wound in which bony fragments may be seen. A fracture may be combined with dislocation of a joint.

A. Types of Fractures

According to the mechanism of trauma, and their appearance on an x-ray, fractures are classified in Table 16.

1. Clinical Signs of a Fracture—Examination

Physicians and EMS personnel should be aware of the typical signs of fractures (Table 17). Every time orthopedic injuries are examined, an evaluation for nerve damage or loss of peripheral circulation should be included. An examination includes checking for pulses, capillary refill, sensation, and motor function.

Table 17 Fracture: Clinical Signs

Typical signs of fractures	Other variable signs of fractures
1) Deformity of the limb	1) Loss of sensation
2) Crepitus by movement. Checking for crepitus causes pain, and should only be performed in unconscious patients.	2) Compromized circulation distal to the injury
3) Shortening	
4) Swelling	
5) Pain	
6) Loss of use	
7) Hematoma and, in open fractures,	
8) Wound with bone ends	

2. Initial Treatment of Fractures—Fracture Reduction

The combination of prehospital fracture reduction and wound management has been shown to result in a reduction in postoperative infections. In open fractures without prehospital care the infection rate was 22%. In those in which prehospital fracture reduction and wound treatment was performed the rate was 4% [10]. Again, fracture reduction should only be performed by trained personnel. Only major deformities should be reduced on the scene of the accident. The procedure is as follows [24] (Fig. 5):

1. Perform gentle longitudinal traction
2. Restore the correct rotation
3. Restore the alignment
4. Check the fracture; check pulses
5. Maintain traction
6. Apply a splint

3. Splinting the Fracture

The main principle of splinting is to immobilize the fracture and the nearest joints. This may be done very simply or with more sophisticated tools. If the injury occurs in remote areas in which ambulance services are not available, simple splints may be made from wooden sticks and carpets. Most ambulances have splints for most common occasions (see below), but these are not always the most appropriate devices.

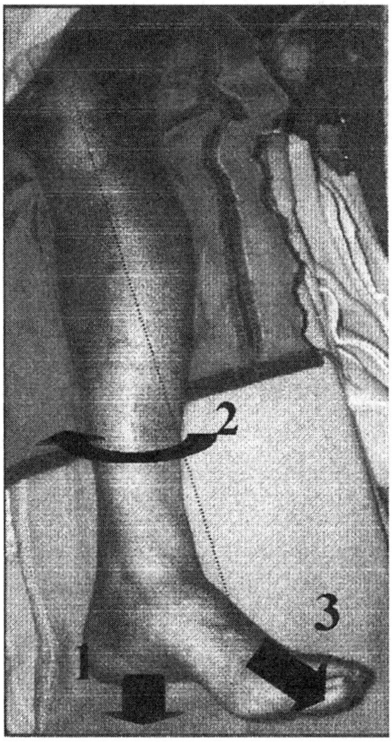

Figure 5 Procedure for reduction of fractures: (1) perform gentle longitudinal traction, (2) restore the correct rotation, and (3) restore the alignment. Dotted lines show the situation after reduction.

The injured limb should be elevated to the level of the heart. Higher elevation should be avoided because it may lead to ischemia and CS [5]. For further discussion on equipment for splinting see the section on Equipment.

B. Wounds

Wounds must be covered with sterile dressings. Cleansing is normally not a part of prehospital treatment, but if there is much contamination with foreign material the wound may be gently irrigated with Ringer's solution or a similar preparation.

Foreign bodies or bone fragments should not be removed. To prevent compression of tissue, a sterile dressing shaped as a doughnut should be used as a bolster around the fragment or foreign body. Wound dressings should not be removed before the patient has reached the operating theater to prevent nosocomial infections [26].

1. Tetanus and Intravenous Antibiotics

If there are long transport times, patients with wounds should receive antibiotics before or during transport (see sec. XVII). Tetanus toxoid may be given when admitted in the hospital.

XI. PELVIC, ACETABULAR, AND LONG BONE FRACTURES

Fractures in pelvic, acetabular, and long bones are associated with mortality rates varying from 7–50% in different materials [27–29]. The high mortality rate in pelvic fractures is associated partly with hemorrhage and partly in combination with other injuries in the head, chest, and abdomen (Table 18). Early intervention for these fractures with wound debridement and fixation has proved to reduce complications such as ARDS (adult respiratory distress syndrome) [30], infection, and pulmonary embolism. Early mobilization reduces lung problems and wound complications [31].

In a study by Johnson et al. the decreased incidence of ARDS was demonstrated in patients who had suffered two major fractures. The largest reduction in incidence was in the group with ISS > 40 (Fig. 6). Early surgery and fixation on this group of fractures is now the policy in most trauma centers.

XII. SPINE INJURIES

A. Epidemiology and Mechanism of Trauma

Estimates from the United States indicate that 10,000 citizens each year survive spine injuries. The incidence ranges from 30 to 50 per 1 million population. Most victims are

Table 18 Cause of Death in Patients With Pelvic Fracture

Hemorrhage (abdominal, pelvic, extremity)
Head injury
Sepsis
Multiple organ system failure
Respiratory failure
Pulmonary embolus

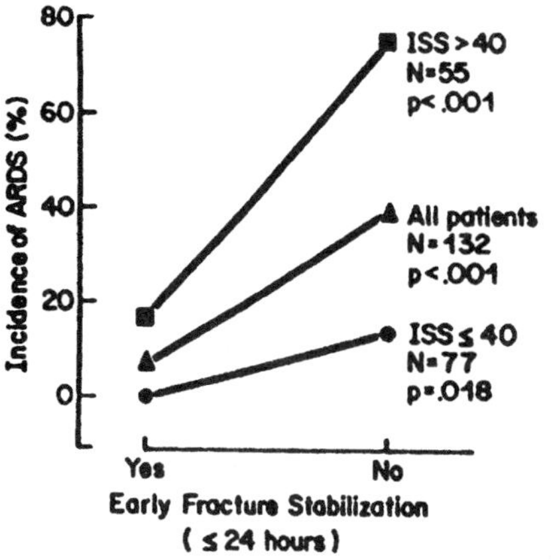

Figure 6 Incidence of ARDS compared with early versus late fracture fixation and injury severity score (ISS). (From Ref. 30.)

male between 10 and 40 years of age. The prevalence is approximately 250,000 [32]. Half of the injuries occur in the cervical region, often leading to quadriplegia.

Spine injury is present in 2–4% of all trauma patients. In contrast to earlier views, there seems to be no difference in incidence between patients with or without traumatic brain injury (TBI) [33,34]. Spinal cord injury is present in 30–70% of cervical spine injuries [35]. Accidents involving motor vehicles cause 50–70% of spine injuries; 15% are related to sporting activities and 16% to falls [36,37]. Although penetrating objects also cause spinal cord damage, most cord damage follows blunt trauma [38]. The main mechanism and complications are described in Table 19.

B. Strategies for Prehospital Treatment

Several cases of poor neurologic outcome caused by suboptimal treatment have been reported [39,40]. This devastating potential has led to a clinical practice whereby trauma patients are immobilized with or without signs of a spine injury.

In 1965, Kossuth was the first physician recognized for proposing protocols for extrication and cervical protection of trauma victims [41]. In 1967–68, Farrington established the concept of prehospital immobilization [42,43], and in 1974 Hare invented the first stiff extrication-type collar [44].

Table 19 Injury Mechanism and Complications by Spinal Cord Trauma

1. A *direct injury* generates a
2. *secondary* process that results in
3. *hemorrhagic necrosis* starting in the central region
4. in severe injuries *progressing* to involve the entire diameter of the spinal cord.
5. The process may be *exacerbated* by hypotension and hypoxia.
6. A catecholamine surge may lead to *pulmonary edema.*
7. Paralysis of sympathetics may for 2 to 3 days lead to *vasoldilatation* and *hypotension.*
8. *Respiratory complications* are common in high-level injuries (hypoventilation, paradoxical ventilation, aspiration, atelectasis, pulmonary embolism).

C. Immobilization or Not?

The diagnosis and clearance of the cervical spine in trauma victims remain a large problem. It is estimated that in the United States 800,000 patients undergo cervical spine radiography each year, at cost of $180 million. Spine injuries are identified in only 10,000 cases [45]. The annual costs of performing spinal immobilization on five million U.S. citizens is estimated to be as high as $75 million, or $15 per person [46].

Small prospective studies have led to the development of so-called clinical cervical spine clearance (CCC) protocols. These protocols are used either prehospital, to exclude patients from immobilization, or in the hospital to exclude patients from radiography. Muhr et al. instructed paramedics to use a spinal clearance algorithm in a prospective study including 281 trauma victims. Spinal immobilization was reduced by one-third [47]. For now larger-scale prospective studies fail, and issued guidelines should still be adopted. The conclusions of a position paper from the National Association of EMS Physicians [48] are shown in Table 20. A study by Hauswald et al. compared two EMS systems, one of them performing no prehospital intervention or immobilization of trauma victims (Malaysia), and one having a full intervention system (USA). The conclusion was that out-of-hospital immobilization has little or no effect on neurologic outcome in patients with blunt spinal injuries [49]. The study has its limitations, but still is a reminder that the common clinical practice is not based on convincing evidence.

Spinal immobilization on a rigid backboard is not an innocuous procedure. Such side effects as respiratory compromise and patient discomfort are described later. In many cases conscious (not sedated) patients themselves resist painful movements and thereby ''self-splint'' their spines with muscular tension.

1. Whiplash Injuries

Whiplash mechanism injuries caused by rear-end collisions of motor vehicles is a common cause of neck injuries. The myofascial injury causes neck pain. Eighty-two percent of patients experience headache acutely. Other symptoms are paresthesias, neuralgia, and dizziness. Some patients experience symptoms after an interval free from symptoms. Most patients recover after 3 months, but 10–30% still have symptoms after 2 years. There is only a minimal association between outcome and trauma energy. Whiplash injuries may result in long-term disability, and all patients with this kind of trauma mechanism should be thoroughly examined by a physician, with follow-up examination after a few days. Also important is a thorough prehospital primary survey of the spine, followed by documentation in the EMS report.

Table 20 Indication for Spinal Immobilization

Spine immobilization is indicated in prehospital trauma patients who: sustain an injury with a mechanism having the potential for causing spinal injury and who have at least *one* of these following clinical criteria:

1. Altered mental status
2. Evidence of intoxication
3. A distracting painful injury (e.g., long bone extremity fracture)
4. Neurologic deficit
5. Spinal pain or tenderness

Source: Ref. 48.

2. Immobilization

The cervical spine is immobilized following the procedure described in the American College of Surgeons manual of ATLS.

D. Prehospital Management

1. Airway Management

A careful evaluation of the airway and respiratory function is important before any attempt at airway management or induction of general anesthesia. The strategy for airway management should be tailored according to each patient's injuries and general condition. Algorithms may not satisfy the needs in every situation [38]. Endotracheal intubation should be performed by an experienced operator, and he should use the technique with which he is most familiar. Sophisticated methods are excellent in the hands of the experienced; in the hands of the inexperienced they may lead to hypoxia, aspiration of gastric contents, or even death.

The first question to be answered is if there a need for immediate endotracheal intubation. In the prehospital setting this question is of even greater importance. On a patient fixed to a backboard the chances of respiratory arrest and aspiration during transport must be weighed against the consequences of a failed intubation. Alternatives to intubation such as cricothyrotomy are always options to be considered.

2. Oral Intubation With Manual In-Line Stabilization

Protracheal intubation is the method of choice in the case of apnea and respiratory distress. Two assistants hold the head, neck, and torso in neutral position. In the standard situation, IV anesthetics and muscle relaxants should be administered. If the vocal cords are not readily visible, cricothrotomy should be considered as a first-line option.

If there is any sign of compromised airway the intubation procedure should be performed on an awake patient, with only light analgesia and topiciliation of the airway with local anesthesia. In the hands of an experienced physician a wake fiberbronchoscopic intubation is elegant and safe. Portable fiberoptic bronchoscopes/laryngoscopes are now available for field use.

The ATLS protocol has traditionally recommended nasotracheal intubation in spontaneously-breathing patients [50]. This strategy is heavily criticized by many clinicians. There are many potential complications: nasal trauma and bleeding, an elevated rate of failed intubation and the risk of penetrating the skull or orbit in case of basilar skull fractures. Figures 7 and 8 are modified ATLS algorithms proposed by Capan et al. [38].

3. Alternatives to Endotracheal Intubation

Some alternatives to endotracheal intubation must be discussed. These devices and methods have advantages and disadvantages, as discussed in Chapter 13.

1. The laryngeal mask airway (LMA). The laryngeal mask is widely used in anesthesia for elective surgery. Its use in emergency medicine, especially in the prehospital setting is still a controversy. To put this airway in the right position in an emergency situation skill and training is needed. When performed by the ''expert,'' the intubation trauma should be minimal. The laryngeal mask airway (LMA) gives no guarantee against aspirating gastric content. The intubating LMA (ILMA) is a device that may be very helpful in cases of failed intubation.

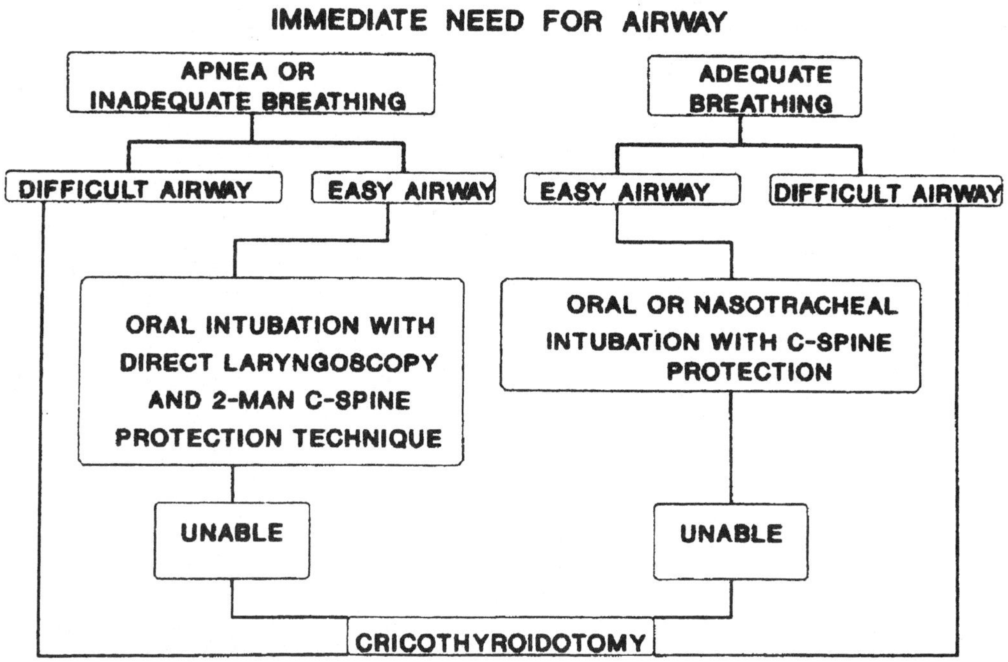

Figure 7 Modified ATLS algorithm for patients with suspected cervical spine injury and immediate need to secure the airway. (From Ref. 38.)

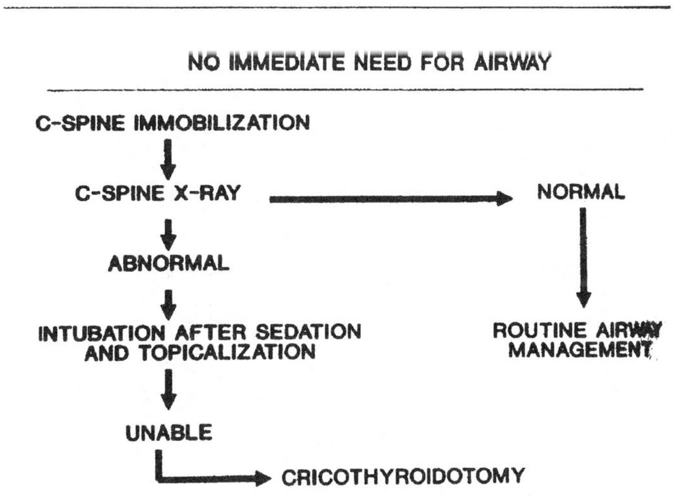

Figure 8 Modified ATLS algorithm for patients with suspected cervical spine injury without an immediate need to secure the airway. (From Ref. 38.)

An endotracheal tube may be inserted through this device blind, with a bougie or with a fiberoptic bronchoscope.

2. The Combitube. This device has two inflatable cuffs and is placed blind in the esophagus or trachea. Unlike the laryngeal mask it is a guarantee against aspiration. The intubation trauma is minimal. The major disadvantage of the combitube is that there are many contraindications for use (portal hypertension, etc.).
3. Chin Lift and Jaw Thrust. In some situations the airway of a patient with spine injuries may be secured with this simple method for a limited time. The neck should not be hyperextended. An experimental study on cadavers with C1-C2 fractures by Donaldson et al. showed chin lift/jaw thrust may cause significant compression of the spinal cord [51].
4. The Haines Recovery Position. For the unconscious trauma patient this position reduces movement of the spine. There is less neck movement and less degree of lateral angulation than when the lateral recovery position is used (Fig. 9).

4. Circulation

Neurogenic pulmonary edema is a consequence of a catecholamine surge occurring in the first few minutes after the spinal cord is injured. The edema is a result of large shunting into pulmonary capillaries. After this the sympathetics are paralyzed for 2 to 3 days, resulting in low systemic and pulmonary pressures, especially in high-level injuries. Hypotension may be misinterpreted as a sign of hemorrhage. Aggressive fluid therapy and infusion with catecholamines may be necessary. The optimal therapy goal centers on aggressive management of blood pressure, normovolemia, and normoglycemia.

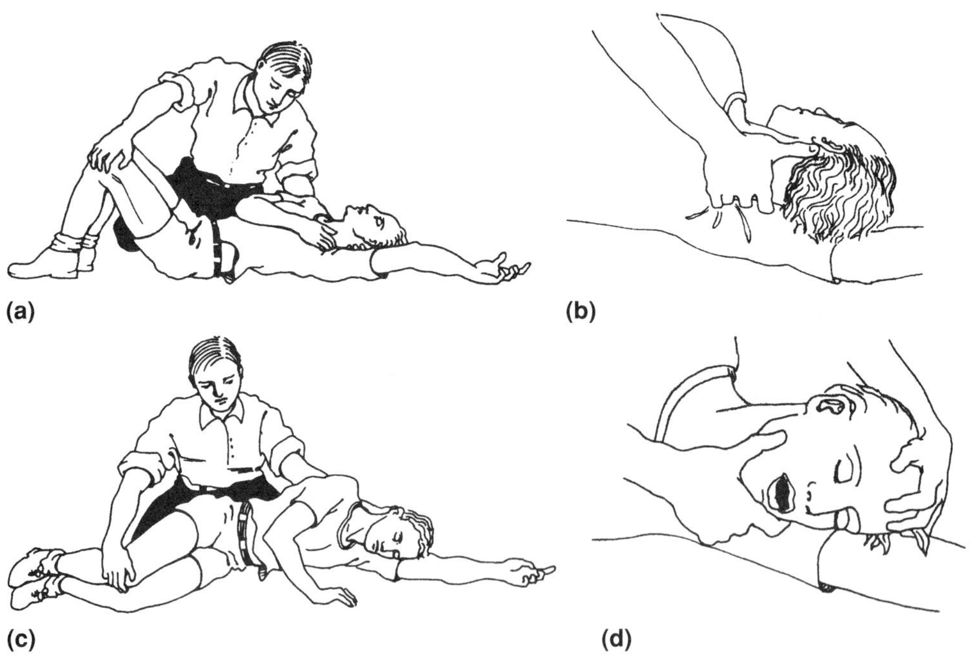

Figure 9 The Haines recovery position. (From Ref. 51a.)

5. Pharmacologic Therapy—Steroids

The 1-year follow-up to the National Acute Spinal Cord Injury Study (NASCIS III) recommends the use of high-dose methylprednisolone. The results are not very impressive, but still the effects are clinically significant. To derive benefit the treatment must be started within 8 hr of injury. If started >3 hr after injury the infusion should be continued for 48 hr.

XIII. SPECIAL ASPECTS OF ORGANIZING MEDICAL SERVICES, SURVEY, AND TREATMENT DURING SPORTING EVENTS

Taking part in emergency medical services during crowded sporting events and championships presents some special challenges to the medical personnel. The medical needs are not always very well defined by the organizers. There are different groups of patients to take care of: the athletes, audience, VIPs, and organizers. The incidence of serious injuries or illness is normally low, but when an athlete gets injured the job of the medical personnel is observed by "the whole world," especially during televised events.

A. Objectives of Treatment

For the organizers and TV producers the objective is to give their customers a production within tight time scedules. Injuries mean delays, and therefore injured persons (according to the author's experience) are to be removed from the competition field without any kind of treatment.

Medical personnel have established standards of treatment and ethics. Our objective is to save lives and reduce suffering and secondary injury. The evacuation of the patient should be done according to established procedures.

The athletes' objective is of course to stay alive and to stay in "business." In some sports such as ice hockey, the athletes have a great tolerance of injuries. Most professional teams have their own medical personnel along.

Conflicts between the different objectives of these groups may lead to difficulties for the medical personnel on-site. In the worst cases such problems may lead to suffering and increased morbidity and mortality.

B. Recommendations

Those responsible for emergency medical services during large sporting events or contests should follow the recommendations given in the Table 21.

Table 21 Planning of Emergency Medical Services During Sporting Events

Take part in the planning from an early stage.
Do not compromise on important medical and ethical principles, and make this clear to the organizers at an early stage.
Treatment and evacuation should be performed without delay, and from every location of the venue (e.g., use of helicopters with hoist) and by specially trained personnel.
Medical personnel should be highly qualified and trained. (Field physicians should be part of the available medical teams.)
Special attention should be given to changing weather conditions (heat/humidity/cold), which may lead to a dramatic increase in the incidence of casualities.

XIV. TREATMENT OF PAIN OUTSIDE A HOSPITAL

A. Opioids

The primary drug for treatment of pain is morphine. For optimal control it should be administered IV. For adults we recommend repeated doses of 5 mg IV. The interval between each dose should be approximately 10 min. In the hands of the anesthesiologist, fentanyl is a good alternative. For non-medical personnel using mixed opioid agonists/antagonists, such as buprenorphine, for sublingual administration may be an acceptable alternative. The author always gives an antiemetic drug together with morphine, for example, Metochlopramide 5 to 10 mg IV.

B. Ketamine

Used in the prehospital setting, ketamine is a drug for the experienced anesthesiologist. It has a broad therapeutic range. In low doses it has analgesic effects with very few side effects, the influence on respiration is usually negligible, and the level of consciousness is hardly changed [52]. In anesthetic doses, side effects such as hallucinations and hypersalivation are more common in adult patients. The recommended dosage for analgesia is 0.25 mg/kg bodyweight IV, or 0.5 to 1 mg/kg IM. To reduce vagal stimulation and salivation, atropine should be given (0.5 to 0.8 mg IV for the adult patient). To prevent hallucinations a benzodiazepine should be given in small doses IV, such as diazepam 2.5 to 5 mg IV.

C. NSAIDs

Nonsteroid anti-inflammatory drugs (NSAIDs) are recommended in soft tissue injuries without fractures, but should not be administered in patients with renal failure or shock. Among the NSAIDs available for parenteral administration are Ketorolac (10 to 30 mg IV/IM (maximum 90 mg per day), and diclofenac 75 mg IM (maximum 150 mg per day). These routes are alternatives when a rapid onset of the effect is needed. The author prefers the IV way. Intramuscular injections are reported (rarely) to cause serious infections [53].

Paracetamol is a possible drug of choice for treatment of moderate pain, often in combination with NSAIDs, as above. For adults, single doses of 1 gram or more po/rectal/IV may be necessary. Paracet is also available in combination with opioids and for IV use. Drugs should only be administered the peroral way when an operation or hospitalization is excluded. There is a well-known series of precautions to take into consideration before giving NSAIDs, especially obtaining any history of gastrointestinal bleeding.

1. Regional Anesthesia

The use of regional anesthesia is not very common in the prehospital setting. Neuraxial blocks of the spine (epidural and subarachnoidal blocks) should only be performed on hemodynamically stable patients. In the prehospital setting it is often impossible to decide whether a serious heamorrhage is developing or not. The author has used regional anesthesia during secondary transports. Epidural blocks or brachial plexus block are established with indwelling catheters in smaller hospitals, and infusion of local anesthetics are continued during transport. These patients may then stay awake during transfer. Induction of general anesthesia with mechanical ventilation during transport may in some cases be avoided.

The use of some simple regional blocks like femoral block or ankle block may be of interest in some special situations, include the following:

Extended entrapment, where general anesthesia is not possible.

Situations in remote areas where general anesthesia may not be continued for the whole extent of the transport. (For example, patient on board a ship with crush injury of the knee, who has to be winched aboard on a helicopter, and therefore, may not be heavily sedated.

In femoral shaft fractures, a femoral nerve block block will give almost immediate pain relief [54].

As is the case with every kind of anesthesia, regional anesthesia is associated with complications and should therefore be left in the hands of an anesthesiologist. Equipment for treating of complications should be available.

XV. PREVENTION OF COMPLICATIONS

A. Embolism

Deep venous thrombosis with pulmonary embolism is a well-known complication after orthopedic injuries and is a leading cause of morbidity and death [55]. In femoral neck fractures deep venous thrombosis near the fracture site is already seen preoperatively in ultrasound studies [56].

B. Prevention

Different strategies for the prevention of thrombosis and embolism, used alone or in combination, are listed in Table 22 [57]. The antithrombotic therapy should be started as early as possible. Some reports have concluded that administering low molecular heparin may increase the incidence of hematoma after spinal anesthesia [58]. The procedure in Norwegian hospitals is therefore to give these injections either at least 2 hr before or directly after spinal/epidural puncture. In a consensus document of the American Society of Regional Anesthesia it is stated that the decision to perform a neuraxial block on a patient receiving low-molecular-weight heparin (LMWH) should be made on individual basis, weighing the risks of spinal hematoma with the benefits of regional anesthesia. In regions with long transport times (>1 1/2 hr) to the hospital, administration of LMWH or dextran should be considered before transport.

XVI. EQUIPMENT AND TECHNIQUES FOR PREHOSPITAL TREATMENT OF ORTHOPEDIC INJURIES

A. Monitors

Monitors constructed for prehospital use should ideally be light, easy to carry and apply, visible from different angles and under different lighting conditions and battery operated,

Table 22 Strategies for Prevention of Thrombosis and Embolism

Early fracture reduction
Early definitive surgery
Early mobilization
Compression stockings
Use of heparin or low-molecular-weight heparin (LMWH)
Infusion of dextrane

with a battery capacity of several hours which allows recharging with 12 or 24/28 V in vehicles. Alarms should be both audible and visual. The monitor should be easily understandable to nonphysicians, and reveal only information from connected equipment (e.g., if no ECG leads are attached it should not show a flat line ECG). Trend recording is desirable. For practical reasons it is desirable to have available as many functions as possible in one monitor; however, the EMS team is then much more vulnerable in case of equipment failure. A backup unit should therefore always be available. We use a multichannel monitor providing ECG, pulse oximetry, automated blood pressure, temperature, and $ETCO_2$, with the possibility for invasive pressure as well.

B. Extrication and Protection: Cervical Collars, Spine Boards, and Scoop Stretchers

Immobilization and extrication are procedures mainly carried out by ambulance or rescue personnel. The extrication phase carries dangers to the patient and challenges to both the physician and nonphysician in the field. The procedure will be considered in detail. Merely lifting the patient out from a damaged vehicle *may* involve the risk of aggravating injuries.

Before extrication is begun, the primary survey and resuscitation phase should be completed as quickly and as much as possible, and during the extrication phase the EMS personnel should continuously support the cervical spine and survey vital functions. In lengthy extrications, it may be necessary before the patient is released to perform one or more of the following procedures:

1. administration of oxygen
2. establishing intravenous access
3. endotracheal intubation
4. induction of anesthesia

Sophisticated portable monitors therefore may be of necessity.

Thorough immobilization includes securing the patient's head and total spinal column in the neutral midline position before moving the patient. Immobilization starts with gentle, manual in-line stabilization of the head during the airway assessment in the primary survey. The head is brought to and kept in the neutral position, except if this procedure results in increased pain, muscular defense (i.e., spasms), spinal injuries, or neurological symptoms, or if it compromises the airway. If life-threatening conditions are excluded, a rigid cervical collar is applied. This reduces the possibility of compression of the cervical spine, but does not preclude its movement [59]. It is of paramount importance that the collar is chosen and adapted according to the size of the patient.

1. The Backboard

With the collar in place the patient is secured to some kind of backboard. Ideally, the whole spine should be immobilized (i.e., from the sacrum to the head), but in sitting patients—as in cars—short spine boards extending from the lumbar spine to the head are applied. In adults, padding between the head and the board may be necessary. In children padding below the scapulae may be required to avoid the large occiput to induce cervical flexion when immobilized on a backboard. After the patient is safely positioned and tightly strapped to the backboard he may be moved.

Backboard fixation has significant side effects: respiratory compromise, risk of aspiration, compression complications, head and back pain, and increased intracranial pressure. Fixation times of more than 30 to 45 min should be avoided. Some authors conclude that backboards should not be the preferred surface for the transfer of patients with spinal injuries [60].

2. The Scoop Stretcher

The scoop stretcher offers good protection against movement in the total spine during transfer [61,62]. The scoop stretcher consists of two separate parts that interlock when applied. It may be slid under the patient virtually without moving the patient, and offers a possibility for carrying or transferring to an ordinary stretcher practically without any movement in the spine.

C. Vacuum Mattress and Vacuum Splinting Devices

The vacuum mattress consists of thousands of tiny isopore balls within a plastic mattress. When air is evacuated from the mattress (by a simple hand- or foot-operated suctioning device) it becomes rigid and may be carried in almost all positions. It is particularly suitable for patients trapped in difficult positions, where the soft, air-filled mattress may be slid under and fit to the body, whereas afterward it may be emptied of air by vacuum and used as a stretcher in extrication and transportation.

The author has used such a mattress for wintertime evacuation of patients in sleds downhill, and from ships into helicopters offshore. During long transports the vacuum mattress can be too stiff and hard, and uncomfortable to the patient. This may be avoided by putting a thin blanket between patient and mattress. There are also mattresses with two chambers, one vacuum and one inflatable, giving the patient more comfort and stability during transport. When securing the patient into the mattress, care should be taken that the knee is not overextended, and that the lumbar spine is not in hyperkyphosis. Vacuum splints for use on the extremities and neck are also available (Fig. 10).

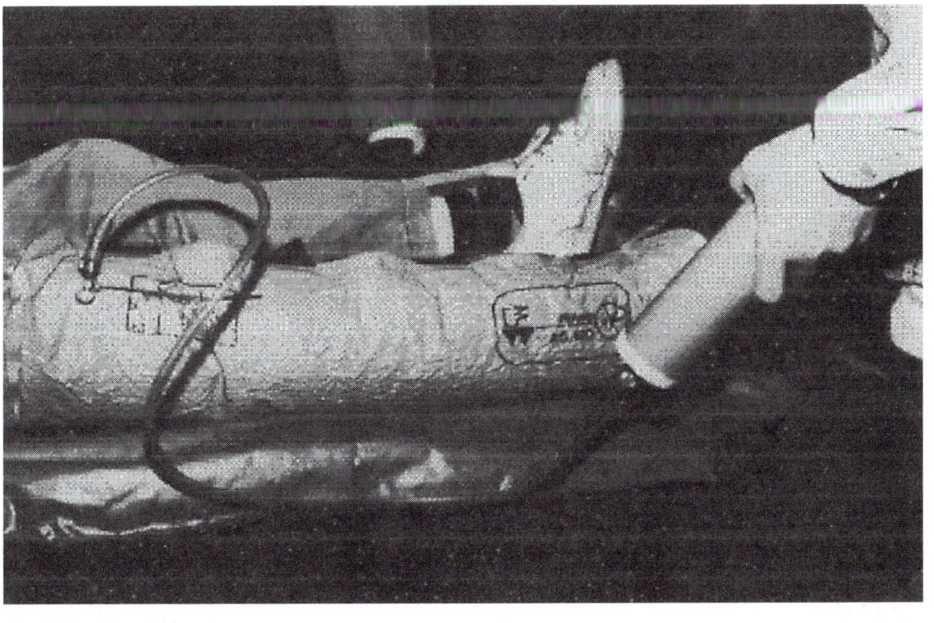

Figure 10 A vacuum splint for limbs.

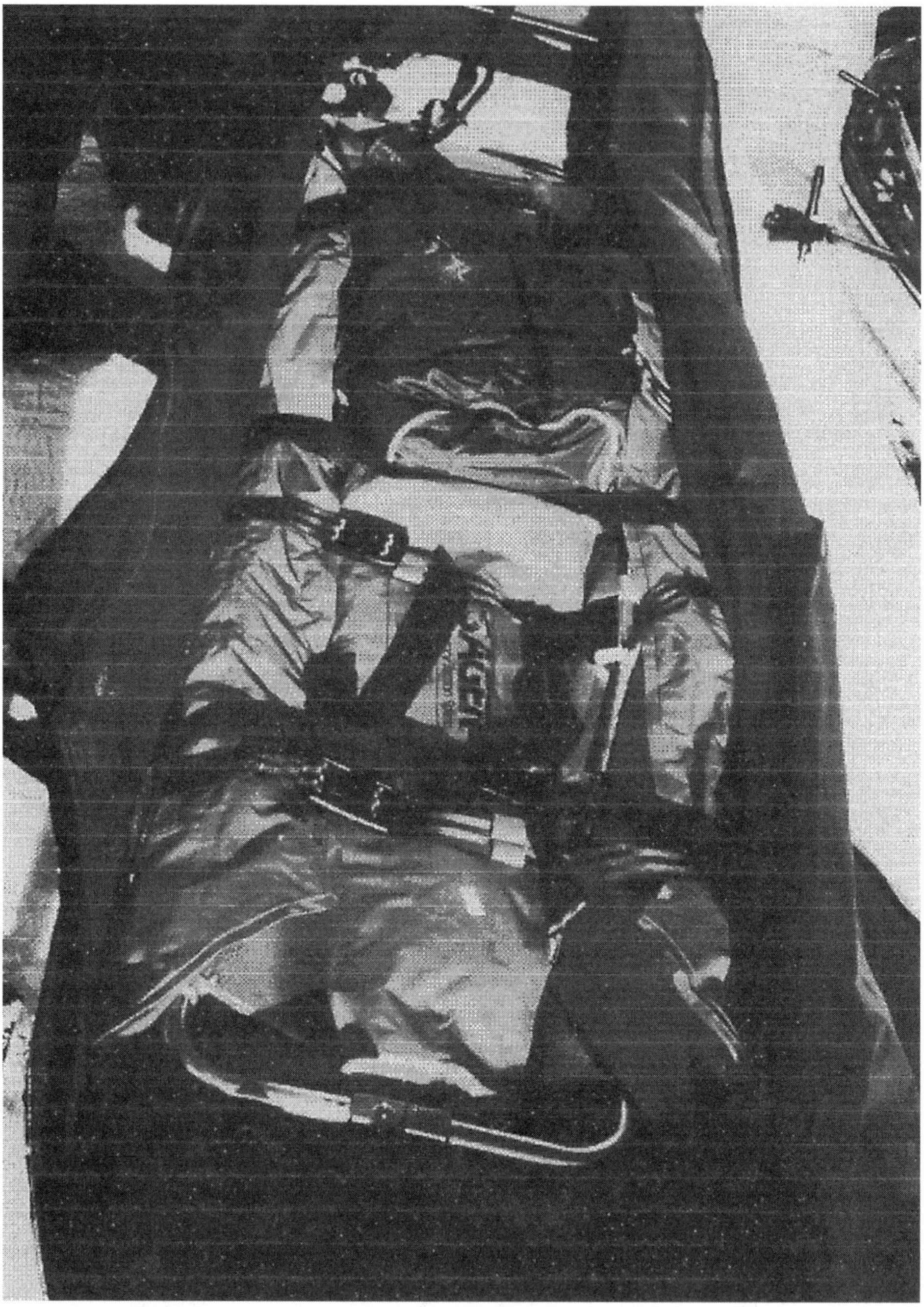

(a)

Figure 11 A sled used during the Winter Olympics in Lillehammer, 1994. (a) The sled has all the necessary equipment for extrication and stabilization and transport; a scoop stretcher, a vacuum mattress, vacuum splints, cervical collars, a Sager splint, equipment for ventilation/intubation, oxygen, and a heating system for patient and infusions. (b) Patient transportation in the lower part of the slope. It is operated by two persons, is extremely stable, and has a safe brake system.

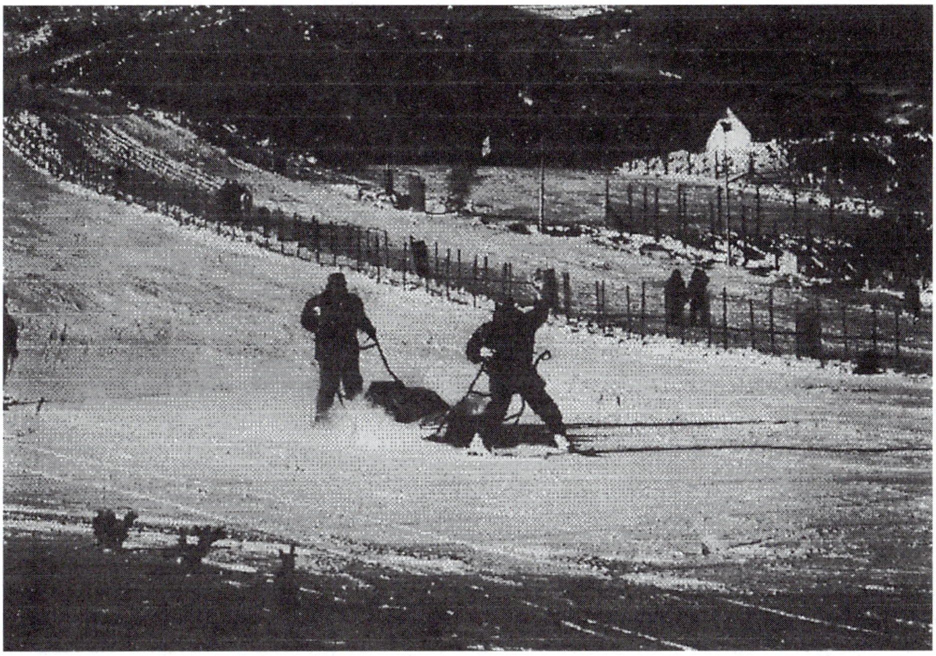

(b)

A transportation and treatment system with a specially constructed sled was used during the Winter Olympics in Lillehammer in 1994. The downhill slope of Kvitfjell is up to 60% steep. The patients were therefore were always fixed to a vacuum mattress (Fig. 11).

D. Pneumatic Circular Splints

These inflatable plastic splints are still rather common. They may be applied around the lower extremity with a semi-extended knee and the upper extremity with the elbow in 90° of flexion. When pumped up they apply a pressure to the whole extremity [63]. Excessive pressure and extended use of pneumatic splints may lead to ischemia, nerve damage, and compartment syndrome. Ashton [64] demonstrated that blood flow to the extremities was greatly reduced when these splints were filled up to a pressure of 30 to 40 mm Hg. In 14 of 15 healthy volunteers the blood flow went to zero when the limb was elevated.

Today, there are a number of good alternatives to this splint. If, in spite of this, it has to be used, it should be used only for a short time, and only with low pressure. It should not be used on open fractures, because of the danger of perforation of the splint and tissue necrosis.

E. MAST/PASG

Military antishock trousers (MAST) or pneumatic antishock garment (PASG) are used as treatment and prevention of shock. The mechanism of this device has been thought to be due to an increase in circulating blood volume and cardiac stroke volume through decreasing the venous pooling in the lower extremities. However, recent reports have failed to document this when applied to patients with abdominal hemorrhage [65]. In thoracic trauma it may even be harmful [66,67]. The National Association of EMS Physicians has

Table 23 Recommendations for Use of PASG

Class I:	Usually indicated, useful, and effective
	Hypotension due to ruptured AAA
Class IIa:	Acceptable, uncertain efficacy, weight of evidence favors usefulness and efficacy
	Hypotension due to suspected pelvic fracture
	Anaphylactic shock (unresponsive to standard therapy)[a]
	Otherwise uncontrollable lower extremity hemorrhage[a]
	Severe traumatic hypotension (palpable pulse, blood pressure not obtainable)[a]
Class IIb:	Acceptable, uncertain efficacy, may be helpful, probably not harmful
	Elderly
	History of congestive heart failure
	Penetrating abdominal injury
	Paroxysmal supraventricular tachycardia (PSVT)
	Gynecological hemorrhage (otherwise uncontrolled)[a]
	Hypothermia-induced hypotension[a]
	Ruptured ectopic pregnancy[a]
	Septic shock[a]
	Urologic hemorrhage (otherwise uncontrolled)[a]
	Assist intravenous cannulation[a]
Class III:	Inappropriate option, not indicated, may be harmful
	Adjunct to CPR
	Diaphragmic rupture
	Penetrating thoracic injury
	Pulmonary edema
	To splint fractures of the lower extremities
	Extremety trauma
	Abdominal evisceration
	Acute myocardial infarction
	Cardiac tamponade
	Cardiogenic shock
	Gravid uterus

[a] Data from controlled trials not available. Recommendation based on other evidence.
Source: Ref. 68.

reviewed literature concerning PASG, giving recommendations according to the principles for evidence based medicine [68]. The conclusions are summarized in Table 23.

The same side effects seen for pneumatic splints are also seen with MAST. Compartment syndrome may be seen after MAST application for more than 1 hr. In some multitrauma situations, such as pelvic fractures, it is still a good alternative.

F. Traction Splints and the Sager Splint

The Thomas splint has been in use since the late 1800s. Its use was credited with reduced mortality in femoral fractures. This splint and its modifications are still in use today. Through tension applied in the longitudinal axis, a fracture will be reduced, pressure on the injured skin and tissue will decrease, and perhaps most important, the patient will experience significant pain relief. The thigh retains its cylindrical shape, leaving less potential for blood loss. A frequently used traction splint in is the Sager splint (Fig. 12a). It is used for fractures of the femur and tibia/fibula. The traction force may

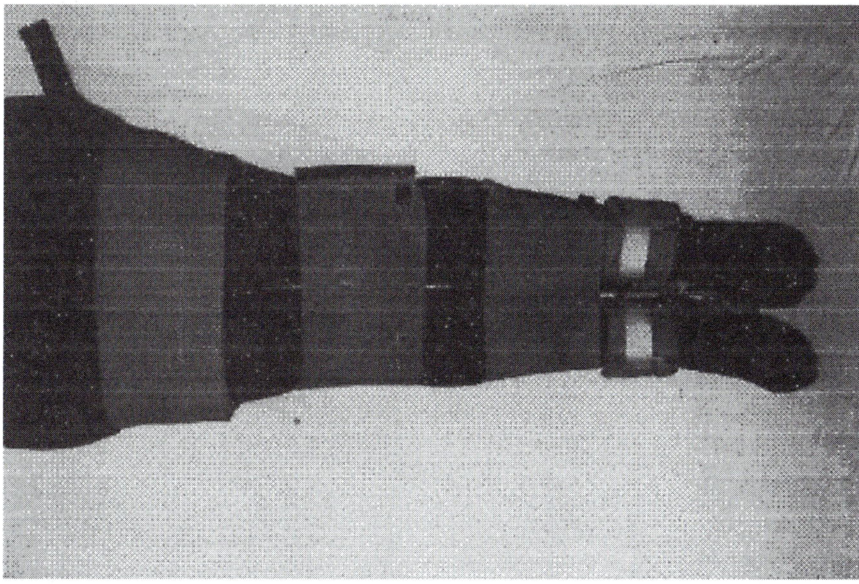

(a)

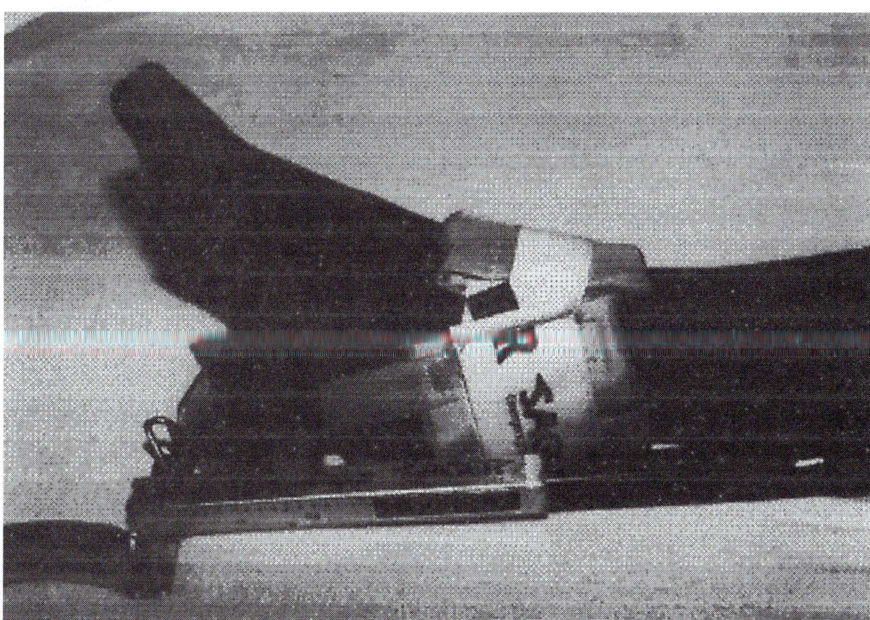

(b)

Figure 12 The Sager splint, an ideal tool for reducing and stabilizing fractures, with pain relief as a result. (a) The bilateral Sager splint applied on a patient. (b) The traction scale makes it possible to perform a quantifiable dynamic traction.

Table 24 Using the Sager Splint

1. The proximal part is placed between the patient's legs. Be careful not to compress urogenital organs.
2. After the distal part is fixed to the ankles, increasing traction force is performed through pulling the handle.
3. Stop pulling when pain is significantly reduced, by approximately 10% of body weight. Never exceed 6.8 kg (15 lb).
4. Check peripheral circulation and sensation continuously *before* and *during* transport.

be quantified on a scale (Fig. 12b). The splint is easy to use, but every user (including physicians) needs to be trained. The instructions for users must be carefully followed (see Table 24).

A case of skin necrosis of the foot (dorsum pedis) has been reported after 14-hr use of the Sager splint (personal communication, Regional Hospital, Trondheim, Norway, 1994). In this case, the splint was also used after transport (in the hospital as the patient waited for his operation). Care should therefore be taken by using this splint over a long period. There are also reported injuries of the urethra with the Thomas splint [69].

G. Case: Skier With Open Fracture of the Femur

Patient: A Swedish skier, 18 years old, male.

History: The patient is doing powder-snow downhill skiing. After 12.30 hr he falls. The left ski gets stuck in the snow, and does not release during the fall. This causes a rotating injury of the femur.

Status at the scene: Severe pain, awake, normal respiration and circulation. Fracture of the left femur with the following clinical signs: (1) deformity of the limb, (2) crepitus by movement, (3) shortening, (4) swelling, (5) pain, (6) loss of use, (7) hematoma. The fracture is closed with no wound or bone ends. There is no loss of sensation or circulation.

Treatment at the scene: Volunteer personnel from the Red Cross arrive with a snowmobile a few minutes after the accident. No reduction attempt is started. The fracture is stabillized with a vacuum splint. The patient is transported 10 min to the local district physician's office.

Treatment by local physician/EMS: Due to strong pain the patient receives morphine 10 mg IV, diazepam 5 mg IV. X-ray shows a spiral fracture of the femur (Fig. 13a). The fracture is reduced with a Sager splint. This reduction is followed by immediate pain relief. For further stabilization a vacuum mattress is used during transport to the hospital (2 hr transportation time).

Treatment during transport: morphine 2.5 mg IV diazepam 2.5 mg IV, oxygen 2 liters on a nasal catheter. Ringer's solution 2 liters IV.

Treatment in the hospital: He reaches the hospital at 16:00 hr. The surgery, which lasts 2 hr, 10 min, is performed promptly (Fig. 13b). Epidural anesthesia is administered peri- and postoperatively. There are no complications. A fracture of a tooth is treated (glued) by a dentist. The patient is transferred to the hospital in his home city after 5 days.

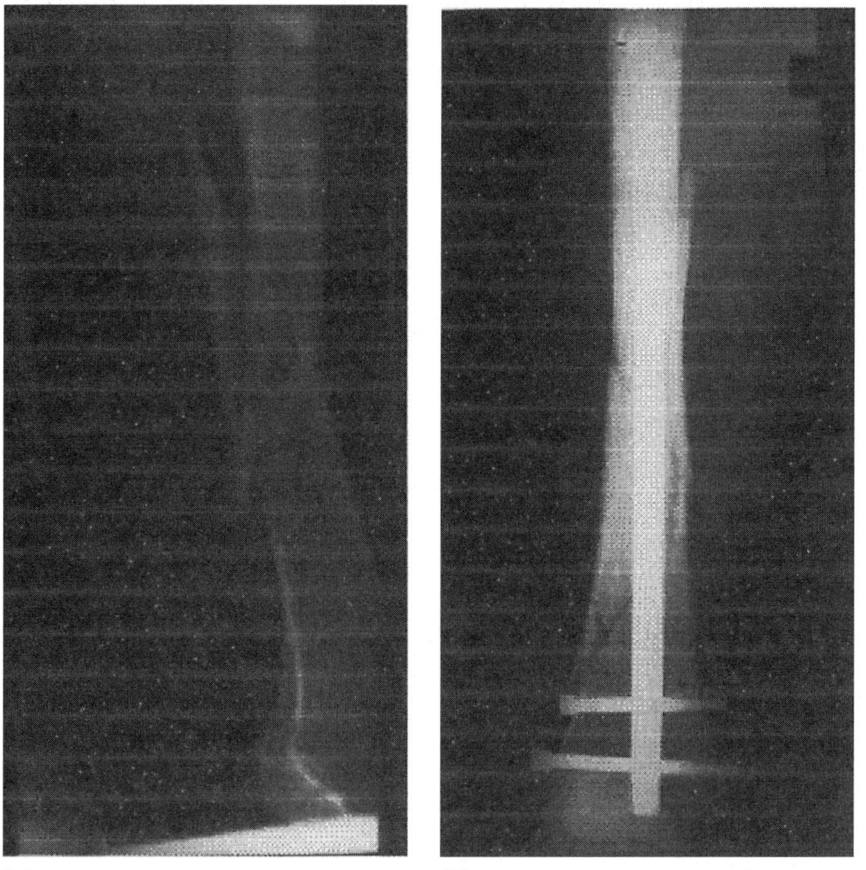

(a) (b)

Figure 13 A fracture of the femur. (a) X-ray before reduction with Sager splint, (b) X-ray after the operation.

XVII. TRAUMATIC AMPUTATION AND REPLANTATION

A. Epidemiology

Amputation injuries occur with a peak between 20 to 40 years of age, and men predominate over women by 3 or 4 to 1. In the nonwar population, distal injuries are more frequent than the proximal. Incomplete and complete amputations occur with the same frequency [70]. The mechanism of injury ranges from ''clean'' guillotine amputations to avulsion injuries.

Today, replantation surgery is rather common, and during the last 30 years has reached success rates up to 90% [71]. The outcome from replantation of whole limbs, especially the lower extremeties is more moderate [72]. The goal of surgery is the restoration or reconstruction of a functional limb. Proper prehospital treatment of the patient and his amputated limb is essential for good results.

With some exceptions, *all* amputated parts should be considered for replantation. The final decision to perform a replantation attempt is made by the microvascular surgeon. The patient and amputated body parts must therefore be taken to a hospital where this is

Table 25 Indications and Contraindications for Replantation

Good outcome	Contraindicated, relatively poor outcome
1. Multiple digits	1. Amputations in unstable patients secondary to other life-threatening injuries
2. The thumb	2. Multiple-level amputations
3. Wrist or forearm	3. Self-inflicted amputations
4. Sharp amputations with minimal to moderate avulsion proximal to the elbow	4. Single digit amputations proximal to the flexor digitorum superficialis insertion
5. Single digits amputated between proximal interphalangeal joint and distal interphalangeal joint	5. Warm ischemia more than: 6 hr involving muscle 16 hr for hand and digit amputation
6. Amputations in children	6. Frozen amputation part
7. Appropriate emergency department care	7. Serious underlying disease such as vascular disease, complicated diabetes mellitus, congestive heart failure
8. Experienced team	8. Extremes of age

Source: Refs. 15, 71.

possible. Amputated parts not used for replantation may be used as a source for bone, skin, vessels and nerves. Indications and contraindications for replantation are listed in Table 25.

B. Survival Time of the Tissue

Muscle and connective tissue tolerate ischemia relatively poorly. Amputated parts with large amounts of muscle tolerate less ischemia time (proximal amputations). Preservation of amputated parts at room temperature is called warm ischemia, and may be tolerated up to 6 to 8 hr. With cold ischemia this time increases up to 24 hr [73,74].

C. Survey and Treatment in Traumatic Amputation

Patients with amputation injuries must undergo the same systematic survey and treatment as every other trauma victim. Serious and dramatic limb injuries must not distract from securing the delivery of oxygen to vital organs: free airways, adequate ventilation, and restoration of acceptable circulation.

1. History

Important factors that may influence the outcome of an eventual replantation should be recorded according to Table 26.

2. Survey

The examiner should at this stage decide whether or not there is a possibility for replantation attempts. It is important to make contact with the microvascular surgeon at an early stage in order to avoid time loss and transport to the wrong hospital.

D. Treatment

Manipulation of the wounds in the injured limbs and amputated parts must be reduced to an absolute minimum.

Table 26 History and Clinical Findings to Be Recorded in Amputation Injuries

1.	Mechanism of trauma (sharp cut, dull cut, crushing cut, cut and avulsion, avulsion, crush avulsion)
2.	Exact time and place of amputation
3.	Condition of the amputated part and the stump
4.	Degree of contamination
5.	Hand dominance (right vs left)
6.	General condition of the patient
7.	Other injuries
8.	Coexisting diseases (e.g., medical diseases)

1. Hemorrhage

Limb injuries are rarely lifethreatening initially, except when causing exsanguination. Clean guillotine injuries often show little hemorrhage because of vascular spasm and vessel contraction. Partial amputations, blunt degloving injuries, crush wounds, and penetrating injuries may cause severe bleeding. Bleeding is best controlled by direct pressure [14]. Tourniquets should be avoided except in cases with entrapment and no access to the injured limb.

2. Wound Cleansing and Dressing: Antimicrobial Therapy

If there is much foreign material and dirt, the wound may be gently irrigated with Ringer's solution or sterile saline. Debridement should not be done on the scene. Soap, disinfectants, and antiseptics may cause further tissue damage and are therefore banned. The wound should be covered with sterile dressings. These should be slightly irrigated with saline or Ringer's solution. If necessary, a pressure dressing or an elastic bandage should be applied. Compression with a rubber bandage may in some cases be necessary. Be aware that when applying a constraining wrap it is important to ensure greater pressure distally than proximally.

Bulky bandages may hide severe hemorrhage, and should be avoided. The bandage should be observed during transport to detect bleeding. Antimicrobal therapy is compulsory in all amputation injuries (see below).

3. Care of the Amputated Part

All amputated parts must be collected. If a part is not replanted, it may be used as a donor for tissue. The amputated parts should be wrapped in saline-soaked gauze. Sharp edges from bone should be bolstered. The author received an 18-year-old girl in the emergency room, with amputation of her right forearm. Bone had perforated the plastic of the transportation bag, and the arm was soaked with ice water. It could not be used for replantation. The National Orthopedic Centre in Norway does not recommend cooling when replantation is possible within 4 to 6 hr [75].

The best storing temperature has proved to be about 4°C, but a practical goal should be about 10°C. Freezing of the body part during transport must be avoided. For preserving the amputated limb the two-package technique is recommended (Fig. 14). The package with the amputated limb should be tied to the patient, to avoid it ''disappearing'' during transport.

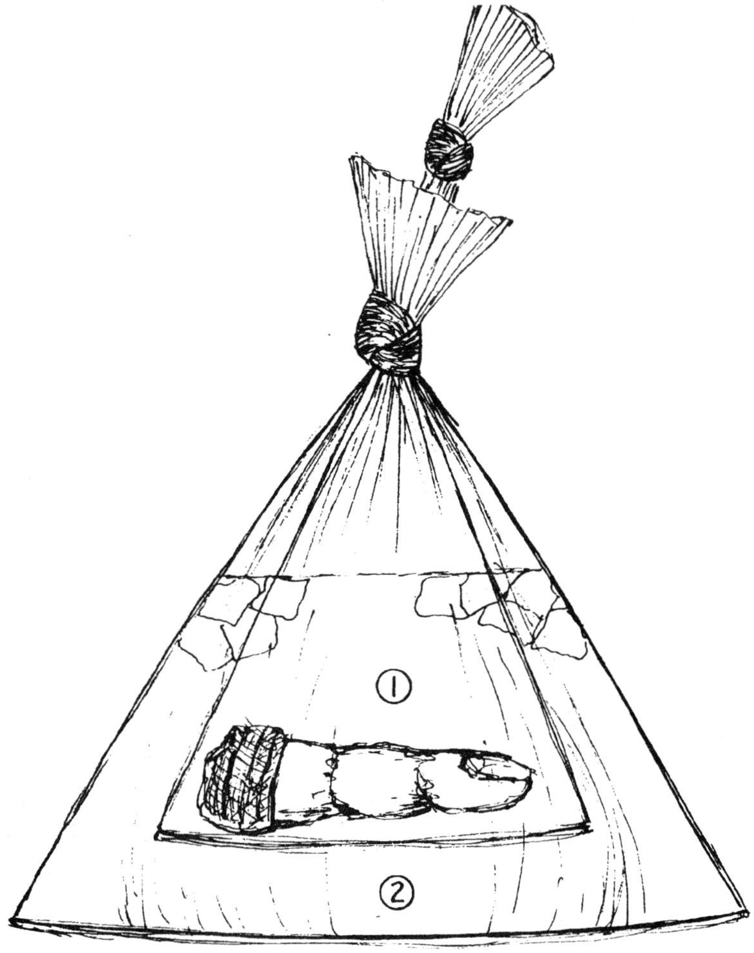

Figure 14 The two-package technique. Taking care of the amputated parts. The temperature should be about 4°C. The amputated part must not freeze! (1) Ice/water. (2) Inner bag, body part, bandaged with gauze soaked in sterile saline. (Courtesy of Kjell Arne Borge.)

E. Incomplete Amputation

If the distal part of an incomplete amputated limb has no pulse, no capillary refill and no bleeding, this part should be cooled by the same method as for complete amputations as Schlenker and Koulis recommend in a review article [71].

The amputated part should be splinted to avoid rotation and further movement. Care should be taken in attempts to reduce the fracture. Malrotation may cause ischemia and nerve damage.

F. Emergency Amputation

In cases in which the patient is entrapped, and his/her general condition is poor, an emergency amputation may be considered. The same considerations must be made if the patient is entrapped aboard a ship at sea or in very remote areas.

An amputation should be performed with general anesthesia, or at least with profound analgesia. If the patient is in bad condition, a tourniquet should be used during the procedure. In the Norwegian Air Ambulance helicopters we carry a small surgical kit and a normal simple wire saw (''Rambo-type''). As much as possible of bone, skin, and other tissue must be preserved. The amputated part should be cooled as described above. Definitive surgery must be performed in the hospital.

XVIII. INJURIES FROM EXPLOSIVES AND SHOT WOUNDS

A. Explosions—Blast Injuries

Injuries caused by explosions are not only confined to military activity. Terrorist bombings and industrial explosions also frequently cause blast injuries. Explosion victims with amputations or other injuries to the musculoskeletal system should always be considered having blast primary injuries. Most deaths are caused by head trauma resullting from secondary and tertiary blast injuries [77].

1. Primary Blast Injury (PBI)

Primary blast injury (PBI) is caused by direct blast to the body. A PBI may kill the casualty by causing barotrauma to gas-containing organs of the body. These organs are more vulnerable to pressure differences compared to fluid-filled or solid organs [78].

Respiratory Tract

The most common injuries are pulmonary contusions, with or without laceration, barotrauma with pneumothorax, and interstitial/mediatsinal/subcutaneous emphysema.

Gastrointestinal Tract

These injuries occur in the same prevalence as lung injuries and involve mostly the gas-filled organs. Subcapsular haematomas may occur in the liver, spleen, and kidneys.

Auditory System

The blast injury may cause damage to both the middle and inner ear. Typical signs are hearing loss, tinnitus, and vertigo.

2. Secondary Blast Injury

Secondary blast injuries are caused by flying debris.

3. Tertiary Blast Injury

Tertiary blast injuries cause trauma through displacement of the body and its impact with stationary objects.

4. Survey and Treatment

History

To assure correct treatment it is important to compile a history in which the following information is included:

Distance from explosion
Was the victim underwater or in an enclosure?
Was body armor used?
Exposure to chemical or burning substances (binary exposure)

Survey

The examiner should search for typical signs of a blast injury such as the following:

Ruptured tympanic membrane
Hypopharyngeal petechiae or ecchymoses
Fundoscopic evidence of retinal air embolism
Subcutaneous emphysema

The respiratory function should be surveyed by checking the following items:

Cyanosis, tachypea, and hemoptysis
Decreased breath sounds, abnormal percussion sounds
Thoracic pain

Respiratory support with mechanical ventilation is associated with a significant risk in these patients and should therefore be considered thoroughly.

The extent of abdominal injuries is difficult to determine. The clinical signs are often vague.

Treatment

Oxygen should be administered liberally
Pain treatment
Intravenous access

Signs of inhalation of chemicals, burning substances, or hot gases should be checked.

B. Shot Wounds

The physician performing the primary survey of a patient with gunshot wounds should have a basic knowledge of ballistics [79]. When a missile strikes the body, energy ($E = 1/2\ mv^2$) is transferred to the tissue along the wound track and causes different degrees of damage. When high-energy missiles (bullets with high speed) penetrate the skin, large amounts of energy are released and cause an expanding cavity. Supersonic missiles cause shock waves that may lead to damage of tissue and bone at a distance from the wound itself [80]. Low energy missiles cause damage along their wound track mostly through laceration and crushing. The shape and size of the missile is important in assessing the extent of the damage.

1. History

When taking care of patients with gunshot wounds, EMS personnel must always assure themselves that there is no chance of further shooting. From time to time tragic accidents involving physicians and ambulance personnel occur. During the prehospital survey the physician should determine which kind of weapon was used, from what distance it was fired and the exact time of shooting.

2. Survey

Normal principles for trauma management must be followed. The patient should be thoroughly examined for more wounds and to check if the missile has left the body again. Often the patient has been penetrated by more than one missile. Hemorrhage and wounds should be treated as for amputations, and fractures should be splinted. Sensation and circulation distal to the wound must be checked.

XIX. STAB WOUNDS

Stab wounds to the extremities may be life-threatening when involving proximal arteries. Hemorrhages must be promptly treated by point control, as for amputations. Foreign bodies and knives remaining in the wound should not be removed on the scene. The patient should be examined for further wounds.

XX. ANTIMICROBAL THERAPY IN ORTHOPEDIC INJURIES

Intravenous antibiotics and tetanus toxoid IM should be given as early as possible in amputations, crush injuries, and open fractures. Together with early fracture reduction and surgery this reduces the risk of serious infection [76]. *Staphylococcus aureus, Streptococci* and *gram negative bacilli* are the most common species. In cases of human bites *Eiknella corrodens* also must be considered.

The choice of antibiotics for IV administration may vary considerably according to local traditions and bacterial resistance patterns. Some authors recommend an infusion of penicillin or a first-generation cephalosporin. In the military setting there is a tradition for the combination of penicillin and chloramfenicol. Injection with tetanus toxoid should be compulsory. When the immunization status is unknown, administration of of human tetanus immunglobulin should be considered [14].

XXI. SPECIAL SITUATIONS

A. The Elderly Patient With Orthopedic Trauma

Orthopedic injuries in the elderly is an increasing health problem in industrial countries, causing suffering and death. These injuries also create a burden to the health care system. Bone mass decreases after a peak is reached in the third decade. Bone mass is less in women than men at all ages. Muscle mass and bone mass share a constant relationship. Hip fractures are more common in elderly people with an abnormal decrease in bone density [81]. Hip fractures are associated with more deaths, disability, and medical costs than all other osteoporotic fractures. The total number of hip fractures has doubled with 17-year increment. The main cause is the dramatic increase in the number of elderly people. From the age of 70 years the incidence doubles with each 5-year increment [82].

Mortality rates by fractured hips vary in different surveys, but an increased mortality rate has been shown with increasing age, poor medical condition (comorbidity), and American Society of Anesthesiologists physical status classification 3 or 4 [83]. When surveying the elderly trauma patient on the scene, the physician should therefore pay close attention to coexisting medical diseases. In some cases the direct cause of the fall may, for example, be a myocardial infarction, a hypotensive episode, an arrythmia episode, or a stroke. The patient should be carefully examined for the medical conditions listed in Table 27.

1. Treatment

The extent of prehospital treatment and monitoring should be selected according to the general state of the patient. The dosage of opioids should be given divided IV to prevent hypoventilation or hypotension. Oxygen should be routinely administered. To avoid pulmonary edema, IV fluids should be administered with care. The same care should be taken

Table 27 Medical Conditions to Be Examined in the Elderly

Heart disease: angina, former myocardial infarction, heart failure, arrythmias
Lungs: asthma, previous episodes of dyspnea
Neurologic disorders: stroke, multiple sclerosis, Parkinson's disease, dementia

in the use of MAST. Placing a patient with an advanced heart disease into supine position may cause dyspnea and decompensation.

2. Observation and Monitoring

The level of monitoring should be increased in this group of patients and involves the airway, respiratory rate, pulse, and capillary refill. Use of multichannel ECG monitoring makes it possible to detect arrythmias or severe coronary ischemia.

B. The Child With Orthopedic Trauma

Survey and treatment of an injured child is somewhat different from that for adults, as their physiology and pathophysiology is different. The circulation compensates for blood loss longer than in adults (no drop in BP [84]). Thus, the decompensation appears without warning. The child does not always see the advantages of co-operating with his helpers, and frightened parents often create extra pressure on their work. The following could be helpful reminders when approaching injured children.

1. Endotracheal Intubation and General Anesthesia in Children

Airways should be secured and adequate ventilation provided before transportation. If respiration is unstable or with stridor, consider immediate intubation and general anesthesia. This should only be performed prehospital by an experienced anesthesiologist. All equipment and drugs for dealing with complications should be accessible. Monitoring the child under general anesthesia during transportation is extremely demanding.

Induction of anesthesia may be performed with the following drugs:

Atropine: 0.01 to 0.02 mg/kg IV
Thiopenthon: 3 to 4 mg/kg IV (in hypovolemia 1 to 2 mg/kg) *or* Ketamine 2.0 mg/kg IV (if circulation is unstable)
Succinylcholine: 2 mg/kg IV

General anesthesia may be continued with

Morphine: 0.1 mg/kg
Diazepam: 0.05 to 0.1 mg/kg IV
Pancuronium: 0.1 mg/kg IV

2. Treatment of Pain in Children

Treatment of pain in children is somewhat different than for adults. Soft tissue injuries should be treated after the ICE rule. Fractures should be stabilized. This will give pain reduction. The injured child should initially not receive drugs (or others) po.

Morphine: 0.05 mg/kg IV (or IM)

Ketamine: 0.25 to 0.5 mg/kg IV (or 0.5 to 1.0 mg/kg IM)

For minor pain, paracetamol: 15 mg/kg rectal (not more than 65 mg/kg/24 hr)

3. Fluid Therapy in Children

Injured children often look healthier than they really are! Estimate blood loss. Estimate age and weight of the patient, and calculate the blood volume. Establish an IV line if possible. Initially this may be easier than later, when hypovolemic shock has developed.

The circulation should be stabilized before transportation, unless uncontrolled internal hemorrhage is suspected. The same principles as for adults are useful, but the child's blood volume should be estimated to avoid overhydration.

4. Where and How to Transport the Child

The child with severe injuries should be taken to a trauma center, with a staff trained in taking care of pediatric trauma patients. Injured children should be accompanied by experienced personnel. If there are severe injuries, an experienced physician, if possible, should take care of the young patient during transportation.

XXII. SUMMARY AND CONCLUSIONS

Adequate prehospital treatment of orthopedic injuries is important for outcome and survival.

In the primary survey the principles for ATLS should be followed. Life-threatening symptoms have first priority for treatment.

Arterial hemorrhages will normally be brought under control through direct compression.

Early prehospital fracture reduction and wound treatment has been shown to decrease mortality. The combination of prehospital fracture reduction and wound management has been shown to result in a reduction in postoperative infections.

When the primary survey is completed and the patient demonstrates no uncontrolled hemorrhage, he is examined thoroughly for orthopedic injuries.

EMS personnel should be properly trained in procedures for reducing fractures and dislocations. This includes training in the use of devices for splinting.

For fractures in the lower limb the Sager splint or similar devices are preferred. These splints perform tension in the longitudinal axis so that the fracture will be reduced, resulting in pain relief.

Dislocations of the hip and knee should be reduced at the scene of the accident if transport time to the hospital is long.

Soft tissue injuries of the joints are initially cooled (ice), bandaged (compression), and elevated (to prevent edema).

Outcome of replantation of limbs by traumatic amputation is good, especially by amputation of the hand and fingers. All amputated parts should be collected on the scene, and cooled, but not frozen, before transport.

Survey and treatment of an injured child is somewhat different from that in adults.

Incidence of fracture increases with age. An increased mortality rate has been shown with increasing age. In the elderly with orthopedic injuries special attention should be taken to coexisting medical diseases.

Analgesia is an important part of prehospital treatment. First choice is morphine administered IV. For the anesthesiologist ketamine is a more potent alternative. By unstable respiration and circulation, endotracheal intubation and general anesthesia should be performed, but only by the experienced personnel.

The use of NSAIDs should be considered in injuries without fractures.

Every EMS should have a good system for documentation. The EMS report form should be as simple as possible. Documentation of medical examination, findings, treatment, and the condition of the patient during transport is mandatory. The GCS [85] and RTS should be included in the form. Documentation of problems and complications in treatment is important for quality assurance purposes.

REFERENCES

1. D Skinner, P Driscoll, R Earlam. ABCs of Major Trauma. London: BMJ, 1991.
2. National Safety Concil: Accident Facts, 1993 ed., Chicago, National Safety Council, 1993.
3. JS Jensen, E Tondevold. Mortality after hip fractures. Acta Orthop Scand 50:161, 1979.
4. Lauritzen et al. Effect of external hip protectors on hip fractures. Lancet 341:11–13, 1993.
5. G Teasdale, B Jennet. Assessment of coma and impaired consciousness. A practical scale. Lancet 2:81–83, 1974.
6. HR Champion, WJ Sacco, WS Copes, DS Gann, TA Genarelli, ME Flanagan. A revision of the Trauma Score. J Trauma 29:623–629, 1989.
7. American College of Emergency Physicians: Trauma care system quality improvement guidelines. Ann Emerg Med 21:736–739, 1992.
8. G Muhr, H Tscherne. Bergung und Erstversorgung beim Schwerverletzten. Chirurg 49:593–600, 1978.
9. KM Willett, H Dorrell, P Kelly. Management of limb injuries. In: D Skinner, P Driscoll, R Earlam, eds. ABCs of Major Trauma. London: BMJ 1991, pp. 57–61.
10. H Tscherne, L Gotzen. Fractures with Soft Tissue Injuries. New York: Springer Verlag, 1984.
11. W Hammerschmidt. Narkosenkomplikationen und Narkosenzwischenfälle im Rettungsdienst. In: GH Engelhart, ed. Rettungsdienst im Wandel. Edewecht: Stumpf und Kosseney, 1992, pp. 41–58.
12. SH Miller, G Price, D Buck, et al. Effects of tourniquet ischemia and post-ischemic edema on muscle metabolism. J Hand Surg 4:547, 1979.
13. Pillgram-Larsen, S Mellesmo, R Peck. Injuries from mines. Tidskr Nor Laegeforen 12:2183–2187, 1992.
14. S Mellesmo, J Pillgram-Larsen. Primary care of amputation injuries. JEUR 8:131–135, 1995.
15. DL McGee, WC Dalsey. The mangled extremity. Compartment syndrome and amputations. Emerg Med Clin North Amer 10:783–800, 1992.
16. WH Bickell, SP Bruttig, GA Millnamow, J O'Benar, CE Wade. The detrimental effects of intravenous crystalloid after aortotomy in swine. Surgery 10:529–536, 1991.
17. SA Stern, SC Dronen, P Birrer. Effect of blood pressure on hemorrhage volume and survival in near-fatal hemorrhage model incorporating a vascular injury. Ann Emerg Med 22:155–163, 1993.
18. WH Bickell. Are victims of injury sometimes victimized by attempts at fluid resuscitation? Ann Emergency Med 22:256–266, 1993.
19. E Skogvoll, I Kirkeby-Garstad, AM Kvam. Pulmonary edema after prehospital fluid therapy. NA Forum, Høstmøte, Norway, 1993 (in Norwegian).
20. SA Gould, L Sehgal, HL Sehgal, GS Moss. Hypovolemic shock. Crit Care Clin 9:239–246, 1993.
21. PR Williams, ID Russel, WJ Mintowt-Czyz. Compartment pressure monitoring—current UK orthopedic practice. Injury 29(3):229–232, 1998.
22. A Ekeland. Treatment of skiing injuries. Nord Med 109:38–39, 1994.

23. NL Caroline. Emergency Care in the Streets. Boston: Little, Brown and Company, 1981, p. 384.
23a. V Schumpelick, NM Bleese, U Mommsen. Chirurgie. Stuttgart: EnkeVerlag, 1986, p. 644.
24. KM Willett, H Dorrell, P Kelly. Management of limb injuries, ABC of Major Trauma. D Skinner, P Driscoll, R Earlam, eds. London: BMJ, 1991, pp. 57–61.
25. DL McGee, WC Dalsey. The mangled extremity. Compartment syndrome and amputations. Emerg Med Clin North Amer 10:783–800, 1992.
26. L Kinzl. Erstversorgung von Fracturen. In: FW Ahnefeld, W Dick, J Kilian, HP Schuster, eds. Notfallmedizin. Berlin: Springer Verlag, 1986, pp. 91–94.
27. BS Davidson, GT Simmons, PR Williamson, et al. Pelvic fractures associated with open peroneal wounds: A survivable injury. J Trauma 35:36, 1993.
28. D Bironi, E Steinmann, EM Utiyyama, et al. Open pelviperineal trauma. J Trauma 30:492, 1990.
29. RE Kuminsky, I Shbeeb, G Makos, et al. Blunt pelviperineal injuries. An expanded role for the diverting colostomi. Dis Colon Rectum 25:787, 1982.
30. KD Johnson, A Cabambi, B Seibert. Incidence of respiratory syndrome in patients with multiple musculoskeletal injuries: Effect of early operative stabilization of fractures. J Trauma 25: 375, 1985.
31. JN LaDuca, LL Bone, RW Seibel, et al. Primary open reduction and internal fixation of open fractures. J Trauma 20:375, 1985.
32. SR Garfin, MED MER Katz, Marshall LF. Prehospital care of spinal cord injuries. Topics Emerg Med 9:37–44, 1987.
33. P Bayless, VG Ray. Incidence of cervical spine injuries in association with blunt head trauma. Amer J Emerg Med 7:139–142, 1989.
34. J Williams, D Jehle, E Cottington, C Shufflebarger. Head, facial and clavicular trauma as a predictor of cervical-spine injury. Ann Emerg Med 21:719–722, 1992.
35. R Riggins, J Kraus. The risk of neurologic damage with fractures of the vertebrae. J Trauma 17:126–133, 1977.
36. GR McLatchie. Injuries to the neck and spine. In: GR McLatchie, ed. Essentials of Sports Medicine. Edinburgh: Churchill Livingstone, 1993, pp. 265–275.
37. EJ Kennedy, ed. Spinal Cord Injury. The Facts and Figures. Birmingham: University of Alabama Press, 1986, p. 1.
38. LM Capan, SM Miller, RM Sommer. Perioperative anesthetic management of spine injuries. Prob Anesth 8:377–400, 1994.
39. B Jeanneret, F Magerl, JC Ward. Overdistraction: A hazard of skull traction in the management of acute injuries of the cervical spine. Arch Orthop Trauma Surg 110:242–245, 1991.
40. DJ Muckart, Bhagwanjee, et al. Spinal cord injury as a result of endotracheal intubation in patients with undiagnosed cervical spine fractures. Anesthesiology 87:418–420, 1997.
41. LC Kossuth. Removal of injured personnel from wrecked vehicles. J Trauma 5:704–705, 1965.
42. JD Farrington. Death in a ditch. Bull Amer Coll Surg 52:121–130, 1967.
43. JD Farrington. Extrication of victims—surgical principles. J Trauma 8:492, 1968.
44. T Dick, R Land. Spinal immobilization devices. J Emerg Med Serv 7(12):26–30, 1982.
45. JR Hoffman, AB Wolfson, K Todd, WR Mower. Selective cervical spine radiography in blunt trauma: Methodology of the national emergency X-radiography utilization study (NEXUS). Ann Emerg Med 32:461–469, 1998.
46. P Orledge. Out-of-hospital spinal immobilization: Is it really necessary? Acad Emerg Med 5: 203–204, 1998.
47. MD Muhr, DL Seabrook, LK Wittwer. Paramedic use of a spinal injury clearance algorithm reduces spinal immobilization in the out-of-hospital setting. Prehosp Emerg Care 3:1–6, 1999.
48. RM Domeier. The National Association of EMS Physicians Standards and Clinical Practice Committee. Prehosp Emerg Care 3:251–253, 1999.

49. M Hauswald, G Ong, D Tandberg, X Omar. Out-of-hospital spinal immobilization: Its effect on neurologic injury. Acad Emerg Med 5:214–219, 1998.
50. American College of Surgeons, Committee on Trauma. Advanced Trauma Life Support Student Manual. Chicago, American College of Surgeons, 1999.
51. WF Donaldson III, BV Heil, VP Donaldson, VJ Silvaggio. The effect of airway maneuvers on the unstable C1-C2 segment. A cadaver study. Spine 22(11):1215–1218, 1997.
51a. BD Gunn, N Eizenberg et al. How should an unconscious person with a suspected neck injury be positioned? Prehosp Disas Med 4:239–244, 1995.
52. M Brandt, W Dick. Ketamin als Analgetikum in der Notfallmedizin. In: FW Ahnefeld, E Pfenninger, eds. Ketamin in der Intensiv- und Notfallmedizin. Berlin: Springer Verlag, 1989, pp. 61–64.
53. T Rygnestad, AM Kvam. Streptococcal myositis and tissue necrosis with intramuscular administration of diclofenac (Voltaren®). Acta Anaesth Scand 39:1128–1130, 1995.
54. R McGlone, H Sadhra, DW Hamer, et al. Femoral nerve block in the initial management of femoral shaft fractures. Arch Emerg Med 4:163, 1987.
55. JE Dalen, IS Ockene, J Hirsch. Venous thromboembolism: Scope of the problem. Chest 89: 370, 1986.
56. EW Salzman, WH Harris. Prevention of venous thromboembolism in orthopedic patients. J Bone Joint Surg 581:903, 1976.
57. MH Marshall. Perioperative issues related to thromboembolic phenomena. Problems in Anesthesia 8:473–488, 1994.
58. Norwegian Association of Anesthesiologists (NAF). Consensus—Regional anesthesia by bleeding disorders/prophylaxis against thrombosis, 1999 (in Norwegian).
59. JR Cline, E Scheidel, EF Bigsby. A comparison of methods of cervical immobilisation used in patient extrication and transport. J Trauma 25:649–653, 1985.
60. PW Main, ME Lovell. A review of seven support surfaces with emphasis on their protection of the spinally injured. J Accid Emerg Med 13:34–37, 1996.
61. KJ Abrahams, JP Nolan, CM Grande. Trauma anesthesia: anesthesiology's oldest speciality reborn. Anesth Clin North Amer 9:44–49, 1994.
62. SA Lord, WC Boswell, JS Williams, JW Odom, CR Boyd. Airway control in trauma patients with cervical spine fractures. Prehosp Disaster Med 9:44–49, 1994.
63. P Rommens, KP Schmitt-Neuerburg. De preklinische versorgung van zwaargekwetsten, Tijdschr Geneesk 43:379–385, 1987.
64. H Ashton. Effect of inflatable plastic splints on blood flow. BMJ 2:1427–1430, 1966.
65. KL Mattox, WH Brickell, PE Pepe, J Burch, D Feliciano. Prospective MAST study in 911 patients. J Trauma 29:1104–1111, 1989.
66. B Honigman, SR Lowenstein, EE Moore, K Roweder, P Pons. The role of the pneumatic antishock garment in penetrating cardiac wounds. JAMA 266:2398–2401, 1991.
67. J Ali, B Vanderby, C Purcell. The effect of the pneumatic antishock garment (PASG) on hemodynamics, hemorrhage, and survival in penetrating thoracic aortic injury. J Trauma 31: 846–851, 1991.
68. RM Domeier, RE O'Connor, et al. Use of the Pneumatic Anti-shock Garment (PASG). Prehosp Emerg Care 1:32–35, 1997.
69. JR Corea, AW Ibrahim, M Hegazi. The Thomas splint causing urethral injury. Injury 23:340–341, 1992.
70. WC Dalsey. Management of amputated parts. In: JR Roberts, Hedges, eds. Clinical Procedures in Emergency Medicine. Philadelphia: WB Saunders, 1985, pp. 599–606.
71. JD Schlenker, CP Koulis. Amputations and replantations. Emerg Med Clin North Amer 11: 739–753, 1993.
72. J Dorrler, PC Maurer, S von Sommoggy, J Ingianni. Subtotal and total traumatic extremity amputation—when replantation, when amputation? Langenbecks Arch Chir Suppl Li Verh Dtsch Ges Forsch Chir 651–654, 1989.

73. JW Hayhurst, BM O'Brien, H Ishida, et al. Experimental digital replantation after prolonged cooling. Hand 6:134, 1974.
74. W May Jr. Successful digital replantation after 28 hours of cold ischemia. Plast Reconstr Surg 67:566, 1981.
75. A Reigstad. Storing of Amputates. National Centre for Orthopedic Surgery, Kronprinsesse Märthas Institutt, Oslo, Dec. 1993 (in Norwegian)
76. JD Schlenker, CB Koulis. Amputations and replantations. Emerg Med Clin North Amer 11: 742–743, 1993.
77. ER Frykberg, JJ Tepas. Terrorist bombing: Lessons learned from Belfast to Beirut. Ann Surg 208:569–576, 1988.
78. YY Phillips, JT Zajtchuk. The management of primary blast injury in conventional warfare: Ballistic, blast and burn injuries. In: Office of the Surgeon General, Textbook of Military Medicine. Washington, DC, 1991, Vol 5, Part 1, pp. 295–331.
79. Z Stanec, S Skrbic, I Dzepina, et al. High-energy war wounds. Ann Plast Surg 2:97–102, 1993.
80. KG Swan, RC Swan. Principles of ballistics applicable to the treatment of gunshot wounds. Surg Clin North Amer 71:221–239, 1991.
81. LJ Melton, HW Wahner, LS Richelson, et al. Osteoporosis and the risk of hip fracture. Am J Epidemiol 124:254, 1986.
82. JS Jensen. Trochanteric fractures: An epidemiological, clinical and biochemical study. Acta Orthop Scand 52(suppl 188):9, 1981.
83. BL White, WD Fisher, Laurin. Rate of mortality for elderly patients after fracture of the hip in the 1980s. J Bone Joint Surg 69A8:1335–1339, 1987.
84. FW Ahnefeld. Notfallmedizin. Berlin: Springer, 1986, pp. 266–270.
85. G Teasdale, B Jennet. Assessment of coma and impaired consciousness. A practical scale. Lancet 2:81–83, 1974.

29

Burns

SØREN LOUMANN NIELSEN

Rigshospitalet, Copenhagen University Hospital, Copenhagen, Denmark

Throughout history fires have made clear marks on society. Today, we still face a relatively large number of burn victims whose injury or death is caused by either inhalation of smoke or direct thermal cutaneous/mucosal injury. The vast majority of burn patients have minor burns that can be treated safely in the emergency room. The burn mortality among adults in New Zealand was recorded over a 10-year period. In 1988, hospital admission frequency was 251/million/year, a figure comparable to those from the United States, Canada, and Finland. Mortality was 19.2/million/year [1].

I. THE INCIDENT SCENE

Anyone who has been a spectator at a large fire must admit that it is a spectacular but frightening sight. The extreme forces involved make it a dangerous scene. The roof may fall, the windows may blast outward, and victims may jump from heights in panic (Fig. 1).

When attempting to rescue a victim of an electrical accident, the rescuer/prehospital care provider must be aware of the possibility of the electrical current not being switched off (Fig. 2).

In contrast to most other emergency responses, the prehospital personnel responding to a fire might not be able to enter the incident scene (e.g., a burning four-story building). The prehospital care provider must depend on firefighters to conduct the process of search and rescue. It is an extremely difficult task to find and rescue entrapped victims during a fire.

After arriving at the scene, prehospital care providers must quickly estimate the magnitude of the incident and if necessary notify the hospital service of the magnitude and possibility of a fire on the magnitude of a disaster. The triage area must be situated

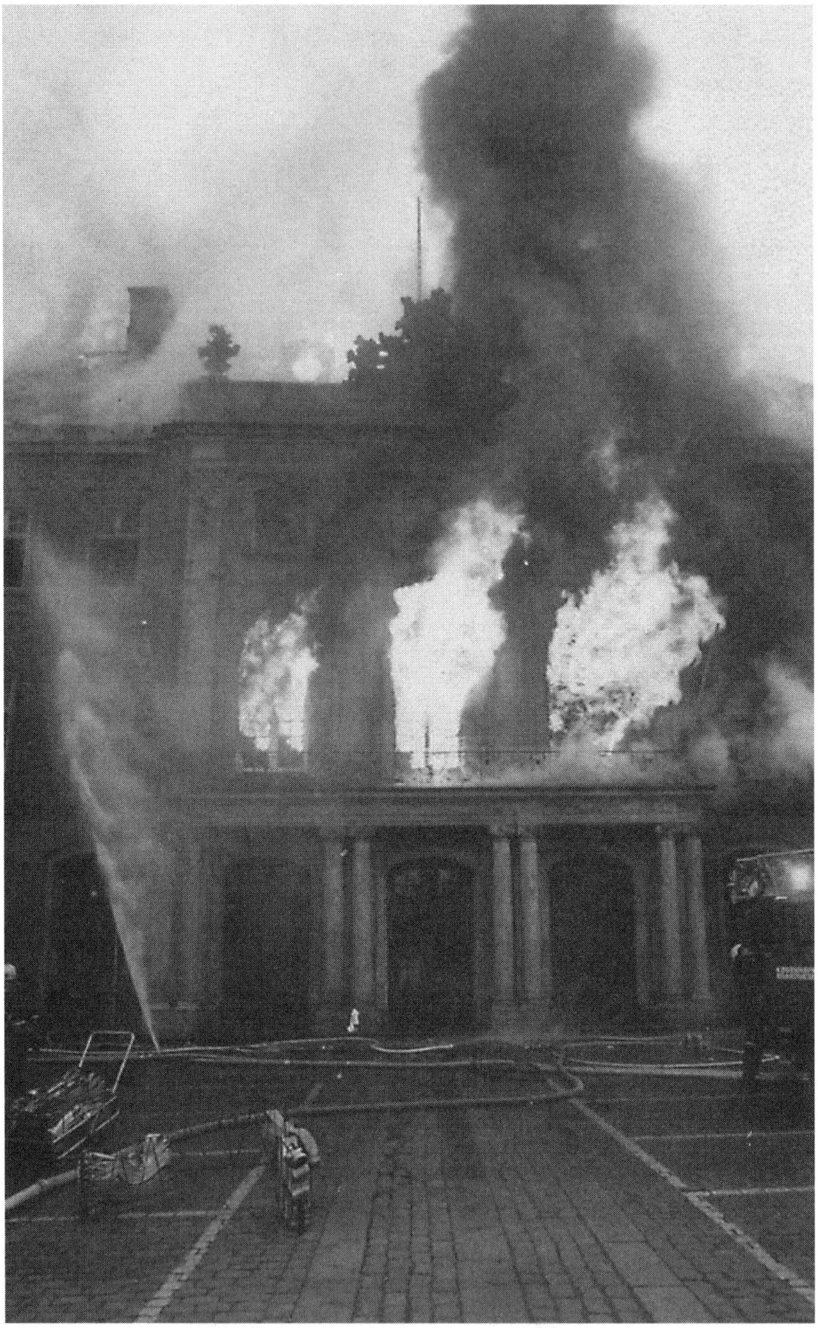

Figure 1 Falling tiles chopping hoses. (Photo courtesy of G. Jensen.)

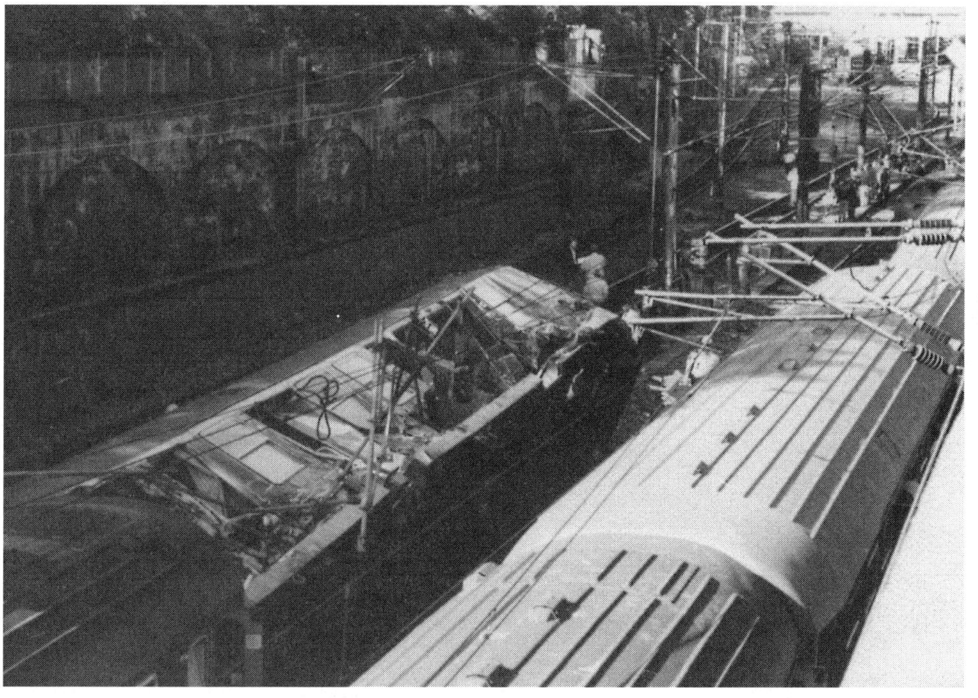

Figure 2 Railroad crash with power lines hanging down. The 20,000-V current has been switched off. (Photo courtesy of S. Weiss.)

so as to protect victims from further injuries while allowing a free flow of ambulances to and from the scene.

II. PATHOPHYSIOLOGY OF BURNS

The three-dimensional microscopic appearance of a burn presents three zones. A zone with coagulation necrosis is located centrally. Peripheral to this is the zone of stasis, where the circulation is impaired. Under unfavorable conditions necrosis may develop. Peripheral to the zone of stasis lies the zone of hyperemia. As part of the inflammatory response, this zone is characterized by generalized vasodilatation (Fig. 3).

The macroscopic correlate is classified according to the depth of the burn and is divided into the following three types (Fig. 4):

First degree: Erythema; not considered a burn despite intense pain
Second degree: Partial thickness; can be divided into superficial and deep
Third degree: Full thickness; loss of all epidermal and dermal tissue elements

Edema develops in all burned surfaces of the skin as well as the mucosa. Fluid transport at a capillary level is governed by the Starling equation.

$$J_v = K_f[(P_c - P_{if}) - \sigma(\pi_c - \pi_{if})]$$

J_v is the transvascular fluid flux, K_f is the filtration coefficient, P_c and P_{if} are the hydrostatic pressures in the capillaries and interstitial fluid, respectively, σ is the macromolecular

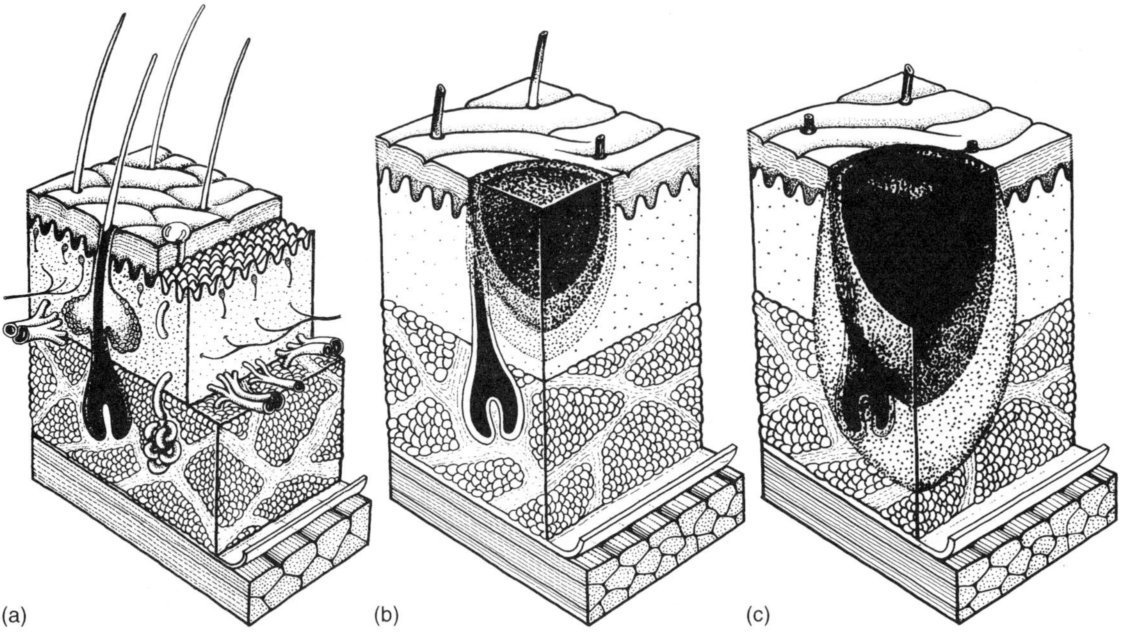

Figure 3 (a) Schematic outline of the microscopic appearance of normal skin. (b) Schematic outline of the microscopic appearance of a second-degree burn. (c) Schematic outline of the microscopic appearance of a third-degree burn. (Courtesy of P. G. Skanning, M.D.)

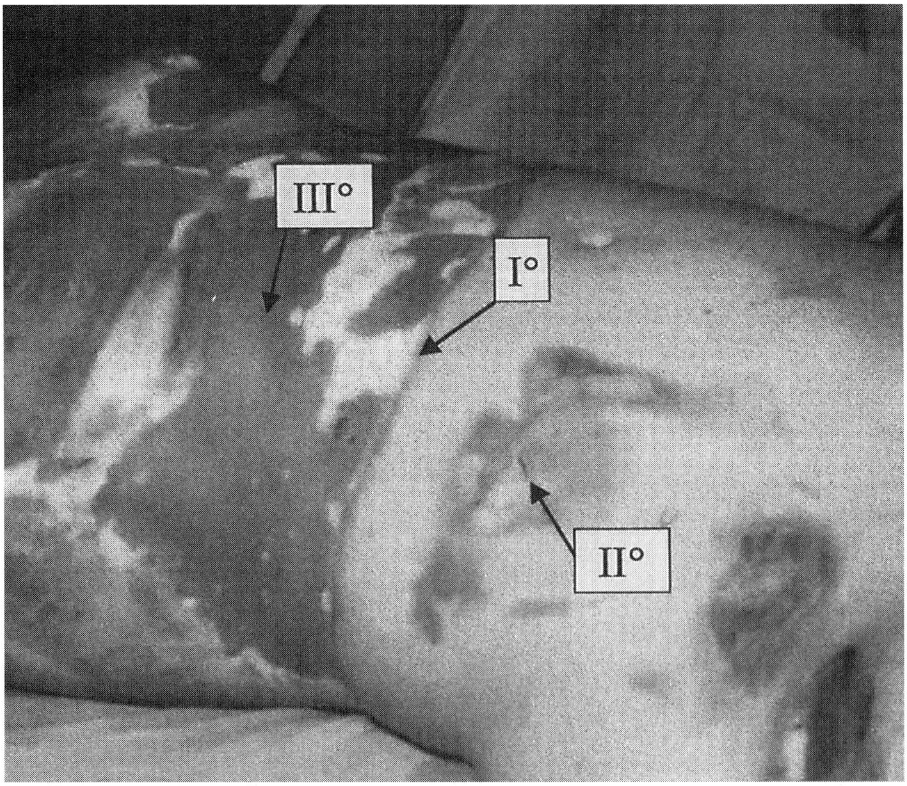

Figure 4 Macroscopic appearance of first-, second-, and third-degree burns.

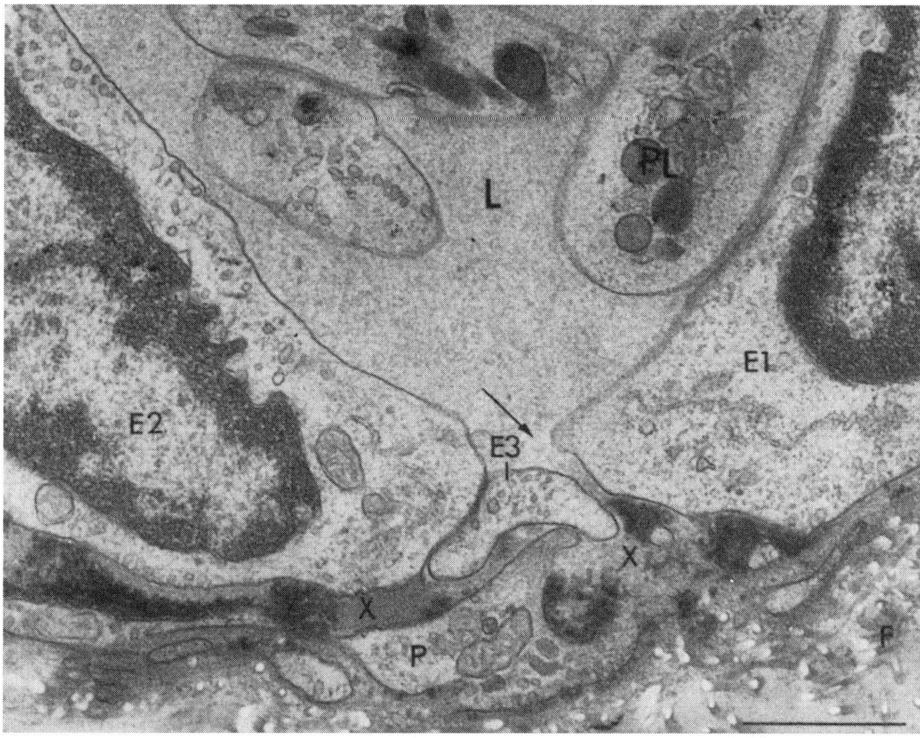

Figure 5 Electron micrograph showing the gap between endothelial cells (arrow). (From Ref. 1a.)

reflection coefficient, and π_c and π_{if} are the colloid osmotic pressures in the capillaries and interstitial fluid, respectively.

All factors in this equation are changed in the direction of favoring the production of edema, as the lymphatic drainage capacity is overwhelmed. The endothelial cells literally slip apart, as shown in Fig. 5. The most important factors are a decrease in σ, leading to net out-filtration of plasma proteins, and highly negative P_{if}, resulting in a ''vacuum effect'' because of the denaturation of subcutaneous collagen [2,3].

Water accumulation also occurs in unburned tissues because of systemic spillover of permeability-increasing substances such as histamine and cytokines produced in the burned tissues [4]. Burn shock in the early phase is mainly a hypovolemic shock, which can largely be corrected by infusion of (crystalloid) fluid. In an in vitro guinea pig model involving extensive burns (>65%), Baxter and Shires [4] were able to show that the plasma of some of these individuals contained a ''cardiac depressant factor.'' In a comparable group Martyn et al. was not able to correct right ventricular dysfunction by low dose dopamine infusion [5].

III. PATHOPHYSIOLOGY OF INHALATION INJURY

In addition to thermal lesions, fires pose an imminent danger of cellular hypoxia due to inhalation of asphyxiating fumes and the low pO_2 in the environment. Smoke consists of fumes, gaseous mists, and hot air.

In the supraglottic area, inhalation injury is of both thermal and toxic origin. Edema may develop within minutes after the incident and progress over the first 24 hr. In the lower airways, a toxic reaction to smoke leads to sloughing of the mucosal surface, decreased ciliary function, and plugging of bronchioli. This results in a decrease in airflow conduction and a decrease in the exchange of gases, primarily oxygen. Although a myriad of substances have been identified, the most important gases contained in smoke are carbon monoxide (CO) and hydrogen cyanide (CN).

A. Carbon Monoxide

All fires produce CO. Most victims found dead on the scene have succumbed to CO intoxication. Carbon monoxide has an affinity 200 times that of O_2 for hemoglobin and binds with cytochrome A and P-450, resulting in an inability to use the small amounts of oxygen available (Fig. 6, Table 1).

Despite a correct curve with a dicrotic notch, pulse oximetry *is not* a reliable picture of the capillary oxygen content as the absorption spectra of HBO_2 and HBCO coincide. Furthermore, intoxication with CO often coincides with exposure to cyanide.

B. Cyanide

Fires involving polyurethane and polyamide produce substantial amounts of CN. This compound acts to synergistic effect with CO as cytochrome oxidase (Fe^{3+}) is inhibited by cyanide [6]. Hydrogen cyanide is highly toxic and reaches toxic levels within minutes

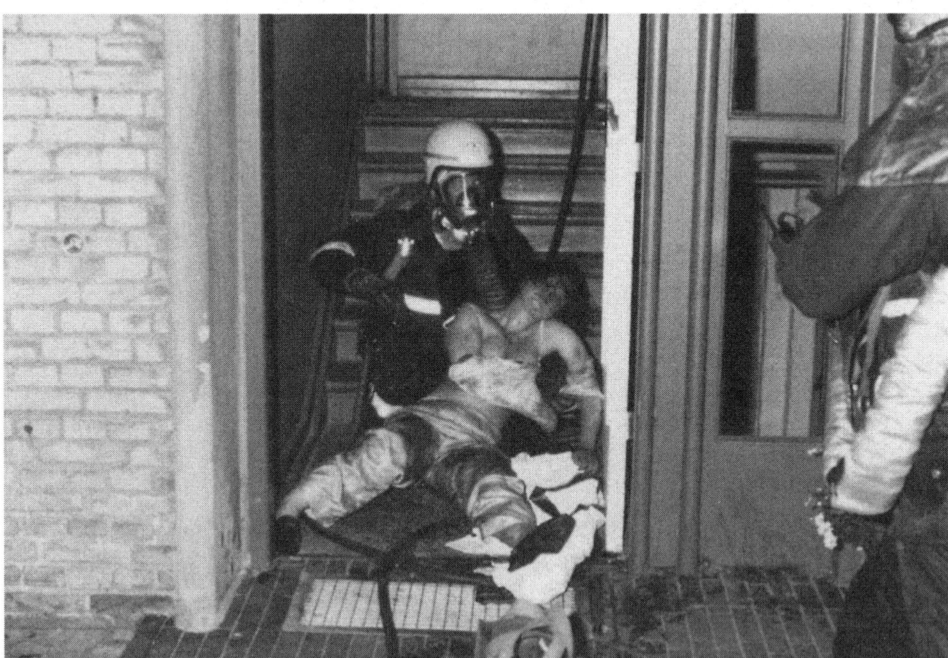

Figure 6 Surviving young female, heavily smoke intoxicated, rescued from burning apartment by fireman equipped with a helmet and a closed-circuit breathing apparatus; no burns. (Photo courtesy of S. Weiss.)

Table 1 Signs and Symptoms of Carbon Monoxide Poisoning Related to Hemoglobin of CO

HBCO	Symptoms
<10%	No symptoms (normal among smokers)
10–30%	Headache, dizziness, disorientation, decreased concentration, irritability
30–50%	Confusion, ataxia, angina, arrhythmia, hyperventilation
>50%	Cardiac arrest, coma

Note: The correlation between HBCO level and symptoms is poor.

after ignition. Most of its victims die at the scene. Evidence of cyanide poisoning is largely based on the history from the scene and persisting acidosis not explained by the level of carboxyhemoglobin (HBCO) [6]. Some antidotes (sodium thiosulfate and amylnitrate) are known, but their uses are limited because of their toxic side effects. A new atoxic cyanide-binding drug, hydroxycobolamin (HC), has been developed. The mechanism seems to be that cyanide has a higher affinity for HC than for cytochrome oxidase [7].

IV. PATHOPHYSIOLOGY OF ELECTRIC INJURY

Approximately 3% of patients who have sustained burn injury and need hospitalization are victims of electrical forces [8]. The distribution by age has two peaks. One appears in children <6 years of age who are usually injured as a result of oral contact with electrical sockets. The other incidence peak is among young male adults, reflecting the male dominance in the construction and electrical industries. The overall fatality rate is 3–15% [9]. The lesions are divided into low-voltage and high-voltage injuries. Somewhat arbitrarily, the dividing line is set at 1000 V. The basic pathophysiology is poorly understood, and the theories about pathogenesis are controversial. Electric energy E in joules is generated according to the following formula:

$$E = I^2 R t$$

where I is current in A, R the resistance in Ω, and t is the time of contact in seconds. One theory is that energy is transformed into heat and dissipated in the tissue, leading to necrosis [10]. Another theory is that the progressive tissue necrosis is secondary to a primary vascular lesion. Vessels and nerves are known to have low resistance, which in turn will lead to a large amount of current [11]. Household accidents are caused by contact with AC 110 to 380 V at 50 to 60 Hz. They may result in tetanic muscle contractions, prolonging the time the victim is exposed to the current, and thus increasing the damage. Low-voltage lesions mimic thermal burn [12]. Death in this situation is attributed to induction of cardiopulmonary arrest. The current is thought to spread throughout the body; as little as 100 μA may induce ventricular fibrillation.

In high-voltage injuries the pattern is different. The victim may be thrown, causing multiple blunt injuries. Skin lesions may be deceptively minor, but beneath apparently uninjured skin, as far as 25 cm from the current entrance site, a devastating muscular compartment syndrome may develop because of extensive muscular necrosis.

A. Prognosis

The prognosis of patients with burn injuries has improved progressively during the past 50 years. The first achievements came with aggressive fluid resuscitation. This evidence is still valid, as patients not sufficiently fluid resuscitated in a disaster situation have a far higher mortality compared with fully fluid-resuscitated patients [13].

In the United States data collected from 1991 to 1993 show that the *total body surface area* (TBSA) percentage survived by 50% (LD_{50}) of the total population with burns *without* inhalation injury is 75%. The same figure in patients *with* inhalation injury is 55%. The overall mortality rate in patients with inhalation injury is 29%. Sixty-two percent of all nonsurvivors had inhalation injury. Eleven percent of all burned patients exhibited an inhalation injury. The improvement is seen primarily in the younger age groups. Burns in elderly people still have a higher mortality (LD_{50} >70 years is a TBSA of 30%) [8].

V. INITIAL ASSESSMENT: ABCs

A. Airway/Breathing

Spine protection is important for burned patients, as for all other trauma patients. Airway and breathing should be assessed as soon as possible. Marked edema of the upper airway may develop during the first 12 to 24 hr and may compromise the airway within a very short time. Signs, symptoms, and information from the scene that correlate with the development of an inhalation injury are listed in Table 2.

Burns (even extensive ones) *not affecting the face, neck, or airway* do not per se require intubation. On the other hand, patients with burns involving the neck and the oral vicinity may require immediate intubation because the airway may be lost even in situations without signs of inhalation injury. If the patient urgently needs a permanent airway, the orotracheal route is preferred. Careful consideration should be given to securing a patent airway. During a 3-year period and while serving 1 million citizens, the Emergency Physician System of Cologne, Germany, treated 41 burned children and 221 burned adults, and they intubated five children (12%) and 45 adults (20%) [15].

Direct thermal injuries are rarely seen below the larynx. All burn patients must receive 100% oxygen via a venturi mask, preferably with a reservoir. Unconscious burn victims should receive 100% oxygen via a tight-fitting face mask or preferably be intubated as soon as possible, especially if CO and/or CN intoxication is suspected. Patients in whom a high degree of suspicion of inhalation injury exists or who need *long* (>1 hr)

Table 2 Signs, Symptoms, and Information from the Scene That Correlate With the Development of an Inhalation Injury

1. Stridor
2. Hoarseness
3. Use of accessory respiratory muscles
4. Facial burns
5. Singeing of the eyebrows
6. Soot or redness of the mucosa in the mouth or in the pharynx
7. Carbonaceous sputum
8. Accident in a confined space

Source: Modified from Ref. 15a.

transport by air or by road, especially under difficult conditions for advanced airway management, should be intubated prior to transport using liberal indications and a low threshold based on a high degree of suspicion. Longitudinal thoracic escharatomy may be needed in patients with circumferential truncal burns.

1. Problems and Pitfalls in Airway Management

In blast injuries burns may be *combined with skeletal and/or soft tissue lesions* that may progress rapidly to serious airway compromise. Insertion of an orotracheal airway may not be possible at all. The prehospital care provider might also encounter patients with *closed head trauma* whose low Glasgow coma scale score [3–8] may be mistaken for a manifestation of CO or CN poisoning, and in whom nasal intubation is contraindicated because of concerns about an undisclosed basilar skull fracture. A surgical airway through burned skin should be used only as a last resort, because the risk of devastating intrathoracic infection is increased.

2. Early Indications for Intubation

As with any other trauma patient, an impending loss of airway warrants intubation. Intubation is indicated if *stridor* is present at first contact with a patient with an obvious inhalation injury. In case of *hoarseness* or early or increasingly *troublesome work of breathing* with use of accessory respiratory muscles, intubation should be seriously considered.

B. Circulation

Intravenous access may be very difficult to obtain. Veins on the hands and arms on unburned skin are preferable. External jugular and femoral veins are also very suitable be-

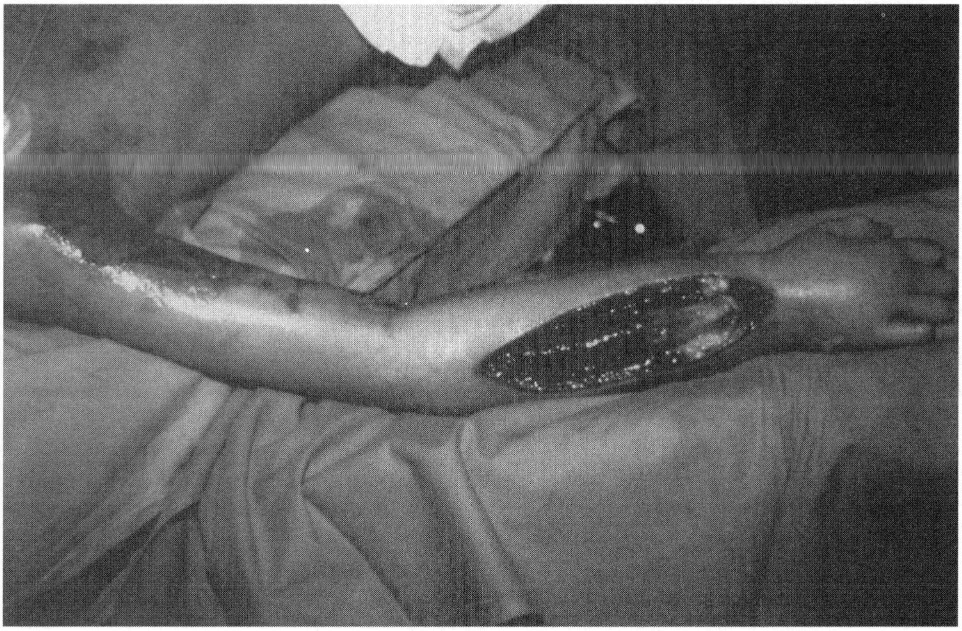

Figure 7 Electrical lesion requiring fasciotomy of forearm in a young boy. (Photo courtesy of B. F. Alsbjorn, M.D.)

cause they easily accommodate large-bore intravenous cannulas. Other central veins (internal jugular and subclavian) should be used only when in desperate need, which is rarely encountered under prehospital conditions. In children <7 years old intraosseus access in the proximal tibia can be used as an emergency vascular access.

In this early phase (<1 hr) hypotension is *not* burn-induced hypovolemia. Other causes such as blunt abdominal or thoracic trauma or neurogenic shock should be sought. If vascular access is not achieved after a few attempts in the prehospital setting, further attempts should not delay transport to the nearest facility, where surgical vascular access can be achieved. In patients with high-voltage injuries not only escharotomy but also fasciotomy should be considered before transfer over a longer distance (Fig. 7).

VI. PAIN MANAGEMENT

Lukewarm tap water provides excellent pain therapy. With a water atomizer the burned area can be soaked constantly with water, minimizing the risk of profound hypothermia, while the patient is transferred to an ambulance with the full heat turned on (approximately 25°C) as soon as possible (Fig. 8).

It is generally agreed that the intense pain after a burn injury in the acute phase should be treated with small doses of opioids given intravenously. Administration subcutaneously or even intramuscularly may lead to unpredictable absorption because of the impending hypoperfusion. Chambers and Guly described the safe and successful prehospital use of intravenous nalbuphine administered to burn patients by trained paramedics [16]. It seems as if benzodiazepines (e.g., lorazepam) may have a place as an adjunct to opioid

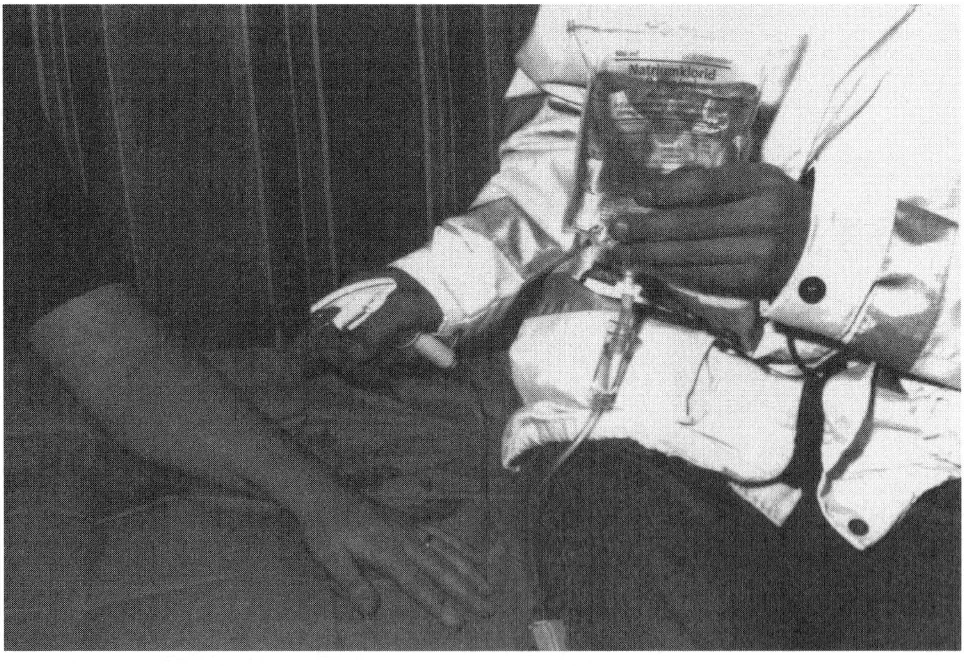

Figure 8 Cooling burned forearm with water from atomizer. (Photo courtesy of M. Nielsen, Copenhagen Fire Department.)

analgesics in the treatment of burn pain [17]. Some patients with limited thermal skin injury may benefit from entonox (50% N_2O, 50% O_2).

A. Local Skin Therapy

Edema formation is caused in part by histamine release from mast cells in the early phase after the burn. Histamine release is inhibited by (water) cooling [18,19]. This cooling treatment may also limit the injury in depth. It is used throughout Europe, but is not recommended in advanced trauma life support (ATLS) training [20]. The use of ice is not recommended.

VII. INITIAL FLUID THERAPY

The Lund–Broder chart gives a rough estimate of TBSA (the rule of nines; Figs. 9, 10).

Children's heads are also relatively larger, representing 18% in infancy, with a de-

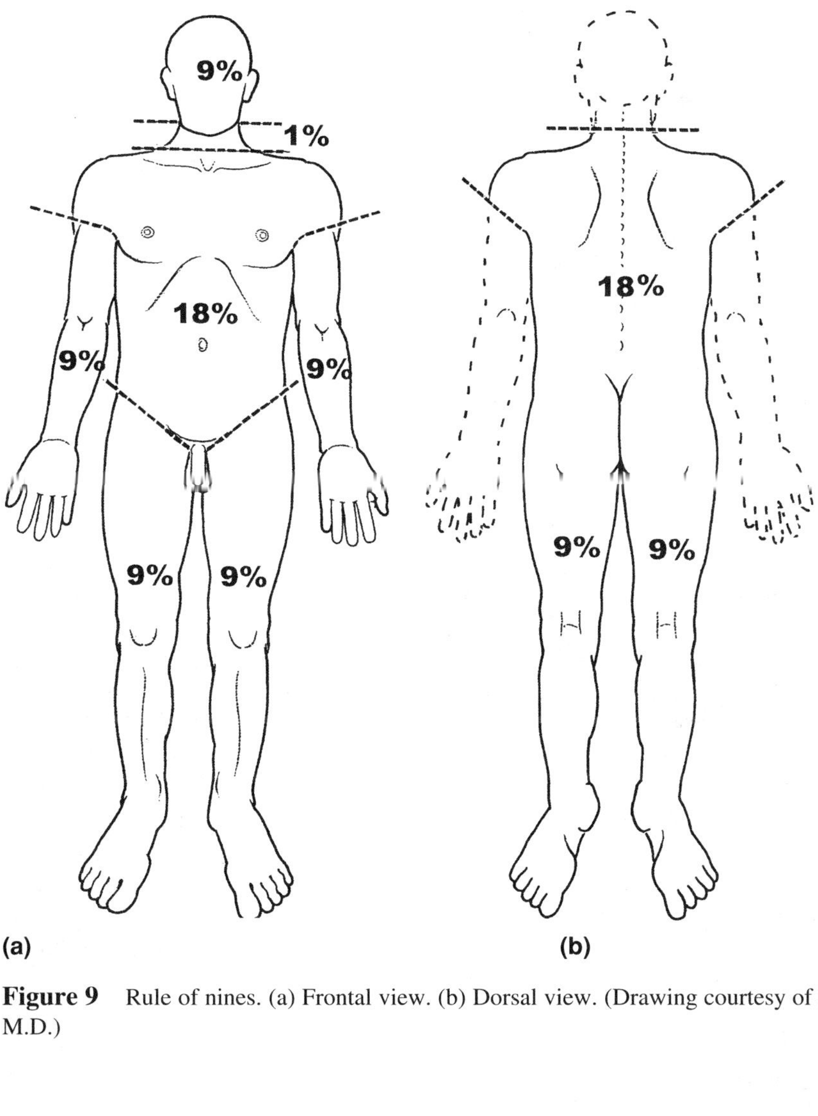

(a) (b)

Figure 9 Rule of nines. (a) Frontal view. (b) Dorsal view. (Drawing courtesy of P. G. Skanning, M.D.)

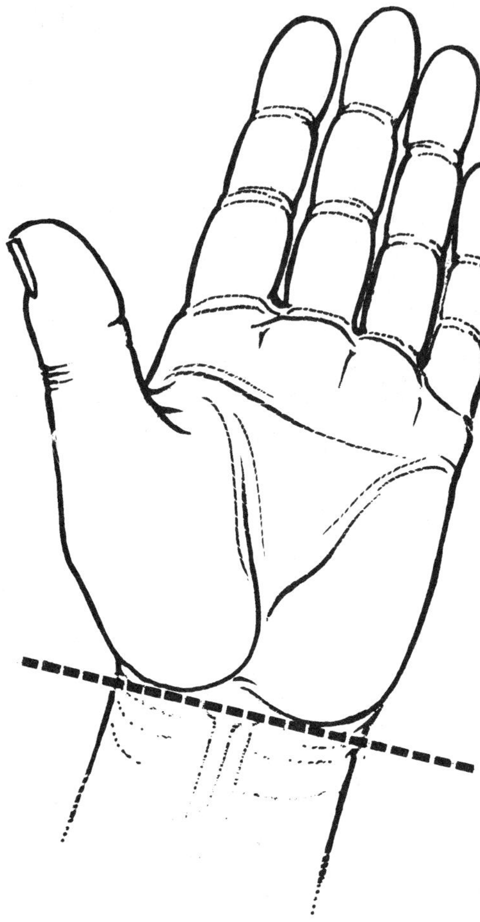

Figure 10 A child's hand, from wrist to fingertips, is approximately 1% of total surface area. (Drawing courtesy of P. G. Skanning, M.D.)

creasing proportion with age. The amount of resuscitation fluid is estimated on the basis of TBSA. In the past, several regimens have been used. A randomized but not blinded trial of dextran versus lactated Ringer's solution showed that resuscitation could be accomplished with both solutions and with equal mortality, but the Ringer's group had a significantly higher urinary output [21]. According to Gunn et al., hypertonic sodium lactate offers no advantage compared with normotonic lactated Ringer's (LR) solution [22]. Combination of hypertonic saline *and* dextran (HSD) versus LR showed in an experimental situation that the volume required to restore cardiac output and oxygen delivery was significantly lower in the HSD group [23]. At a later stage (24 hr) some formulas incorporate such colloids as dextran, albumin, or hydroxyethyl starch. Early administration of colloids (pentastarch, albumin) carries the risk of increased and prolonged interstitial edema [24]. In spite of all these possibilities, the most popular formula by far is the Parkland formula, which is used worldwide and recommended by ATLS.

4 ml/kg/TBSA/24 hr of LR

Table 3 Criteria for Contact With a Burn Center

1. Second- or third-degree burns >10% TBSA in children <10 years of age or adults >50 years of age
2. Second- or third-degree burns >20% TBSA in other age groups
3. Third-degree burns >5% TBSA
4. Second- or third-degree burns involving face, hands, feet, genitalia, perineum, and major joints
5. Electrical burns, including those caused by lightning
6. Chemical burns
7. Burns with inhalation injury
8. Burns in patients with significant coexisting disease or trauma
9. Whenever second opinion is sought.

Source: Modified from Ref. 24a.

Based on observation of 51 patients with proved inhalation injury, Navar et al. concluded that the amount of LR needed to maintain urine output of 30 to 50 ml/hr was 40% higher than in patients without inhalation injury [25].

If the rehydration process is not carefully monitored, there is a risk of inducing congestive heart failure.

VIII. WHO NEEDS TO GO TO A BURN CENTER OR HYPERBARIC CENTER?

Criteria for transfer to or at least contact with a burn center are shown in Table 3. If the transportation distance is more than moderate (>½ hr), it is recommended that the patient be taken to the nearest facility for stabilization in order to determine the magnitude of the burn, secure the airway, and establish vascular access. In inexperienced hands there is a tendency to overestimate the extent of the burn and to underestimate the severity of scalds [19].

Several trials have supported the efficacy of (HBO) therapy in the treatment of CO intoxication [26,27]. In 1999 Scheinkestel et al. published the results a well-conducted randomized double-blind trial involving 191 patients in which neurologic sequelae were assessed in patients with CO poisoning after treatment with hyperbaric oxygen versus normobaric oxygen (NBO). They found a worse outcome *after HBO as compared to NBO* [28]. This area awaits further investigation until changes in recommendations are generally accepted (Table 4). The treatment of thermal injuries within HBO has yielded conflicting

Table 4 Conditions Associated With CO Intoxication Requiring Treatment With Hyperbaric Oxygen (HBO)

1. History of loss of consciousness, presumably due to CO toxicity
2. Neurologic symptoms other than slight headache
3. Cardiac ischemia on ECG or clinically
4. Carboxyhemoglobin (HBCO) >25% after 2 hr breathing normobaric oxygen
5. Pregnancy with HBCO > 10% or signs of fetal distress

evidence [29,30]. The data presented so far *do not* support direct referral of burn patients to a facility with an HBO unit.

IX. MASS BURN CASUALTIES

Even though fire disasters have been an uncommon experience during the past 20 years, they demonstrate that planning and policy making need to be done *prior* to the incident. There are striking differences as to whether a disaster occurs outdoors or indoors. Outdoor fire disasters are characterized by a large number of victims with a small number of fatalities on the scene, therefore a large number of patients will reach the hospital with a significant late mortality rate. Indoor fire disasters cause a large number of deaths because of inhalation of CO and CN^-. In terms of treatment, the majority of the wounds are <30% TBSA or >70% TBSA [13].

X. TRIAGE

The key concept in triage is making the best use of the available resources with respect to the medical possibilities, the possibility of saving of an individual versus saving the group, and the amount and the quality of transportation available. The triage of large numbers of burn victims remains a highly complex problem. Planning must include expert triage, as only a minority of the victims will need rapid transfer to a burn unit [13].

XI. CONCLUSION

1. In patients with facial or neck burns inhalation injury should be anticipated. The situation may progress within minutes into respiratory insufficiency.
2. For burns >15% TBSA, infusion of intravenous lactated Ringer's solution is instituted.
3. Prompt cooling with water is a excellent pain treatment and may reduce the depth of the burn.
4. All opioid analgesics should be given intravenously.
5. In the prehospital situation hypotension *is not* caused by burn shock. Hypovolemia due to thoracic or abdominal lesion is the most likely explanation.
6. Avoid overhydration, especially in elderly burn patients.
7. Despite conflicting evidence, hyperbaric oxygen therapy is still indicated in CO intoxication.

REFERENCES

1. AE Waller, SW Marshall, JD Langley. Adult thermal injuries in New Zealand resulting in death and hospitalization. Burns 24:245–251, 1998.
1a. RS Cotran et al. The delayed and prolonged vascular leakage in inflammation II. An electron microscope study of the vascular response after thermal injury. Am J Pathol 46:589–620, 1965.
2. T Lund, H Wiig, RK Reed. Acute postburn edema: Role of strongly negative interstitial fluid pressure. Am J Physiol 255:H1069–H1074, 1988.
3. T Lund, H Onarheim, H Wigg, RK Reed. Mechanisms behind increased dermal imbibition pressure in acute burn edema. Am J Physiol 256:H940–H948, 1989.

4. CR Baxter, T Shires. Physiological response to crystalloid resuscitation of severe burns. Ann NY Acad Sci 150:874–894, 1968.
5. J Martyn, RS Wilson, JF Burke. Right ventricular function and pulmonary hemodynamics during dopamine infusion in burned patients. Chest 89:357–360, 1986.
6. PH Breen, SA Isserles, J Westley, MF Roizen. Combined carbon monoxide and cyanide poisoning: A place for treatment? Anesth Analg 80:671–677, 1995.
7. JE Cottrell, P Casthely, JD Brodie, K Patel, A Klein, H Turndorf. Prevention of nitroprusside-induced cyanide toxicity with hydroxycobolamin. New Eng J Med 298:809–811, 1978.
8. JR Saffle, B Davis, P Williams. Recent outcome in the treatment of burn injury in the United States: A report from the American Burn Association Patient Registry. J Burn Care Rehab 16:219–232, 1995.
9. RS Lee. Injury by electrical forces: Pathophysiology, manifestations and therapy. Curr Prob Surg 34:684–764, 1997.
10. JL Hunt, AD Mason, TS Masterson, BA Pruitt. The pathophysiology of the acute electrical injuries. J Trauma 16:335–340, 1976.
11. B Ponten, U Erikson, SH Johansson, et al. New observation on tissue changes along the pathway of the current in an electrical injury. Scand J Plast Reconstr Surg 4:75–80, 1970.
12. LC Labarge, PA Ballard, RK Daniel. Experimental electrical burns: Low voltage. Ann Plast Surg 13:185–190, 1984.
13. G Arturson. Analysis of severe fire disasters. In: M Masellis, SWA Gunn, eds. The Management of Mass Burn Casualties and Fire Disasters: Proceedings of the First International Conference on Burns and Fire Disasters. Dordrecht/Boston/London: Kluwer Academic, pp. 24–33, 1992.
14. AKM Khoo, ST Lee, WT Poh. Tracheobronchial cytology in inhalation injury. J Trauma 42: 81–85, 1997.
15. A Lechleuthner, A Schmidt-Barbo, B Bouillon, W Perbix, J Holzki, G Spilker. Prehospital care of burns: An analysis of 3 years use of the emergency physician system (EPS) Cologne. Burns 19:153–157, 1993.

15a. AKM Khoo, ST Lee, WT Poh. Tracheobronchial cytology in inhalation injury. J Trauma 42: 81–85, 1997.

16. JA Chambers, HR Guly. Prehospital intravenous nalbuphine administered by paramedics. Resuscitation 27:153–158, 1994.
17. DR Patterson, JT Ptacek, GJ Carrougher, SR Sharar. Lorazepam as an adjunct to opioid analgesics in the treatment of burn pain. Pain 72:367–374, 1997.
18. JV Boykin, E Eriksson, MM Sholley, RN Pittman. Cold-water treatment of scald injury and inhibition of histamine-mediated burn edema. J Surg Res 31:111–123, 1981.
19. JWL Davies. Prompt cooling of burned areas: A review of benefits and the effector mechanisms. Burns 6:1–6, 1982.
20. GM Beer, P Kompatscher. Standardization of the first aid treatment of burn injuries in Vorarlberg, Austria. Burns 22:130–134, 1996.
21. KV Hall, B Sørensen. The treatment of burn shock: Results of a 5-year randomized, controlled clinical trial of Dextran 70 v. Ringer lactate solution. Burns 5:107–112, 1979.
22. ML Gunn, JF Hansbrough, JW Davies, SR Furst, TO Field. Prospective randomized trial of hypertonic sodium lactate versus lactated Ringer's solution for burn shock resuscitation. J Trauma 29:1261–1267, 1989.
23. SM Milner, MP Kinsky, SC Guha, DN Herndon, LG Philips, GC Kramer. A comparison of two different 2400 mOsm solutions for resuscitation of major burns. J Burn Care Rehab 18: 109–115, 1997.
24. K Waxman, R Holness, G Tominaga, P Chela, J Grimes. Hemodynamic and oxygen transport effects of pentastarch in burn resuscitation. Ann Surg 209:341–345, 1989.

24a. American Burns Association. Hospital and prehospital resources for optimal care of patients with burn injury: Guidelines for development and operation of burn centers. J Burn Care Rehab 11:97–104, 1990.

25. PD Navar, JR Saffle, GD Warden. Effect of inhalation injury on fluid requirements after thermal injury. Am J Surg 150:716–720, 1985.
26. SR Thom, RL Taber, II Mendiguren, LM Clark, KR Hardy, AB Fisher. Delayed neuropsychologic sequelae after carbon monoxide poisoning: Prevention by treatment with hyperbaric oxygen. Ann Emerg Med 25:474–480, 1995.
27. JI Ducasse, P Celsis, JP Marc-Vergnes. Non-comatose patients with acute carbon monoxide poisoning: Hyperbaric or normobaric oxygenation? Undersea Hyperbar Med 22:9–15, 1995.
28. CD Scheinkestel, M Bailey, PS Myles, K Jones, DJ Cooper, IL Millar, DV Tuxen. Hyperbaric or normobaric oxygen for acute carbon monoxide poisoning: A randomised controlled clinical trial. Med J Aust 170:203–210, 1999.
29. AL Brennan, J Still, M Haynes, H Orlet, F Rosenblum, E Law, WO Thompson. A randomized prospective trial of hyperbaric oxygen in a referral burn center population. Am Surg 63:205–208, 1997.
30. JA Niezgoda, P Cianci, BW Folden, RL Ortega, JB Slade, AB Storrow. The effect of hyperbaric oxygen therapy on a burn wound model in human volunteers. Plast Reconstr Surg 99: 1620–1625, 1997.

30

Emergency Management of Injury from the Release of Toxic Substances: Medical Aspects of the HAZMAT System

DAVID J. BAKER

Hôpital-Necker Enfants Malades, Paris, France

HANS-R. PASCHEN

Amalie Sieveking-Krankenhaus, Hamburg, Germany

I. INTRODUCTION

There is growing awareness by emergency medical system (EMS) personnel of the problems of managing of the injured following the release of toxic substances [1,2]. Although such incidents are relatively rare, when they do occur they may cause mass casualties and can rapidly overwhelm the existing medical services [3]. The management of toxic trauma differs from conventional physical trauma since, although many of the injuries may be immediate and accompanied by burns and blast trauma, there may be insidious development of toxic injury far beyond the site of the incident. There is also a risk of toxic injury to the EMS responders through contamination from the site and the patients themselves. Thus, EMS personnel must be familiar with the characteristics of toxic release, protocols for containment of toxic substances, individual, and site safety, safe casualty decontamination, treatment, and evacuation. They must above all be able to work as part of a coordinated response involving other emergency services.

II. HAZMAT

A toxic substance or agent may be defined as any substance that is injurious to health in an uncontained state. There are many thousands of such substances in civil life that are under the control of the United Nations Hazardous Materials Convention (HAZMAT). HAZMAT provides an internationally recognized system for (1) the recognition of toxic substances in production, storage and transport, (2) a database of properties and management of toxic agents, (3) the medical effects and treatment protocols, (4) containment and decontamination procedures, and (5) the types of protection required for safe operations. All EMS personnel should be aware of the essentials of the HAZMAT system [4,5].

III. PLANNING FOR HAZMAT INCIDENTS

Preplanning for HAZMAT incidents must take place in conjunction with other emergency services, notably the fire department, which usually has overall control in a toxic release incident. The following points are of importance in the consideration of planning for toxic mass casualties [6]:

1. The aim should be to minimize adverse health effects.
2. Public health authorities are recognized as having the lead role in many countries, but they do not necessarily have the required expertise in the primary management of casualties.
3. A multidisciplinary approach is necessary and should involve the health ministries, the local fire department, local and regional health authorities, members of the health professions, hospitals and other treatment centers, EMS responders, and pharmacists.
4. There should be an assessment of the practical resources available, their location, and who has authority for their release.
5. Information and communications are of vital importance.
6. There is a need for a good reporting system for the scale of the incident and its likely consequences.

IV. RECOGNITION OF A HAZMAT INCIDENT

Release of HAZMAT agents may take place due to a leakage or an explosion that may or may not be accompanied by fire. Therefore, depending on the nature of the incident, the toxic hazard may be revealed or concealed and its nature identified or not identified. Local visual clues may provide the first warnings, and EMS responders should maintain a high level of caution before entering the site. If a tanker is involved in a road accident with a leak of a noxious substance, the HAZMAT nature of the incident will be clear, particularly if there is a HAZMAT placard visible on the tanker. Similarly, an accident in an industrial setting should arouse suspicions, particularly if HAZMAT placards are visible. Unexplained signs and symptoms in casualties may often be the first indication of a HAZMAT incident [7].

V. RESPONSE

If a HAZMAT incident is evident it must be declared quickly and steps taken immediately to cordon off the area and warn those in danger of downwind contamination. Normally these steps will be taken by the controlling fire services, but it is possible that an EMS crew may arrive at the scene first. If this is the case the fire authorities should be alerted.

Table 1 Goals of the HAZMAT Responder

Protect yourself. Approach the scene cautiously arriving upwind. Maintain a safe distance and inspect the scene from a nearby elevated area such as a hill. Inspect the established exclusion zones and resist the temptation to rush in to attempt a rescue. If a command post has been established, report to the incident commander.
Identify the chemical. Be familiar with the Department of Transportation (DOT) placard system and the National Fire Protection Association (NFPA) hazard labeling system, material safety data sheets (MSDS), and shipping papers.
Consult the appropriate protocol and local sources to obtain information about the chemical, its health effects, and medical treatment.
Determine the potential for secondary contamination (transmissibility). Understand the risk to yourself and others in the support zone, ambulance, or hospital if decontamination is not completed at the scene.
Perform appropriate and thorough decontamination.
Provide basic and toxic advanced life support (TOXALS).
Transport victims to an appropriate medical facility as quickly as possible.

Source: Modified from Ref. 5.

The EMS team should follow the standard goals of the HAZMAT responder (Table 1) and should take all reasonable actions to avoid becoming the next casualties. In many countries, there is an information service provided by the chemical industry to assist fire and other emergency response services. In addition, large chemical companies run their own fire services and are able to send special teams to the site of a toxic incident.

VI. HAZARD IDENTIFICATION

HAZMAT information is available from many sources in the form of reference manuals, and printed and electronic databases. Toxic compounds are divided into nine groups, depending on their physicochemical and pathophysiological properties. Each substance has a U.N. code number, which allows rapid determination of its nature and properties. In addition, special information cards carried in the transport vehicle provide detailed information from the manufacturer. These and database sources provide information on the identity of the compound, and its class, as well as methods of fire fighting and control, decontamination and medical treatment. HAZMAT placards seen on transporters and buildings in which hazardous materials are stored provide an immediate alert to the presence of HAZMAT. The exact nature of the placard varies nationally, and readers are advised to consult the exact system operating in their own country [4]. Figure 1 shows examples of HAZMAT warning placards used in the United States and Europe.

VII. INCIDENT ORGANIZATION

Emergency medical system personnel arriving at an incident at which there are indications of a toxic release should inform the fire and police departments immediately and remain clear of the site (uphill and upwind if possible) until a fully protected medical response team is available. After a HAZMAT incident has been declared the first task of the incident commander is to ensure the identification of contaminated (hot), decontaminated (warm),

The Kemmler Plate

The numerical hazard lists the primary hazard first, then the lesser hazards. If a number is repeated, this means the hazard is intensified. For example

3	Flammable liquid
33	Highly flammable liquid
333	Spontaneously flammable liquid
333X	Spontaneously flammable liquid which reacts violently with water

HAZMAT classes

1	Explosives
2	Gas under pressure
3	Flammable liquids
4	Flammable solids
5	Oxidizing agents
6	Poisons
7	Radioactive substances
8	Corrosive agents
9	Miscellaneous

Hazard identification by class
U.N. Product Number

The UKHIS Plate or HAZCHEM Placard

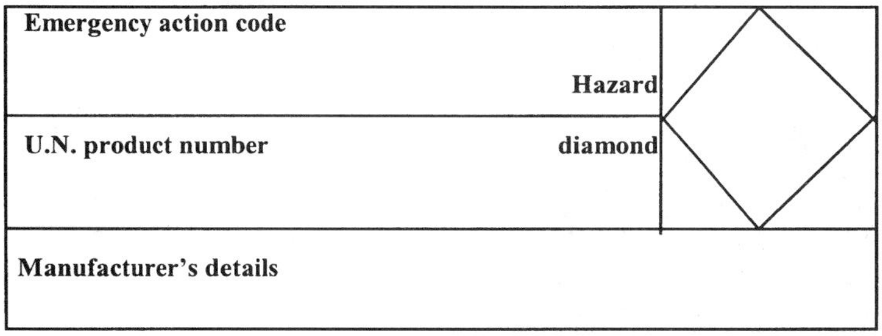

There are 4 elements:
1. The emergency action code
2. The U.N.'s product number
3. The hazard diamond
4. Manufacturer's details

The first figure of the emergency action code tells the fire service how to fight the fire, whether with jets, fog, foam, or dry agent. The middle letter indicates what protective clothing must be worn when dealing with the hazard, and whether it must be contained or can safely be washed into the storm drains. If the letter "E" is present at the end of the code, this means "consider evacuation." The medical team should stay clear until it is safe to approach.

Figure 1 HAZMAT identification plates. Hazardous materials are identified by a toxic class and identification code. There are national variations in the way this information is presented. Examples are shown from European Union.

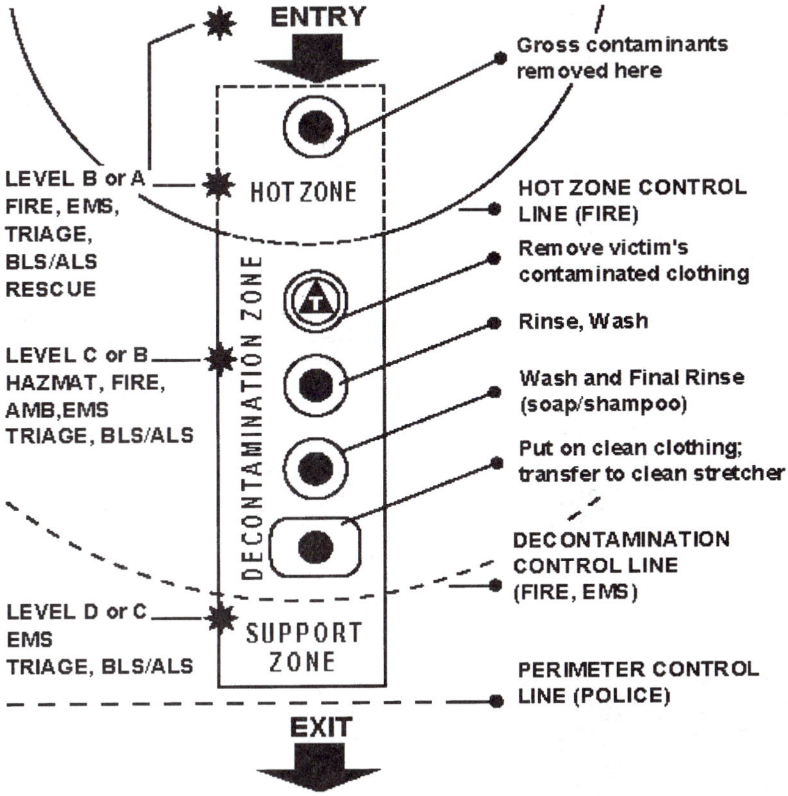

Figure 2 The organization of a HAZMAT incident. (From Ref. 5.)

and decontaminated (cold) zones (Fig. 2) [5]. These will need careful enforcement through a cordon since many persons caught inside the zones will try to get as far away from the accident as possible. In many cases they will present themselves, undecontaminated to the nearest medical facility, thereby exposing the medical staff to risk. Emergency medical system personnel may only enter the decontamination zone wearing suitable protective equipment to avoid injury to themselves. When a persistent toxic hazard has been released casualties will require decontamination. If the exact nature of the release is in doubt the requirement for decontamination should be assumed. There may be life-threatening delays in removing victims through decontamination from the hot zone, and so medical care may be required in the decontamination zone by specially trained and equipped personnel. Medical responders should, therefore, know how to use protective equipment and understand procedures for decontamination.

VIII. PROTECTIVE AND DECONTAMINATION PROCEDURES

Personal protective equipment used in HAZMAT incidents is graded according to four levels A—D (Table 2); ordinary street clothing is designated as level D [1]. Fire personnel will use a level A suit, which includes a self-contained breathing apparatus for the most toxic hazards or where identity of the hazard is uncertain (Fig. 3). Emergency medical

Table 2 Protection Levels in HAZMAT Incidents

Level	Personal protective equipment (PPE)
A	Positive-pressure self-contained breathing apparatus (SCBA). Fully encapsulating chemical-resistant suit. Double layer of chemical-resistant gloves. Chemical-resistant boots. Airtight seal between the suit, and the gloves and boots.
B	Positive-pressure self-contained breathing apparatus (SCBA). Chemical-resistant, long-sleeved suit. Double layer of chemical-resistant gloves. Chemical-resistant boots.
C	Full-face, air purification device (respirator). Chemical-resistant suit. Chemical-resistant outer gloves. Chemical-resistant boots.
D	Equipment does not provide specific respiratory or skin protection and usually consists of regular work clothes.

Source: Ref. 1.

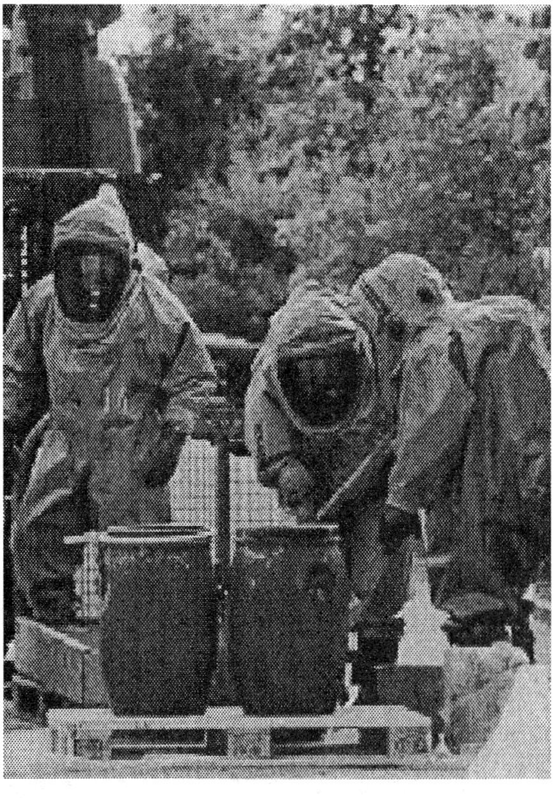

Figure 3 Responders to HAZMAT incident wearing level A protective suit. (Courtesy of the Hamburg Fire Service, Hamburg, Germany.)

system personnel working on patients in the decontamination zone will wear level C protection, which includes a protective suit and gloves and a facemask with a device to filter the ambient atmosphere.

IX. EXTRICATION, DECONTAMINATION, AND TRIAGE

The victims will be extracted wherever possible from the high-risk hot zone by fire personnel and moved the start of the decontamination zone. Decontamination starts with the removal of gross contaminants followed by a multistage decontamination in the decontamination zone. The question of integration of decontamination with triage of casualties has recently been considered in some detail by the Parisian fire service as part of an urban response plan to toxic terrorist attack [8].

X. ADVANCED LIFE SUPPORT IN THE CONTAMINATED ZONE: TOXALS

The enforced delay due to decontamination and evacuation of toxic casualties may cause increased morbidity or mortality. There is thus a need to bring ALS as far forward as possible in the HAZMAT management scheme. This concept has been designated by ITACCS as toxic advanced life support (TOXALS) [9,10] which may be defined as the application of advanced life support procedures in a contaminated or potentially contaminated environment by specially trained and protected emergency personnel.

The protocols of TOXALS may be summarized by an extension of the familiar ABC system for emergency life support which are shown in Table 3.

Table 3 Toxic Advanced Life Support (TOXALS) Protocols

A: Assessment and airway. Assessment must be of both the environment and of the patient through a primary survey, remembering that physical injury may accompany toxic trauma. Before entry to a contaminated zone the nature of the hazard must be determined if possible from the HAZMAT placards and other information. If reliable information is not available a persistent, transmissible threat must be assumed.

B: Breathing. The assessment of breathing in toxic trauma relies on rate, form, and depth. Because of the need for personal protection, normal respiratory assessment by auscultation will not normally be available. There must therefore be special reliance on observation and palpation. Modern level C equipment allows good voice communication through the protective mask, and it will be possible to ask the patient simple questions and assess the response.

C: Circulatory support. This will be necessary following haemorrhage and dysrhythmlas which result from a number of toxic hazards. It may be necessary to gain intravenous access during decontamination which will require practice beforehand wearing gloves.

D: Decontamination. The requirement for decontamination depends on the persistency of the toxic hazard. Patients affected by gases and vapors will not normally require decontamination [1]. In cases in which the nature of the toxic release is in doubt all patients should undergo full decontamination.

Disability. Disability from both toxic and traumatic causes must be assessed from a primary survey, which will allow triage.

E: Evacuation. This will be initially from the contaminated to the decontamination zones. Triage of the patients is required after entry to the decontamination zone. After decontamination is complete transfer will be possible to the clean (decontaminated) zone and then to hospital care.

XI. PRACTICAL ASPECTS OF TOXALS

A. Airway Management

The immediate life-threatening aspects of toxic trauma arise principally from the effects on the respiratory system. Damage is possible at all levels of the respiratory tract with varying latency, depending on the nature of the hazard. Many toxic hazards are very irritating and produce a massive outpouring of secretions and upper airway blockage. In addition, there may be laryngeal, bronchial, and bronchiolar spasm. There may be a reduction in compliance and development of pulmonary edema. Clearance of secretions and vomitus will require an efficient suction device. A Guedel airway should be inserted initially and the patient placed in the lateral position if possible since the risk of vomiting and inhalation is high in toxic incidents. Endotracheal intubation must be regarded as the most desirable option, both for the protection of the airway and for efficient controlled ventilation later. Use of the laryngeal mask airway may be an acceptable compromise given the difficult operating circumstances presented by a toxic release incident, and may provide a useful aid to subsequent intubation [11].

B. Ventilation in a Toxic Environment

If available, oxygen should be given by mask immediately after attention to the airway at the highest achievable concentration. Oxygen availability and resupply may be limited in a contaminated zone, however. Intermittent positive pressure ventilation will be required for developing or complete respiratory failure. The practical possibilities in a contaminated zone are for the use of a modified bag–valve–mask (BVM) device or an automatic ventilator. A suitable BVM must incorporate a filter system. Various versions of filters are available commercially and can be selected according to the hazards faced. It is important to note that unless they are specially prepared, most filters are ineffective against carbon monoxide. The BVM provides an effective first response, but has the disadvantage of the unprotected airway and therefore potentially gastric insufflation since there may be a tendency to overventilate by hand in an emergency [12].

Controlled automatic ventilation is a better solution, particularly for ventilation during possibly prolonged periods of decontamination and evacuation. A portable gas-powered ventilator which is a volume preset flow generator with a peak flow rate of 40 litres/min. and an appropriate inspiratory time gives better ventilation in conditions of decreasing compliance and increasing resistance, and results in less gastric insufflation when used with a pharyngeal mask [13]. There are two possibilities for emergency automatic ventilation in a toxic environment: (1) to deliver 100% oxygen using a conventional gas-powered automatic emergency ventilator, or (2) to use a ventilator capable of filtering the ambient atmosphere and using it as a driving gas. The first option is limited by the need for a resupply of bottled oxygen, which may be difficult in a HAZMAT incident. Recently a portable emergency ventilator capable of operation in a contaminated zone through filtration of the ambient atmosphere by a battery-powered internal compressor supplemented by bottled oxygen has been produced from a military design [13]. It should be noted that many portable ventilators offer an air-mix mode delivering approximately 50% oxygen by entraining ambient air. This mode should never be used for ventilation in a contaminated environment.

C. Monitoring and Further Assessment

Even basic patient monitoring may be difficult in the contaminated zone (the monitors used must be capable of decontamination), but monitoring should be started if possible after transfer to the decontaminated zone. Pulse oximetry and end-tidal CO2 should be measured in patients undergoing continued emergency ventilation. After decontamination and transfer to the cold zone the patient can be examined (with careful auscultation), and full conventional monitoring can be attached.

D. Pharmacological Support

Pharmacological support is important in the management of toxic injury, particularly for the respiratory effects, and may be started inside the contaminated zone. Guided by the HAZMAT database [4], correct measures will reverse the compliance and resistance changes and improve the ventilation. Specific antidotes are available for certain intoxications. Organophosphate (OP) poisoning, either from pesticide or military nerve agent release, is treated with anticholinergics and oximes. To antgonize the muscarinic effects of OP poisoning patients should receive 2 mg atropine IV every 15 min until adequate atropinization has been established. The pediatric dosage is 0.05 mg/kg repeated every 15 min as necessary.

Oximes can regenerate acetyl choline esterase in cases of pesticide poisoning and following exposure to some nerve agents [14]. Pralidoxime is the oxime most widely spread throughout the world and has been used extensively in developing countries. However, in vitro and in vivo studies of toxigonin have indicated that this oxime may be more effective in pesticide poisoning [15] but should be used in higher doses than previously indicated. The dosage of pralidoxime is 1 gram IV given over 30 to 60 min with a maximum infusion rate of 0.5 grams per min for adults and 20 to 50 mg/kg over 30 to 60 min with a maximum infusion rate of half the total dose per minute in children. Oxime therapy should be started as soon as possible after exposure to organophosphates. In many armed forces around the world autoinjector devices containing atropine, oxime, and diazepam as an anticonvulsant are available for immediate postexposure use.

Many HAZMAT compounds give rise to toxic pulmonary edema and bronchospasm, and the place of systemic and inhaled corticosteroids has been the subject of considerable debate. Although steroids have proved to be of value in the management of severe bronchospasm their role in preventing the onset of pulmonary edema is less clear. On balance, however, certain authors feel that the use of high-dose methyl prednisolone given as soon as possible after exposure is of value in phosgene poisoning, and this may also apply to other pulmonary edemagens [16].

There are many differences in the availability and use of antidotes around the world, and the reader is advised to consult specialized national formularies for further details. Many countries operate online poison information services that can provide information in addition to that available from the HAZMAT sources.

XII. CONTINUING CARE

There are many aspects of toxic trauma that develop some time after injury. The development of toxic respiratory failure and pulmonary edema may be latent, and therefore special care should be taken to monitor patients during evacuation to the hospital and inside the hospital department itself. All patients who have been exposed to potentially toxic edema-producing compounds should rest and be monitored for at least 24 hr with usual respiratory radiographic and physiological respiratory investigations. Early and effective emergency management may lead to a reduced risk of developing adult respiratory distress syndrome (ARDS) later. Hospital management should also take account of developing neurological and neuromuscular lesions and critical care facilities will be required for the most seriously injured [17].

XIII. CONCLUSIONS

Injury from mass toxic release is increasingly likely, given the large quantities of toxic compounds currently being produced and transported, and EMS personnel should be aware of the risks and correct management.

The U.N. HAZMAT system provides an internationally recognized classification of toxic hazards with a coding system that allows rapid identification and access to information concerning protection, decontamination, and treatment.

EMS personnel should be familiar with the organization of a HAZMAT incident and essential protective procedures if they are to avoid becoming the next casualties.

Suitably trained and protected EMS personnel will be able to provide essential life support for patients in a contaminated zone (TOXALS).

Through good planning and awareness, the special problems of toxic release incidents, although relatively rare, may be handled with confidence by medical responders working in conjunction with other special emergency services.

REFERENCES

1. J Borak, M Callan, W Abbott. Hazardous Materials Exposure: Emergency Response and Patient Care. NJ: Prentice Hall, 1991.
2. HW Levitin, HJ Siegelson. Hazardous materials disaster medical planning and response. Emer Med Clin North Am 14:327–349, 1996.
3. Calamity at Bhopal. Lancet 1378–1379, 1984.
4. AC Bronstein, PL Currance. Emergency Care for Hazardous Materials Exposure. 2nd ed. Mosby Lifeline, 1994.
5. U.S. Dept. of Health and Human Services, Public Health Services Agency for Toxic Substances. Managing Hazardous Materials Incidents. vols. 1–3, 1995.
6. TMM Moles. Emergency medical services systems and HAZMAT major incidents. Resuscitation 42:103–116, 1999.
7. T Okumura et al. The Tokyo subway sarin attack: Disaster management. Part 2: Hospital response. Ann Emerg Med 618–624, 1998.
8. JF Laurent, F Richter, A Michel. Management of the victims of urban chemical attack: The French approach. Resuscitation 42, 1999.
9. DJ Baker. Advanced life support for toxic injury (TOXALS): Eur J Emerg Med 3:256–262, 1996.
10. DJ Baker. Management of respiratory failure in toxic disasters. Resuscitation 42:103–116, 1999.
11. RM Levitan, EA Ochroch, S Stuart, JE Hollander. Use of the intubating laryngeal mask airway by medical and nonmedical personnel. Am J Emerg Med 18:12–16, 2000.
12. G Updike, VN Mosesso Jr, TE Auble, E Delgado. Comparison of bag-valve-mask, manually triggered ventilator, and automated ventilator devices used while ventilating a nonintubated mannikin model. Prehosp Emerg Care 2:52–55, 1998.
13. DJ Baker. The CompPac: A new approach to field and general emergency ventilation. Internat Rev Armed For Med Serv LXXI (10/11/12):284–287, 1998.
14. J Tafuri, J Roberts. Organophosphate poisoning. Ann Emerg Med 16:193–202, 1987.
15. F Worek, M Baecker, H Thiermann, et al. Reappraisal of indications and limitations of oxime therapy in organophosphate poisoning. Human Exper Toxicol 16:466–472, 1997.
16. WF Diller. Therapeutic strategy in phosgene poisoning. Toxicol Ind Health 1:93–99, 1985.
17. JL de Bleeker. The intermediate syndrome in organophosphate poisoning: An overview of experimental and clinical observations. J Toxicol Clin Toxicol 33:683–686, 1995.

31

Near-Drowning

WALTER HASIBEDER and WOLFGANG SCHOBERSBERGER

The Leopold Franzens University of Innsbruck, Innsbruck, Austria

I. DEFINITIONS

Drowning has been defined as death by submersion in a liquid. In contrast, near-drowning is survival or at least temporary survival of a patient beyond 23 hr following a submersion accident. Unfortunately, a variety of other modified definitions exist in the medical literature, which in the authors' opinion cause confusion more than adding important information to the problems surrounding drowning accidents. Depending on the presence or absence of lung pathophysiology a differentiation has been made between dry and wet drowning. Secondary drowning has been defined as an accident in which death occurs some time after initial resuscitation because of severe acute lung injury due to fluid aspiration. In the German literature the term secondary drowning is used for patients developing acute lung injury with a time delay after fluid aspiration, regardless of their outcome. To help alleviate the confusion caused by differences in terminology the term near-drowning should be reserved for patients surviving a submersion accident beyond 23 hr, regardless of the presence or absence of fluid aspiration and acute lung injury.

II. EPIDEMIOLOGY

It is estimated that 3.5 deaths per 100,000 population are caused by drowning accidents worldwide. In the United States approximately 8000 people drown per year and death caused by submersion represents the second most common cause of accidental death in children, exceeded only by motor vehicle accidents [1,2]. In the years 1971 to 1988, 45,680 unintentional, nonboat-related drowning deaths were reported among children through 19-years-old in the United States [2]. Drowning is the third leading cause of death in children between 1 and 14 years of age, and the leading cause of injury death among toddlers aged 1 and 2 years [2].

Regarding the location of submersion accidents, adolescents and teenagers are more likely to drown in natural bodies of freshwater. Alcohol consumption and risk-taking behaviors often seem to be associated with these accidents. Toddlers most often drown in residential swimming pools, bathtubs, whirlpools, hot tubs, and buckets [2]. Body part entrapment and hair entanglement in pool and spa drains with suction fittings sometimes play a role. The vast majority of victims drown in their own backyards. Epidemiological studies have shown that the peak time for submersion accidents in children is on warm summer weekends between 3 and 6 P.M. [3]. In most cases parents were occupied with normal household routine at the time of accident. Approximately 40% of infant drowning occurs in bathtubs [2,3]. In unsupervised toddlers 50% of all drowning accidents occur between the ages of 0 and 4 years, although the highest rate is reported in children between 1 and 2 years. One has to keep in mind that especially in infants, drowning may also portray homicide, abuse, or neglect rather than unintentional causes.

An important risk factor for drowning and near-drowning accidents is the presence of a seizure disorder. Patients with epilepsy represent a population with a four to five times higher risk of drowning compared with the normal population [3].

Near-drowning is also the major cause of death from diving accidents [4]. Unfortunately, the pathophysiology of drowning accidents in divers is frequently unknown. Nitrogen anesthesia, panic behavior, or carbon dioxide or carbon monoxide poisoning may all be involved.

III. PATHOPHYSIOLOGY

A. The Lung

The events surrounding drowning accidents in men were described almost 40 years ago by Noble and Sharpe [5]. Victims of drowning accidents usually show an initial phase of panic struggling and swimming movements. Apnea and breath holding occur during the submersion phase and are often followed by the victim's swallowing large amounts of fluid with subsequent vomiting, gasping, and fluid aspiration. Ultimately severe hypoxia leads to unconsciousness, loss of airway reflexes, and further movement of water into the lungs.

In autopsy studies, however, approximately 10% of patients demonstrate no evidence of fluid aspiration. On hospital admission approximately 20% of patients demonstrate no radiographic signs of fluid aspiration [6]. In these patients aspiration was prevented by complete closure of the upper airways. This "laryngospasm" may persist well beyond the death of drowning victims.

In drowning victims two patient populations can therefore be distinguished. First, the majority of patients with fluid aspiration usually develop acute lung injury, often progressing to severe ARDS within a very short time. In these patients severe respiratory failure and hypoxia independent of submersion time may develop at the scene and intubation, mechanical ventilation with positive end expiratory pressure, has to be instituted without delay to prevent hypoxic cardiovascular arrest. The second group of patients are those without aspiration for whom ventilatory support is usually not a major problem in the emergency situation.

Acute lung injury and severe ARDS can be initiated by even small amounts of aspirated fluids. It has been estimated that the volume of aspirated fluids seldom exceeds

3 to 7 ml × kg^{-1} BW in men [7]; therefore in a 70-kg person as little as 350 ml of fluid entering the lung, which has an estimated alveolar surface area that approximates half of a soccer field, may produce severe lung failure.

Freshwater aspiration primarily affects surfactant phospholipids [8]. Inactivation of surfactant renders alveoli unstable and leads to alveolar collapse and atelectasis, thus increasing the amount of absolute shunt area within the lung. In addition, hypotonic fluids may exert a direct cell toxic effect on alveolar and vascular endothelial cells, leading to cell swelling and probably rupture of cell membranes, and thus promoting interstitial and alveolar edema formation. Aspiration of seawater leads to development of acute alveolar edema due to drainage of protein-rich fluids from the intravascular space into the alveoli. Edema formation is due to seawater hypertonicity, which exceeds three to four times the tonicity of blood [8,9]. Seawater does not change the surface tension properties of a pulmonary surfactant, but it does reduce the concentration of surfactant within alveoli [8]. The introduction of fluids into the airways usually results in bronchospasm, leading to an increase in relative shunt areas. These pathophysiologic events result in various degrees of hypoxemia, decreased lung compliance, and increased work of breathing (Fig. 1). Rupture of alveolar septa and development of acute emphysema in parts of the lung have been reported to occur in some drowning victims in autopsy studies [10]. It is believed that forceful exhalation against a fluid column aspirated into the upper airways during submersion can produce dramatic increases in alveolar pressure in some areas of the lung, thus producing mechanical disruption of fragile alveolar structures. In addition to the patho-

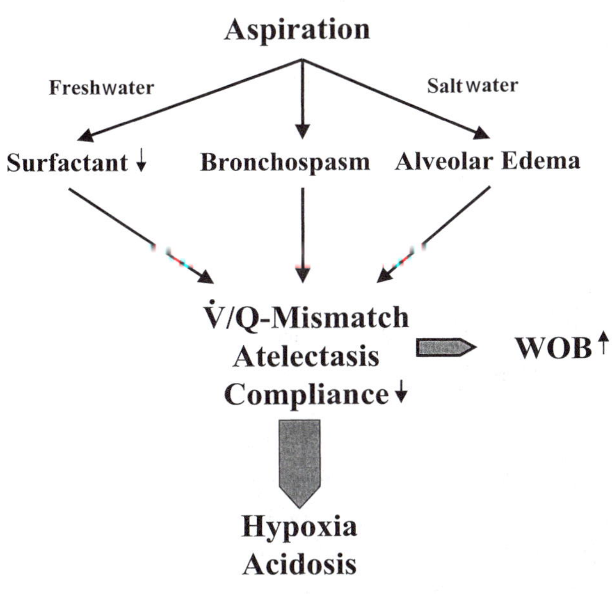

Figure 1 Lung pathophysiologic changes with fluid aspiration. Freshwater aspiration destroys pulmonary surfactant, leading to alveolar instability and alveolar collapse. In contrast, because of hypertonicity saltwater aspiration promotes plasma leakage into alveoli and pulmonary edema. Fluid aspiration may cause intense bronchospasm. Atelectasis, increases in pulmonary ventilation/perfusion mismatch, impair gas exchange, leading to hypoxia and progressive acidosis. At the same time, the work of breathing (WOB) is significantly increased and may contribute to a major part of whole body oxygen consumption.

physiologic events arising from fluid aspiration it has been demonstrated that as many as 70% of drowning victims aspirate foreign material, such as mud, algae, and vomitus [10]; therefore the hospital stay of near-drowned patients may be complicated by the development of lung infections [11].

Figure 2 presents the chest X-ray and CT scan from a near-drowned diver who aspirated freshwater during an emergency ascent in a mountain lake. In the chest X-ray only a few aerated lung areas can be detected. The pathophysiology of fluid aspiration seems to affect the whole lung quite homogeneously. In contrast, the CT scan reveals

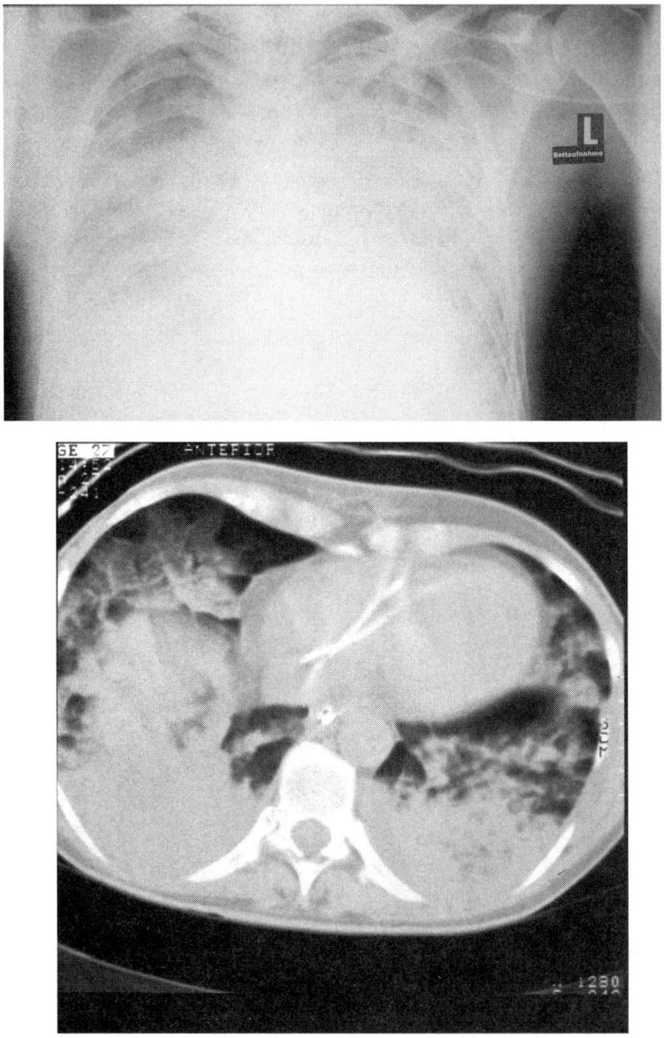

♂;Age = 46

Figure 2 Lung chest X-ray and CT scan after near-drowning in a diver a few hours after an accident. The chest X-ray demonstrates ''milky'' homogeneous infiltration of both lungs. In contrast, the CT scan reveals massive dorsal atelectasis and interstitial lung edema in nondependent areas of both lungs.

complete atelectasis of dependent lung areas in conjunction with pronounced interstitial edema in nondependent lung areas, a picture that has been described as typical for severe acute respiratory distress syndrome [12].

B. The Cardiovascular System

The pathophysiology of the cardiovascular system in submersion accidents is determined by the extent and duration of hypoxia, the derangement of acid-base status, the magnitude of stress response, coexisting hypothermia, and the presence or absence of a ''diving reflex.'' The latter may significantly influence the overall cardiovascular response to hypoxia and may be beneficial with regard to hypoxia tolerance during submersion [13,14]. Under normal conditions low arterial oxygen tension stimulates arterial chemoreceptors located in the glomerular carotid bodies at the carotid bifurcation. Stimulation leads to activation of the sympathoadrenergic and parasympathetic nervous system, causing bradycardia and intense vasoconstriction in ''nonvital'' organs (e.g., skin and splanchnic area; Fig. 3). Because of simultaneous apnea the inhibitory effects of lung mechanoreceptors on

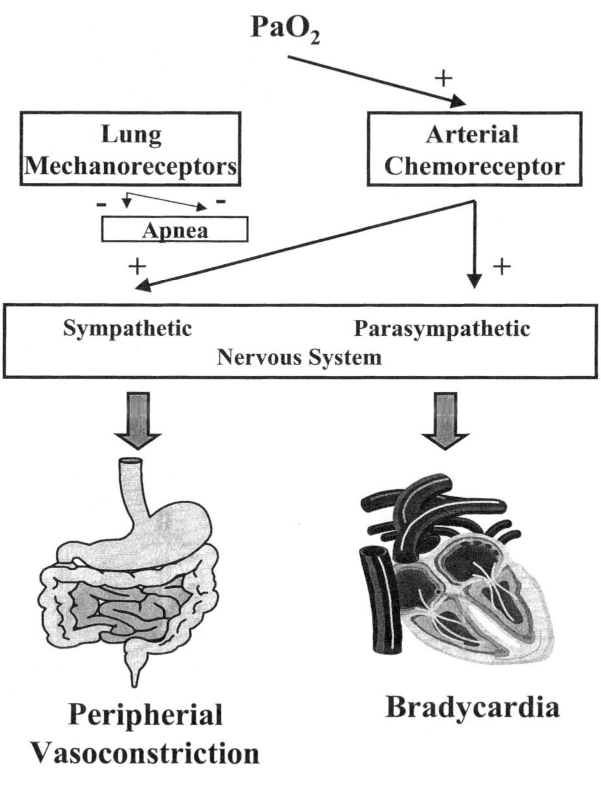

Figure 3 Proposed physiological mechanisms of the ''diving reflex'' in man. Hypoxemia stimulates arterial chemoreceptors, leading to activation of sympathetic and parasympathetic nervous system via the central cardiovascular control system (+). During spontaneous breathing the effects of arterial chemoreceptors are opposed by afferent signals originating from lung mechanoreceptors (−). With apnea, the effects of lung mechanoreceptors are eliminated, resulting in intense peripheral vasoconstriction and bradycardia. The diving reflex can be initiated by face submersion in cold water and is augmented by high lung volumes before submersion.

chemoreceptor-mediated activation of the cardiovascular control center within the medulla oblongata is lost. As a result, redistribution of blood flow from nonvital organs to the heart and central nervous system together with bradycardia, which reduces myocardial oxygen consumption, may significantly prolong hypoxia tolerance. In small children and to a lesser extent in adults an identical cardiovascular reflex can be mediated by simple face contact with cold water [15]. This reflex is triggered via sensory fibers of the trigeminal nerve. In addition, this reflex seems to be augmented in cold water and when the subject has taken a deep breath of air before facial submersion [16].

Severe hypoxia, together with life-threatening stress during initial submersion, causes massive catecholamine release with intense vasoconstriction in most tissues. Vasoconstriction in extremities may be so intense that a pulse pressure is hard to detect. High catecholamine levels together with severe hypoxia and acidosis may cause cardiac failure with consecutive decreased systemic oxygen delivery. In animal models of drowning, focal myocardial necrosis has been identified at autopsy. These lesions resemble those observed in pheochromocytoma patients who succumbed because of catecholamine crisis [17]. In a population of pediatric patients, a characteristic cardiovascular pattern similar to cardiogenic shock, characterized by low cardiac index, elevated right and left ventricular filling pressures, elevated systemic and pulmonary vascular resistance indices, and decreased systemic oxygen delivery and consumption, were described after generalized hypoxic-ischemic injuries [18]. In addition, cardiovascular depression with low cardiac output and decreased systemic perfusion pressure, making catecholamine support necessary, was reported in a majority of pediatric patients after severe near-drowning accidents [19]. In our institution most patients need excess volume during the first 24 to 48 hr after a severe submersion accident. In addition, approximately two-thirds of the patients need some form of catecholamine, mostly vasopressor support to achieve hemodynamic stability. These findings stress the major importance of hypoxia as the primary cause of cardiovascular failure in patients with submersion accidents.

In former times it was believed that functional cardiovascular arrest in drowning patients was due to severe electrolyte disturbances associated with large volumes of fluid aspiration. These electrolyte abnormalities were thought to cause arrhythmias, ventricular fibrillation, and finally heart arrest. The evidence was mainly based on animal experiments in which the volume of aspirated fluid exceeded 22 ml $\times$ kg^{-1} [1]. Today, however, it seems clear that the amount of aspirated fluid in men seldom exceeds 3 to 7 ml $\times$ kg^{-1}. Only 15% of both fresh- and saltwater drowned patients demonstrate significant electrolyte disturbances [20], therefore cardiac rhythm disturbances and finally cardiac arrest mainly result from uninterrupted hypoxia, severe acid-base disturbances, catecholamine stress, and sometimes hypothermia. With regard to cardiac electrophysiology, any type of cardiac arrhythmia can be observed in near-drowned patients. During hypothermia, sinus bradycardia and atrial fibrillation are most common [1]. Concerning the ECG ST-segment elevations or depression, changes in T-wave amplitude, increased P-R interval, and widening of QRS complex have been described.

C. Electrolytes, Hematology, Acid-Base Status, and the Kidney

As pointed out earlier, aspiration of more than 3 to 7 ml $\times$ kg^{-1} BW of fluids is unusual in humans, and it has been suggested that more than 22 ml $\times$ kg^{-1} of fluid aspirate are required to produce significant serum electrolyte changes [1]. Electrolyte disturbances after near-drowning may occur in certain situations, however. Yagil et al. reported life-threatening changes in serum levels of calcium and magnesium in patients near-drowned in the Dead Sea [21].

Because of the limited amount of aspirated fluid, near-drowned patients develop hemolysis with significant changes in hemoglobin concentration or hematocrit only on very rare occasions [6]. In addition, severe renal dysfunction is also uncommon [10]. Quite similar coagulopathy and especially disseminated intravascular coagulation (DIC) are sparse, and if present suggest prolonged severe diffuse hypoxic injury [22].

Even after limited submersion times, significant alterations concerning the acid-base status of near-drowned patients can be expected. The effects of airway obstruction with subsequent apnea on arterial oxygen tension and acid-base balance was demonstrated in dog experiments [23]. Arterial carbon dioxide tension ($PaCO_2$) increased by approximately 6 mmHg $\times$ min^{-1} (= 0.8kPa $\times$ min^{-1}), while arterial pH decreased by 0.05 U $\times$ min^{-1}. Within 5 min of apnea mean arterial pH had decreased to 7.15 and mean $PaCO_2$ had increased to 70 mmHg (= 9.3 kPa). Even more dramatic were changes in arterial oxygen tension (PaO_2), which decreased from a baseline of 90 mmHg (= 12kPa) to 40 mmHg (= 5.3kPa) within 1 min and to 10 mmHg (= 1.33kPa) within 3 min. After 5 min PaO_2 was only 4 mmHg (= 0.53 kPa). It has to be pointed out that despite extreme hypoxemia 80% of the animals were successfully resuscitated by a brief period of positive pressure ventilation, and in some cases additional closed-chest cardiac massage.

D. Central Nervous System and Outcome

Primary severe hypoxic injury of the central nervous system leading to severe debilitation or brain death is the most important factor related to outcome and subsequent quality of life in near-drowning victims [1,3,9]. The factors determining final neurological injury are complex. Ambient water temperature, body isolation, level of stress during submersion, submersion time, presence or absence of the "diving reflex," and coexisting cardiovascular and neurologic disease may all influence neurological outcome. Some investigators hypothesized that aspiration of cold water might be beneficial for survival by promoting central hypothermia. This hypothesis lacks clear evidence [14], however. In addition, the development of adult respiratory distress syndrome and infectious complications significantly increases subsequent mortality after fluid aspiration [6,11].

Investigators sought clues for the prognosis of near-drowned patients that might help guide initial management and define patients for whom further intensive care treatment may not be reasonable and cost-efficient. No convincing correlation could be demonstrated [24,25], however, between outcome and initial values of pH, electrolyte concentrations, arterial oxygen tension, EEG recordings, duration of submersion, initial body core temperature, initial resuscitative measures, and the need for mechanical ventilation.

The level of consciousness at the time of hospital admission provides some prediction of outcome. Conn et al. studied 56 children after submersion accidents according to their initial neurologic presentation [26]. Fifty-three percent of patients were awake, 6% showed blunted consciousness, and 31% were comatose. All patients presenting awake or with only blunted consciousness survived with normal brain function. Even in the group of comatose patients, 33.5% survived without obvious neurologic deficit, 23% survived with some form of brain injury, and 33.5% died in the hospital. Modell et al. reported the outcome of 121 patients, including adults and children [27]. Sixty-one patients were alert at admission, and all patients recovered with normal brain function. Out of the 31 patients admitted with blunted consciousness, 90% survived without deficit. Twenty-nine

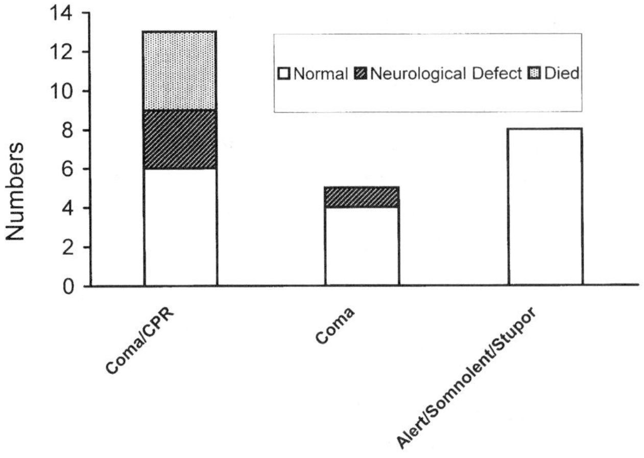

Figure 4 Prognosis of near-drowning in a mixed pedriatic (n = 6) and adult patient (n = 19) population from our institution over a 5-year period (1992–1997). Forty-six percent of patients with coma and cardiopulmonary resuscitation survived neurologically intact. All patients initially presented alert, somnolent, or with stupor survived. Only 1 out of 5 patients presenting with coma but with the presence of cardiopulmonary function survived with a neurological deficit. Note: n = 25.

patients were admitted in coma. Fifty-five percent recovered with normal brain function, 10% survived with some neurologic deficit, and 34% died in the hospital. Between 1992 and 1997 25 near-drowned patients, including children and adults, were admitted to our intensive care unit. Of 13 patients admitted in coma and after cardiopulmonary resuscitation, 46% survived neurologically intact, 15% survived with neurological deficits, and 31% died (Fig. 4). Of those patients with coma but without cardiovascular arrest at the scene 75% survived neurologically intact. All patients initially presenting alert, somnolent, or with stupor survived without neurological defect. In a recent investigation on prognosis of unwitnessed out-of-hospital cardiac arrest, near-drowning appeared to be an independent factor related to survival [28]. These findings strongly suggest that aggressive resuscitative measures, including interruption of hypoxia and cardiovascular stabilization, should be instituted urgently in most near-drowning victims regardless of clinical presentation.

IV. EMERGENCY TREATMENT

Hypoxia is the major cause of death in near-drowned patients, therefore the primary goal of treatment is to restore adequate oxygen delivery to tissue. Immediate rescue from the water is of utmost importance. Coexisting trauma to the cervical spine and head injuries must be anticipated, especially in patients with submersion accidents in shallow water. In these patients unnecessary movements of the cerebral spine have to be avoided, and mechanical stabilization should be initiated as soon as possible. In hypothermic patients wet clothes should be removed and further temperature loss prevented by isolating the patient with dry blankets and aluminium foil, if available.

Neurologic and cardiopulmonary presentation may guide correct initial treatment (Fig. 5). Alert patients without clinical signs of pulmonary insufficiency should receive supplemental oxygen by mask or a nasal catheter. In these patients pulmonary function

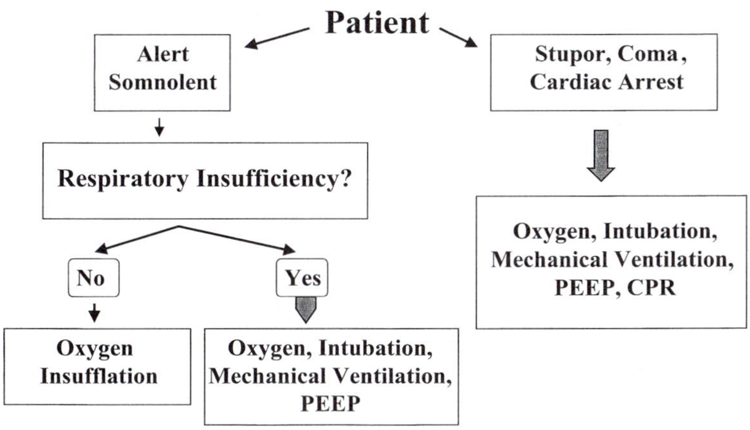

Figure 5 Emergency decisions in near-drowning patients. Neurologic status and clinical signs of respiratory insufficiency at presentation should guide management decisions. Alert patients without clinical signs of pulmonary insufficiency receive supplemental oxygen by mask or nasal catheters. In case of progressive deterioration of respiratory function intubation and mechanical ventilation with positive end expiratory pressure (PEEP) and 100% oxygen are mandatory. Patients presenting with stupor or coma should be intubated and mechanical ventilation with 100% oxygen and PEEP should be started at the scene. Aggressive CPR is indicated in most patients presenting without vital signs.

should be observed in a hospital for further 12 to 24 hr. A recent study in childhood drowning victims reported that patients with a Glasgow coma scale ≥13, normal chest X-ray, lack of clinical signs of respiratory distress, and normal room air oxygen saturation can be safely discharged home 4 to 6 hr after emergency room presentation [29].

Patients presenting awake or somnolent but with clinical signs of respiratory distress (e.g., tachypnea, dyspnea, cyanosis, rales, and cough, sometimes producing bloody, fruity sputum) receive oxygen at high inspiratory concentrations. In an emergency this can only be accomplished by a tight-fitting mask combined with reservoir bag and an oxygen source.

In case of progressive deterioration of respiratory function, intubation and mechanical ventilation with positive end expiratory pressure and 100% oxygen are mandatory. Although never investigated systematically in near-drowned patients, initial treatment with positive end expiratory pressures of 8 to 12 mm H_2O using a PEEP valve connected to a resuscitator bag and/or ventilator may be expected to prevent or attenuate the development of atelectasis after fluid aspiration and therefore significantly improve arterial oxygenation.

Emergency intubation should be performed with cricoid pressure and muscle relaxation using a rapid-onset relaxant (e.g., succinylcholine). Near-drowning patients have a high risk of vomiting and subsequent aspiration of gastric contents because they usually have swallowed large amounts of water during submersion. After intubation the institution of a nasogastric tube may adequately decompress a full stomach and aid bag or mechanical ventilation. There is no use in attempting to drain water from the lungs, as these procedures have been shown to be highly ineffective [3].

Comatose patients need immediate tracheal intubation and mechanical or bag ventilation with positive end expiratory pressure and 100% oxygen. Asystoly and ventricular fibrillation warrant aggressive cardiopulmonary resuscitation, as the prognosis still is not dismal. Numerous case reports have been published demonstrating that especially immersion in cold water is compatible with long-term survival, even when the period of immersion is relatively long. Unfortunately cardiopulmonary resuscitation is still underutilized for victims of submersion accidents [30]. A recent study from Scotland has shown that even members of emergency services often fail to either initiate prehospital resuscitation or continue this to the hospital for victims of witnessed cold water drowning accidents.

On some occasions it may be necessary to start artificial ventilation while the patient is still in the water. Although mouth-to-mouth or mouth-to-nose ventilation is beneficial in apneic patients with intact cardiovascular function this maneuver is extremely difficult to perform in water and especially during swimming, therefore transport to the ground should not be delayed under these conditions.

Patients of submersion accidents usually are hypovolemic and need adequate volume resuscitation. Rapid infusion of 1500 cc crystalloid or 500 cc colloid solution via an IV line can be performed without delay. There is no systematic evidence to support the usefulness of prophylactic antibiotic or steroid therapy in the emergency setting in order to decrease or attenuate the incidence and severity of ARDS or infectious complications.

V. SUMMARY

Near-drowning is a frequent, preventable accident with significant morbidity and mortality in a previous healthy population. Prompt resuscitation and aggressive respiratory and cardiovascular treatment are crucial for optimal survival. In most patients the primary injury is pulmonary, resulting in severe arterial hypoxemia and secondary damage to other organs. Damage to the central nervous system is most critical in terms of patient survival and subsequent quality of life. Immediate interruption of hypoxia is of utmost importance in the emergency situation. Accurate neurologic prognosis cannot be predicted from initial clinical presentation, laboratory, radiological, or electrophysiological examinations, therefore aggressive initial therapeutic efforts are indicated in most near-drowning victims. All near-drowned patients should be evaluated and observed in the hospital.

REFERENCES

1. JS Olshaker. Near drowning. Environ Emerg 10:339–350, 1992.
2. RA Brenner, GS Smith, MD Overpeck. Divergent trends in childhood drowning rates: 1971 through 1988. JAMA 271:1606–1608, 1994.
3. AI Fields. Near drowning in the pedriatic population. Crit Care Clin 8:113–129, 1992.
4. A Spira. Diving and marine medicine review part II: Diving diseases. J Travel Med 6:180–198, 1999.
5. CS Noble, N Sharpe. Drowning: Its mechanism and treatment. Can Med Assoc J 89:402–405, 1963.
6. JH Modell, SA Graves, A Ketover. Clinical course of 91 consecutive near-drowning victims. Chest 70:231–238, 1976.
7. MG Harries. Drowning in man. Crit Care Med 9:407–408, 1981.
8. ST Giammona, JH Modell. Drowning by total immersion: Effects on pulmonary surfactant of destilled water, isotonic saline, and sea water. Amer J Dis Child 114:612–616, 1967.
9. JP Orlowski. Drowning, near drowning, and ice-water submersion. Pediat Clin North Am 34: 75–91, 1987.

10. RH Fuller. The 1962 Wellcome prize essay. Drowning and the postimmersion syndrome. A clinicopathologic study. Mil Med 128:22–36, 1963.
11. GA Kennedy, RK Kanter, LB Weiner, et al. Can early bacterial complications of aspiration with respiratory failure be predicted? Pediat Emerg Care 8:123–125, 1992.
12. L Gattinoni, P Pelosi, G Vitale, et al. Body position changes redistribute lung computed-tomographic density in patients with acute respiratory failure. Anesthesiology 74:15–23, 1991.
13. L Manley. Apnoeic heart responses in humans: A review. Sports Med 9:286–310, 1990.
14. BA Gooden. Why some people do not drown: Hypothermia versus the diving response. Med J Aust 157:629–632, 1992.
15. N Hayashi, M Ishihara, A Tanaka, et al. Face immersion increases vagal activity as assessed by heart rate variability. Eur J Appl Physiol 76:394–399, 1997.
16. LB Campbell, BA Gooden, JD Horowitz. Cardovascular responses to partial and total immersion in man. J Physiol (Lond) 202:239–250, 1969.
17. SB Karch. Pathology of the heart in drowning. Arch Path Lab Med 11:697–700, 1983.
18. SE Lucking, MM Pollack, AL Fields. Shock following generalized hypoxic-ischemic injury in previously healthy infants and children. J Pediat 108:359–364, 1986.
19. ChA Hildebrand, AG Hartmann, L Arcinue, et al. Cardiac performance in pedriatic near-drowning. Crit Care Med 16:331–335, 1988.
20. JH Modell, JH Davis. Electrolyte changes in human drowning victims. Anesthesiology 30: 414–420, 1969.
21. Y Yagil, R Stalnikowics, J Michaeli, et al. Near drowning in the Dead Sea: Electrolyte imbalances and therapeutic implications. Arch Intern Med 145:50–52, 1985.
22. RM Culpepper. Bleeding diathesis in fresh water drowning. Ann Intern Med 83:675–678, 1975.
23. JH Modell, EJ Kuck, BC Ruiz, et al. Effect of intravenous vs. aspirated distilled water on serum electrolytes and blood gas tensions. J Appl Physiol 32:579–584, 1972.
24. JM Lavelle, KN Shaw. Near drowning: Is emergency department cardiopulmonary resuscitation or intensive care unit cerebral resuscitation indicated? Crit Care Med 21:368–373, 1993.
25. MA Nichter, PB Everett. Childhood near-drowning: Is cardiopulmonary resuscitation always indicated? Crit Care Med 17:993–995, 1989.
26. AW Conn, JE Montes, GA Barker, et al. Cerebral salvage in near-drowning following neurological classification by triage. Can Anaesth Soc J 27:201–210, 1980.
27. JH Modell, SA Graves, EJ Kuck. Near-drowning: Correlation of level of consciousness and survival. Can Anaesth Soc J 27:211–213, 1980.
28. M Kuisma, K Jaara. Unwitnessed out-of-hospital cardiac arrest: Is resuscitation worthwhile? Ann Emerg Med 30:69–75, 1997.
29. AL Causey, JA Tilelli, ME Swanson. Predicting discharge in uncomplicated near-drowning. Am J Emerg Med 18:9–11, 2000.
30. JP Wyatt, GS Tomlinson, A Busuttil. Resuscitation of drowning victims in south-east Scotland. Resuscitation 41:101–104, 1999.

32

Accidental Hypothermia and Avalanche Injuries

PETER MAIR

The Leopold Franzens University School of Medicine, Innsbruck, Austria

I. INTRODUCTION

Accidental hypothermia is an unintentional reduction in body core temperature below 35°C. This is an arbitrary definition. Many patients already demonstrate symptoms of mild accidental hypothermia (e.g., shivering) at a core temperature of 36°C. On the other hand, a body core temperature of 35°C is just within the range of the diurnal variations in core temperature observed in some healthy adults [1,2].

The major problem in patients with mild and moderate accidental hypothermia (body core temperature between 35°C and 28°C) is the danger of a further decrease in core temperature during rescue and initial resuscitation, the so-called afterdrop phenomenon [3–5]. To avoid this sometimes life-threatening complication, patients who are already suffering from mild and moderate accidental hypothermia need a specialized diagnostic and therapeutic approach in the prehospital environment. An additional problem in patients with severe accidental hypothermia (body core temperature less than 28°C) is the highly irritable myocardium, which is prone to ventricular fibrillation [1,3,4,6].

Severe accidental hypothermia offers potent protection from ischemic tissue injury, therefore successful resuscitation and full neurological recovery are possible in arrested patients with severe accidental hypothermia even after prolonged cardiac arrest and resuscitation efforts lasting for several hours [7–9]. The arrested hypothermic heart often does not respond to electrical or pharmacological therapy unless it is rewarmed [1,3,4,10]. Because of the profound protection from ischemic cerebral injury and the inability to restore spontaneous circulation, the diagnosis of death is difficult during hypothermia. Death in a hypothermic patient is mostly defined as "the failure to revive with rewarming," and it is commonly accepted that "nobody is dead unless warm and dead" [1,3,4].

Table 1 Main Causes of Accidental Hypothermia

Exposure to cold in a healthy individual submerged in snow or ice water
Exposure to cold in a healthy individual either trapped or intoxicated in a cold environment
Exposure to moderate cold in an individual with severely impaired thermoregulation

II. INCIDENCE AND MAIN REASONS FOR ACCIDENTAL HYPOTHERMIA

Hypothermia is not only a problem of northern countries with cold winters or a problem of mountain areas. Accidental hypothermia and hypothermia-related deaths also occur in regions with milder climate. Hypothermia is possible in an ambient temperature range between 10°C and 15°C whenever the ability of a patient to maintain his or her body core temperature is altered (e.g., drug abuse, alcohol intoxication, neurological disorders) [2]. A low body core temperature is often not detected, and therefore accidental hypothermia is undoubtedly an underdiagnosed problem. A recent publication from the United States reports an annual death rate of 0.3/100,000 inhabitants per year [11].

The main causes for hypothermia are listed in Table 1. The three main causes of accidental hypothermia are different with respect to the rate of cooling, resulting in some characteristic differences in pathophysiology and in-hospital therapy, therefore Lloyd [1] has suggested classifying hypothermia according to the underlying reason, into ''immersion,'' ''exhaustion,'' and ''urban hypothermia'' (Table 2). For the prehospital environment, however, a classification of hypothermia according to severity is perhaps more useful. (See Table 3.)

Table 2 Classification of Hypothermia

	Immersion hypothermia	Exhaustion hypothermia	Chronic urban hypothermia
Duration of cooling	Within 1 hr	A few hours	Many hours
Cold stress	Overwhelming	Severe	Only mild
Pathophysiological changes			
Endogenous heat production	Overwhelmed	Exhausted	Exhausted
Vasoconstriction	+++++	++++	++
Fluid shifts	little, none	+++++	+++++
Main reasons	Near-drowning, avalanche accident, exposure in injured/intoxicated victim	Prolonged exposure	Malnutrition, inadequate housing, elderly victims
Main problems	Concomitant asphyxia	Hypovolemia, exhaustion	Cerebral and pulmonary edema with rewarming, concomitant diseases
Optimal rewarming technique	Active rewarming	Active rewarming	Passive rewarming

++ = minimal; ++++ = maximal; +++++ = substantial.
Source: Ref. 1.

Table 3 Classification of Accidental Hypothermia According to Severity

	Accidental hypothermia safe zone	Accidental hypothermia danger zone	Accidental hypothermia cardiorespiratory arrest
Motor function	Involuntary shivering	Muscle rigidity	Muscle rigidity or atonic muscles
Cerebral function	Conscious	Unconscious	Deep coma
Pupils	Normal	Perhaps fixed, dilated	Fixed, dilated
Cardiocirculatory function	Strong central pulses easy to detect	No peripheral pulses central pulses palpable often hard to detect	No central pulses
Respiratory function	Hyperventilation	Hypoventilation, or only occasional gasps	No spontaneous respiration
Body core temperature	Tp ≥ (30°C to 32°C)	(30°C to 32°C) > Tp	Tp ≤ 30°C

III. PATHOPHYSIOLOGY OF ACCIDENTAL HYPOTHERMIA RELEVANT FOR PREHOSPITAL MANAGEMENT

Body core temperature is regulated closely to 37°C (±0.2°C). Even minor decreases in body core temperature immediately activate protective mechanisms that counteract further cooling. The human thermoregulatory system maintains body core temperature primarily by two mechanisms, sympathetic stimulation and shivering [1,2].

Sympathetic stimulation causes intense peripherial vasoconstriction and reduces heat loss from the skin (body insulation increased by a factor of 6). Sympathetic stimulation also increases metabolic heat production and cardiac output to four to five times the resting values, resulting in a marked increase in body oxygen consumption. The unintentional muscle contractions associated with shivering further enhance endogenous heat production, but also tissue oxygen consumption. Sympathetic stimulation and shivering may be blunted by coexisting problems. Sedatives, narcotics, and vasoactive drugs interact with the thermoregulatory vasoconstriction and thereby significantly enhance body cooling. Hypoglycemia and intoxication with narcotic drugs are the two most common reasons for the absence of shivering in a hypothermic patient [2].

Later, during cooling (with a body core temperature below 30°C), the direct depressive effects of the cold on the cardiovascular and metabolic system outweigh the stimulatory effects of sympathetic activation. Increased metabolic heat production is replaced by a state of *vita minima*, with reduced metabolism and reduced respiratory and cardiac function. Heart rate, arterial pressure, and cardiac output are decreased, and shivering disappears. Muscles and joints become stiff and rigid.

The intense vasoconstriction triggered by cooling causes a considerable temperature gradient between the core (heart, brain, lungs) and the surface (extremities, skin, fat tissue) of the body. The skin temperature is up to 20°C lower than visceral temperature. This helps the body to maintain a temperature as high as possible for the heart and the brain. This temperature gradient, however, may cause a further sudden decrease in core temperature during rescue and initial treatment, whenever cold blood from the periphery of the body returns to the core (afterdrop phenomenon). Movements and postural changes during rescue are one important reason for the mobilization of large amounts of cold (also acidotic and desaturated) blood from the peripherial areas of the body [3,5]. Another important mechanism is vigorous efforts at active external rewarming in patients with a core temperature below 30°C.

At a core temperature below 30°C the myocardium is highly irritable and prone to ventricular fibrillation (VF). The increased likelihood for VF in association with therapeutic interventions during rescue, transport, and initial prehospital treatment has been well known for decades. The phenomenon is referred to as ''hypothermic sudden cardiac death'' or ''sheltering death.'' The ventricular irritability of the hypothermic heart has been attributed to excessive sympathetic stimulation, temperature gradients within the myocardium, electrolyte and acid base disturbances, myocardial hypoxia, and hypothermia-induced disturbances in myocardial electrical conduction [2]. Cardiopulmonary arrest after ice water immersion has been attributed to a sudden loss of hydrostatic pressure on the human body after removal from water (''postimmersion collapse'') [12].

The capacity of hypothermia to protect tissue from ischemic injury is well documented. The most important protective mechanism is undoubtedly a reduction in metabolism and oxygen requirement of approximately 7% (±2%) per 1°C decrease in core temperature. More recently, an additional protective mechanism of even mild hypothermia has been proposed, namely the reduced release of mediator substances (e.g., glutamate) responsible for cerebral ischaemia/reperfusion injury [13]. During intentional hypothermia (with core temperature below 20°C) cardiac arrest is tolerated without neurological injury up to 60 min in children and up to 40 min in adults.

IV. CLINICAL SYMPTOMS AND CLASSIFICATION OF ACCIDENTAL HYPOTHERMIA

Clinical symptoms of hypothermia depend predominantly on body core temperature, but to some extent also on the rate of cooling. Slow cooling is associated with less intense vasoconstriction but more pronounced fluid shifts. Fluid shifts, on the other hand, play no major role in patients with rapid cooling (e.g., after ice water immersion; Table 2). Concomitant trauma or diseases can significantly change clinical presentation. Furthermore, there are wide variations in the individual response to cold, and a particular symptom may be absent in one patient but pronounced in another. In general, accidental hypothermia is classified into mild (35°C to 32°C), moderate (32°C to 28°C), and severe (<28°C) accidental hypothermia and accidental hypothermia with cardiopulmonary arrest (<30°C).

A. Mild Hypothermia (Core Temperature 35°C to 32°C)

The most characteristic clinical finding in mild accidental hypothermia is extensive involuntary muscle shivering. Heart rate and blood pressure are increased, and the patient typically hyperventilates. He feels stressed and intensely cold and is often agitated. Although conscious, intellectual impairment and impairment of motor coordination are common. Sometimes hallucinations occur, and inappropriate behavior must be expected. This places the patient at a high risk for accidents in exposed areas (e.g., mountains), and he should never be left alone or unsecured. A few patients feel paradoxically hot, and the phenomenon of paradoxical undressing has been reported.

B. Moderate Hypothermia (Core Temperature 32°C to 28°C)

With moderate accidental hypothermia, thermogenic shivering gradually disappears. The Disappearance of shivering indicates that protective mechanisms to maintain the core temperature are overwhelmed and a more serious level of cooling has been reached. Consciousness becomes increasingly depressed, and at a core temperature below 30°C to 28°C the hypothermic patient is typically comatose. During moderate hypothermia arrhythmias occur frequently, most often supraventricular tachyarrhythmias. In general, it is already difficult to obtain peripheral pulses or to measure blood pressure because of the intense vasoconstriction. Muscles and joints become rigid.

C. Severe Hypothermia (Core Temperature <28°C)

At a core temperature below 28°C the patient is typically in a deep coma. The pupils become fixed and dilated. Cerebral response to hypothermia can vary, however, and some patients (in particular, chronic alcoholics) are still conscious at a core temperature of 26°C to 28°C.

When the core temperature falls below 28°C the heart becomes bradycardic. Central circulatory reflexes are not functioning, and myocardial contractility is considerably reduced. The heart rate is about 10 per min at a temperature below 24°C. During severe accidental hypothermia multifocal extrasystoles and ST-T segment changes sometimes produce a bizzare ECG pattern, which is often mistaken as cardiac arrest. The severely hypothermic heart is highly irritable, and VF occurs after even minor stimulation. Movements during evacuation, endotracheal intubation, insertion of a gastric tube, insertion of an esophageal temperature probe, and central venous catheterization all have been reported as possible triggers for VF. Ventricular fibrillation indicates witnessed cardiac arrest caused by external stimulation, whereas asystole indicates a very low body core temperature or concomitant asphyxia. Hypothermic cardiopulmonary arrest caused by VF therefore has a far better prognosis than cardiopulmonary arrest caused by asystole. Respiration is reduced (volume and rate) and in general only a few occasional gasps are found at a core temperature below 24°C. Increased bronchial secretion and reduced mucociliary clearance, as well as increased lung water, are associated with hypothermia and are of clinical importance in patients with slow cooling and prolonged hypothermia. They result in reduced lung compliance, increased lung resistance, and pulmonary hypertension. Adequate tissue oxygen supply in hypothermic patients depends not only on respiratory and cardiovascular function; it is also endangered by a decreased blood viscosity and a leftward shift of the oxyhemoglobin dissociation curve (Fig. 1). This is typically outweighed, however, by the rightward shift associated with acidosis, which should not be corrected vigorously.

In general, at a core temperature below 20°C respiration stops and asystole occurs. The EEG is isoelectric at a core temperature below 20°C.

In patients with a core temperature below 28°C and prolonged cooling and hypothermia (urban hypothermia; Table 2) considerable disturbances in the acid base status, electrolyte status, and the intravascular volume must be expected. They are the consequence of hypothermia-induced diuresis (central hypervolemia due to intense vasoconstriction,

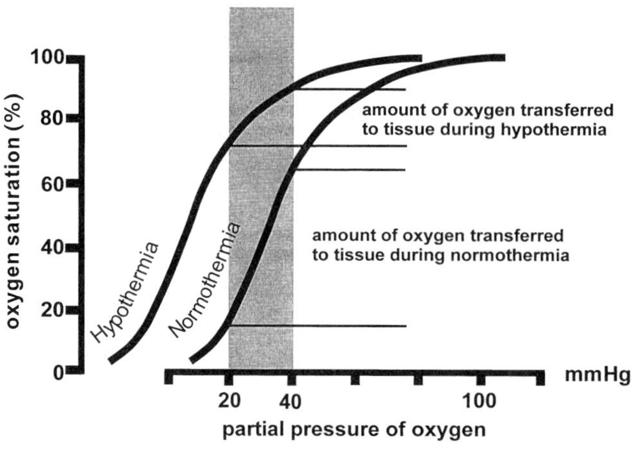

Figure 1 Leftward shift of the oxyhemoglobin dissociation curve associated with hypothermia and its consequences on tissue oxygen supply. The range of partial pressure of oxygen (pO_2) values normally found at the level of tissue capillaries (20 mmHg to 40 mmHg) is shifted from the steep to the flat aspect of the dissociation curve, resulting in a smaller amount of oxygen dissociated from hemoglobin and transferred to the tissue with a given decrease in tissue pO_2. This effect of hypothermia may be outweighed by a rightward shift of oxyhemoglobin dissociation curve associated with acidosis.

reduced response to antidiuretic hormone, tubular dysfunction). Water and electrolytes shift into the intracellular compartment. Patients with lengthy exposure to the cold have significant dehydration, hypokalemia, high lactate levels, and metabolic and respiratory acidosis. Victims of urban hypothermia with a core temperature below 28°C should be rewarmed only slowly while extensively monitored in an intensive care unit.

D. Hypothermia and Cardiopulmonary Arrest (Core Temperature <30°C)

Hypothermia markedly changes the pathophysiology and prognosis of cardiac arrest when the core temperature falls below 30°C. Successful resuscitation with full neurological recovery has been repeatedly reported [9,14–16] in the extremities for arrested hypothermic patients (Table 4). A major problem is the prehospital diagnosis of cardiac arrest.

Table 4 Hypothermic Patients With Cardiac Arrest in Extremities: Clinical Parameters Still Associated With Successful Resuscitation

	Successful resuscitation after
Submersion in ice water	40 min
Cardiac arrest without CPR	66 min
External chest compression	6.5 hr
Body core temperature as low as	
Intentional hypothermia	9°C
Accidental hypothermia	13.7°C

The heart rate is slow, and even central pulses are usually weak and can be easily missed. Respiration is slow and often reduced to a few occasional gasps when the core temperature is below 28°C. It is therefore important to thoroughly search for pulses and respiration for at least 1 min not to miss signs of life in a hypothermic patient. If external chest compression is started in patients with extreme bradycardia it will most likely induce VF and thereby convert a state of low but sufficient blood flow to cardiac arrest. A portable ECG to detect a perfusing rhythm is often helpful. Sometimes, however, it is difficult to obtain an adequate ECG signal with regular pads or electrodes because of the wet or frozen skin, and needle electrodes can be helpful.

V. PREHOSPITAL DIAGNOSTIC APPROACH FOR HYPOTHERMIC PATIENTS

A diagnostic approach to guide prehospital therapy can be done adequately based on clinical symptoms (Fig. 2). According to the presence or absence of shivering, the level of consciousness, and the cardiopulmonary status hypothermic patients can be classified into "hypothermia in the safe zone" (core temperature >30°C to 32°C), "hypothermia in the danger zone" (core temperature <28°C to 30°C), and "hypothermia with cardiopulmonary arrest" (Table 3). Clinical assessment can sometimes be obscured by accompanying neurological disease, intoxication, or cerebral trauma.

Prehospital measurement of body core temperature is therefore often desirable. It should be available in all emergency medical systems (EMS) regularly confronted with hypothermic patients. Prehospital measurement of body core temperature is best done with an electrical thermistor probe. Rectal and esophageal measurement are cumbersome in the prehospital environment, while measurements in the mouth and nose often do not represent core temperature. Tympanic temperature has been validated as a good marker

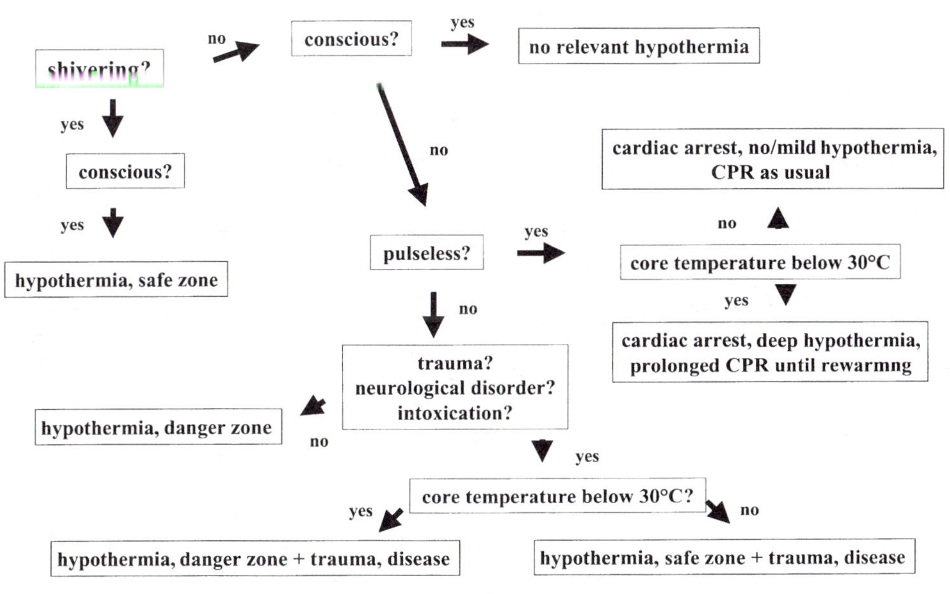

Figure 2 Diagnostic approach to a casualty with suspected accidental hypothermia.

of body core and cerebral temperature [17]. The usefulness and reliability of infrared emission tympanic thermometers in the prehospital environment, however, has been questioned [18]. Tympanic thermography is nevertheless widely used in Central European EMS, as it is convenient and safe. In general, problems encountered with tympanic temperature measurement are few—predominantly false low readings caused by ice water or snow in the ear.

VI. THERAPY OF ACCIDENTAL HYPOTHERMIA IN THE PREHOSPITAL ENVIRONMENT

A. General Considerations

No prospective, randomized data support the therapeutic principles of prehospital management of accidental hypothermia. Many of the therapeutic recommendations are primarily based on case reports, small case series, and the experience gathered with the in-hospital treatment of accidental and intentional hypothermia. Therapeutic strategies vary between different EMS systems, and they often have a rather weak scientific basis.

One cornerstone in the prehospital management of patients with accidental hypothermia is the strict avoidance of any further heat loss. Cooling during rescue and evacuation occurs not only by conduction, but significant heat loss is also secondary to convection, radiation, evaporation, and respiration (Table 5). The patient must be protected from wind, and wet clothing should be removed. He should be insulated with dry, warm clothes and wrapped in aluminum foil. Convection is a major source of heat loss that is often neglected. Moving the layer of air surrounding the patient increases heat loss several times. This phenomenon is referred to as the wind chill factor. It is responsible for the fact that an ambient temperature of 0°C without wind is equal to an ambient temperature of −8°C with a wind of 5 meters/sec, and equal to an ambient temperature of −18°C with a wind of 15 meters/sec.

Avoiding any active or passive movement during rescue is another uniformly recommended measure to prevent a further decrease in the core temperature during rescue by the afterdrop phenomenon. Such a rapid decrease in core temperature can cause sudden cardiac death in hypothermic patients in the danger zone (i.e., sheltering death).

Table 5 Possible Sources for Heat Loss and Methods to Avoid Them

Source	Measure to avoid	Comments
Conduction	Insulation with dry clothes/blankets	Minor source of heat loss (15–20%); do not forget the head, particularly in children; 20 to 30 times enhanced when immersed in water
Evaporation	Remove wet clothes; dry the skin (drowning)	Cut clothes to avoid unnecessary movements
Radiation	Wrap in aluminum foil	Major source of heat loss (50–60%); do not forget the head, a major source for heat loss by radiation
Respiration	Airway rewarming if available	Minor source of heat loss (10%)
Convection	Protect from wind	Moving the layer of air around the body enhances heat loss several times, so-called wind chill factor

Metabolic heat production is greater than the heat loss of the human body in case of complete insulation. Metabolic heat production can therefore passively rewarm the body (estimated maximum rewarming rate: 2°C/hr). Good insulation results in a slow, passive rewarming of a hypothermic patient in the safe zone. Passive rewarming, however, is too slow and inefficient in patients with a core temperature below 30°C (danger zone) because of the markedly reduced metabolic heat production. Whether active rewarming of a hypothermic patient in the danger zone should be initiated while still in the prehospital environment is controversial.

In cases of lengthy exposure to cold (urban hypothermia) and whenever rapid evacuation is possible, active prehospital rewarming should be avoided in hypothermic patients in the danger zone. Instead, therapy should be supportive and aimed at avoiding major complications such as afterdrop and hypothermic sudden cardiac death. In remote areas when evacuation will be delayed for several hours, however, initiation of prehospital rewarming is sometimes reasonable.

Basically, active rewarming of a hypothermic patient can be accomplished by two different methods.

Active external rewarming: any rewarming technique with exposure of the patient's skin to an exogenous heat source

Active internal rewarming: all methods delivering heat internally directly to the core of the body

In the prehospital environment, basically three methods of active rewarming are practical and widely used.

Active external rewarming with chemical hot packs
Active internal rewarming with airway rewarming
Active internal rewarming with 40°C warmed intravenous solutions

Recently an additional method for prehospital rewarming has been introduced, combining the application of subatmospheric pressure and heat to the forearm and hand (''negative pressure rewarming'').

No scientifically valid data prove the efficiency or safety of any of the methods in the prehospital environment. Most authors nevertheless suggest that active external rewarming with chemical hot packs should be used only in patients with a core temperature above 30°C to 32°C [10]. Airway rewarming can be used at any core temperature, but its major effect is most likely the prevention of further heat loss by respiration rather than efficient active internal rewarming [20]. Infusion of warmed fluids is often cumbersome or even impractical in the prehospital environment. It is efficient, theoretically, only if solutions are applied through a central venous catheter (Table 6).

The correct choice of an adequate hospital facility for a hypothermic patient while at the scene can avoid unnecessary delays in adequate in-hospital therapy. Only patients with hypothermia in the safe zone may be transported to the ''nearest hospital.'' Patients with hypothermia in the danger zone should be specifically transported to a hospital experienced in the treatment of accidental hypothermia and having methods of invasive active internal rewarming readily available [21] (peritoneal lavage, thoracic lavage, or hemofiltration). Whenever possible, hypothermic patients with cardiopulmonary arrest or profound hemodynamic instability should be transported to a medical center with extracorporeal circulation directly from the scene. Immediate circulatory support and rapid rewarming with extracorporeal circulation is the preferred method of treatment for these patients. If

Table 6 Possible Methods of Active Rewarming in the Prehospital Environment

	Hot packs	Airway rewarming	Warmed infusion	Negative pressure rewarming
Mechanism	Active external	Active internal	Central venous: active internal; peripheral: active external!	Subatmospheric pressure combined with heat applied to forearm and hand
Practicality	Excellent, commercially available, or self-made	Good, portable device commercially available	Poor, difficult to warm solutions and insulate administration set	Portable, commercially available device in development
Advantages	Easy and cheap; universally available	Preferential core rewarming; preferential brain rewarming?	Theoretically best rewarming rate: 0.6°C/liter 40°C solution	Theoretically optimal efficient method in a preliminary clinical evaluation
Disadvantages	Preferential rewarming of the surface of the body; danger of afterdrop circulatory collapse if applied <30°C; thermal injury of the skin	Low efficiency; theoretical rewarming rate: 0.03°C/hr	Central venous line necessary?! Increased preload for the heart	Only limited, preliminary clinical data available, efficiency not proven yet

transport to a medical center with extracorporeal circulation is not possible within a reasonable period of time, successful in hospital resuscitation is sometimes possible using methods of active internal rewarming during ongoing cardiopulmonary resuscitation.

B. Specific Therapeutic Considerations

The specific prehospital management of patients with accidental hypothermia depends on the level of consciousness, the cardiopulmonary function, and the body core temperature [19]. There are marked differences between safe and danger zone hypothermia (Tables 7 and 8).

The cornerstone of the therapy of safe zone hypothermia is complete insulation of the patient to avoid further heat loss and to enhance spontaneous rewarming. Active external rewarming with hot packs, as well as airway rewarming, may be used if available. Hot drinks without alcohol enhance rewarming in conscious patients (about 0.6°C core temperature increase per liter of hot drink). Immobilization is mandatory to avoid an afterdrop in core temperature secondary to active and passive movements during rescue [19].

For hypothermic patients in the danger zone immobilization is of the utmost importance. Postural changes and even minor movements during rescue may induce hypothermic sudden cardiac death. More recent publications still report a high rate of VF during rescue

Table 7 Therapy of Hypothermia (Safe Zone)

- Basic life support
  - Complete insulation to avoid further cooling
    - Do not forget to remove wet clothes
    - Do not forget to protect from wind
  - Avoid any unnecessary movement
    - Do not allow casuality to walk
    - Evacuate in a supine position, whenever possible
  - Expect inappropriate behavior and impaired motor coordination
    - Secure casuality in exposed mountain areas
  - Active rewarming, in particular if prolonged evacuation from remote area
    - Warmed blankets
    - Chemical hot packs
    - Airway rewarming if available
    - Hot drinks in conscious patients
  - Transport to the nearest hospital, as no specialized treatment necessary
- Advanced life support
  - ECG monitoring and intravenous access difficult to establish, and in general not necessary
  - Treat concomitant trauma or diseases as usual
  - Normal reaction to drugs can be expected
  - Volume replacement in case of traumatic shock
    - Warmed fluid whenever possible
    - Cautious volume replacement

and initial therapy (60% of all hypothermic patients admitted with cardiac arrest to a Swiss center) [6]. Obviously, precautions to avoid hypothermic sudden cardiac death are often neglected. Most experts recommend avoiding active external rewarming with hot packs in patients with danger zone hypothermia in the prehospital setting. Only active internal rewarming with airway rewarming, together with complete insulation, may be used [20].

Advanced life support in hypothermic patients in the danger zone is controversial in many aspects. Endotracheal intubation may induce VF [3,16]. Several larger case studies, however, have demonstrated that VF after endotracheal intubation is rare [4]. The advantages of a secure airway and adequate oxygenation far outweigh the potential risk of VF secondary to endotracheal intubation in most patients. Performed with a cautious technique in a deeply sedated patient to avoid any stress, endotracheal intubation is a safe procedure recommended by most experts in any unconscious hypothermic patient.

Even extreme bradycardia may generate a blood flow sufficient for the reduced metabolic demands during severe hypothermia. Low systemic arterial pressure is in general well tolerated even for prolonged periods, therefore many experts suggest that pharmacological interventions to increase the heart rate or blood pressure should usually be avoided in the prehospital environment as long as a perfusing rhythm is present on the ECG. Whether prophylactic administration of antiarrhythmic drugs, such as bretylium or lidocaine, can avoid hypothermia-induced arrhythmias or hypothermic sudden cardiac death is controversial [22]. The hemodynamic side effects of antiarrhythmic drugs in general outweigh their potential benefits. Noninvasive transcutaneous pacing in animals with hypothermia-associated bradycardia was safe, and significantly improved hemodynamics in an experimental animal model [23]. Its use in humans has not been reported so far.

Table 8 Therapy of Hypothermia (Danger Zone)

- Basic life support
  - Complete insulation to avoid further cooling
    - Remove wet clothes only if possible without movement
    - Isolate from wind avoiding unnecessary movements
  - Avoid any movements, as they may induce ventricular fibrillation
  - Evacuate in a supine position only
  - Avoid active external rewarming in the prehospital setting
    - Danger of afterdrop
    - Danger of hemodynamic collapse
  - Consider active external rewarming of the trunk if prolonged evacuation expected
    - Warmed blankets
    - Chemical hot packs
  - Active internal rewarming with airway rewarming may be used if available
  - Transport to a hospital with an intensive care unit and personnel experienced in the treatment of hypothermic patients, availability of invasive core rewarming techniques within the hospital necessary, extracorporeal circulation desirable
- Advanced life support
  - Continuous ECG monitoring mandatory, peripheral intravenous access whenever possible
  - Continuous temperature monitoring (tympanic) desirable
  - Endotracheal intubation to secure airways if Glasgow coma scale ≤ 7
    - Use sedation and cautious technique
  - Symptoms of concomitant trauma or diseases are obscured
  - An altered response to drugs must be expected
    - Catecholamines
    - Vasopressors
  - Avoid volume administration in the prehospital setting
  - Therapeutic interventions may induce ventricular fibrillation
    - Endotracheal intubation under deep anesthesia only
    - Avoid invasive pacing, central venous lines

C. Therapeutic Considerations in Arrested Hypothermic Patients

Many aspects of cardiopulmonary resuscitation in patients with severe accidental hypothermia are controversial (Table 9). It is often difficult to detect spontaneous circulation in a severely hypothermic patient without ECG or invasive blood pressure monitoring. It is therefore difficult to decide when external chest compression should be started. Even extreme bradycardia and weak ventricular contractions may provide a blood flow sufficient for the reduced demands during hypothermia. Most clinicians suggest avoiding external chest compression in the prehospital environment whenever a coordinated electrical myocardial activity is present, even in an apparently dead patient. External chest compression is performed as usual by most clinicians [24], although experimental animal data suggest that higher compression forces may be needed because of a decrease in thoracic and myocardial compliance [25]. A reduction in the frequency of external chest compression to 40 per min has also been proposed, but scientific support for such a recommendation is completely missing [2].

At a core temperature below 30°C the arrested hypothermic heart typically does not respond to electrical or pharmacological therapy, therefore many clinicians restrict prehospital advanced life support to three attempts at defibrillation [10]. If not successful,

Table 9 Therapy of Hypothermic Patients With Cardiac Arrest

- Basic life support
  - Check for pulses and respiration for at least 1 min. Do not initiate CPR in a patient with any sign of life
    - Do not start CPR in presence of bradycardic pulse
    - Do not start CPR in presence of occasional gasps
    - Do not start CPR in presence of spontaneous movements
  - Insulation to avoid further cooling during prolonged resuscitation efforts
  - Do not use active external or internal rewarming in the prehospital setting
  - Artificial ventilation and external chest compression may be performed as usual
    - Or reduce frequency of chest compressions (controversial)
    - Or reduce ventilatory rate (controversial)
    - Or increase force of compression (controversial)
  - Continue resuscitation until rewarming >30°C, if necessary for several hours
  - Transport to a hospital with extracorporeal circulation, even when choice of hospital considerably prolongs prehospital time
- Advanced life support
  - ECG monitoring mandatory
    - Often only ECG definitely detects/excludes a perfusing rhythm
  - Temperature monitoring (tympanic) desirable
  - Endotracheal intubation sometimes difficult due to muscle rigidity
    - Blind nasotracheal intubation
  - Recommendations for advanced life support are controversial and often have a poor scientific basis
    - No epinephrine (controversial)
    - Reduced dose of epinephrine, no repetitive doses (controversial)
    - Limit defibrillation attempts to three (controversial)
  - Continue resuscitation until complete rewarming in all patients except
    - Primarily asphyxiated avalanche victims
    - Trauma incompatible with survival

the patient is transported to an appropriate hospital for extracorporeal rewarming as fast as possible. In some hypothermic patients, however, spontaneous circulation can be restored despite a core temperature below 30°C. It may therefore be justified to repeatedly defibrillate a hypothermic patient.

In some case reports, restoration of spontaneous circulation was reported in close correlation with the administration of epinephrine [3,14,21]. Most clinicians do not administer epinephrine during hypothermic cardiopulmonary resuscitation, however, and the American Heart Association does not recommend epinephrine for patients with a core temperature below 30°C [10]. Repeatedly administered epinephrine may accumulate to toxic levels, and thus repeat doses of epinephrine should be given at longer than standard intervals. Scientific valid data concerning the necessity of epinephrine or the optimal dose of epinephrine during hypothermic resuscitation are completely absent. Whether such antiarrhythmic drugs as lidocaine or bretylium can prevent sudden ventricular fibrillation or facilitate successful defibrillation in patients with severe accidental hypothermia is also controversial and not well studied.

No matter if a modification of standard resuscitation technique is used or not, it is essential to continue resuscitation efforts until rewarming above 30°C [3,10]. Due to the significant protection from ischemic cerebral injury, successful resuscitation with full neurological recovery is possible even in the extremities. Termination of resuscitation efforts in the prehospital environment is justified only in case of trauma obviously incompatible with survival, or signs of asphyxia in an avalanche victims [26] (no "air pocket," snow in mouth and nose; see Sec. VII).

In summary, hypothermia becomes life-threatening when the body core temperature falls below 30°C. Because of characteristic pathophysiological changes, however, accidental hypothermia necessitates a specialized therapeutic approach even in the case of a mild or moderate decrease in the body core temperature. Major problems may complicate rescue and prehospital treatment of patients with accidental hypothermia. A marked decrease in body core temperature may occur early during rescue and prehospital therapy, the so-called afterdrop phenomenon. Cold blood is shifted from the surface to the core of the body by movements during rescue or by efforts at rapid external rewarming. In addition, with a body core temperature of less than 28°C, the myocardium is highly irritable, and even minor stimulations of the hypothermic heart can cause VF.

In general, rewarming in the prehospital environment is indicated only in cases of delayed or prolonged evacuation. Active external rewarming with chemical hot packs, active internal rewarming with 40°C warmed intravenous solutions, or active internal rewarming with airway rewarming may be used. Only limited, preliminary clinical data are available for negative pressure rewarming, another promising method of active rewarming suitable for the prehospital environment.

Severe accidental hypothermia markedly changes the pathophysiology and prognosis of concomitant cardiac arrest. Hypothermia offers profound protection from ischemic cerebral injury, and successful resuscitation with full neurological recovery is possible even after prolonged cardiac arrest and resuscitation efforts lasting for several hours. On the other hand, in general the hypothermic heart does not respond to pharmacological or electrical therapy unless rewarmed above 32°C. It is therefore difficult to diagnose death in a hypothermic patient, and most experts consider nobody dead unless warm and dead.

VII. AVALANCHE ACCIDENTS

A. Epidemiology and Incidence of Avalanche Accidents

The exact number of annual avalanche victims is unknown, as international registries include only data from mountain rescue services in Europe and North America. Avalanche accidents in less developed countries are not registered. Only when they bury densely inhabited areas and an extraordinarily high number of people die are avalanches recognized in less developed countries (e.g., 284 avalanche victims in southeast Turkey in 1992 or 183 avalanche victims in Kashmir in 1995). The registry of the International Commission for Alpine Rescue includes data from 17 European and American countries [27]. This registry demonstrates that approximately 150 victims die each year under an avalanche. About four times that number are involved in an avalanche accident each year and survive. In developed countries avalanche accidents are almost exclusively due to mountaineering and skiing activities (tourist avalanches). Avalanche accidents in inhabited areas (disaster avalanches) occur only rarely. The number of avalanche victims is steadily increasing in the United States, whereas the number remains unchanged in European countries. The unchanged number of avalanche victims in European countries is at least partly the result of intensified efforts by avalanche information services to inform and educate the public about the danger of avalanches and how to avoid them.

B. Probability of Survival and Cause of Death

If a skier or mountaineer is caught by an avalanche, the probability that he will be buried by the snow mass is about 50%, as half of the victims remain on the surface of the avalanche. The overall survival rate when completely buried under snow is about 30% [27]. By contrast, more than 95% of all victims survive, when the head and the thorax remain outside the snow masses. Autopsy findings in avalanche victims demonstrate that the major cause of death in avalanche victims is asphyxia (60–80% of all fatalities) [28]. Trauma is an uncommon reason for death in avalanche victims, accounting for less than 10% of all casualties (causing death predominantly in victims remaining on the surface of the avalanche). In contrast to previous assumptions, hypothermia is also a rare and uncommon cause of death when buried under a snow avalanche, accounting for less than 10% of all fatalities [26,28,29].

It has been assumed for almost three decades [27] that survival in an avalanche depends predominantly on the depth and the duration of burial under the snow mass. An almost linear correlation between the time the victim was buried under the avalanche and his or her probability of survival was assumed. According to these assumptions, about 50% of all casualties are alive 60 min after avalanche descent. Avalanche victims alive after 1 hr may have cooled to a core temperature of less than 30°C. If extricated after prolonged burial, cardiac arrest may be secondary to accidental hypothermia, and potent protection from ischemic brain injury can be assumed.

Consequently, aggressive resuscitation and rewarming efforts using cardiopulmonary bypass were the ''gold standard'' in the therapy of arrested hypothermic avalanche victims during the 1980s [5,26,30]. In 1994, Brugger and Falk [26] recalculated the probability of survival when buried under a snow avalanche, analyzing data from 332 avalanche victims in Switzerland between 1981 and 1989 (Fig. 3). Their results have significantly changed attitudes toward the probability of survival when buried under a snow avalanche. Brugger and Falk did not find a linear correlation between the time buried under snow and the probability of survival. The type of snow and the depth of burial had no major impact on the probability of survival. Probability of survival is 92% within the first 15 min under the snow avalanche, but rapidly decreases to 30% during the following 20 min. Most of the victims alive under the avalanche survive the following 60 min. All obviously have a patent airway, free of snow, and an air pocket around the mouth and the nose, allowing respiration. Thereafter, most of the avalanche victims that are still alive die within a short period of time (Fig. 3). The reason for that second rapid decrease in the probability of survival remains unclear. Perhaps the wall of the air pocket becomes iced due to the warm air expired, and oxygen diffusion across the wall of the air pocket is no longer possible.

These new data concerning the probability of survival when buried under an avalanche have had a major impact on the rescue strategies in avalanche accidents and the therapeutic management of arrested hypothermic avalanche victims [26,30]. Obviously 60% of all avalanche victims die from asphyxia between 15 and 30 min under the snow, therefore predominantly rapid extrication from the avalanche by uninjured companion mountaineers using avalanche transceivers will save the life of an avalanche victim. Only

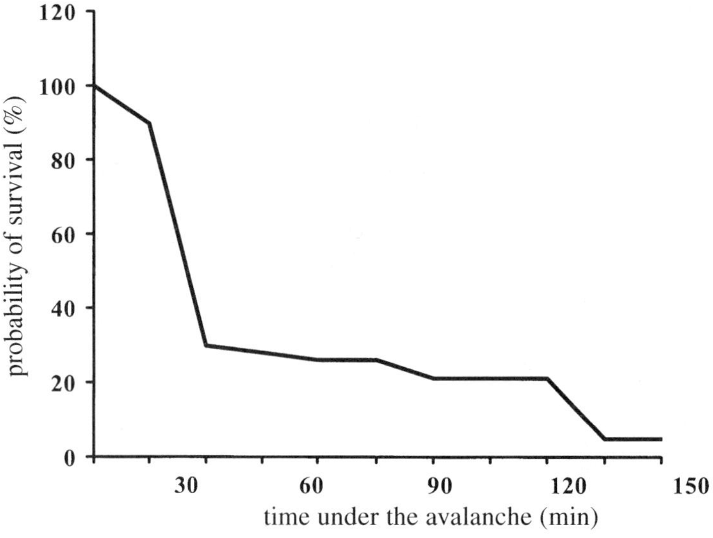

Figure 3 Probability of survival when buried under a snow avalanche. Probability of survival is 92% within the first 15 min and rapidly decreases to 30% during the following 20 min, therefore rapid extrication from the avalanche by uninjured companion mountaineers using avalanche transceivers will save the life of the victim when buried under snow. (Adapted from Ref. 26.)

a few patients survive long enough to become profoundly hypothermic (about 5–10%). Most arrested avalanche victims extricated hypothermic after prolonged burial have died from asphyxia within the first 30 min and cool only thereafter. This is in accordance with the poor survival rates reported for aggressive resuscitation efforts in hypothermic arrest victims after avalanche accidents [30]. Aggressive resuscitation and rewarming efforts with extracorporeal circulation are obviously indicated only in a few selected avalanche victims with hypothermic cardiac arrest.

C. Search Strategies in Avalanche Accidents

The probability of survival is 92% if extricated within 15 min. It dramatically decreases during the following 20 min. A timely activation of mountain rescue services after avalanche accidents is possible nowadays, and with the widespread use of cellular phones, even in remote mountain areas. Even with the rapid transport of rescue personnel and rescue dogs by helicopters, organized help will rarely arrive at the scene of an avalanche accident within the first 15 min after avalanche descent. During the time period with the highest probability of survival, the only possibility to extricate an avalanche victim is by experienced companion mountaineers using avalanche transceivers (Table 10). An analysis of avalanche accidents in Central Europe, however, has demonstrated that the widespread use of avalanche transceivers did not markedly reduce the overall mortality of avalanche victims (33% survival rate in avalanche victims carrying a transceiver versus 25% in those not carrying an avalanche transceiver) [27]. With the present status of education in the use of avalanche transceivers, it is not possible to extricate a considerable number of avalanche victims within the first 15 min after avalanche descent essential for

Table 10 Possible Rescue Strategies in Avalanche Accidents

Strategies to avoid burial under the snow masses
Avalanche air bag
Strategies for immediate use by companion mountaineers
Avalanche transceivers
Strategies for organized rescue efforts by the mountain rescue services
Rescue dogs
Search with avalanche probes
Digging the avalanche

survival. Training mountaineers in a rapid search technique and pointing out the importance of the additional equipment necessary for immediate extrication (portable shovel, avalanche probe) can perhaps reduce the mortality in avalanche accidents in the next few years.

The widespread use of avalanche transceivers resulted in only a small reduction of mortality in avalanche victims, thus much attention has been paid to alternative techniques, focusing on equipment to help to avoid burial of the head and the thorax. The avalanche air bag is one of these techniques, now commercially available and more widely used. The avalanche air bag is a gas-filled balloon mounted on a commercial backpack that inflates automatically within a few seconds after manual initiation (Fig. 4). Experience with avalanche air bags is limited, however promising. In several test series and a few

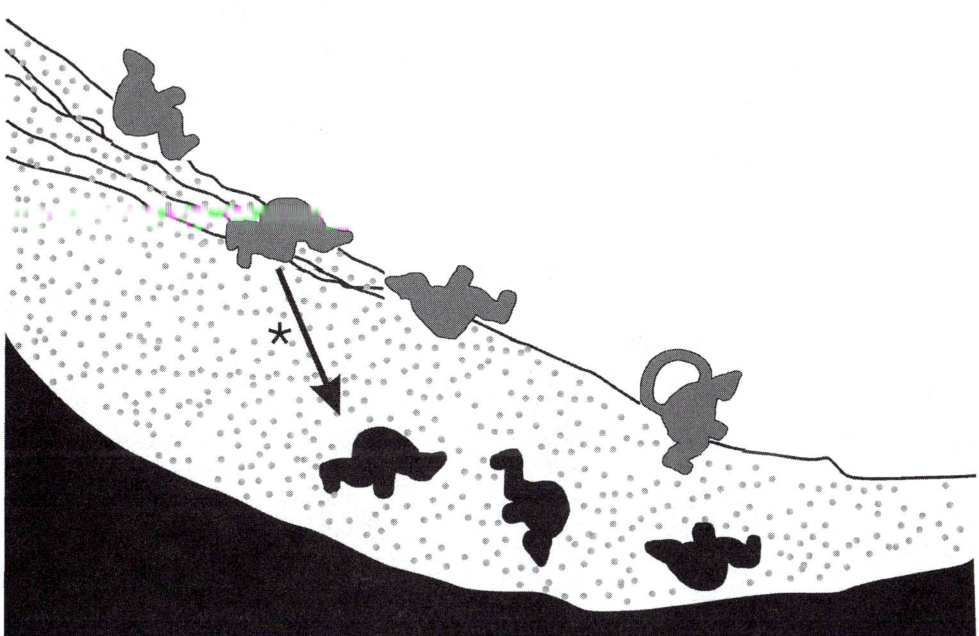

Figure 4 Simulated avalanche accident. Avalanche air bag prevents burial under the snow masses. *Victim without the 150 l gas-filled balloon integrated in a backpack is buried by the snow masses.

Table 11 Efficiency of Different Search Strategies

	Search with a rescue dog	Search with avalanche probes (20 rescuers)	Success rate
Initial search	5–10 min	30 min	Partially and superficially buried victims
Standard search	30 min	4 hr	80% of all victims
Extended search	2 hr	20 hr	95% of all victims

Note: mean times necessary to search an avalanche.
Source: Avalanche Handbook. Tyrolean Avalanche Information Service, Innsbruck, Austria.

occasional avalanche accidents the air bag reliably prevented complete burial of the victim under the snow masses. The major problem is the necessity for manual initiation of the filling process of the balloon.

The probability of survival when extricated from the avalanche by organized rescue efforts will be only 30%. A survival rate of 30% is possible only when the victim is extricated within 90 min after the avalanche occurs (Fig. 3). The possible search techniques for avalanche victims not carrying an avalanche transceiver are search with rescue dogs, search with avalanche probes, and digging into the avalanche (Tables 10, 11).

Whenever well-trained rescue dogs are available they are the fastest and best method of search. They make possible the extrication of a considerable number of casualties within 90 min; therefore, searching the avalanche with probes is generally used only later during the rescue mission (Fig. 5). Digging the avalanche normally results in the extrication of dead casualties after several hours.

The basis for most successful organized rescue efforts is the use of helicopters to reach even remote mountain areas within a short period of time. The inability to land the helicopter near the site of the accident does not exclude helicopter rescue missions. Rescue dogs and rescue personnel can be released with the help of a winch (Fig. 6).

D. Therapy of Avalanche Victims After Extrication

The diagnostic and therapeutic approach to avalanche victims extricated within 45 min after avalanche descent is shown in Fig. 7. Many avalanche victims rescued within a few minutes after avalanche descent are either unconscious or already in respiratory arrest when extricated from the snow masses. When their airways are freed from snow and with a short period of ventilation (mouth-to-mouth ventilation by companion mountaineers), spontaneous respiration starts and most victims awake within a few minutes. Although trauma is rather uncommon in avalanche victims, a thorough evaluation of the conscious avalanche victim is mandatory in order not to miss life-threatening injuries (focusing in particular on compression trauma to the chest and the abdomen, cervical spine injury, and head injury).

Beside postischemic coma, head injury should also be considered in those avalanche victims remaining unconscious after initial resuscitation. Endotracheal intubation, artificial ventilation, volume resuscitation, and catecholamine therapy should be initated immediately in any unconscious avalanche victim to assure cerebral oxygenation and an adequate cerebral perfusion pressure. If present, accidental hypothermia is usually only mild in an adequately dressed mountaineer. In the case of prolonged cardiopulmonary arrest unre-

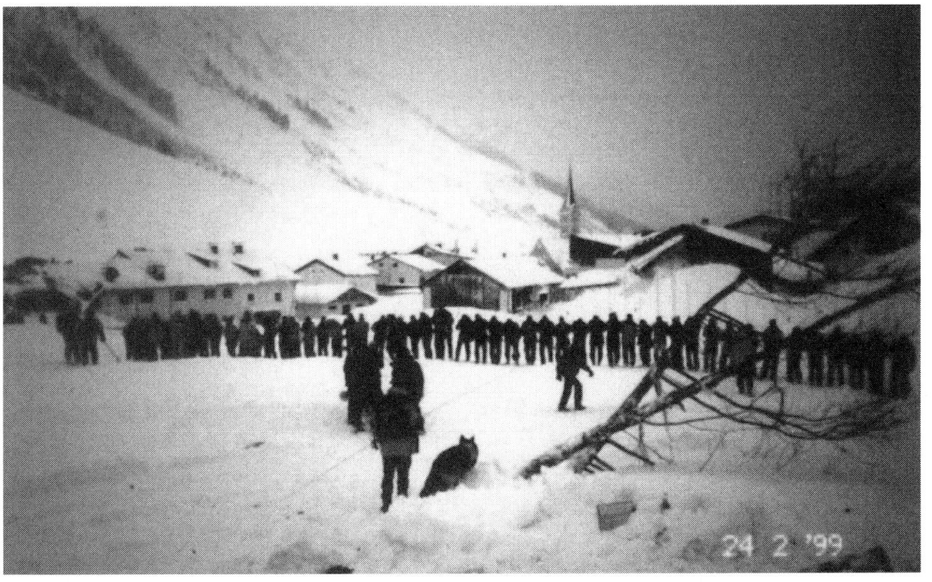

Figure 5 Mountain rescue team searching the disaster avalanche of Galtür, February 1999. Standing shoulder to shoulder and inserting the probe once every step forward results in an 80% probability of a successful search. Searching the avalanche with rescue dogs is about eight times faster than searching the avalanche with probes.

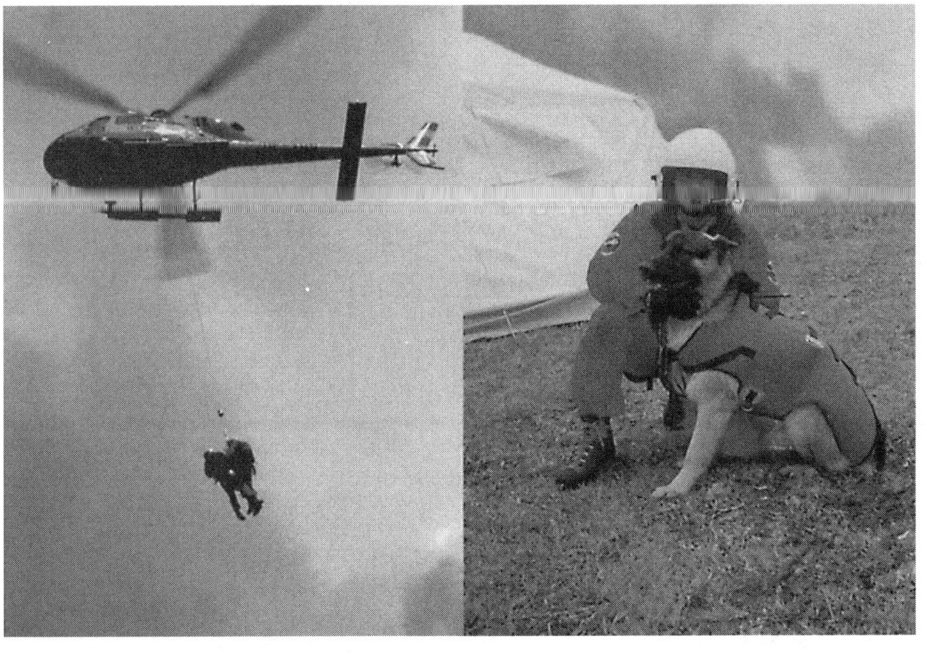

Figure 6 If landing the helicopter is not possible directly at the scene of an avalanche, accident rescue personnel can be transported to the scene with the help of a winch or a fixed tow (left). Rescue dogs are transported in a special belayer accompanied by their dogmaster (right).

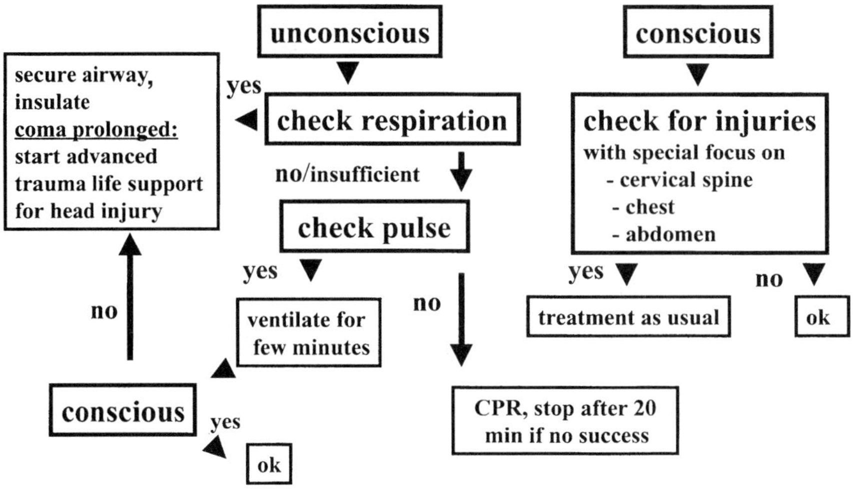

Figure 7 Therapeutic approach to an avalanche victim extricated within less than 45 min. Accidental hypothermia is not present after this short period of time when buried under snow; prolonged resuscitation efforts in case of resistant cardiac arrest are not indicated.

sponsive to advanced life support, resuscitation may be stopped at the scene [26]. Cooling is markedly enhanced after extrication from the avalanche (wind, wet and snow-covered clothes), and complete insulation is essential.

The diagnostic and therapeutic approach to the avalanche victim extricated more than 45 min after avalanche descent is shown in Fig. 8. Early recognition and adequate therapy of accidental hypothermia (often moderate or severe after prolonged burial under

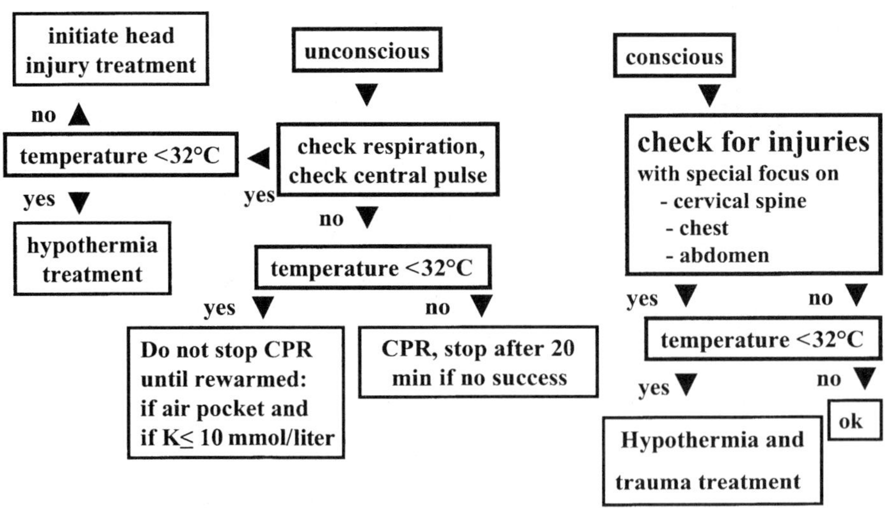

Figure 8 Therapeutic approach to an avalanche victim extricated after more than 45 min. Accidental hypothermia can be expected after this period of time when buried under snow; resistant cardiac arrest may be secondary to accidental hypothermia and prolonged resuscitation efforts until complete rewarming may be indicated.

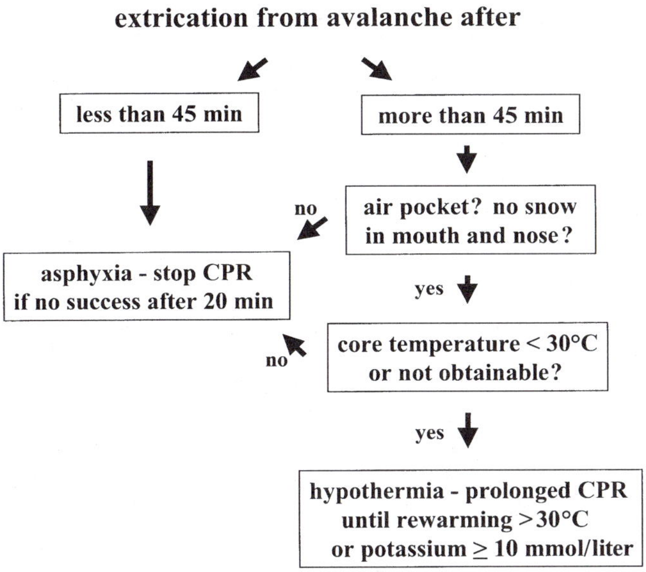

Figure 9 Management of the asystolic avalanche victim after extrication; differentiation of cardiac arrest secondary to asphyxia from cardiac arrest secondary to accidental hypothermia.

the snow masses) and differentiation between primarily asphyxiated arrest victims and patients with cardiac arrest secondary to accidental hypothermia [26] are the two major problems in these patients.

One problem of the prehospital therapy of avalanche victims is the differentiation between primarily asphyxiated asystolic avalanche victims from casualties who have arrested secondary to severe accidental hypothermia (Fig. 9). The duration of burial under the snow mass and the presence and absence of an air pocket are the key points in this differential diagnosis (Fig. 8). Victims buried under snow masses for less than 45 min are not profoundly hypothermic. Although varying over a wide range between 1°C/hr and 8°C/hr in extremities, avalanche victims cool between 3°C/hr to 6°C/hr on average [27]. Respiration under an avalanche always necessitates an air pocket (sometimes a small one) around the mouth and nose [27]. Absence of such an air pocket or snow in the mouth and the nose indicate immediate respiratory arrest after avalanche burial, and asphyxia must be expected. If the differential diagnosis between asphyxia and hypothermia is not possible based on clinical parameters alone, a plasma potassium determination may be extremely helpful. Many avalanche victims primarily asphyxiated before cooling have extraordinarily high plasma potassium levels (≥10 mmol/liter) [16,26,30].

The rescue and treatment recommendations described before may be realized only in areas with a sophisticated mountain rescue service and sophisticated resources, which are present only in a few European and North American countries. In countries without emergency medical helicopter systems and rescue dogs on call, mortality rates in avalanche accidents will be almost 100%.

E. Disaster Avalanche

Disaster avalanches burying inhabited areas rarely occur in Europe and North America. Medical problems in victims from disaster avalanches are markedly different from those

Table 12 Key Points in Search and Rescue After Disaster Avalanches

Large number of victims and limited medical resources
Less developed countries
Remote, poorly accessible areas
Limited air and ground transport capabilities
Trauma an important cause of morbidity and mortality
Prepare for prehospital trauma care at the scene
Hypothermia common in a large number of victims
Prepare for prevention of hypothermia after extrication
Prepare for treatment of accidental hypothermia at the scene
Organize in-hospital treatment for a large number of patients with severe hypothermia (including extracorporeal circulation)

encountered in tourist avalanches (Table 12). Trauma is an important cause of morbidity and mortality in victims caught in destroyed cars and houses. Asphyxia is a less common cause of death, as many victims are surrounded by a large air pocket. Victims are often buried for prolonged periods, and therefore accidental hypothermia is common when extricated after several hours. The major problem in the treatment of victims of disaster avalanches is not only the large number of patients encountered; in addition, these patients must often be treated for several hours at the scene, as evacuation is impossible because of the danger of further avalanches (roads closed) or poor weather conditions (no helicopter transport available).

VIII. CONCLUSIONS

In summary, more recent data markedly changed our knowledge about the probability of survival when buried under a snow avalanche. Most avalanche victims die from asphyxia shortly after avalanche descent. Trauma and hypothermia are rare causes for death in avalanche victims. Predominantly rapid extrication from the avalanche by uninjured companion mountaineers using avalanche transceivers will save the life of an avalanche victim. If cardiac arrest is diagnosed after extrication from the avalanche, it is rarely secondary to accidental hypothermia, therefore prolonged resuscitation efforts and in-hospital rewarming with extracorporeal circulation are indicated only in a few hypothermic patients after avalanche accidents.

REFERENCES

1. EL Lloyd. Accidental hypthermia. Resuscitation 32:111–124, 1996.
2. PE Lonning, A Skulberg, F Abyholm. Accidental hypothermia: A review of the literature. Acta Anaesth Scand 30:601–613, 1986.
3. MG Larach. Accidental hypothermia. Lancet 345:490–498, 1995.
4. DF Danzl, RS Pozos. Multicenter hypothermia survey. Ann Emer Med 16:1042–1055, 1987.
5. U Althaus, B Aeberhard, B Schuepbach, BH Nachbur, W Muehlemann. Management of profound accidental hypothermia with cardiorespiratory arrest. Ann Surg 195:492–495, 1982.
6. BH Walpoth, BN Walpoth-Aslan, HP Mattle, BP Radanov, G Schroth, L Schaeffler, AP Fischer, L Segesser, U Althaus. Outcome of survivors of accidental deep hypothermia and circulatory arrest treated with extracorporeal blood warming. New Eng J Med 337:1500–1505, 1997.
7. E Roggero, H Stricker, P Biegger. Severe accidental hypothermia with cardiopulmonary arrest: Prolonged resuscitation without extracorporeal circulation. Schweiz Med Wochenschr 122: 161–164, 1992.

8. K Lexow. Severe accidental hypothermia: Survival after 6 hours 30 minutes of cardiopulmonary resuscitation. Artic Med Res 50 suppl. 6:112–114, 1991.
9. M Gilbert, R Busund, A Skagseth, PA Nilsen, JP Solbo. Resuscitation from accidental hypothermia of 13.7°C with circulatory arrest. Lancet 355:201–202, 2000.
10. W Kloeck, RO Cummins, D Chamberlain, L Bossaert, V Callanan, P Carli, J Christenson, B Connoly, JP Ornato, A Sanders, P Steen. Guidelines 2000 for cardiopulmonary resuscitation and emergency cardiovascular care. International consensus on science. Hypothermia. Circulation 102(suppl 1):229–232, 2000.
11. Center for Disease Control and Prevention. Hypothermia related deaths—Virginia, November 1996–April 1997. JAMA 279:102, 1998.
12. MD Stoneham, SJ Squires. Prolonged resuscitation in acute deep hypothermia. Anaesthesia 47:784–788, 1992.
13. F Sterz, A Zeiner, I Kurkciyan, K Janata, M Mullner, H Domanovits, P Safar. Mild resuscitative hypothermia and outcome after cardiopulmonary resuscitation. J Neurosurg Anaesth 8: 88–96, 1996.
14. C Winegard. Successful treatment of severe hypothermia and prolonged cardiac arrest with closed thoracic cavity lavage. J Emerg Med 15:629–632, 1997.
15. DF Vretenar, JD Urschel, JCW Parrot, HW Unruh. Cardiopulmonary bypass resuscitation for accidental hypothermia. Ann Thor Surg 58:895–898, 1994.
16. MG Hauty, BC Esrig, JG Hill, WB Long. Prognostic factors in severe accidental hypothermia: Experience with the Mt. Hood tragedy. J Trauma 27:1107–1112, 1987.
17. BH Walpoth, J Galdikas, F Leupi, W Muehlemann, P Schlaepfer, U Althaus. Assessment of hypothermia with a new tympanic thermometer. J Clin Mon 10:91–96, 1994.
18. IR Rogers, DL O'Brien, C Wee, A Smith, D Lopez. Infrared emission tympanic thermometers cannot be relied upon in a wilderness setting. Wild Environ Med 10:201–203, 1999.
19. E Kornberger, P Mair. Important aspects in the treatment of severe accidental hypothermia: The Innsbruck experience. J Neurosurg Anesth 8:83–87, 1996.
20. AD Weinberg. The role of inhalation rewarming in the early management of hypothermia. Resuscitation 36:101–104, 1998.
21. AJ Ireland, VI Pathi, R Crawford, IW Colquhoun. Back from the dead: Extracorporeal rewarming of severe accidental hypothermia victims in accident and emergency. J Accid Emerg Med 14:255–257, 1997.
22. RM Elenbaas, K Mattson, H Cole, M Steele, J Ryan, W Robinson. Bretylium in hypothermia-induced ventricular fibrillation in dogs. Ann Emerg Med 13:994–999, 1984.
23. RG Dixon, JM Dougherty, LJ White, D Lombino, RR Rusnak. Transcutaneous pacing in a hypothermic-dog model. Ann Emerg Med 29:602–606, 1997.
24. P Mair, E Kornberger, B Schwarz, M Baubin, C Hoermann. Forward blood flow during cardiopulmonary resuscitation in patients with severe accidental hypothermia: An echocardiographic study. Acta Anaesth Scand 42:1139–1144, 1998.
25. PA Maningas, LR DeGuzman, SJ Hollenbach, KA Volk, RF Bellamy. Regional blood flow during hypothermic arrest. Ann Emerg Med 15:390–396, 1986.
26. H Brugger, B Durrer, L Adler-Kastner. On-site triage of avalanche victims with asystole by the emergency doctor. Resuscitation 31:11–16, 1996.
27. H Brugger, M Falk, L Adler-Kastner. Avalanche emergency: New aspects in the pathophysiology and therapy of buried avalanche victims. Wi Kli Wo 109:145–159, 1997.
28. H Stalsberg, C Albretsen, M Gilbert, M Kaerney, E Mostue, L Nordrum, M Rostrup, A Orbo. Mechanism of death in avalanche victims. Virchows Archiv A Pathol Anat 414:415–422, 1989.
29. MD Grossmann, JR Saffle, F Thomas, B Tremper. Avalanche trauma. J Trauma 29:1705–1709, 1989.
30. P Mair, E Kornberger, W Furtwaengler, H Antretter, D Balogh. Prognostic markers in patients with severe accidental hypothermia and cardiocirculatory arrest. Resuscitation 27:47–54, 1994.

33

Diving Injuries and Hyperbaric Medicine

GUTTORM BRATTEBOE

Haukeland University Hospital, Bergen, Norway

ENRICO M. CAMPORESI

State University of New York Upstate Medical University, Syracuse, New York

I. INTRODUCTION

Decompression sickness (DCS), arterial gas embolism (AGE), and barotrauma are syndromes precipitated by a rapid change in pressure to which the body is exposed. It has been proposed that the term decompression illness (DCI) should be used to encompass all manifestations of decompression barotraumas and/or DCS (Table 1) [1–3]. The most frequent cause for this pathology, which is caused by a change in pressure (dysbarism), is an insufficient decompression time after exposure to elevated pressures, such as after diving underwater or a similar sudden reduction of environmental pressure at high altitude in aviators who fly in compressed cabins. Astronauts can also be exposed to very low pressure in their habitat aboard a space capsule, both in preparation for and by accident during extravehicular activities. In all cases, the pathology of dysbarism is similar and is caused by the elevated partial pressure of inert gas in tissues, usually nitrogen, coming out of solution and forming bubbles in tissues or even in the bloodstream. For such a bubble formation to happen in oversaturated tissue the pressure must rapidly be reduced by 50%, therefore a strict distinction between DCS and AGE might be blurred during the clinical exposure. It has been hypothesized that both diseases are often present simultaneously, but with different manifestations. Barotrauma occurs when there is sufficient pressure differential across a tissue–air interface within the body to cause injury. Gas-containing spaces in the body shrink with compression and expand during decompression according to Boyle's law, and the largest volume variations occur near the surface, as shown in Figure 1.

Table 1 Classification of Decompression Illness

Decompression sickness
Type 1
Musculoskeletal
Skin
Lymphatic
Fatigue
Type 2
Neurological
Cardio respiratory (''chokes'')
Vestibulary/auditory
Shock
Arterial gas embolism
Barotrauma
Lung
Sinus
Inner ear
Middle ear
Dental
Gastrointestinal

Source: Refs. 1–3.

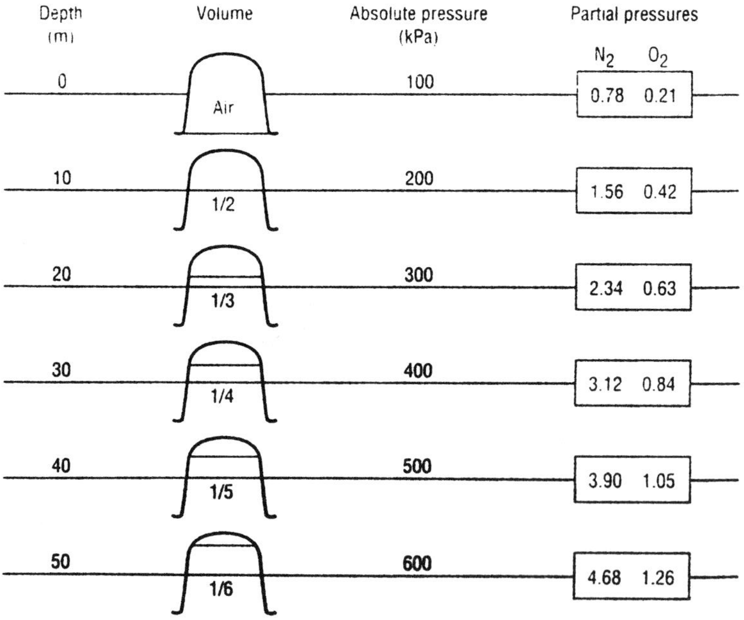

Figure 1 Volume pressure changes as a function of depth with corresponding partial pressures of nitrogen (N_2) and oxygen (O_2) in ata (1 ATA = 101 kPa = 1 bar = 760 mmHg). (From Ref. 3a.)

An understanding of the various forms of DSIs and of the evolution of treatment can be best gleaned from its history. Briefly, French physicians in the latter half of the nineteenth century described the sharp joint pain in the knees and shoulder in compressed air workers upon and after decompression, and demonstrated the beneficial effects of acute recompression to the original pressure followed by more gradual ascent. In 1878 Paul Bert demonstrated in animals that the cause of DCS was dissolved nitrogen becoming gaseous during decompression and that the bubbles formed were responsible for the ''bends'' [4]. It was not until 1909 that the value of recompression therapy at the work site was statistically demonstrated during the construction of the Hudson River tunnel in New York [5].

II. PATHOPHYSIOLOGY OF DCI

Equilibration of blood and tissue compartments with the respired gases during exposure to a raised pressure environment continue until equilibrium is reached and all tissues are saturated. During exposure to compressed air in a high-pressure work environment (''caisson''), or while breathing from compressed air tanks during SCUBA (self-contained underwater breathing apparatus) diving, nitrogen equilibrates with different tissues in relation to solubility and perfusion rate of each compartment (e.g., like anesthetic gases). Like blood, ''fast'' tissues can equilibrate in minutes, while ''slow'' tissues, like adipose areas or myelinated nerves, can take up to 12 hr to equilibrate. When the diver or the compressed air worker leave maximum exposure pressure, they may not have been exposed long enough to absorb sufficient gas to provide a clinically important risk of sufficient bubble formation, and therefore they can return safely to the surface without so-called decompression stops. This is commonly called a ''nonstop dive.'' If, however, the diver stays at pressure beyond a certain threshold combination of depth and time, a direct decompression is no longer safe, and progressive ''stops'' at various shallower depths are required. Several versions of these diving tables are in use, based upon different mathematical models and modifications by experience (Fig. 2). Moreover, personal computers are also available today to calculate predicted decompression stops from a given dive profile.

Additional factors contributing to the manifestation of DCI are whether or not a significant degree of pulmonary barotrauma was suffered during ascent or decompression.

Depth (feet)	Bottom time (min)	Time first stop (min:sec)	Decompression stops (feet) 50	40	30	20	10	Total decompression time (min:sec)
90	30						0	1:30
	40	1:20					7	8:30
	50	1:20					18	19:30
	60	1:20					25	26:30
	70	1:10				7	30	38:30
	80	1:10				13	40	54:30
	90	1:10				18	48	67:30
	100	1:10				21	54	76:30
	110	1:10				24	61	86:30
	120	1:10				32	68	101:30
	130	1:00			5	36	74	116:30

Figure 2 U.S. Navy standard air decompression table for a dive to a maximum depth of 90 feet (30 meters). As one can see from the table the diver can only make a nonstop dive to this depth if the time from descent is started until start of ascent is less than 30 min. (From Ref. 5a.)

Pulmonary barotrauma is caused by intra-alveolar air entering as small bubbles into the arterial circulation through the disruption of lung parenchyma. An additional factor is related to ''silent'' bubbles that may form from the dissolved gases during a no-decompression ascent, which are usually transported from the venous blood into the lungs. These bubbles are able to diffuse into the alveoli and therefore are filtrated from the lung and are not present in the arterial side of the lung circulation. The situation may be different if a simultaneous right-to-left cardiac shunt is present anatomically within the heart of the diver, as these bubbles may then pass across into the arterial circulation from the right ventricle to the left ventricle. Additional complexity is added to the clinical manifestation of DCI from the adaptation that can arise from regular daily decompression in compression air workers and divers; it is well known that this ''acclimatization'' is rapidly lost during a break from regular daily work and may manifest itself suddenly when resuming diving, even with minimal decompression profiles. It has been shown that occasional divers, such as sport divers making several dives deeper than 10 meter sea water (msw) during a 1-week vacation, tend to run into trouble later in the week, often about the fourth or fifth day. Possibly this is due to the progressive accumulation of dissolved gas in slow tissues which eventually cannot be off-gassed before the next dive exposure. Exposure to lower ambient pressures (during mountaineering or high altitude) after several dives or after deep dives may also precipitate DCI. Factors predisposing to the onset of the symptoms are listed in Table 2. All these factors favor accumulation of inert gas in slow tissues, and may contribute to the rapid onset of symptomatology after surfacing.

Often the clinical manifestations first presenting to the physician are a mixture of DCS, AGE, and barotrauma, although no clear etiology of pulmonary barotrauma can be evidenced by the exposure. In fact, AGE can be a neurological complication of a pulmonary overpressure accident, sometimes heralded by additional manifestation of extravascular gas such as pneumothorax, pneumomediastinum, or other subcutaneous gas presence in soft tissues. Pulmonary barotrauma and AGE have been reported after very shallow dives (e.g., 2 meters), while the diver must have been deeper than 10 meters for DCS to occur.

Decompression bubbles can distribute anywhere within the body and can be found both extra- and intravascularly. The most accepted mechanism is that bubbles will cause deleterious effects by simple, mechanical expansion and by surface interaction with the blood at the blood–gas and endoltheliurn interface [6]. It has been hypothesized that bubbles in the region of muscle tendinous insertions can cause pressure on nerve endings and be responsible for local sharp pain in some cases of ''limb-bends.'' Furthermore, platelet aggregation and the release of intravascular mediators is one example of the effect of

Table 2 Predisposing Factors for Decompression Illness

Exercise before the dive, during bottom time, after the dive
High partial pressure of CO_2
Cold during decompression
Obesity
Age
Alcohol
Dehydration
Recent local injury

Source: Ref. 3.

blood–gas interaction. Complement activation and activation of platelet and other enzyme groups can lead to hemorheological changes and the development of rapid-onset hypovolemic shock in serious DCI. Finally, embolic bubbles, which obstruct capillaries or small-size arterioles, will completely obliterate vascular segments and will cause embolic symptoms. Even transitory passage of bubbles across the endothelial vessel surface will eventually result in subsequent circulatory disturbance in the specific affected vascular bed, however. This is particularly evident in the central nervous system (CNS) and the subsequent distribution of extravascular fluid.

III. MANIFESTATIONS OF DECOMPRESSION DISORDERS

The traditional classification of DCI is listed in Table 1. A classic distinction has been made between type 1 DCS (mild) and type 2 DCS (serious), due to ''peripheral'' manifestations versus ''central nervous system'' manifestations. In practical terms this distinction has an operational rationale in that it supports that type 2 DCS must be treated immediately, and in the U.S. navy does not require the presence of a medical officer. This concept has been extended from the navy to the field of compressed air workers and to diving contractors. Treatment of severe DCI in a resort facility following sports diving without the presence of a physician is still practiced around the world. From the neurologist point of view, however, even mild symptoms of bubble embolization in a peripheral vascular system can and often are accompanied by the simultaneous presence of subtle neurological injury due to showering of emboli in specific areas of the brain or spinal cord, therefore, a sharp distinction between type 1 and type 2 DCS can be blurred in clinical practice. It is recommended, however, that in the case of a suspected DCI the information listed in Table 3 be recorded.

IV. MUSCULOSKELETAL PAIN

The widest known manifestation of DCS is the ''bends,'' indicating peripheral limb pain, most commonly in the knees, the shoulders, or other large synovial joints. Joint pain may be the presenting symptom, but at times peripheral limb pain is not limited to joints. In a large series of 1249 cases of DCI, pain was the initial symptom in 41% of the cases [2]. Often limb pain may be associated with more serious neurological manifestations, which might be less obvious.

The pain from the bends varies in presentation but is often very sharp and defined, up to the point of having been described as ''incapacitating,'' even in experienced divers. The joint pain in DCI tends to be somewhat relieved if the joint is held in an anatomical

Table 3 Information to be Recorded in the Case of Suspected Decompression Illness

Clinical manifestation(s)
Time to onset of each manifestation and its pattern of evolution (progressive, static, spontaneous improving, relapsing)
Tissue inert gas burden (depth–time profile)
Whether or not there is evidence of barotrauma
Other dives during previous 24 hr

Source: Refs. 1–3.

neutral position or if a pressure cuff is inflated around the joint. When not treated by recompression, the pain may change in characteristic and even disappear, but most often it dissolves over several days.

V. CARDIORESPIRATORY DECOMPRESSION SYMPTOMS ("CHOKES")

A particularly severe form of DCS presents with a large buildup of venous gas emboli in the pulmonary circulation and the associated liberation of vasoactive products from the lungs. This is a seldom-occurring condition, requiring a high tissue inert-gas burden, but it has also been described following a relatively short, deep exposure. The onset is typified by sharp onset of retrosternal pain, which limits inspiration and dry cough, at times accompanied by circulatory collapse. The symptoms may resemble those of drowning, but a careful history may differentiate between the two entities. Rapid treatment by recompression is mandatory to save the diver's life [7].

VI. NEUROLOGICAL DECOMPRESSION SYMPTOMS

Neurological symptoms are extremely common in DCI, and drivers often seek medical advice on paresthesias with or without objective hypesthesia. Also, a degree of fatigue or tiredness disproportionate to the amount of physical exercise preceding the diving activity is present. This fatigue can be accompanied by other symptoms (transient) from the CNS (e.g., headache) and requires attention. One should also be aware of the fact that often there are patchy areas of reduced sensibility, not always following the anatomical dermatomes. Although neurological DCI most often seems to affect the spinal cord, careful investigations have revealed signs of supraspinal sequela in a proportion of such patients [8].

The classic manifestation of gas embolism due to pulmonary barotrauma is immediate loss of consciousness upon surfacing, often leading to a significant neurological focalization such as hemiplegia or monoplegia accompanied by circulatory collapse or vertigo. Most often the symptoms are labyrinthine (the ''staggers'') or an ascending paraplegia (''spinal bends''). Central nervous system dysfunction can present as a variable feeling of visual disturbances, a change in consciousness, and sometimes even psychosis. The onset of tingling, difficulty in moving the feet, and the progression within minutes into complete paraplegia are the classical presentation of AGE. Neurological examination will also reveal multiple neurological defects, with loss of discrimination between sharp and blunt, hot and cold, reduced vibratory sense in the distal limb, loss of urine and feces, and impotence. The progression of spinal decompression disease may advance to quadriplegia and produce significant cardiocirculatory collapse. This syndrome is rare and will not totally regress spontaneously if recompression treatment is not rapidly initiated. Barotrauma to the inner ear may result in hearing loss or tinnitus.

VII. DIAGNOSIS OF DCI

The diagnosis of DCI often can only be made from patient history and dive profile, and often it is impossible to elicit any physical sign directly in the patient. It is important

Table 4 Emergency Phone Numbers to Divers Alert Network (DAN) Worldwide

DAN America International Headquarters	+1-919-684-8111 or +1-919-684-4326 (accepts collect calls)
DAN America-Mexico	+52-5-629-9800 code 9912935 or +52-5-328-2828 code B5100
DAN Australia (DES)	+1-800-088-200 +61-8-8212-9242 (from overseas)
DES New Zealand	+64-9-445-8454
DAN S.E.A.P. Philippines	+63-2-815-9911
DAN Singapore	+65-750-5546
DAN Europe	+41-1-383-1111
DAN Japan	+81-3-3812-4999

to remember that any person seeking medical advice who has been diving during the last 24 hr should initially be regarded as having a diving-related condition. A careful history and a proper clinical examination is mandatory. Also, note that it is possible to get medical advice from discussing the case with colleagues with competence in diving medicine (phone numbers in Table 4). In some cases the need for immediate recompression treatment may mean obtaining only short neurological examination, but when time permits, a complete neurological evaluation must follow. If a multiplace chamber (a pressure chamber with space for more than one person) is available, it is useful in severe cases for the physician to recompress with the patient in the chamber and to perform the neurological examination in depth. A well-documented neurological examination will provide a baseline from which to judge the evolution and the resolution of the symptoms over the next hours and days of treatment. If hospital facilities are available, it is also useful to obtain a chest X ray. It is not diagnostically useful to do other studies at the time symptoms are appearing, but later specialist neurological examination accompanied by electroencephalographic studies can be useful in the diagnosis of DCI of the CNS [9].

VIII. INITIAL TREATMENT AND TRANSPORT OF INJURED DIVERS

For the diver who has signs of DCI, the early start of oxygen therapy and rapid, safe transport to a hyperbaric chamber is the most important measure. By administration of high-flow 100% oxygen the hypoxemia can be reversed and the nitrogen diffusion gradient from saturated tissues will increase, hereby enhancing the elimination of gas from peripheral tissues. The progression of a DCI can thus be halted or even reversed [10]. It was found in an analysis of over 2000 diving accidents that 68% of the divers who have been given oxygen while under transport to a hyperbaric facility showed partial or complete resolution of their symptoms, compared to only 40% of those who didn't receive supplemental oxygen [11]. It is the time from injury until recompression treatment is instituted, however, that is the most important factor for determining whether or not complete relief after treatment can be obtained (Fig. 3).

In most diving casualties, drowning is though to be the cause of death, following either procedural or technical problems at depth, or severe DCI. As recreational

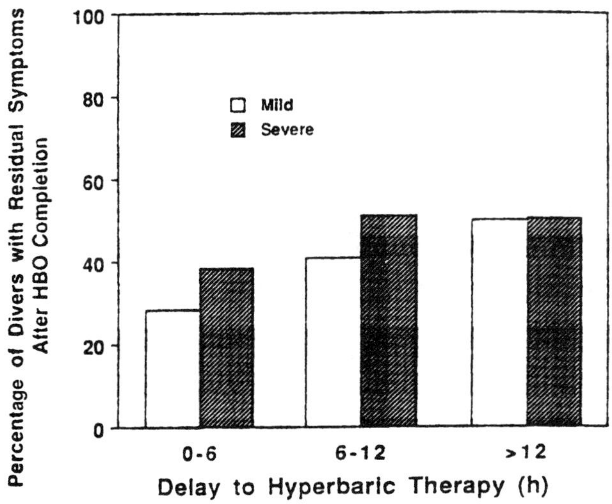

Figure 3 Relation between delay to hyperbaric therapy of DCI and residual symptoms after completion of recompression therapy. Results from 1274 diving accidents reported to the Divers Alert Network. Mild cases include those with pain, numbness, tingling, fatigue or dizziness. Severe cases include those with motor weakness, difficulty walking, cerebral symptoms, or alteration in consciousness. Whereas those treated within 6 hr are less likely to experience residual symptoms, delay to treatment of over 12 hr results in complete relief in half of all cases. (From Ref. 2.)

divers tend to go deeper, the result of equipment problems (e.g., icing of the mouthpiece) can be fatal. If the diver was able to release his buoyancy vest before losing consciousness he or she can be found floating on the surface, or the diver can be brought to the surface by dive mates. If a diver surfaces in severe respiratory distress or is unconscious, one cannot easily know what the reason for the acute situation is. The resuscitation in this case follows the same guidelines, however, regardless of the exact pathological reasons.

IX. AIRWAY AND BREATHING

Maintenance of airways, restoration of ventilation with oxygen-enriched air, and circulation support/bleeding control is most important. One must also bear in mind the possibility of underwater trauma and carbon monoxide (CO) poisoning from polluted breathing gas in addition to drowning and severe DCI. When treating an unconscious diver, spine control must be maintained and foreign bodies/water/secretions removed from the mouth and oropharynx. If the diver is not breathing, cardiopulmonary resuscitation, with controlled ventilation with bag-valve-mask or endotracheal tube, following the advanced cardiac life support (ACLS)/advanced trauma life support (ATLS) protocols, depending on whether there is trauma or not must be done [12].

When assessing airways and breathing one should always listen for breath sounds on each side of the chest, as a pneumothorax can be present, either as a result of barotrauma or from other types of trauma. If a pneumothorax is suspected needle decompression in the midclavicular line above the third rib must be performed and later a drain should be placed, preferably under sterile conditions. The drain must be safely secured and fitted with a Heimlich valve if active suction cannot be used. It is especially important to decompress a pneumothorax before evacuation by aircraft, since low cabin pressure at altitude can cause the gas volume to enlarge.

Ventilation with high concentrations of oxygen is mandatory and is the most important specific treatment of DCI in addition to recompression in a hyperbaric chamber. The oxygen can be delivered via a tight-fitting face mask at flow rates 10 liters min, or via an on-demand mask. In remote areas in which limited oxygen is available this can represent a major problem, but even industrial oxygen (e.g., used for welding) can be used in emergency situations. It can be delivered through the mouthpiece from the diving equipment if it is possible to connect, for example a welding oxygen hose to the second stage on the regulator. In the case of administration of 100% oxygen for more than 4 hr it is recommended that a 5 min air break be introduced for every 25 min of oxygen exposure to diminish the possible side effects on the lungs.

X. CIRCULATION AND REHYDRATION

When assessing the circulatory status of the patient's heart rate and rhythm, and the pulse pressure must be recorded. Bleeding from extremity wounds is controlled by positioning the extremity above heart level while applying pressure and a sterile dressing. The use of tourniquets should be discouraged, as this will not control the bleeding properly [12]. If possible the continuous recording of ECG, intermittent noninvasive blood pressure, pulse oximetry, and temperature is advocated (Table 5). Close clinical supervision by skilled personnel is most important, however. Sufficient peripheral circulation with dry and warm skin in the extremities should be re-established.

As divers with DCI tend to be dehydrated, a largebore venous catheter must be placed so that intravenous infusion of crystalloids (normal saline or Ringer's solution) can be given at a rate of 500 to 1000 ml/hr [13]. When microcirculation is good this

Table 5 Physiological Parameters for Monitoring and Documentation of Patients with Suspected Decompression Illness or Arterial Gas Embolism

RR
SaO_2
HR
Pulse
BP
EKG
Core temperature
Blood glucose
Urine output
Peripheral neurology
GCS
Fluids and medication given

facilitates gas transport from the peripheral tissues to the lungs. The use of glucose-containing solutions should be avoided since the patient may have injury to the CNS [14]. The only use for glucose-containing solution in this situation is to treat a proven hypoglycemia. Likewise, there is no scientific evidence for advocating the use of dextrans or hydroxyethyl starch (HES) rather than crystalloids, although some hyperbaric centers use dextran 40 (Rheomacrodex) because it is believed that this should preserve the microcirculation [15]. The rationale is that a well-functioning microcirculation will enhance the elimination of dissolved nitrogen from the peripheral tissues.

The goal is to re-establish an optimal hydration and volume status. The hydration status can be monitored by blood pressure (BP) readings, skin texture, capillary refilling, and mental status. A urinary output of more than 1.0 mg/kg body weight (BW)/hr is the target. Placement of a urinary bladder catheter is thus mandatory in a paralyzed or unconscious diver. Likewise, a gastric tube can be useful in these patients to decompress the ventricle.

Oral solutions remain a possibility if there is no intravenous fluid available. Oral rehydration can be tried at a rate of 1000 to 2000 ml/hr, given that the diver is conscious and able to drink it without problems. A palatable oral rehydration solution can be prepared by mixing one part orange or apple juice with two parts water, adding 1 teaspoon of table salt per liter solution. If salt is not available, one part seawater and nine parts water can be mixed with the juice [13].

XI. NEUROLOGICAL ASSESSMENT

When the A, B, and C are under control it is important to make a rapid neurological assessment of the diver. This includes Glasgow coma scoring, motor and sensory function assessment, ability to pass urine, and preferably reflexes. The findings must then be documented on the patient's case notes, with the appropriate time of observation. Patients with DCI can deteriorate under transport, but some of them can show resolution of symptoms (completely or partly) after having received oxygen for some time. It is therefore important to be able to show the progression/regression of symptoms over time.

XII. EXPOSURE AND ENVIRONMENT

As in other trauma cases, a diver with suspected barotrauma must be examined for other injuries, which include a thorough clinical examination of the whole body after having removed the diving suit and other clothing. Wet clothes may also represent an additional health threat to the injured diver, because hypothermia can develop even in quite warm environments. Hypothermia will also retard the washout of nitrogen because peripheral circulation decreases. On the other hand, the CNS may tolerate slight hypothermia better than hyperthermia, and fever should be treated symptomatically. If possible, the core temperature should be recorded.

XIII. PHARMACOTHERAPY

Besides oxygen and intravenous fluid there is no evidence for advocating other pharmacological interventions in the treatment of divers with suspected DCI. If a diver has paralysis, however, the use of low molecular weight heparin can be necessary to avoid thromboembolic complications caused by muscular inactivity and supine bed rest. The use of glucocorticoids as adjuvant therapy in the treatment of DCI has had variable results. Case histories have indicated some effect, although a retrospective analysis of AGE cases did not show any benefit [16,17]. High doses of methylprednisolone administered within 8 hr of traumatic spinal cord injury can slightly improve the long-term result, but this has not been shown for DCI. On this basis, there is not sufficient evidence for advocating this at present. The same rationale applies to the recommendation of routine use of lidocaine or nonsteroide anti-inflammatoric drugs (NSAIDS) in divers with suspected DCI [13]. Analgesics should be used with care, because they can make it difficult to assess the response to recompression therapy, but acetylsalicylates or paracetamol can be used if the patient develops a fever.

XIV. TRANSPORT TO A HYPERBARIC FACILITY

As mentioned earlier, the best treatment for DCI is recompression as soon as possible. Transport to the nearest hyperbaric facility must be initiated as fast as possible after the accident. Information on the geographic location of this facility can be obtained from the Divers Alert Network (DAN, for phone numbers see Table 4). Depending on local factors, one must also decide if surface transport should be used or if air evacuation is possible. In some parts of the world emergency helicopter services can be used, while in other remote places one must rely on boat or road transport. In either instance, if air evacuation is chosen the maximum cabin altitude should be not higher than 300 meters (1000 feet) above sea level, and oxygen should be given throughout the transport. A diver with suspected DCI should be transported in the supine position, as there is no evidence for keeping the head low in an attempt to avoid bubbles traveling to the head/CNS. If there is impaired consciousness, placement on the side (lateral recovery position) will protect the airways better. There is also need for close monitoring by skilled personnel at all times, who can detect and treat any deterioration of the vital signs and functions that may ensue during transport.

XV. DOCUMENTATION

During the transport of a diver with suspected DCI it is important to document the case history, symptoms, initial clinical findings, and progression in addition to the specific treatment given. Concerning the history, dive profiles, duration, multiple dives, and any problems with special emphasis on the initial presentation of symptoms must be recorded. A regular anesthetic record, completed by an anatomical drawing of a figure with the dermatomes (Fig. 4) can be used. If there have been violations of a dive table, other dive mates who have been subjected to the same dive profile, although asymptomatic, ought to come along to the hyperbaric facility for recompression. The reason for this is that they might develop DCI at a later stage or even have subclinical neurological manifestations. The evolution of neurological symptoms must also be recorded (e.g., twice an hour) during transport.

If the diver has been using a dive computer this should accompany the diver to the recompression treatment so that a printout of the dive profile can be produced. It can be smart to take along the diving equipment as well (e.g., if there is a suspition of CO pollution of the breathing gas) for medicolegal reasons.

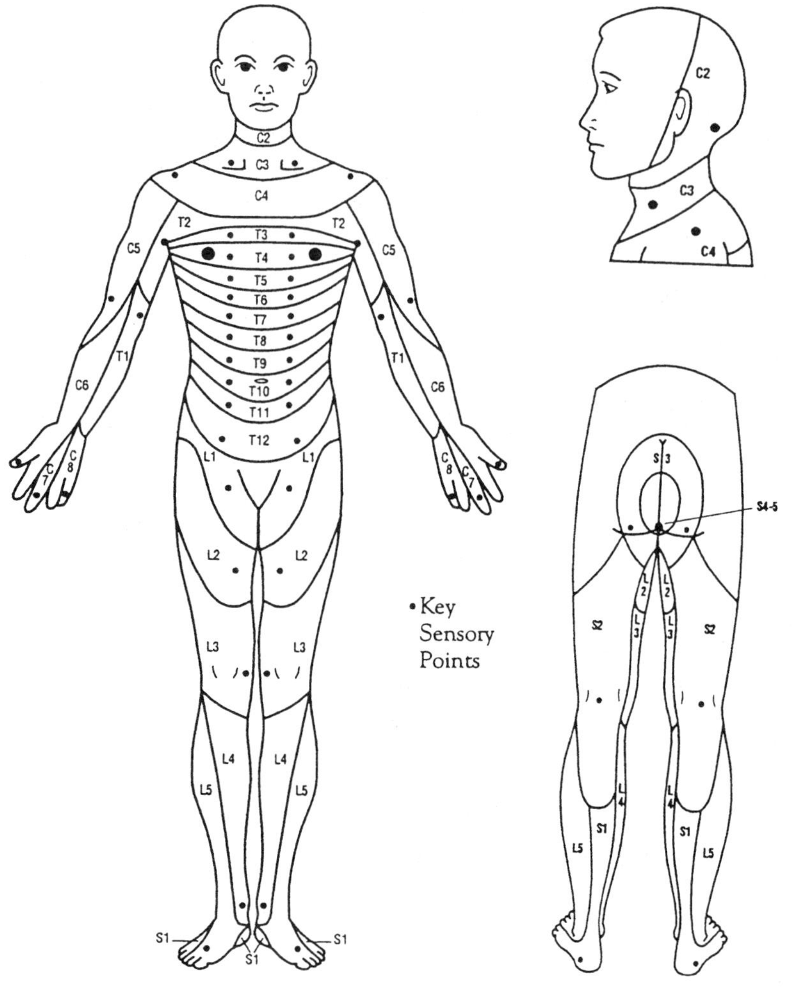

Figure 4 Anatomical figure with dermatomes for documentation of sensory abnormalities. (From Ref. 13a.)

XVI. RECOMPRESSION TREATMENT OF DCI

The appropriate treatment for DCS is rapid recompression on 100% oxygen to a pressure equivalent to 18 msw (282 kPa) for a given period of time. The most frequent pressure time combination scheme has been named ''Table 6'' from the time it was published by the U.S. Navy (Fig. 5). The oxygen breathing periods of this treatment table can be increased at both 18 msw and 9 msw. In a multiplace chamber, the patient will be breathing through a helmet or an oronasal mask, while in a monoplace chamber the patient breathing directly from the oxygen flowing inside the chamber. At all times the patient must be closely monitored and accompanied by experienced personnel. If paraplegia or hemiplegia is present, the patient must be positioned carefully to avoid pressure points and possible venous thromboembolism.

In the case of suspected AGE (dramatic developing symptoms after a rapid or uncon-

Table 6 Indications for Hyperbaric Oxygen Therapy Recommended by the Undersea and Hyperbaric Medical Society (UHMS)

Air or gas embolism
Carbon monoxide poisoning
Gas gangrene
Crush injury and compartment injury
Decompression sickness
Enhancement of healing in selected problem wounds
Exceptional blood loss
Intracranial abscess
Necrotizing soft tissue infections
Refractory osteomyelitis
Delayed radiation injury
Skin grafts and flaps (compromised)
Thermal burns

Source: Ref. 20.

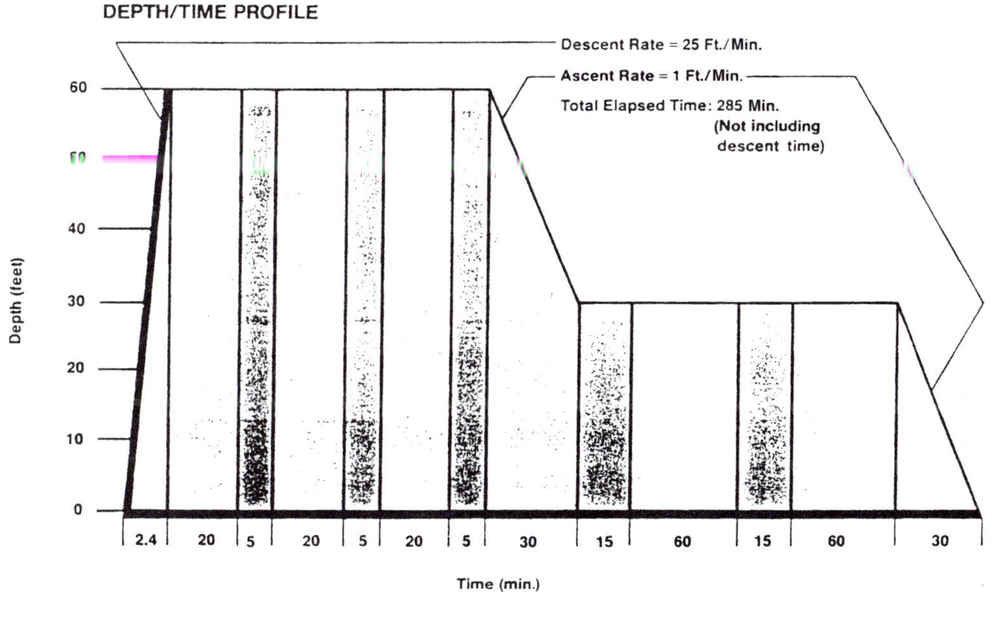

Figure 5 U.S. Navy oxygen treatment Table 6 normally used for treating decompression sickness. In the Norwegian Navy the oxygen periods on 30 feet (9 meters) are divided into 20 min with 5-min air breaks to reduce the possibility for oxygen convulsions. (From Ref. 5a.)

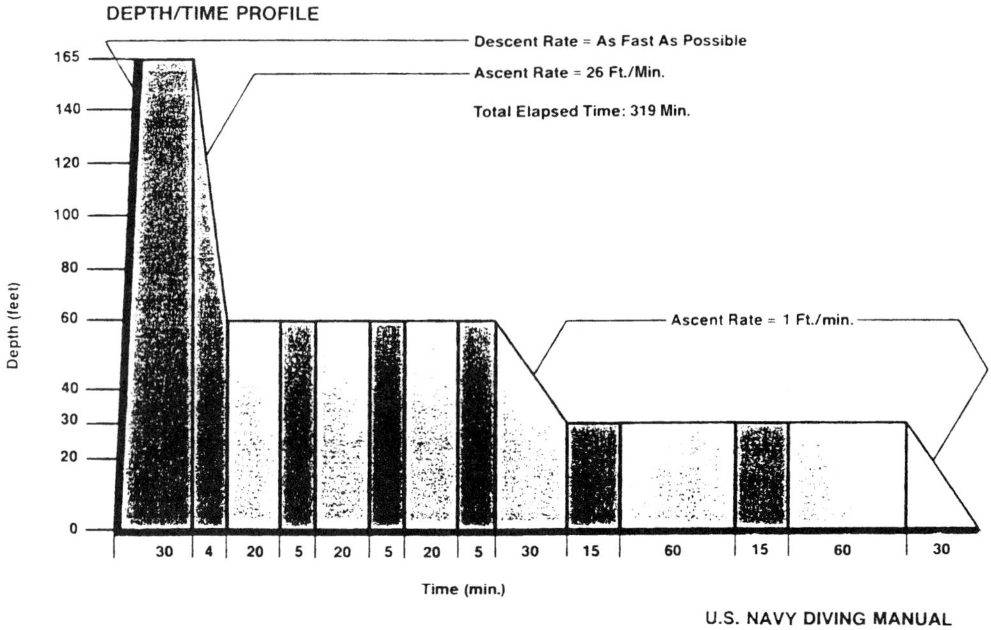

Figure 6 U.S. Navy oxygen treatment Table 6A normally used for treating AGE. The initial treatment pressure is higher to reduce the size of the emboli. The treatment gas in the deep phase is air to avoid oxygen convulsions. In the Norwegian Navy the oxygen periods on 30 feet (9 meters) are divided into 20 min with 5-min air breaks to reduce the possibility for oxygen convulsions. (From Ref. 5a.)

trolled ascent) the initial recompression is to a higher pressure than in DCS, as shown in Fig. 6. Recompression is rarely immediately successful, and symptons may be relieved following a silent interval at pressure.

XVII. FURTHER TREATMENT AND FOLLOW-UP

Most frequently the diver does not return to an asymptomatic state after a single treatment; often residual symptoms are visible for several days. In those cases, additional treatment sessions can be recommended after 8 to 12 hr. These sessions can be with a shallower or shorter table. The therapy guidance is that as long as improvement continues, oxygen at pressure will be considered beneficial. There are suggestions that improvement can in fact continue for several days, up to 2 weeks following the initial injury. Recompression treatment or hyperbaric oxygen therapy (HBO_2) has few side effects, but prolonged treatment for several days can result in lung damage, although this seldom is a clinical problem. Other rare but significant side effects are convulsions due to acute oxygen toxicity to the CNS, claustrophobia, and barotrauma to the ears. Convulsions are treated by discontinuation of the oxygen breathing, and eventually treatment with, e.g., diazepam.

Finally, flying after recompression for neurological decompression illness should be avoided for several days because of the possibility of reinjuring borderline oxygenated tissues in the so-called ischemic penumbra. If significant neurological residuals are detected, diving should not recommence, and long-term outcome can only be reasonably proposed after extensive studies and informed discussion with the patient. Patients who only had limb pain and were successfully treated in the chamber could resume diving after 24 hr, however.

XVIII. IN-WATER RECOMPRESSION AND PORTABLE CHAMBERS

It has been argued that in very remote locations in which it is not practically possible to transport a diver with suspected DCI to recompression in a hyperbaric facility, the use of in-water recompression may be used as a last option. This may look easy and straightforward in theory, but in practice this is not the case. The procedure includes taking an injured diver who possibly can develop seizures or reduced consciousness into the water again and placing him or her at, for example, 6-meter, and 3-meter, depths for rather long periods. First, the diver can lose consciousness and drown. Second he or she needs to be exactly at a certain depth for the chosen time. Third, he or she needs continuous close supervision of consciousness. Fourth, he or she can readily end up becoming hypothermic even in fairly warm waters. Finally, he or she needs a large supply of breathing gas. In summary, the final result may be a drowned and dead diver instead of slight peripheral neurological sequela. It should be mentioned, though, that in-water recompression treatment has been done in northwest Australia using a full face mask with communication equipment and 100% oxygen as treatment gas [18]. The safest alternative, however, remains surface oxygen therapy at atmospheric pressure (1 ATA) en route to a hyperbaric facility.

A promising alternative to the usual steel chambers is the so-called Chamberlite 15 bag. This is a collapsible bag developed from the Gamow bag, which was originally constructed for treating high-altitude illness. The bag has been reinforced to withstand greater pressure, however, and has been used for regular hyperbaric oxygen therapy. This may be a much better alternative for treating DCI in remote areas than in-water decompression. Until now only one paper is listed in Medline [19]. Small steel chambers also have been constructed, but these are so heavy that it is not easy to transport them, and the size is so small that it is not possible to monitor the patient safely. Because of this background the use of these chambers is not encouraged.

XIX. OTHER MEASURES

A patient who has been diving during the last 24 hr should not receive nitrous oxide as part of general anesthesia, because this anesthetic gas may diffuse into gas bubbles containing nitrogen, thereby making a DCI worse. A general anesthetic is thought to be the best solution, because regional techniques in a patent with possible spinal injury cannot be recommended.

XX. RESOURCES ON THE WORLD WIDE WEB

There are several high-quality diving and hyperbaric medical resources on the World Wide Web. The links below can serve as a starting point for the interested reader:

http://www.uhms.org/
http://www.brooks.af.mil/web/hyper/
http://www.gulftel.com/~scubadoc/
http://www.mtsinai.org/pulmonary/books/scuba/

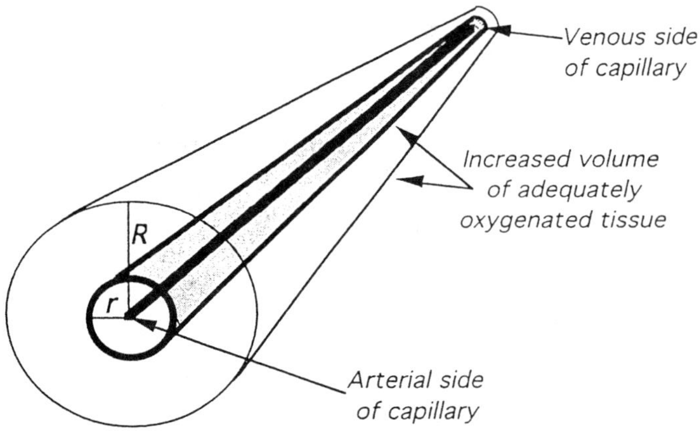

Figure 7 Relative increase in the tissue volume that is adequately oxygenated by an increase in the partial pressure of oxygen. The thin dark cylinder (line) represents a capillary. The two cones with radii r and R represent the normal and increased oxygenated tissue volumes, respectively. (From Ref. 21a.)

XXI. HYPERBARIC MEDICINE

The therapeutic use of oxygen under high pressure (HBO_2) is not limited to treatment of divers, but has been used for a number of other diseases for many years. The main effect of HBO_2 is a substantial increase in the oxygen supply to the tissues because the partial pressure of oxygen is raised to supernormal levels, which cannot be attained under normobaric pressure (Fig. 7). Under such conditions the amount of oxygen present in a physical solution (in addition to the amount bound to hemoglobin) in the plasma is sufficient for covering a substantial part of metabolic demands of the cells. In marginally circulated tissues, the ''tissue cylinder'' that each capillary then can oxygenate is substantially increased. This is of special interest in anaerobic infections, such as gas gangrene, which is caused by *Clostridium welchi (perfringens)*. Table 6 lists the conditions in which there is international consensus that HBO_2 may play a significant part of the treatment. This hyperoxia has several other effects, including a marked reduction in edema. In relation to trauma the most important conditions in which HBO_2 can be useful are CO intoxication and smoke inhalation, crush injury and compartment syndromes, and thermal burns. It is outside the scope of this book to explore this in detail, hence the interested reader can consult other sources [1, 20, 21, http://www.uhms.org].

XXII. CONCLUSIONS

Persons who are presenting with a medical problem within 24 hr after diving must be regarded as having a diving-related condition. A careful history and clinical examination with special attention to the nervous system is mandatory.

In the case of suspected decompression illness, oxygen therapy must be started as soon as possible and continue during the transport to a place in which recompression therapy can be safely undertaken.

When air evacuation is used a cabin pressure of less than 300 meters (1000 feet) should be avoided.

Rehydration with IV or oral fluids should be started to ensure sufficient circulation.
Medically competent personnel must accompany the patient at all times.
Hyperbaric oxygen therapy can be of value in the treatment of other acute conditions, such as carbon monoxide poisoning, crush injury, and gas gangrene.

REFERENCES

1. TJR Francis, D Smith, eds. Describing Dysbarism. Bethesda, MD: Undersea and Hypebaric Medical Society, 1991.
2. DH Elliott, RE Moon. Manifestations of the decompression disorders. In: PB Bennett, DH Elliott, eds. The Physiology and Medicine of Diving. 4th ed. London: Saunders, 1993; pp. 481–505.
3. F Faralli. Decompression illness. In: G Oriani, A Marroni, F Wattel, eds. Handbook on Hyperbaric Medicine. Berlin: Springer, 1996; pp. 135–182.

3a. P Wilmhurst. Diving and Oxygen. Br J 317:996–999, 1998.

4. P Bert. La Pression Barométrique: Recherches de Physiologie Experimentale. Paris: G. Mason, 1878.
5. FL Keays. Compressed Air Illness with a Report of 3,692 Cases New York Vol. 2 Dept. Med. Publ. Cornell University Medical College 1909; pp. 1–55.

5a. U.S. Navy Diving Manual, Revision 2. Flagstaff, AZ: Best Publishing, 1988.

6. TJR Francis, DF Gorman. Pathogenesis of the decompression disorders. In: PB Bennett DH Elliott, eds. The Physiology and Medicine of Diving. 4th ed. London: Saunders, 1993, pp. 454–480.
7. A Greenstein, D Sherman, Y Melamed. Chokes—Favorable response to delayed recompression therapy: A case report. Aviat Space Environ Med 9:559–560, 1981.
8. BH Peters, HS Levin, PJ Kelly. Neurological and psychologic manifestations of decompression illness in divers. Neurology 27:125–127, 1977.
9. SA Sipinen, J Ahovuo, J-P Halonen. Electroencphalography and magnetic resonance imaging after diving and decompression incidents: A controlled study. Undersea Hyperbar Med 26: 61–65, 1999.
10. DF Gorman. Management of diving accidents. In: DH Elliott, PB Bennett, eds. The Physiology and Medicine of Diving. 4th ed. London: Saunders, 1993.
11. RE Moon. Adjuvant therapy for decompression illness. [illegible]
12. Advanced Trauma Life Support (ATLS) student manual. Chicago: American College of Surgeons, 1997.
13. RE Moon. Treatment of decompression sickness and arterial gas embolism. In: AA Bove, JC Davis, eds. Diving Medicine. 3rd ed. Philadelphia: Saunders, 1997, pp. 184–204.

13a. American Spinal Injury Association. International Standards for Neurological and Functional Classification of Spinal Cord Injury. Chicago: American Spinal Injury Association, 1994.

14. AM Lam, HR Winn, BF Cullen, et al. Hyperglycemia and neurological outcome in patients with head injury. J Neurosurg 75:545–551, 1991.
15. AT Cocett, RM Nakamura. Treatment of decompression sickness employing low molecular weight dextran. Rev Physiol Subacuat 1:2133–2140, 1968.
16. RR Pearson, RF Goad. Delayed cerebral edema complicating cerebral arterial gas embolism: Case histories. Undersea Biomed Res 9:283–296, 1982.
17. DF Gorman. Arterial gas embolism as a consequence of pulmonary barotrauma. In: J Desola, ed. Diving and Hyperbaric Medicine. Barcelona: European Undersea Biomedical Society, 1984, pp. 348–368.
18. C Edmonds. Underwater oxygen treatment of DCS. In: RE Moon, PJ Sheffield, eds. Treatment of Decompression Illness. Kensington, MD: Undersea and Hyperbaric Medical Society, 1996, pp. 255–266.

19. H Shimada, T Morita, F Kunimoto, S Saito. Immediate application of hyperbaric oxygen therapy using a newly devised transportable chamber. Am J Emerg Med 14:412–415, 1996.
20. NB Hampson, ed. Hyperbaric Oxygen Therapy: 1999 Committee Report. Kensington, MD: Undersea and Hyperbaric Medical Society, 1999.
21. G Oriani, A Marroni, F Wattel, eds. Handbook on Hyperbaric Medicine. Berlin: Springer, 1996.
21a. EM Camporesi, MF Mascia, SR Thom. Physiological Principle of hyperbaric oxygenation. In: G Oriani, A Marroni, F Wattel, eds. Handbook of Hyperbaric Medicine. Berlin: Springer, 1996, pp. 35–58.

34

Snake, Insect, and Marine Bites and Stings

JUDITH R. KLEIN

UCSF–San Francisco General Hospital, San Francisco, California

PAUL S. AUERBACH

Stanford University School of Medicine, Stanford, California

Humans coexist with a vast array of snakes, insects, and sea-dwelling organisms that may bite or sting if disturbed or threatened. Some of these species are aggressive in their interactions with man. Others assume a defensive posture when they perceive harm to themselves or to their offspring. It is critical for medical personnel to familiarize themselves with regional creatures that can pose a threat to the local population, because recognition of the agent of a bite or sting is the first step in prompt and appropriate treatment.

In all cases of snake, insect, or marine bites or stings, the immediate approach to care is the same. First to be addressed are airway, breathing, and circulation (the ABCs). Life-threatening physiologic perturbations should be managed before local wound issues. In some cases, an antivenin is the cornerstone of definitive therapy. Only in an extreme circumstance should antivenin be administered outside a strictly monitored setting (emergency department, intensive care unit) given the incidence and dangers of anaphylactic reactions. Generally speaking, the goals of field treatment are rapid stabilization and expeditious transport to an appropriate medical facility. With these goals in mind, morbidity and mortality can be minimized.

I. SNAKEBITES

Worldwide, more than 3000 species of snakes are responsible for approximately 300,000 human bites each year. Of all snake species, only 375 are known to be venomous. Their habitats range from sea level to timberline and from land to aquatic to arboreal environs.

While mortality from snakebite is low in the United States and other nations with highly developed medical care systems, snakebite and venom-related deaths are quite common in India, Southeast Asia, sub-Saharan Africa, and tropical America. An observational study in Nigeria revealed 497 bites per 100,000 population in rural areas, with a 12.2% mortality [1].

A. Species Identification and Geography

Distinguishing venomous from nonvenomous species is critical in areas in which human interactions with snakes are common. As illustrated in Figures 1 and 2, nonvenomous snakes in the United States tend to have round pupils (an exception: the venomous coral snakes); small teeth, not fangs; and in the case of pit vipers, a double row of subcaudal plates. In addition, bite marks from nonvenomous snakes appear as parallel rows of four scratches rather than as one or more puncture marks.

Medically important terrestrial venomous snake species fall into three families: *Viperidae, Elapidae*, and *Atractaspididae*. As outlined in Table 1, the family *Viperidae* comprises the crotalids (pit vipers) and the old world vipers. The pit vipers are distinguished by the presence of heat-sensing facial pits that assist in detecting prey. Of the pit vipers, rattlesnakes are responsible for 60% of venomous snake bites in the United States. The eastern diamondback rattlesnake is the largest and most dangerous snake in the United States. Other crotalids, such as the cottonmouth and the copperhead, inflict less severe bites. In contrast to pit vipers, old world vipers lack heat-sensing pits. Of the 40 species in Africa, Europe, Asia, and South and Central America, Russell's viper and the *Bothrops* species distinguish themselves with the lethality of their venom.

The second family of venomous snakes, the elapids, consists of coral snakes, cobras, mambas, kraits, and the vast majority of venomous snakes in Australia. The coral snake is common in tropical America and is readily identifiable by the bright red, yellow, and

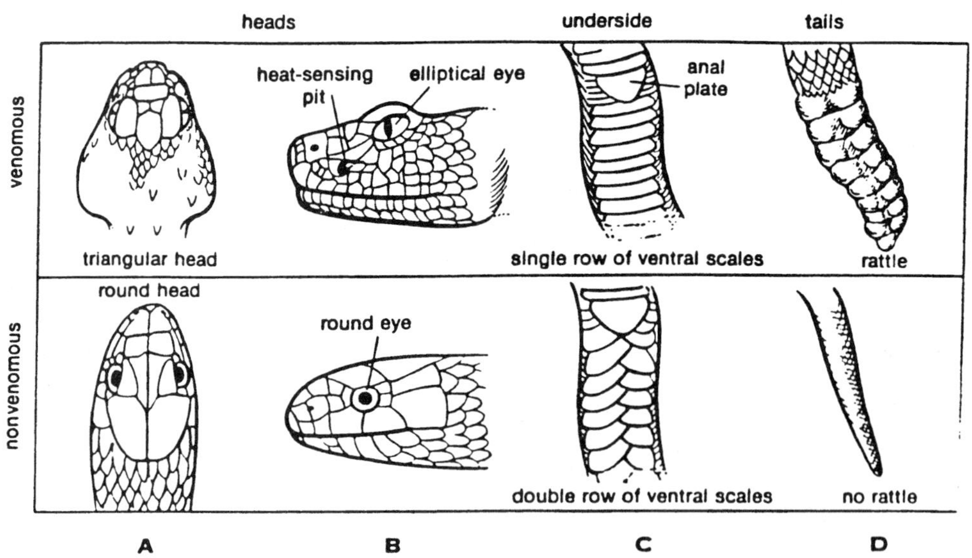

Figure 1 Identification of venomous pit vipers in the Americas (exception: coral snakes are similar in appearance to nonvenomous pit vipers). (From Ref. 1a.)

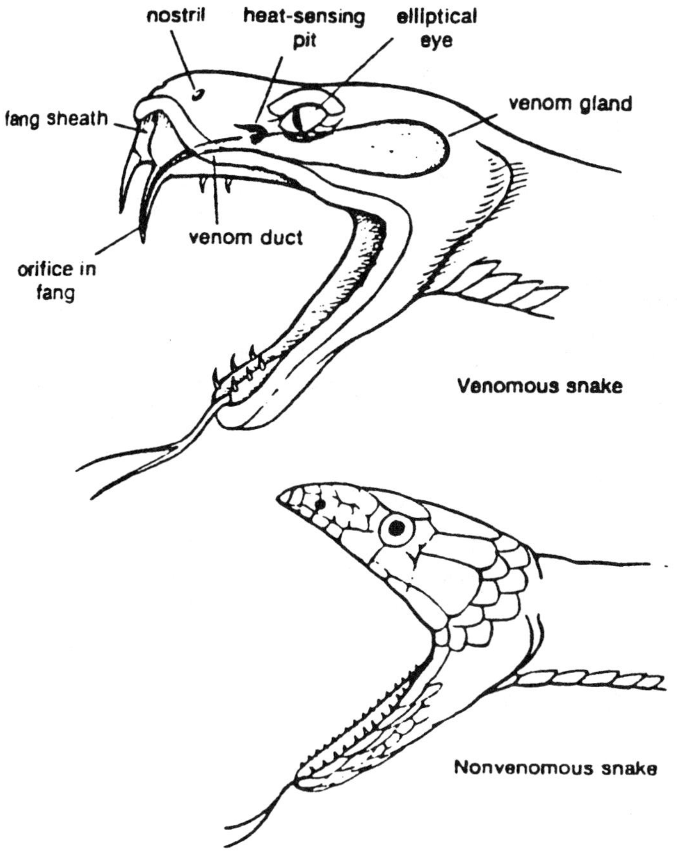

Figure 2 Mouth and venom apparatus of pit viper vs. mouth of nonvenomous snake or coral snake. (From Ref. 1a.)

Table 1 Venomous Snake Species of the World

Family	Subfamily	Species	Habitats
Viperidae	Crotalid	Rattlesnake, cottonmouth, copperhead	North and South America and Asia
	Viperinae	Russell's viper, Bothrops	Africa, Europe, Asia, South/Central America
Elapidae		Coral snake, cobra, mamba, krait, Australian elapids (taipan, death adder, tiger snake)	Tropical and warm temperate regions worldwide
Atractaspididae			Forest to semidesert areas of sub-Saharan Africa and the Middle East

black bands that encircle its body. The cobras of Africa and subtropical Asia are notable for their size (1.5 to 5 meters), and for their ability in some cases to ''spit'' venom at their prey. The Australian elapids, notably the coastal taipan, death adder, and tiger snake, vary greatly in size, but all possess highly toxic venom.

The burrowing asps are the predominant species in the third family of venomous snakes, *Atractaspididae*. Inhabiting the soils of Africa and the Middle East, these snakes bear large maxillary fangs that penetrate the skin of victims with a backward stabbing motion.

B. Modes of Envenomation

Most snake bites occur in the summer during the evening in areas marked by seasonal temperature variations. In more equatorial regions, they may occur at any time. Most wounds are inflicted on the victims' feet and ankles, and less frequently on their fingers and hands. The venom apparatus of pit vipers consists of paired venom glands, compressor muscles, ducts, and retractable canalized fangs. The viper strikes at a rate of 2.5 meters per sec, utilizing heat-sensing pits and ground vibration to localize its victim. With a rattlesnake, 25–75% of the venom gland volume is injected, depending upon the victim's perceived size. With its lengthy fangs, a rattlesnake can penetrate rubber or leather boots. In contrast, elapids have fixed, short, tubular fangs that do not retract. Elapids do not strike; rather, they hang on and chew, instilling venom within their victims about 40% of the time. The burrowing asps have large canalized fangs similar to those of vipers, but can use them one at a time in a backward stabbing motion. They are capable of biting with their mouths virtually closed.

C. Pathophysiology and Clinical Manifestations

The venom of the pit viper is extremely varied among species, with cytotoxic, neurotoxic, and hemolytic components. The venom initially produces local tissue and microvascular damage that proceeds to regional tissue necrosis, hemorrhage, and extravasation of intravascular volume. The venom spreads through the lymphatics and bloodstream to generate severe coagulopathy and multiorgan system involvement. At the site of the bite, fang marks are usually visible, but the size of such marks does not correlate with the degree of envenomation. Approximately 20% of the time, the pit viper bite is ''dry''; that is, no venom is instilled. If envenomation has occurred, bleeding, local pain, burning, and dramatic subcutaneous edema occur within 5 to 30 min. Rarely, these symptoms may be delayed for up to 4 hr, but in the vast majority of cases, if no significant local symptomatology is observed within 30 min no significant envenomation has occurred. As viper venom spreads, the victim may experience nausea; vomiting; weakness; fever; chills; a minty, rubbery, or metallic taste in the mouth; and paresthesias of the scalp and distal extremities (severe envenomation). This can progress to autonomic instability; hemorrhage due to coagulopathy; hypotensive shock due to bleeding, third spacing, and decreased systemic vascular resistance; paralysis (diamondback and Mojave rattlesnakes, non-North American vipers); seizures; and death.

In contrast, elapid venom is predominantly neurotoxic, causing nondepolarizing blockade at postsynaptic nerve receptor sites or inhibition of acetylcholine release from presynaptic vesicles. Fang marks may be difficult to appreciate, and pain may be minimal or absent at the site of the bite. With the exception of some myonecrosis and edema sometimes seen with Australian elapid and cobra bites, regional symptoms are generally limited to lymphadenopathy. Dry bites occur about 50% of the time. With envenomation, systemic neurotoxic symptoms ensue within 8 to 10 hr; thereafter progression is extremely rapid, with nausea and vomiting, salivation, paresthesias, fasciculation, descending paralysis, seizures (children), and respiratory failure.

With burrowing asp envenomation, local symptoms may be mild or severe with single or dual fang puncture marks, pain or numbness, swelling, and occasional local necrosis. This may progress to vomiting, diaphoresis, coagulopathy, and—as demonstrated in experimental *Atractaspididae* envenomation in animals—coronary vasospasm.

D. Severity of Envenomation and Grading

Along with identification of the species, assessing the severity of the envenomation is critical in determining the appropriate management and mode of transport. The degree of envenomation is determined by several factors, including the victim's age, size, general health and sensitivity to venom, and the depth (subcutaneous vs. intravenous) and location of the bite. Bites proximal to the proximal interphalangeal joint result in more severe clinical manifestations in humans than those distal to this joint [2]. Other significant factors include the species, size, and sex of the snake, and the quantity of venom discharged. Pit vipers tend to be more generous in the quantity of venom transferred to the victim. Finally, as testimony to the importance of appropriate field management, the amount of physical activity that the victim engages in following the bite and the methods utilized to prevent venom spread may markedly affect the progression of symptoms.

In grading a snake bite, frequent reassessment is vital, as symptoms can be quite dynamic. While several grading systems have been devised for crotalid envenomation, most notably by Dart and colleagues at the Rocky Mountain Poison Center in Colorado, these scores are intended for research purposes and are quite complex; they are therefore of limited utility in the field setting [3].

E. Field Management

The central tenets of prehospital care for snake bite injuries are the same regardless of species or locale: remain calm, reassure the victim, put the victim to rest, transport expeditiously, and *primum non nocere* (first, do no harm). Oral suction of wounds, topical alcohol, (ingested or applied), surgical incisions, electric shock, tourniquets, and cryotherapy have never been proven to be efficacious. In fact, many of these techniques have been shown to have markedly deleterious effects [4]. While identification of the snake is important, the victim or prehospital care provider should not put himself at risk or delay prompt transport in order to capture the snake. The victim and bystanders should move out of striking distance of the snake (approximately the length of the snake) and should remember that even dead or decapitated snakes can continue to envenom for up to 60 min.

Once out of range of the snake, the time of envenomation should be firmly established. The victim should be kept at rest with the bitten extremity at or below the level of the heart. Minimizing activity, avoiding the consumption of stimulants (e.g., caffeine), and calming the victim will limit tachycardia, which may promote venom spread via the circulation. All jewelry, which can serve as a tourniquet as limb edema progresses, should be removed. Local wound care should be limited to soap and water scrub. Avoid contact with extremely cold liquids or ice, which can drive venom components deeper into the tissue, causing further ischemia, or induce a frostbite-variant tissue injury.

While many techniques for the extraction of venom and the limitation of venom spread have been touted, few have actually been shown to be efficacious in controlled studies. Three techniques with supportive evidence will be discussed in detail. Incision and oral suction was long held as an important method of removing venom from tissue. This technique is no longer recommended, because experience and study have demonstrated significant rates of secondary infection and nonhealing without measurable beneficial effects. The use of *mechanical suction*, however, with the Sawyer extractor (Long Beach, CA, Fig. 3), has been shown in animal studies to safely remove up to 30% of crotalid venom if applied within 3 min and maintained for a period of 30 to 60 min following a bite [5]. This device is capable of generating approximately 1 atmosphere of negative pressure when properly applied.

Local compression and immobilization is another technique first developed by Sutherland and colleagues in Australia for use in elapid bites [6]. By wrapping a wide crepe or elastic bandage firmly over the bite and then proximally for the length of the extremity, the intent is to occlude venous and lymphatic flow and delay central circulation of venom (Fig. 4). Distal pulses should remain palpable and must be checked frequently. Excessively tight wrapping may result not only in limb ischemia, but also in marked pain and associated limb movement that can increase lymphatic distribution of venom [7]. The wrapped extremity is immobilized with a splint for up to 6 hr. While significant delay in onset of systemic symptoms has been demonstrated in multiple studies with Australian elapids, the use of this technique is highly controversial with vipers. Theoretically, compression

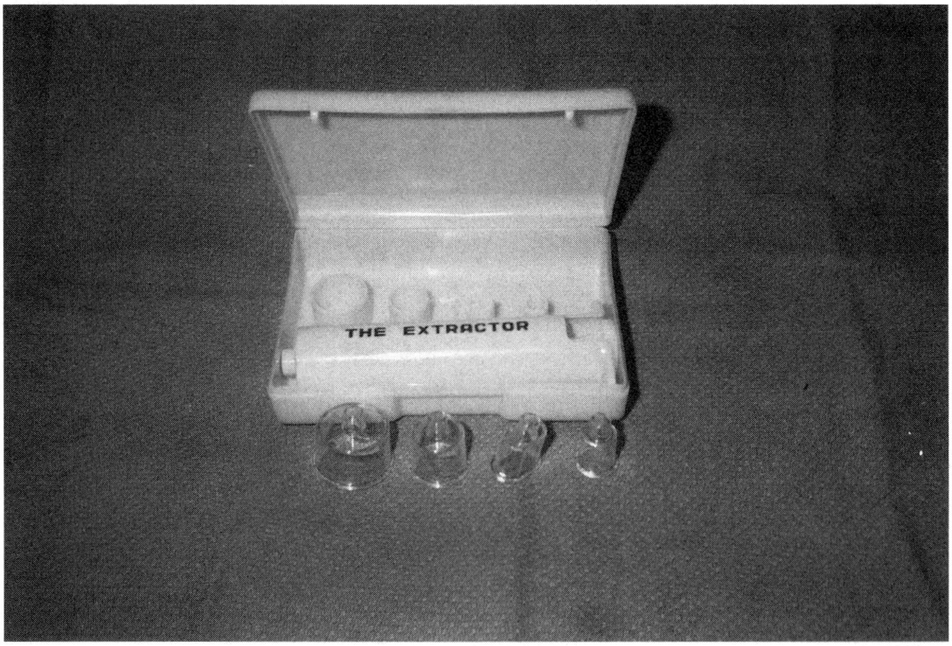

Figure 3 The Sawyer extractor for application of mechanical suction and removal of venom.

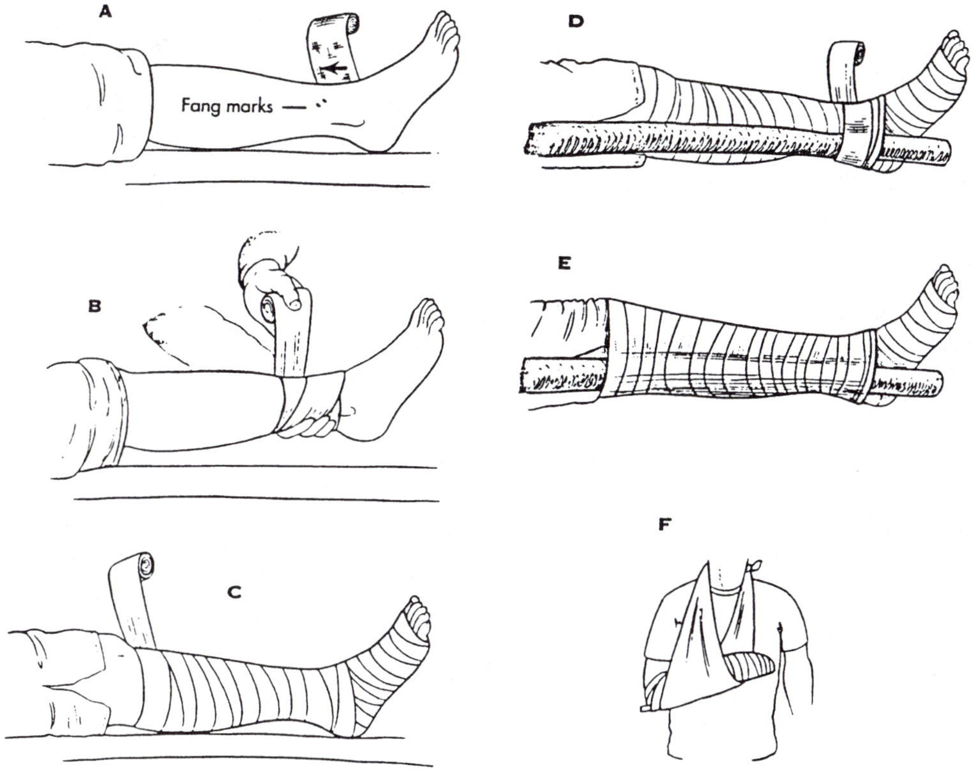

Figure 4 The Australian compression and immobilization technique. (From Ref. 8a.)

could exacerbate local tissue necrosis associated with viper venom and accelerate the development of compartment syndrome [8]. Compression and immobilization, however, may buy valuable time in staving off severe systemic symptoms following viper envenomation [9,10].

The final technique with the most limited supportive evidence is the *lymphatic constriction band* (Fig. 5). In an animal study of crotalid envenomation, the use of a 5- to 7-cm-wide band proximal to the bite site and placed tightly enough to occlude lymphatic and superficial venous flow but not arterial flow, delayed systemic spread of venom without worsening local edema [11]. While using a constriction band has not been proven efficacious in humans, many experts recommend its use for certain envenomations [8].

A general approach to snake bite envenomations is shown in Table 2 In order to determine how best to limit venom spread, one can divide bites into those with significant known or apparent local effects and those without local effects (Table 3). Utilization of compression/immobilization would be indicated in an elapid or other bite with few local symptoms, whereas lymphatic constriction bands with immobilization might be preferable with viper or other bites in which local tissue damage may be significant. While not proven efficacious in all types of envenomation, mechanical suction may be useful with snake bites if implementation does not result in significant delay to transport or definitive care.

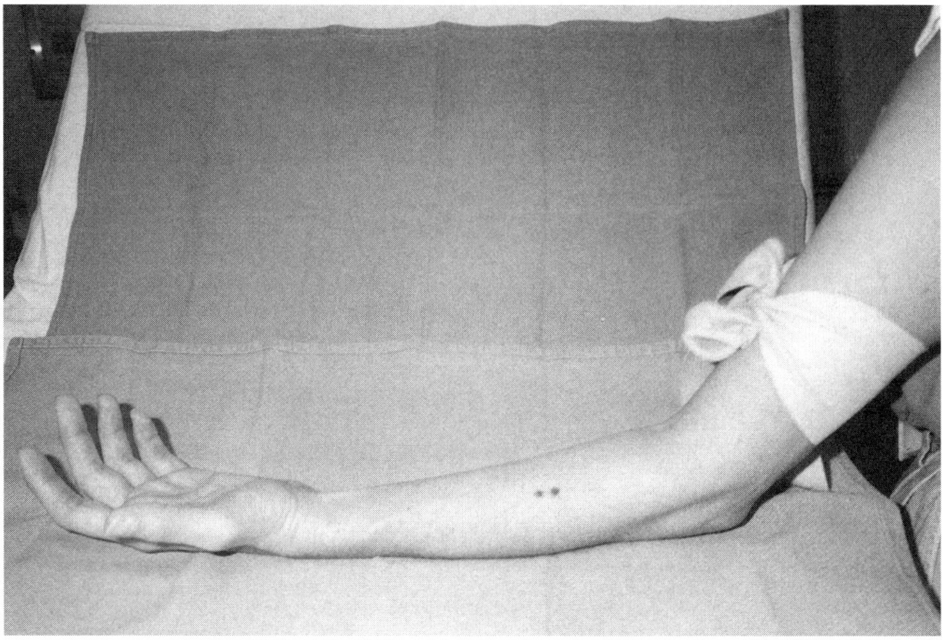

Figure 5 The lymphatic constriction band technique.

Attention should also be focused on the treatment of observed effects. Bites that occur on the neck or upper trunk may result in airway compromise; endotracheal intubation for airway management may be indicated. If possible, an intravenous line should be established to administer fluids and support intravascular volume. If administering an analgesic, an acetaminophen or a narcotic is preferable to aspirin or a nonsteroidal anti-inflammatory agent, given the antiplatelet effects of the latter medications. Specific agents, such as

Table 2 Approach to Venomous Snakebites in the Field

Remain calm and reassure victim
Safely identify snake, if possible
Establish time of envenomation
Remove potential tourniquets
Put victim to rest and splint extremity at or below heart level
Apply mechanical suction
Species specific venom containment (see Table 3)
Supportive care: ABCs pain control
Transport victim expeditiously and immobilized if possible
Avoid:
Ice
Elevating extremities
Tourniquets
Incision and oral suction

Table 3 Snakebite Clinical Manifestations and Venom Containment

Family	Local effects	Systemic effects	Venom containment
Viperidae	Pain/burning, bleeding, ecchymosis, edema, paresthesias	Nausea/vomiting, weakness, fever/chills, coagulopathy, hemorrhage, paralysis, shock/death	1. Mechanical suction 2. Immobilize at heart level 3. Lymphatic constriction band
Elapidae	Minimal pain or edema (see text for exceptions)	Nausea/vomiting, salivation, paresthesias, descending paralysis, seizures (children)	1. Compression and immobilization 2. Mechanical suction 3. Mobilize below heart level
Atractaspididae	Pain or numbness, edema, rarely local necrosis	Nausea/vomiting, hemorrhage, respiratory distress, coronary vasospasm	1. Compression and immobilization 2. Mechanical suction 3. Immobilize below heart level

edrophonium, may also be useful in reversing neurotoxic effects of elapid and certain viper (Russell's viper) venoms [12].

F. Transport and Antivenin Therapy

As stated previously, the goals of the prehospital care of snake bites are to limit the spread of venom, stabilize the victim, and transport the victim safely and expeditiously for definitive care. All transport should be performed with the victim as immobile as possible. Even short periods of walking after upper or lower extremity envenomation can increase the systemic spread of venom [7]. The bitten extremity should be maintained at or below the level of the heart throughout transport. All viper bites should be transported to a medical facility to assess the need for antivenin therapy, the only proven efficacious intervention for viper envenomation [13]. Victims of viper bites should be observed in such a facility for at least 6 to 8 hr, but may be released if no local or systemic symptoms become apparent. All persons with symptomatic viper envenomations should be hospitalized.

Elapid bites should be treated with antivenin if systemic symptoms develop [14]. Given the delayed onset of systemic manifestations, all victims of elapid bites should be transported for observation. Although antivenin therapy is unavailable, bites from burrowing asps also merit transport to a medical facility for observation and admission as needed for supportive care.

While antivenin therapy is clearly the cornerstone of treatment for many otherwise highly toxic or lethal snake envenomations, the use of antivenin in the field is strongly discouraged, given the limited ability to closely monitor patients. While new, highly purified Fab-based antivenins with significantly fewer systemic reactions are being studied, current antivenins have a substantial incidence of anaphylaxis [15]. Table 4 provides a list of manufactures of snake antivenins currently available worldwide.

An assessment of the need for antivenin and appropriate monitoring for administration is best performed in an emergency department or intensive care setting. Mortality

Table 4 Manufacturers of Snake Antivenins Worldwide

Continent	Country/manufacturer
North America	Mexico: Gerencia General de Biologicos y Reactivos, Grupo Pharma S.A., Laboratorio Zapata, Laboratorios ''MYN S.A.''
	USA: Merck, Sharp and Dohme Ltd. Wyeth-Ayerst
Central/South America	Argentina: Ejercito Argentino, Instituto Nacional de Microbiologia
	Brazil: Fundacao Ezequiel Dias, Instituto Butantan
	Colombia: Instituto Nacional de Salud
	Costa Rica: Instituto Clodomiro Picado
	Ecuador: Instituto Nacional de Higiene y Medicina Tropical
	Peru: Insituto Nacional de Higiene
	Venezuela: Universidad Central de Venezuela
Europe	Bulgaria: Institute of Epidemiology and Microbiology
	Czechoslovakia: Chemapol Foreign Trade Co. Ltd., Institute of Sera and Vaccines, SEVAC, Institute for Sera and Vaccines
	England: Lister Institute of Preventative Medicine
	France: Institut Merieux, Laboratoires Lelong, Pasteur-Merieux Serum et Vaccins
	Germany: Behringwerke AG, Twyford Pharmaceuticals GmbH
	Italy: Instituto Sieroterapico Vaccinogeno Toscano
	Russia: Ministry of Public Health, Research Institute of Vaccine and Serum
	Spain: Centro de Estandarizacion de Venenos y Antivenenos
	Switzerland: Institut Serotherapique et Vaccinal Suisse
	Turkey: Refik Saydam Central Institute of Hygiene
	Yugoslavia: Institute of Immunology
Asia	Burma: Industrie and Pharmaceutical Corp,
	China: Ministry of Public Health, Shanghai Institute of Biological Products, Shanghai Vaccine and Serum Institute
	India: Central Research Institute, Haffkine Biopharmaceutical Co. Serum Institute of India
	Indonesia: Perum Bio Farma (Pasteur Institute)
	Japan: Chemo-Sero-Therapeutic Research Institute, Chiba Serum Institute, Japan Snake Institute, Kitasato Institute, Research Foundation for Microbial Diseases, Takeda Chemical Industries
	Pakistan: National Institute of Health
	Phillipines: Serum and Vaccine Laboratories
	Thailand: Thai Government Pharmaceutical Organization, Thai Red Cross Society
Australia	Commonwealth Serum Laboratories
Africa	Middle East: Al Algousa Sharea, Egypt; Department of Zoology, Tel Aviv University, Israel; Ministry of Health Department of Laboratories, Israel; Rogoff Medical Research Institute, Israel; Institut d'Etat des Serums et Vaccins, Razi, Iran
	North Africa: Institut Pasteur, Algeria, Tunisia, Morocco
	South Africa: Fitzsimons' Snake Park, South African Institute for Medical Research

from snake bite is uncommon in the developed world, with less than 0.5% of all bites in the United States resulting in death Ninety-five percent of all snake bite-related deaths occur in underdeveloped nations; undoubtedly, folk treatment regimens, poor means of transport, a dearth of appropriate medical facilities, and the limited availability of antivenins contribute significantly to this unfortunate statistic.

II. INSECT BITES AND STINGS

Insects are the most common forms of multicellular life on Earth. As a consequence, interactions between humans and insects are frequent. Some insects feed on human blood and tissue fluids, injecting salivary secretions containing toxins and pathogens. Other insects bite or sting aggressively or defensively when faced with a threat to themselves or their progeny. The mechanical impact of these bites, coupled with the effects of toxins and the human immune response, can lead to substantial morbidity.

A. Arthropods: Hymenoptera

1. Identification and Pathophysiology

Hymenoptera are the most dangerous insects in the world, causing more deaths than any other group of insect. Hymenoptera are a subset of arthropods composed of the vespids (yellow jackets, hornets, wasps), apids (honeybee and bumblebee), and ants (fire ants). Generally speaking, hymenoptera sting only when provoked or startled. The so-called killer bees, or Africanized honeybees require significantly less provocation to attack. Initially introduced in Brazil, these bees are identical to European honeybees in appearance and venom content, but are more aggressive and will attack enmasse. As a group, they are capable of inflicting the 300 to 500 stings estimated necessary to deliver a lethal dose of venom [16].

When they sting, apids and occasionally vespids detach their stingers along with a venom sac that continues to pump venom even after separation from the insect. This venom consists of multiple vasoactive amines, such as histamines, serotonin, and dopamine, along with peptides and hyaluronidase that facilitate tissue spread. In contrast, fire ant venom consists predominantly of insoluble alkaloids. Individual stings, which the fire ant accomplishes by grasping the victim's skin with its powerful mandibles and then stinging multiple times, are relatively nontoxic. Like Africanized bees, however, fire ants attack in large numbers when provoked.

2. Clinical Manifestations

There are three types of reactions that can be generated by hymenoptera stings: local, systemic, and toxic. *Local reactions* consist of varying degrees of pain, erythema, and edema that can spread to neighboring joints. If a sting is on the neck, airway obstruction can occur even in the absence of anaphylaxis. Bites on the eyelid can penetrate through to the eye and cause severe ocular damage. *Systemic reactions* are the result of a type I hypersensitivity (or allergic) response to hymenoptera venom. A victim who has been previously sensitized to the venom of the stinging species or by another species of hymenoptera to which his immune response cross-reacts can develop an anaphylactic reaction. Symptoms typically develop within 15 min, but may be delayed up to 6 hr. These symptoms include itchy eyes, facial flushing, urticaria, stridor, bronchospasm, vomiting, abdominal cramping, and hypotension. Death from anaphylaxis can occur extremely rapidly.

Finally, *toxic reactions* are similar in appearance to systemic or anaphylactic reactions, but are not allergic in nature. They occur as a result of multiple (>50) stings and tend to result in gastrointestinal symptoms, fever, headache, and muscle spasms without urticaria or bronchospasm.

3. Field Management

In the field, the first priority is to remove the stinger as quickly as possible. Previously, it was felt that stingers should be scraped off and not pinched off to avoid squeezing venom from the venom sac into the victim. As Vissher and colleagues demonstrated, rapid removal of the stinger is far more important than the method of extraction, because the venom sac continues to pump venom into the victim as long as it is in place [17]. Within 20 sec, 90% of the venom sac contents are discharged into the victim, and 100% within 1 min [18]. Following stinger removal, the area should be washed gently with soap and water. Pustules from fire ant stings should be left intact. Ice, nonsteroidal anti-inflammatory agents, histamine receptor-1 and -2 blockers, and topical anesthetics are useful for symptomatic relief.

Systemic and toxic reactions are difficult to distinguish from each other and should be treated in the same manner. Any victim who develops severe urticaria, respiratory distress, or hypotension should be treated with subcutaneous epinephrine: 0.3 to 0.5 mg (0.3 to 0.5 cc of 1:1000 aqueous concentration) for an adult or 0.01 mg/kg for a child. This dose may need to be repeated in 15 to 20 min. Along with epinephrine, histamine-1 and -2 receptor blockers, steroids, and inhaled nebullized beta-adrenergic agonists (2.5 mg of albuterol solution in 2.5 cc normal saline) should be administered to counteract the anaphylactic response. Endotracheal intubation should be performed early for impending airway obstruction. Intravenous fluids should be administered aggressively to treat hypotension caused by a decrease in systemic vascular resistance. Symptoms and management of hymenoptera envenomation are summarized in Table 5. All victims demonstrating sys-

Table 5 Symptoms and Field Management of Hymenoptera Envenomation

Reaction type	Symptoms	Treatment
Local	Pain, erythema, edema, local joint spread	1. Remove stinger rapidly 2. Wash gently with soap/water 3. Ice to bite site 4. Nonsteroidal anti-inflammatory agents 5. Histamine 1 and 2 blockers
Systemic/anaphylactic	Itchy eyes, facial flushing, urticaria, stridor/bronchospasm, vomiting, abdominal cramping, hypotension	Same as above plus 1. Subcutaneous epinephrine (.01 cc/kg of 1:1000 up to .5 cc/dose) 2. Steroids 3. Inhaled beta agonists 4. Intubation as needed 5. Intravenous fluids for hypotension
Toxic	Fever, vomiting, abdominal cramping, muscle spasms	Treat as systemic reaction

temic or toxic reactions should be transported to the emergency department promptly for further treatment and observation.

B. Arthropods: Spiders

There are 30,000 species of spiders worldwide. Fifty of these are considered medically important because they are capable of inducing toxicity in humans. Spiders transfer toxins to their prey via piercing fangs connected by ducts to venom glands. Many spiders that bear venom are unable to deliver it to humans because their fangs cannot penetrate human skin.

Generally speaking, spiders can be divided into hunters and trappers. Hunters actively seek prey and have neurotoxic and proteolytic components in their venom in order to immobilize and digest their catch. Trappers spin elaborate webs which they use to envelop their prey. As a consequence, few trappers have toxic venom; they simply allow their catch to die.

1. Widow Spider (*Latrodectus*)

Identification

The widow spiders account for the vast majority of spider-related deaths. The most well known, the ''black widow,'' *Latrodectus mactans*, is the prototype for these spiders and is found in North and South America, Europe, Australia, and the Middle East. The female is dark black, with a 2-cm body, 4- to 5-cm leg span, and an hourglass-shaped, red marking on its ventral surface. In contrast, the male is only 3 to 5 mm with white stripes along the abdomen. Other species of widow spiders vary in color: the red-legged widow, *L. bishopi*; the red-backed widow, *L. hasselti*, found in Australia and New Zealand; the North American brown widow, *L. geometricus*; and the African widow, *L. indistinctus*.

Envenomation and Clinical Manifestations

The toxic venom component, *alpha latrotoxin*, is the same in all widow spider species. This chemical is a potent neurotoxin that stimulates cataclysmic release of neurotransmitters, specifically acetylcholine and norepinephrine, thereby depleting synaptic vesicles of their contents. The clinical result is muscle fasciculation and spasm, followed by paralysis. Only the female of the species is capable of delivering venom, as the male is too small to bite through human skin. The female spins a web in dark, sheltered corners, most notoriously in outdoor privies, leaving an egg case in the center. The black widow is one of the few trapper spiders that in aggressively guarding its eggs will envenom an intruder who disturbs the web.

Latrodectus bites typically cause minimal local symptomatology. The bite may feel sharp but is often unnoticed. Minimal swelling, warmth, and/or blanching with surrounding induration and erythema typically disappear in 30 to 60 min. Within 2 hr, systemic symptoms may develop and follow a waxing and waning course. A dull ache at the bite site progresses to large muscle group myalgia and spasm, followed by excruciating cramping pain involving the shoulders, back, and abdomen. A rigid abdomen may mimic an acute surgical emergency, but there is no rebound tenderness and the victim is restless, not still, as with peritoneal irritation. Autonomic instability due to massive neurotransmitter release is common. Hypertension, tachycardia, diaphoresis, and fever may be dramatic. Ultimately, respiratory muscle weakness and paralysis can lead to respiratory arrest and death. If untreated, severe symptoms may last for days, but pain is typically at its zenith 8 to 12 hr following envenomation.

Field Management and Transport

Ice may be applied to the bite site to effect pain relief. The victim should be put to rest to limit the spread of the venom and minimize tachycardia and hypertension. Further field management involves close monitoring of the ABCs. Endotracheal intubation may be necessary to manage respiratory insufficiency. Narcotics and benzodiazepines should be used to control pain and muscle spasms. Intravenous calcium gluconate (1 gram) may also be utilized for treatment of muscle spasm, but the effects are usually transient. It may serve a useful diagnostic function if the source of envenomation is in question, however; calcium gluconate is not typically effective in inducing muscle relaxation with other insect envenomations [19].

Antivenin against *Latrodectus* venom blocks the binding of alpha latrotoxin to synaptic membranes, thereby interrupting the massive neurotransmitter release. It is useful with severe envenomations (respiratory arrest, seizures, uncontrolled hypertension) in the very young and elderly, as well as in pregnant victims. As with snake antivenin, widow spider antivenin can precipitate anaphylaxis and should only be administered in a monitored setting, such as an emergency department or intensive care unit. Any victim with systemic symptoms or one that satisfies the criteria for antivenin administration should be transported rapidly to a medical facility. Despite the severe nature of the effects of *Latrodectus* envenomation, mortality from a black widow bite is less than 1% with appropriate supportive care. However, some symptoms, such as pain, may last for months.

2. Brown Spider (*Loxosceles*)

Identification

Like widow spiders, brown spiders of the species *Loxosceles* are found worldwide. *L. reclusa*, the brown recluse spider, is the best known. Fawn to dark brown in color with a 1-cm body and 2- to 3-cm legs, the brown recluse can be identified on the basis of a violin-shaped marking on its dorsal thorax. Unlike the *Latrodectus, Loxosceles* spiders are nocturnal hunters, inhabiting warm, undisturbed areas of human dwellings. They bite when trapped, typically under clothing. Both males and females are capable of delivering venom to humans.

Envenomation and Clinical Manifestations

Brown spider venoms are immunologically distinct, but all have cytotoxic and hemolytic effects. One component, sphingomyelinase, induces endothelial damage in small dermal vessels, resulting in microvascular occlusion with thrombus formation. As a consequence of vascular stasis, tissue infarction ensues, and inflammatory mediators are released. Activation of the host immune response, specifically B cells and the complement cascade, further amplifies the injury. Other components of the venom cause direct hemolytic effects and promote the spread of the venom by digesting the host soft tissue matrix.

The clinical result can be severe dermatonecrosis. Many other spiders and other disease processes (e.g., necrotizing fascitis, septic emboli, trauma, vasculitis) can cause a similar clinical appearance. Further complicating the diagnosis is the fact that in the vast majority of envenomations, the victim is unaware that he has been bitten. Studies of new treatments for loxoscelism are therefore difficult to conduct, for cases are often difficult to confirm in the absence of a spider ''caught in the act.''.

Following a bite, local symptoms consist typically of mild stinging, pruritis, and paresthesias accompanied by edema, erythema, or blanching. Within hours, the area becomes indurated, but the venom effects often do not progress beyond this stage and the induration resolves within days. In a severe reaction however, local ischemia progresses, resulting in worsening pain. Within 12 to 18 hr, a bull's-eye-appearing lesion appears, with a central clear or hemorrhagic vesicle surrounded by a pale ring surrounded in turn by ecchymosis. The vesicle may enlarge and rupture, leaving a sore in the midst of a violaceous discoloration of the skin. Over the next 5 to 7 days, the lesion may become necrotic, leaving a black eschar upon a poorly healing ulcer, which may persist for months. Bites in fatty areas, such as the buttocks, are the most prone to severe necrosis. Systemic reactions (''loxoscelism'') are rare, but may be severe in children. Twenty-four to 72 hr after the onset of cutaneous manifestations, fevers, chills, malaise, nausea, and vomiting can progress to disseminated intravascular coagulation, renal failure, seizures, and coma. Of note, the severity of systemic manifestations does not correlate with the degree of local symptomatology.

Field Management and Transport

Initial field management of brown spider envenomation is similar to that for widow spider envenomation. If possible, the bitten area should be immobilized loosely, elevated, and ice packs applied to limit venom activity. Heat should not be applied. Local wound care with soap and water scrub is critical to decrease the pathogen load at the envenomation site and prevent infection. Pain can be managed with a nonsteroidal anti-inflammatory agent or narcotic analgesic. While many therapies for cutaneous loxoscelism have been suggested, such as electrical shock, dapsone, and hyperbaric oxygen, none has proven effective in controlled studies. Studies in humans and animals have demonstrated that outcome from *Loxosceles* envenomation is as good with supportive care alone (e.g., wound cleansing, debridement) as with aggressive medical management (e.g., dapsone, hyperbaric oxygen) [20,21]. Empirical observations of some experts, however, suggest that some of these may yet prove efficacious. No antivenin for brown spider bite is commercially available at this time.

Transport to a medical facility may be reserved for those victims with rapidly expanding lesions or evidence of systemic toxicity. Conservative management of children with known *Loxosceles* envenomation would dictate evaluation and observation at a medical facility due to the increased risk of systemic reactions. Despite the potential severity of symptoms due to brown recluse venom, death is extremely rare.

3. Funnel Web Spider

Identification

Funnel web spiders are large, aggressive spiders that live predominantly in Australia and other regions of the South Pacific. The most well known of the species, the Sydney funnel web spider, *Atrax robustus*, is extremely dangerous because of the lethality of its venom. The funnel web spider has a 3- to 5-cm black body and a velvety ventral surface bearing a red tuft of hair. While females are larger than males, males are far more aggressive and carry venom five times more potent than that of the female. In fact, all known *Atrax* fatalities have been the result of bites from males. Most funnel web spiders are ground dwellers, living under homes or vegetation, and occasionally in large colonies. *Hadronyche formidabilis*, a species from New South Wales, resides mostly in trees.

Envenomation and Clinical Manifestations

The fangs of funnel web spiders are 4 to 7 mm and vertical in orientation. Funnel web spiders rear back and lift up their bodies to attack. The primary component of their venom, *atraxotoxin*, is neurotoxic. Atraxotoxin generates repetitive action potentials, causing massive neurotransmitter release from presynaptic neurons in both the somatic and autonomic nervous systems.

The victim may experience intense pain at the site of the bite because of the acidity of the venom. The area quickly becomes erythematous and swollen, but no local necrosis occurs. With severe envenomation, systemic symptoms rapidly ensue in a biphasic fashion. In phase I, muscle fasciculations and piloerection extend proximally over the first 20 min. This progresses to fever, marked hypertension, tachycardia, and a severe cholinergic toxidrome, including diarrhea, salivation, diaphoresis, and painful muscle writhing. Laryngospasm and excessive secretions may lead to death during this phase. After a few hours, phase 2 begins and the victim appears to recover. Respiratory and cardiovascular insufficiency may recur, however. Children under the age of 12 years are particularly vulnerable to the effects of funnel web spider envenomation.

Field Management and Transport

Much of the data supporting various aspects of field management with funnel web spider bites have been obtained from studies on monkeys. Based on these studies, it is clear that rapid treatment and transport of the victims is critical, due to the short window between symptom onset and death. While not proven, the use of mechanical suction (e.g., the Sawyer extractor) to remove venom seems logical as long as it does not result in significant delay to definitive care. Compression and immobilization, a technique previously described with elapid envenomation, has been shown to limit dissemination of venom via lymphatic and venous flow, thereby postponing the onset of systemic symptoms [7,22]. If respiratory insufficiency develops, endotracheal intubation may be necessary in the field. A combination alpha- and beta-receptor blocker, such as labetolol, can be administered intravenously for severe hypertension. Atropine for secretion control should be used cautiously, because it can worsen tachycardia.

The victim of a funnel web spider bite should be transported as quickly as possible to a medical facility, by air ambulance if available, in order to administer antivenin. En route, the limb should be immobilized to limit venom spread. Antivenin administration is the most effective intervention against atraxotoxin. Since its introduction in 1980, it has changed the natural history of funnel web spider envenomation dramatically, limiting the severity of symptoms and shortening hospitalization. While adverse reactions are rare, antivenin should be given only in a closely monitored setting.

4. Armed Spider (*Phoneutria*)

Identification

Phoneutria spiders are large, nocturnal, aggressive spiders common in urban areas in South America. *P. nigriventer*, the so-called armed or banana spider, is the largest spider in South America, found mainly in Brazil, Argentina, and Uruguay. Brown to gray in color with a frontal red tuft, the spider is 3 to 4 cm long with a 4- to 6-cm leg span. The female of the species is larger than the male. *Phoneutria* are nocturnal hunters, with potent venom that they deliver via large 4- to 5-mm fangs. Their venom is complex, consisting of proteolytic enzymes, histamine, and at least six neurotoxic peptides. These peptides block sodium channels in somatic and autonomic neurons, leading to action potential potentiation and axonal swelling.

Clinical Manifestations and Field Management

P. nigriventer bites cause severe local pain that radiates up the extremity to the trunk. Within 10 to 20 min, autonomic disturbances include tachycardia, hypertension, hypothermia, priapism, diaphoresis, and visual disturbances. Respiratory paralysis may occur within 2 to 6 hr. Victims at the extremes of age are most susceptible to the effects of envenomation.

Field management of *Phoneutria* bites is predominantly symptomatic. Venom dispersion is too rapid to attempt limitation of venom spread via compression-immobilization or other techniques. Mild envenomations are treated with analgesics alone. Victims of moderate or severe envenomations should be transported to a medical facility for administration of polyvalent antivenin active against *Phoneutria* and *Loxosceles* species. The clinical manifestations and appropriate field interventions for the spiders mentioned above are listed in Table 6.

5. Scorpions

Identification

Scorpions are arthropods found in temperate and desert climates around the world. While there are 650 species of scorpions, only 50 of these, most in the family *Buthidae*, cause harm to humans. Envenomation by scorpions is a significant health problem, particularly among children in the developing world. In India, 50% of children under 4 years of age who are stung by scorpions succumb to the bite.

In the western hemisphere, the habitat of the scorpion extends from the deserts of the southwestern United States through Mexico to South America. In the northern portion of this range, the only medically important species is *Centuroides*, in particular *C. exilicauda*. This scorpion is common in Arizona and northern Mexico and varies greatly, from 1 to 7 cm in length. Yellow-brown in color, it bears a striped dorsum and a small tubercle just proximal to its stinger, by which it can be identified. In South America and the Caribbean, the *Tityus* species of scorpion causes clinically significant bites. It is similar in appearance and behavior to *Centuroides*. In the Eastern hemisphere, dangerous scorpions are found most commonly in North Africa and the Middle East (*Leirus, Androctonus*), India (*Mesobuthus tamulus*), and South Africa (*Parabuthus, Buthotus*; Fig. 6).

Table 6 Symptoms and Field Management of Spider Envenomation

Species	Local effects	Systemic effects	Field management
Black widow (*Latrodectus*)	Minimal edema, warmth, erythema, induration	Dull ache, myalgias, spasms, excruciating crampy pain, autonomic instability, respiratory paralysis	Rest, ice, analgesics, IV calcium gluconate, antivenin for severe symptoms
Brown recluse (*Loxosceles*)	Pruritis, paresthesias, edema, erythema or blanching, induration	Rare	Immobilize extremity, elevate, ice, wound irrigation, analgesics
Funnel web	Severe pain, erythema, edema	Muscle fasciculations, cholinergic toxidrome, fever, laryngospasm	Mechanical suction, compression immobilization, rapid transport, antivenin
Armed (*Phoneutria*)	Severe pain	Autonomic instability, diaphoresis, visual disturbances, respiratory paralysis	Ice, analgesics, antivenin if severe symptoms

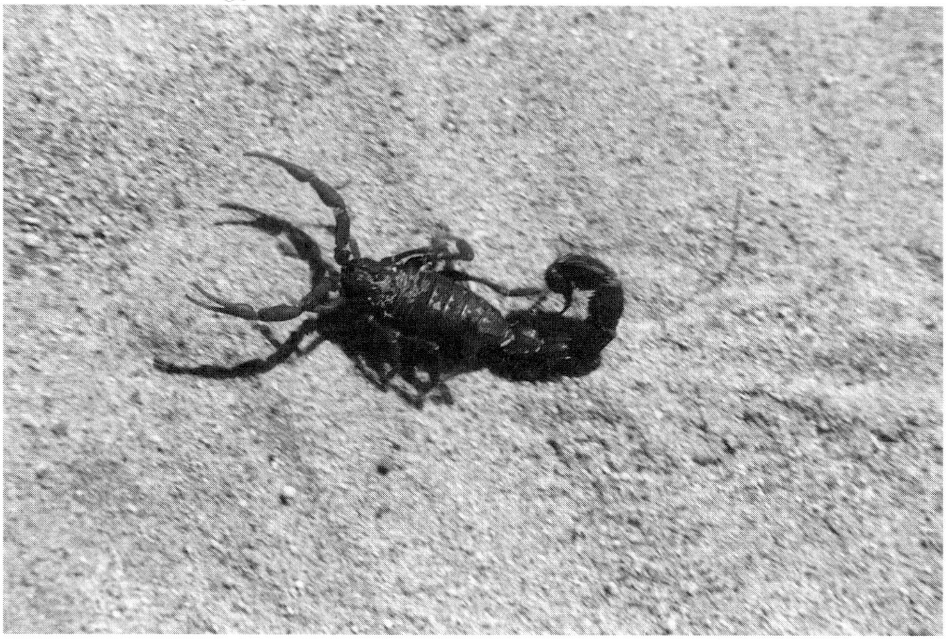

Figure 6 *Parabuthus*: venomous species common in South Africa.

Scorpions are nocturnal, with crablike bodies, two pincers, a five-segment tail, and a terminal stinger attached to a venom gland. They live under debris, in crevices, under clothes, in tents and sleeping bags, and transiently in unoccupied footwear. Although they move about at night, scorpions are only active at temperatures above 25°C (77°F). Guided by chemoreceptors, a scorpion delivers venom by grasping the victim with paired pincers and bringing its stinger-bearing tail over its body.

Envenomation and Clinical Manifestations

Scorpion venom is complex and differs from species to species. The venom of most species contains neurotoxins that stabilize sodium channels in an open or conducting state, causing sustained depolarization and repetitive axonal firing. This results in cranial nerve and somatic neuromuscular dysfunction and massive neurotransmitter (most significantly catecholamine) release. Phospholipases in *Buthotus* and *Parabuthus* venom can produce coagulopathy and intravascular hemolysis. Enzymatic components are not common in scorpion venoms, and hence tissue damage following a sting is minimal.

The majority of *C. exilicauda* stings are minor. Pain may be intense at the sting site and radiate up the extremity. Numbness or hypersensitivity to temperature or pressure is common, but swelling and erythema are minimal if present. Systemic symptoms, more common in children, the elderly, and victims with hypertension, include: blurred vision, dysphagia, tongue fasciculations, slurred speech, laryngospasm, and shaking or jerking of the extremities (pseudo-seizures).

Envenomation can be graded based on the presence of local or radiating bite site pain and cranial and/or somatic nerve dysfunction (Table 7). Grade II envenomations are distinguished from grade I by the extension of local symptoms beyond the immediate bite site. Grade III envenomations are systemic in nature, resulting in either cranial nerve or

Table 7 Grades of Scorpion Envenomation

I	Local pain and paresthesias only
II	Local symptoms extend beyond bite site
III	*Either* cranial nerve or somatic neuromuscular dysfunction
	Cranial nerve: blurred vision, tongue fasciculations, dysphagia, dysarthria, respiratory distress
	Somatic nerves: jerking, restlessness, seizure-like activity
IV	*Both* cranial and somatic neuromuscular dysfunction

somatic neuromuscular dysfunction. Grade IV bites involve both cranial and somatic nerve dysfunction. In severe envenomation, symptoms peak at about 4 hr in an adult and as quickly as 30 min in an infant. The symptoms of milder stings typically resolve within several hours. *Centuroides* species in the United States other than *C. exilicauda* are non-neurotoxic and produce only local effects.

Leirus, Androctonus, Buthotus, Mesobuthus, and *Tityus* stings also cause intense local pain, but edema and erythema are more marked than with stings from *Centuroides*. As venom disseminates rapidly, massive autonomic discharge results in predominantly sympathomimetic effects. Fever, restlessness, severe hypertension, seizures, and tachyarrhythmias are common and may be difficult to control. Cholinergic symptoms may include hypersalivation, excessive secretions, and severe gastrointestinal cramping. In *Parabuthus* stings, venom effects may be delayed for up to 24 hr.

Field Management and Transport

A constriction band to limit lymphatic distribution of venom may be effective in delaying the onset of systemic symptoms, but its use is unproven. If the band is used, it should be placed 10 cm proximal to the sting, and distal pulses must be carefully monitored to avoid creating a tourniquet effect. Local wound care involves gentle cleansing with soap and water. Ice and oral analgesics can be used to reduce pain at the sting site. Narcotics should be avoided because they can potentiate neurotoxic effects. Great care should be taken to maintain normothermia. In a rabbit model, the half-life of venom was longer, and a larger lethal fraction remained in the intravascular space in hypo- and hyperthermic animals [23].

In a severe envenomation, airway management may involve control of secretions and/or endotracheal intubation due to airway obstruction or paralysis. Hypertension may be controlled with a central-acting agent such as clonidine. Tachyarrhythmias should be managed symptomatically. Atropine for control of cholinergic symptoms should be used with caution, given the risks of exacerbation of tachyarrhythmias. Seizures should be treated with a rapidly acting benzodiazepine such as lorazepam.

Species-specific antivenins are available in India, the Middle East, northern and southern Africa, Mexico, the United States, and Brazil, but are not indicated in all cases. With *Centuroides, Parabuthus, and Tityus* stings, antivenin should be used with grade III or grade IV envenomations only. Antivenin is only minimally effective in *Leirus* toxicity because of the slow distribution of specific antivenin to tissues (40 times slower than with *Centuroides*). The focus of treatment is therefore supportive. No antivenin exists for envenomation by *Mesobuthos* species. A summary of the symptoms and field management of medically important scorpion species is provided in Table 8.

Table 8 Symptoms and Field Management of Scorpion Envenomation

Species	Locale	Clinical effects	Field management
Centuroides	Southwestern United States, Mexico	Local pain, numbess, blurred vision, dysphagia, tongue fasciculations, laryngospasm, myoclonus	Constriction band, wound irrigation, ice, oral analgesics (avoid narcotics), clonidine for hypertension, benzodiazepines for seizures, antivenin for grade III–IV envenomations (none for *Leirus* or *Mesobuthus*)
Leirus	Middle East, northern Africa	Local pain, erythema, edema, fever, hypertension, tachycardia, restlessness, seizures, secretions	
Tityus	South America, Caribbean	Same as *Leirus*	
Mesobuthus	India	Same as *Leirus*	
Parabuthus	South Africa	Same as *Leirus*, but up to 24-hr delay	

Transport to a medical facility is indicated in any case in which systemic symptoms are apparent and/or antivenin is indicated. Children, the elderly, and those with significant comorbidities (e.g., hypertension, coronary artery disease) should also be transported, even if systemic symptoms are not immediately apparent. Given the delayed nature of *Parabuthus* venom effects, all victims of *Parabuthus* stings should be transported for observation. While mortality in the United States has been nonexistent since 1968, deaths in the developing world are still common.

III. MARINE BITES AND STINGS

Marine organisms that are hazardous to humans are found predominantly in tropical and warm temperate oceans. The rising number of interactions between humans and the marine environment in the course of work or recreation has inevitably increased the risks of related injuries and illness. Marine hazards include organisms that envenom and those that bite but do not deliver venom to their victims.

A. Envenomations

1. Coelenterates

Coelenterates are a diverse group of invertebrates. Those that are harmful to humans possess venom-containing stinging cells called nematocysts. Coelenterates are capable of delivering venom in an explosive fashion with continuous injection of venom while the nematocysts are in contact with human skin. Dangerous coelenterates include hydrozoans (e.g., fire coral, Portuguese man-of-war), scyphozoans (e.g., box jellyfish), and anthozoans (e.g., anemones).

Fire corals are not true corals. They are sessile bottom dwellers with nematocyst-bearing tentacles that envenom those who accidentally make contact with them. In contrast, the man-of-war *Physalia* lives on the ocean surface with venom-containing tentacles suspended from a nitrogen- and carbon monoxide-filled floating sail. Found in both Atlantic and Pacific waters, the man-of-war's tentacles may reach 30 meters in length and may bear 750,000 nematocysts each. The box jellyfish *Chironex fleckeri* is the most venomous sea creature, capable of causing death within 2 min. It is found predominantly in shallow waters off northern Queensland, Australia. Sea anemones are multicolored, flowerlike sessile creatures with fingerlike tentacles that typically produce a mild to moderate sting, but on occasion an extremely painful one.

The severity of coelenterate envenomation depends upon the species and season; the number of nematocysts triggered; the size of the organism; the size, age, and health of the victim; and the location and surface area of the sting. Mild envenomation causes an immediate stinging sensation and itching, with formation of linear reddish-brown wheals or "tentacle prints" on the skin. Local edema, desquamation, ulceration, and ultimately necrosis may develop with more severe envenomation. If a large number of nematocysts contact the skin (e.g., *P. physalis*) or the venom transferred is particularly potent (e.g., *C. fleckeri*), a systemic reaction may ensue. Symptoms may include vomiting, headache, vertigo, hypotension, dysrhythmias, pulmonary edema, paralysis, and coma. Allergic reactions may play a significant role in the severity of coelenterate envenomation.

Field management of a local reaction involves decontamination and pain control. Nematocysts may be removed immediately by rinsing the wound with a forceful stream of freshwater. Freshwater should not be used in a gentle application or rinse because it will further activate nematocysts, causing greater envenomation. Visible tentacles may be removed with forceps or a gloved hand. Application of 5% acetic acid (vinegar) will inactivate the toxin and should be used liberally with box jellyfish stings prior to attempts to remove the tentacles [24]. Following vinegar application or in the absence of available vinegar, the pressure-immobilization technique (see above) should be applied. While scientific evidence is lacking, consideration should also be given to the use of a constriction band proximal to the envenomation site, particularly in the setting of *C. fleckeri* envenomation. By occluding venous and lymphatic flow without creating a tourniquet, the systemic spread of venom may be retarded without compromising the extremity. Oral and/or intravenous analgesics are often necessary for pain control. Systemic reactions should be treated supportively with endotracheal intubation as needed for respiratory insufficiency and intravenous fluids for hypotension and shock.

Definitive treatment for box jellyfish envenomation is rapid administration of antivenin. In contrast to admonitions to avoid antivenin use in the field with snake and insect envenomation due to the risk of anaphylaxis, death can ensue so rapidly with *C. fleckeri* envenomation that the field administration of antivenin is warranted and common in Australia [25]. One ampule of *Chironex* antivenin (Commonwealth Serum Laboratories, Melbourne, Australia) may be given intravenously or intramuscularly and then repeated every 2 to 4 hr until symptoms no longer progress. Antihistamines and epinephrine should be available to treat anaphylaxis. All victims who exhibit systemic reactions, including the elderly and the young, should be transported to a medical facility for observation and management.

Other fire coral and jellyfish stings may be "decontaminated" with vinegar, bicarbonate, papain, isopropyl alcohol, or household ammonia. Since all species respond differently, one should become familiar with local species and proven remedies.

2. Sea Urchins

Sea urchins are echinoderms with a hard-shelled central body from which protrude spines and/or seizing organs called pedicellariae. Venom-bearing spines are sharp. Once embedded in flesh, they lodge deeply and may be difficult to extract. Non-venom-bearing spines are rounded and less likely to penetrate skin. Pedicellariae seize objects with which they come into contact. They attach and envenom and will be torn from the shell rather than releasing. Sea urchin venom is complex, consisting of proteases, hemolysins, cholinergic agents, and neurotoxins. Envenomation typically occurs as a result of incidental contact by a diver or an individual walking barefoot in a tidal area.

Envenomation causes immediate intense pain, followed rapidly by local erythema, edema, and myalgias. If multiple spines or pedicellariae contact the skin, systemic symptoms may develop. These symptoms include vomiting, abdominal pain, paresthesias, hypotension, syncope, and paralysis with resulting respiratory compromise. Severe synovitis with effusion may develop if a spine enters a joint. Envenomation by pedicellariae typically results in a more severe clinical syndrome with interise local pain and severe circulatory and neurological compromise. Symptoms may persist for up to 6 hr.

Management in the field consists of rapid removal of detached pedicellariae and spines to limit envenomation. Removal of pedicellariae may be accomplished by applying shaving foam to the area, followed by gentle scraping with a razor. Spines may be more difficult to remove because they are brittle and fracture easily. Some embedded spines will dissolve in days to weeks, depending on their size, but may cause infection or granuloma formation. Immersion of the affected area in nonscalding hot water (up to 45°C or 113°F) for 30 to 90 min provides the most effective initial pain relief. Systemic reactions should be managed symptomatically. Transport to a medical facility may be limited to those who manifest systemic symptoms and to those with multiple embedded spines associated with severe pain [26].

3. Starfish

Starfish are stellate echinoderms covered with thorny spines of calcium carbonate. Venomous material produced in the epidermis of the starfish covers the spines. The crown-of-thorns starfish *Acanthaster planci* is a particularly venomous species, with spines of up to 6 cm that can easily penetrate a diving glove. This starfish lives in the coral reefs of the Pacific and Indian Oceans, the Red Sea, the Gulf of California, and the Great Barrier Reef. *A. planci* venom consists of hemolytic, coagulopathic, mycotoxic, and hepatotoxic components.

Penetration of the skin by spines of *A. planci* results in immediate pain, bleeding, and edema that can last up to 2 to 3 hr. Multiple punctures may induce systemic symptoms, including paresthesias, gastrointestinal upset, and muscular paralysis. Previously sensitized victims may experience prolonged local symptoms.

Management of starfish envenomation is supportive. Spines should be carefully removed with forceps and the wound site carefully cleansed. As with sea urchin envenomation, the wound should be immersed in nonscalding hot water for 30 to 90 min or until sustained pain relief has been achieved. Transport to a hospital is indicated for any victim manifesting severe systemic symptoms.

4. Cone Snails

The cone snail is a carnivorous mollusk with a highly developed venom apparatus. Of the 300 species of cone snails, 18 have been found to be dangerous to humans. These are found predominantly in Indo-Pacific waters. Cone snail venom is an amalgam of peptides similar to tetrodotoxin that inhibit neuromuscular transmission by blocking sodium channel function. Venom is injected into the victim via a dartlike tooth thrust through the skin via an extensible proboscis.

A sting typically occurs on a hand or finger and resembles a hymenoptera sting. Local burning or stinging may progress to perioral and peripheral paresthesias, nausea, weakness, ataxia, bulbar dysfunction, and generalized muscular paralysis leading to respiratory failure. Symptoms of a mild envenomation may disappear within a few hours, while those of a severe sting may take weeks to resolve.

While no scientific evidence supports its use in cone snail envenomation, compression and immobilization may be useful in containing the spread of venom until the victim can be transported to a medical facility. Similarly, suction, constriction bands, and hot water immersion have at times been recommended as field therapy, but no supportive evidence exists. If systemic symptoms develop, airway management and intravenous fluids to support failing circulation are the cornerstones of therapy. Edrophonium may be useful as empirical treatment to reverse paralysis.

Rapid transport to a medical facility is indicated in any documented cone snail envenomation.

5. Octopuses

Octopuses are mollusks that lack calcified shells. The most dangerous species, the Australian blue-ringed octopus, *Octopus maculosus*, and the spotted octopus, *O. lunulata*, are usually less than 20 cm in length and found in waters less than 3 meters deep. Bites result in severe, even fatal, envenomations. *O. maculosus* carries a potent and rapidly acting venom in sufficient quantity to paralyze 10 adult humans. The most toxic component, maculotoxin, is identical to tetrodotoxin, which blocks sodium channels and interrupts synaptic transmission. The venom is delivered via strong chitinous jaws capable of tearing skin and soft tissue.

The bite of a blue-ringed octopus is typically a puncture would on the hand that may not be noticed. It is often only mildly painful. Within 10 to 15 min local numbness may progress to facial numbness, bulbar dysfunction, weakness, ataxia, and ultimately flaccid paralysis with respiratory failure. Despite complete paralysis, the well-oxygenated victim may remain alert.

Field therapy of a poisonous octopus bite should focus initially on venom containment. While unproven, the compression and immobilization technique may be useful if the bite is on an extremity. If systemic symptoms develop, endotracheal intubation and mechanical ventilation should be performed early to avoid hypoxia. Symptoms typically improve after 4 to 10 hr, but may take up to 4 days to completely resolve. No antivenin exists. Any victim of a toxic octopus bite should be transported for observation and supportive care.

6. Stingrays

Stingrays are nonaggressive vertebrates that typically rest in calm, shallow areas in tropical waters. They are found partially submerged in sand or mud with only their eyes, spiracles, and tail exposed. When carelessly handled or accidentally stepped on, the stingray whips its tail upward and thrusts one or more of four venomous spines into the victim. Stingray venom contains various toxic fractions, including a cardiotoxin and a respiratory depressant. The strike itself can cause a significant wound with substantial bleeding.

Stingray envenomation typically occurs upon a lower extremity. The victim experiences immediate, severe pain and wound edema. The intensity of the pain peaks at 30 to 60 min, and may last for up to 48 hr. The wound is initially cyanotic but rapidly becomes erythematous, as hemorrhage and necrosis develop in subcutaneous fat and muscle. Systemic symptoms may develop fairly rapidly and include gastrointestinal upset, headache, muscle cramps and fasciculations, tachyarrhythmias, hypotension, seizures, and very rarely, death. Severe pain may result in muscle contractures that mimic paralysis.

In the field, the goals of treatment are to inactivate the venom, prevent infection, and provide pain relief and supportive care [27]. The wound should be irrigated and soaked as soon as possible with nonscalding hot water (45°C or 113°F) to inactivate thermolabile components of the venom, wash out pathogens, and provide analgesia. Retained spine material should be rapidly and carefully removed. As discussed with snake bites, mechanical suction and/or use of a constriction band to occlude venous and lymphatic spread of venom may be useful, but are unproven therapies. Narcotic analgesics or local anesthetics such as 1% lidocaine without epinephrine are also useful. Systemic symptoms should be managed supportively.

Any victim of a stingray strike should be transported to a medical facility for definitive wound care. Systemic symptoms may be delayed for up to 4 hr. Given the severity of potential reactions, observation is indicated.

7. Scorpionfish, Lionfish, and Stonefish

Scorpionfish, lionfish, and stonefish live predominantly in shallow tropical and temperate waters. While lionfish are colorful coral reef fish, scorpionfish and stonefish are well-camouflaged bottom dwellers. All three species carry 12 to 18 dorsal, two pelvic, and three anal spines associated with venom glands. Stonefish venom is particularly potent, likened in toxicity to cobra venom. It contains a neuromuscular toxin that causes an irreversible depolarizing blockade at skeletal, smooth, and cardiac muscle. Envenomation typically occurs when the victim steps on or grasps the fish, resulting in penetration of spines through the skin and injection of venom.

Puncture wounds from the spines of these species result in immediate and intense pain. Local ischemia and cyanosis may progress to erythema and edema involving the entire extremity. Severe envenomation, more common with stonefish than the other species of *Scorpaenidae*, may result in gastrointestinal upset and pain, fever, arthralgias, bronchospasm, hypotension, dysrhythmias, seizures, paralysis and rarely, death.

The wound should immediately be immersed in hot water (45°C or 113°F) in order to inactivate heat-sensitive components of the venom and provide pain relief. Simultaneously, visible spines should be carefully removed to halt any ongoing envenomation, and the wound should be vigorously irrigated. Injection of a local anesthetic without epinephrine or a regional nerve block may be necessary. Multiple topical remedies have been suggested, but none has been proven effective. Systemic reactions should be managed supportively.

Any victim of a stonefish envenomation should be transported for definitive medical care and consideration for stonefish antivenin therapy. Victims of lionfish and scorpionfish punctures require transport only for extensive local symptoms, pain control, or systemic manifestations.

8. Sea Snakes

There are at least 54 species of sea snakes, all of which are venomous. Common in tropical regions of the Indo-Pacific, sea snakes are not found in the Atlantic Ocean or Caribbean

Sea. The largest number of envenomations occurs in Southeast Asia, the Persian Gulf, and the Malay archipelago. Sea snakes are not aggressive and typically attack in self-defense. The fangs of the sea snake are short and easily dislodged. As a consequence, 80% of bites do not result in significant envenomation. When envenomation does occur however, it can be quite severe, for sea snake venom is more toxic than most terrestrial snake venoms. It contains digestive enzymes, along with hemolytic, myotoxic, and potent neurotoxic compounds that cause nondepolarizing neuromuscular blockade.

The diagnosis of a sea snake bite is based on the absence of pain at the puncture site; the presence of fang marks (usually one to four, but as many as 20); the occurrence of the bite while in the water or handling a fishing net; the development of characteristic symptoms; and the identification of the snake. Depending on the volume of venom transferred and the sensitivity of the victim, symptom onset may vary from 5 min to 8 hr. Local symptoms are usually absent. Initially the victim may develop myalgias and stiffness, along with dysphagia and dysarthria. Increasingly severe pain with passive muscle movement is followed by further bulbar dysfunction, ascending spastic or flaccid paralysis, and coma.

Treatment in the field is similar to that for elapid envenomation. The victim should be put to rest and kept calm. A mechanical venom-extracting device such as the Sawyer extractor may be useful if applied rapidly. Thereafter, compression and immobilization of the bite site should be performed as described previously. The extremity should then be immobilized in a dependent position. Compression and immobilization should be maintained until the victim reaches a medical facility, where antivenin therapy can be administered. If the victim deteriorates and systemic symptoms ensue, endotracheal intubation and mechanical ventilation may be necessary to prevent respiratory failure.

Transport for definitive care and antivenin therapy should be swift. Due to the risks of anaphylaxis, antivenin should not be administered outside a strictly monitored setting. The mortality from sea snake envenomation managed without antivenin is up to 25%; with antivenin this is reduced to less than 3%.

Symptoms and field management of the above marine envenomations are summarized in Table 9.

B. Marine Bites

1. Sharks

Marine animals that bite but do not envenom can cause life-threatening wounds that are at high risk for infection. Most notorious among aquatic enthusiasts and among those whose livelihoods depend on the sea is the shark attack. Sharks are typically nonaggressive animals, but some species, such as the great white, tiger, bull, and oceanic white-tip shark, have been observed to attack with little or no provocation. Great white sharks commonly inhabit the warm waters of southern Australia, the east coast of South Africa, and the cool, seal-populated waters of northern California between Tomales Bay and Año Nuevo. Attacks on humans typically occur at the ocean surface within 100 feet of shore and may be the result of an unfortunate similarity between the silhouette of a human near the surface and that of a seal or sea lion. Most attacks are so-called hit and runs involving only a single bite. Initial ''bumps'' by the shark prior to biting may cause severe skin abrasions [28], however.

Lacerations from shark bites are often severe due to the great force and tearing action of shark jaws. While extremities are the most common areas involved, thoracic and abdominal bites may involve massive tissue loss and hemorrhage. Blood loss and

Table 9 Symptoms and Field Management of Marine Envenomation

Species	Clinical manifestations	Field management
Coelenterate (man-of-war, fire coral, box jellyfish, anemone)	Local: stinging, pruritis, edema Systemic (box jellyfish): nausea, vomiting, hypotension, dysrhythmias, paralysis, allergic reactions	Forceful freshwater rinse, vinegar application, consider compression immobilization or constriction band for box jellyfish, antivenin for box jellyfish
Sea urchin	Local: intense pain, erythema, edema Systemic: myalgias, paresthesias vomiting, hypotension	Remove pedicellariae and spines, irrigate and immerse in 45°C (113°F) freshwater
Starfish	Local: pain, bleeding, edema Systemic: paresthesias, GI upset, muscle weakness	Remove spines, irrigate and immerse in 45°C (113°F) freshwater
Cone snail	Local: burning, stinging Systemic: perioral paresthesias, nausea, ataxia, motor paralysis	Consider mechanical suction, compression/immobilization, or constriction band; consider edrophonium for muscle paralysis
Octopus	Local: numbness Systemic: progression of numbness, motor paralysis	Consider compression/immobilization
Stingray	Local: immediate severe pain, edema, bleeding Systemic: muscular cramps and fasciculations, tachycardia, hypotension, seizures	Remove spines, irrigate and immerse in 45°C (113°F) freshwater, control bleeding, consider mechanical suction, constriction band
Scorpionfish, lionfish, stonefish	Local: intense pain, erythema, edema Stonefish: vomiting, fever, bronchospasm, arrhythmia, hypotension, seizure, paralysis	Remove spines, irrigate and immerse in 45°C (113°F) freshwater, consider antivenin for stonefish
Sea snake	Local: none Systemic: myalgias, stiffness, progressive bulbar dysfunction, ascending paralysis, coma	Rest victim, mechanical suction, consider compression/immobilization, antivenin

drowning are the principle causes of mortality in the 15–25% of shark bite victims who expire.

Care in the field consists primarily of treatment of hypovolemic shock. Bitten extremities should be compressed and elevated and rapid fluid resuscitation with intravenous normal saline instituted. Once the victim is hemodynamically stable, the wound(s) should be thoroughly irrigated and foreign bodies removed. Rapid transport to a medical facility is absolutely indicated for proper wound care and treatment of hypovolemia and shock (Table 10).

2. Barracudas

Barracudas are swift, solitary fish who live in the southern Atlantic Ocean, the Caribbean, and Indo-Pacific waters. They are more commonly encountered than sharks. Only the

Table 10 Management of Marine Bites

Copious wound irrigation
Foreign body removal
Control hemorrhage
Fluid resuscitation
Transport for definitive wound care and antibiotics if appropriate

great barracuda, *Sphyraena barracuda*, has been known to injure humans, however. It appears to attack erratically, often out of confusion in turbid waters or in pursuit of shiny objects.

Bites result in straight or V-shaped lacerations, in contrast to the crescent-shaped bite of the shark. Hemorrhage is more moderate and crush injuries less severe than with shark bites. The approach to treatment and indications for transport are identical to those for shark attacks.

3. Moray Eels

Moray eels are bottom dwellers that reside in holes and under coral in tropical and subtropical waters. Generally nonaggressive in nature, morays can attack savagely when cornered or provoked. Older, blind eels may attack without apparent provocation, particularly at night.

The moray's narrow viselike jaws may inflict severe puncture wounds, crush injuries, and lacerations. The moray may bite and hold on to its victim relentlessly, requiring sacrifice of the moray and disarticulation of its jaws. Ripping the moray off the victim may exacerbate the injury. Once the moray disengages (or is forcefully disengaged) from the victim, the wound should be thoroughly irrigated and explored for retained teeth. Given the high risk for infection, transport to a medical facility is indicated in order to definitively cleanse the wound and administer antibiotics [29].

IV. SUMMARY POINTS

The vast majority of snakes, insects, and marine organisms are not aggressive. By taking care not to disturb their habitats, many harmful interactions can be avoided.

Medical personnel should familiarize themselves with regional creatures that can pose a threat to humans, because recognition of the agent of a bite or sting is a critical step in prompt and appropriate treatment.

Attention should focus initially on airway, breathing, circulation, and treatment of life-threatening physiologic derangements prior to addressing local wound issues.

Attempts to limit the spread of venom, such as mechanical suction, compression immobilization, and lymphatic constriction, may be quite useful, but must be administered carefully to avoid causing further harm.

Knowledge of the natural history of a bite or envenomation and the availability of antivenin are important factors in the decision of whether and where to transport a victim.

REFERENCES

1. RN Pugh, RDG Theakston. Incidence and mortality of snakebite in savannah Nigeria. Lancet 2:1181–1183, 1980.

1a. JB Sullivan, WA Wingert, RL Norris. North American venomous reptile bites. In: PA Auerbach, ed. Wilderness Medicine, 3d edition. St. Louis: Mosby, 1995, pp. 684, 685.

2. ST Moss, G Bogdan, RC Dart, SP Nordt, SR Williams, RF Clark. Association of rattlesnake bite location with severity of clinical manifestations. Ann Emerg Med 30(1):58–61, 1997.

3. RC Dart, KM Hurlbut, R Garcia, J Boren. Validation of a severity score for the assessment of crotalid snakebite. Ann Emerg Med 27:321–326, 1996.

4. ME Stewart, S Greenland, JR Hoffman. First-aid treatment of poisonous snakebite: Are currently recommended procedures justified. Ann Emerg Med 10:331–335, 1981.

5. AC Bronstein, FE Russell, JB Sullivan. Negative pressure suction in the field treatment of rattlesnake bite victims. Vet Hum Toxicol 28:485–490, 1986.

6. SK Sutherland, AR Coulter, RD Harris. Rationalisation of first aid measures for elapid snakebite. Lancet 1:183–185, 1979.

7. DM Howarth, AE Southee, IM Whyte. Lymphatic flow rates and first aid in simulated peripheral snake or spider envenomation. Med J Aust 161:695–700, 1994.

8. DL Hardy, SP Bush. Pressure/immobilization as first aid for venomous snakebite in the United States. Herpet Rev 29:204–208, 1998.

8a. SA Minton, RL Norris. Non-North American venomous reptile bites. In: PA Auerbach, ed. Wilderness Medicine, 3d edition. St. Louis: Mosby, 1995, p. 721.

9. RL Norris, SA Minton. Snake venom poisoning: What the herpetoculturist needs to know. Vivarium 6:4–7, 1995.

10. Tun-Pe, Aye-Aye-Myint, Kein-Ei-Han, Thi-Ha, Tin-Nu-Swe. Local compression pads as a first-aid measure for victims of bites by Russell's viper in Myanmar. Trans Roy Soc Trop Med Hyg 89:293–295, 1995.

11. JL Burgess, RC Dart, NB Egen, M Mayersohn. Effects of constriction bands on rattlesnake venom absorption: A pharmacokinetic study. Ann Emerg Med 921:1086–1093, 1992.

12. G Watt, RDG Theakston, CG Hayes, ML Yambao, R Sangalang, CP Ranoa, E Alquizalas, DA Warrell. Positive response to edrophonium in patients with neurotoxic envenoming by cobras (Naja naja philippinensis). New Eng J Med 315:1444–1448, 1986.

13. K Heard, GF O'Malley, RC Dart. Antivenom therapy in the Americas. Drugs 58:5–15, 1999.

14. SK Sutherland, RL Leonard. Snakebite deaths in Australia 1992–94 and a management update. Med J Aust 163:616–618, 1995.

15. RC Dart, SA Siefert, L Carrol, RF Clark, E Hall, LY Boyer-Hassen, SC Curry, CS Kitchens, RA Garcia. Affinity-purified, mixed monospecific crotalid antivenom ovine Fab for the treatment of crotalid venom poisoning. Ann Emerg Med 30:33–39, 1997.

16. RS Vetter, PK Visscher, S Camazine. Mass envenomations by honey bees and wasps. West J Med 170:223–227, 1999.

17. PK Visscher, RS Vetter, S Camazine. Removing bee stings. Lancet 348:301–302, 1996.

18. MJ Schumacher, MS Tveten, NB Egen. Rate and quantity of delivery of venom from honeybee stings. J Allergy Clin Immunol 93:831–835, 1994.

19. RF Clark, S Wethern-Kestner, MV Vance, R Gerkin. Clinical presentation and treatment of black widow spider envenomation: A review of 163 cases. Ann Emerg Med 21:782–787, 1992.

20. S Phillips, M Kohn, D Baker, R Vander Leest, H Gomez, P McKinney, J McGoldrick, J Brent. Therapy of brown spider envenomation: A controlled trial of hyperbaric oxygen, dapsone and cyproheptadine. Ann Emerg Med 25:363–367, 1995.

21. SW Wright, KD Wrenn, L Murray, D Seger. Clinical presentation and outcome of brown recluse spider bite. Ann Emerg Med 30:28–32, 1997.

22. L Hartman, S Sutherland. Funnel web spider (Atrax robustus) antivenom in the treatment of human envenomation. Med J Aust 141:796–799, 1984.
23. M Ismail, MA Abd-Elsalam, AM Morad. Do changes in body temperature following envenomation by the scorpion Leirus quinquestriatus influence the course of toxicity? Toxicon 28: 1265–1284, 1990.
24. J Pearn. Sea, stingers, and surgeons: The surgeon's role in prevention, first aid and management of marine envenomations. J Pediat Surg 30:105–110, 1995.
25. JW Burnett, JE Purcell, DB Learn, T Meyers. A protocol to investigate the blockade of jellyfish nematocysts by topical agents. Cont Dermatitis 4(1):55–56, 1999.
26. JW Burnett, MG Burnett. Sea urchins. Cutis 64:21–22, 1999.
27. PJ Fenner, VA Williamson, RA Skinner. Fatal and non-fatal stingray envenomation. Med J Aust 151:621–625, 1989.
28. JW Burnett. Aquatic adversaries: Shark bites. Cutis 61:317–318, 1998.
29. T Erickson, TL VandenHoek, A Kuritza, JB Leiken. Emergency management of moray eel bites. Ann Emerg Med 21:212–216, 1992.

35

Helicopter Versus Ground Transport: When Is It Appropriate?

DANIEL G. HANKINS

Mayo Clinic and Mayo Medical Transport, Rochester, Minnesota

PÅL MADSEN

Norwegian Air Ambulance Ltd., Høvik, Norway

> If a man is in need of rescue, an airplane could come in and throw flowers on him, and that's just about all. But a direct lift aircraft could come in and save his life.
>
> —Igor Sikorsky, 1967

I. INTRODUCTION

It has been over 50 years since the first rotor-wing rescue of a patient occurred in Burma during the waning stages of World War II. That event set the stage for the further use of helicopters in Korea and the subsequent extensive use of helicopter rescue in Vietnam. This military experience led to the development of civilian helicopter systems around the world. Helicopters have rescued millions of people since 1945, yet they still remain controversial, especially in this era of health care budget cuts. Are helicopters useful and cost-effective or are they expensive flying billboards? Do they save lives or are ground ambulances just as efficacious at transporting the sick and injured? Is it more complex than that (i.e., is one is more useful at one time than another)? Just as with any other modality of treatment or transport in out-of-hospital medicine, the helicopter or ground vehicle each has its own utility and crew capabilities, depending on the circumstances of the event. The proper usage of *any* out-of-hospital treatment requires active physician oversight with continuous quality management and utilization review to continuously attempt to make the system better. An emergency medical services system, including ground, helicopter, and fixed-wing, is a continuously evolving system and not a static entity.

Two of the most important concepts to consider in transportation decisions about patients are: (1) ''stable patients accessible to ground vehicle should be transported by ground vehicle'' [1]; and (2) ''the right crew in the right vehicle needs to be sent to the right patient.'' If time is not a factor and if the patient does not require that out-of-hospital time be minimized, then ground is preferable to rotor-wing. On the other hand, if the patient has a time-dependent injury or illness or requires critical care interventions by highly skilled attendants, then helicopter transport is appropriate. Some patients require that the out-of-hospital time needs to be minimized. There is no doubt that helicopter transport can accomplish this, since a ground ambulance travels at about 1 mile a min, while a helicopter travels 2 miles per min as the bird flies.

The purpose of this chapter is to explore the complex decision-making process that goes into the determination of ''ground versus air'' transport. Among the factors are the skills and training of the ground crews versus air medical crews, cost, and the speed of transport. This process requires total system integration to ensure the optimal use of resources.

II. HISTORY AND BACKGROUND

Although Dominique-Jean Larrey envisioned ''flying dressing stations'' (*ambulances volantes*) during the Napoleanic Wars to reduce morbidity and mortality, he probably did not realize that this literally would happen. It was during the siege of Paris a few decades later that people were first evacuated air via balloon (although it has been said that many of the evacuees were politicians and not sick or wounded patients) [2]. Fixed-wing transport of patients did occur in World War I, although not extensively. Many fixed-wing medical transports occurred in World War II, along with the seminal helicopter transport in Burma mentioned above [3]. The mortality rate for a wounded soldier in World War II was 5.8%. During the Korean War, about 20,000 patients were transported by rotor craft [4]. The average overall transport time ranged from 2 to 4 hr and the mortality rate dropped further to 2.4%. In the period from 1965 to 1969, 370,000 patients were transported in Vietnam, with much shorter transport times and a reduction in mortality to less than 2% [5]. As with many military advances in emergency medical services, the fast transports in Vietnam and the use of paramedical personnel led to advances for civilian EMS around the world. It did not seem right that a soldier wounded in Vietnam had a better chance of survival than a motor vehicle accident victim on the highways of Europe or the United States. Since the first U.S. civilian rotor-wing program started in 1972 in Denver, over 1 million patients have been transported by helicopter. Trauma scene runs average from 10–25% for helicopter services in the United States.

Civilian systems have evolved differently from one country to another. In the United States, the rotor-wing services act as tertiary responders, typically arriving after ground-first responders and ground ambulances are at the scene. In Europe, the rotor-wing services are highly trained first responders that arrive before the ground vehicles do. In both cases the helicopter brings in a crew of highly trained people who can provide sophisticated critical care modalities. In spite of crew differences, whether physician, nurse, or medic, the high level of care provided by the air medical crew members are remarkably alike from country to country. The helicopter brings tertiary care quickly to a situation that would otherwise have basic primary care.

Besides an augmentation of response to a critical scene with more sophisticated medical care, the helicopter crew adds better triage skills, faster evacuation of the most critical patients [6], and the opportunity for air surveillance of the situation if needed by the incident commander on the scene.

A. Vehicles

The nature of a ground ambulance varies from region to region and country to country. In the United States, there are three basic ambulance types.

Type I: a pickup truck cab and chassis with a modular box mounted on the back
Type II: a standard passenger van with an ambulance conversion of the back
Type III: a specialized van cab and chassis with a modular box mounted on the back

The type III ground ambulance is the most widely used in the United States because of the interior room and comfort. Type IIs are also the most expensive to buy and operate, however, so there has been a swing toward ''minimod'' ambulances, a smaller version of the type II.

Helicopters come in a variety of shapes and sizes. The most widely used single-engined EMS helicopter is the Bell 206. Single-engined ships are cheaper to operate, but size and the safety concern of a single engine have swung the pendulum to twin-engined helicopters over the past 10 years. There is more room in the midsized twins with the safety margin of the second engine. Twin-engined helicopters also can be equipped to an IFR (instrument flight rated) configuration, which allows for further safety in expected or unexpected marginal or bad weather conditions. Until the recent advent of a new generation of small to midsized EMS helicopters, the most popular EMS helicopter in the world has been the MBB BK-117. Helicopter programs are continuously looking for the ideal helicopter, which (1) has plenty of room, both to complete the patient care mission and for crew comfort, (2) has two engines for safety and IFR capability, and finally (3) is inexpensive to operate. The ideal helicopter does not yet exist.

B. Crews

Ground ambulances in the United States have crews at several possible skill levels. Rural areas tend to be covered by volunteer services trained to the basic emergency medical technician (EMT-A) level. A basic EMT has about 110 hr of training over and above that of a layperson. There are usually two EMT-As on a basic ambulance—one to drive and one in the back to attend the patient. Busier urban ambulance services have professional paramedics (or emergency medical technician–paramedic [EMT-P]), who have about 1000 hr of training over and above the basic 110 hr. An advanced life support ambulance usually has a crew of two: either an EMT-A with an EMT-P or 2 EMT-Ps.

Rotor-wing crews are also variable. In the United States, about two-thirds of helicopters are staffed by a nurse with either a paramedic (usually) or a respiratory therapist (rarer). About 25% have two flight nurses, and around 6–10% have a physician on board paired with a nurse or paramedic. Flight nurses are highly trained, with a 2- to 4-year degree plus usually at least 10 years of critical care experience and further extensive training in various special areas such as trauma, pediatrics, obstetrics, and cardiology. Paramedics and respiratory therapists have the usual training in their fields, plus must have a depth of background clinical experience, as well as specialty training comparable to the flight nurses.

The role of physicians on air medical helicopters is minimal in the United States and extensive in the rest of the world [7]. There is one paper, a retrospective study from the United States, which suggests that there is no objective difference in the outcome of patients transported by helicopter with a physician or not [8]. This does not mean that physicians are not involved with the helicopter service in the United States; they just don't usually ride in the helicopter. Physicians are actively involved in training and setting guidelines for the medical providers on these services [9].

III. SAFETY/COMFORT ISSUES

A. Helicopter Emergency Medical Service (HEMS) Safety

During the 1980s, commercial emergency medical services (EMS) helicopter activity increased sharply. Unfortunately, so did the accident rate. After a series of fatal EMS helicopter accidents in 1985 and 1986, the safety record of these operations became a great concern in the United States and Europe. Critics insisted that this mode of transportation was not just expensive, but risky as well. Confronted with the unacceptable accident trend, the issue was investigated thoroughly. The National Transportation Safety Board (NTSB) in Washington, D.C., undertook a safety study [10] to examine the accident rates and safety factors relating to this industry. The study period was from 1978 through 1986. The accident rate for EMS helicopters involved in patient transports was approximately twice the rate experienced by nonscheduled helicopter air taxis and 1.5 times the rate for all turbine-powered helicopters. Most accidents were night and weather related, and human error was attributed as the most frequent cause. This and other studies gave basis to safety recommendations, and the accident rate seemed to have been reduced [11]. In 1999 and early 2000, however, there seemed to be an upswing in rotor-wing accidents [12].

Underlying human factors, company management attitude, and CRM (crew resource management) principles are being appreciated to an increasing extent.

B. Ground Ambulance Safety

Comparison of HEMS safety to ground ambulance safety is hampered by methodological problems in obtaining accurate data. Emergency driving with lights and siren, is by no means without risks, however. The typical accident is a collision with another vehicle at intersections, and the high speed increases the incidence of serious injury and fatal outcome. Norwegian data [13] suggest that ambulance emergency driving represents an eightfold increase of accident risk, compared to regular ambulance driving. Forty-five percent of the injured and killed are patients or passengers in the rear compartment of the ambulance. Transport authorities focus on emergency vehicle driver training, warning systems, and vehicle colors. Passenger restraints reduce the risk of severe injury significantly.

C. Patient Influences During Transport

Transport imposes stress to most patients, regardless of the mode. In addition to the concern of being ill or injured and the fear of a prospective hospital stay comes the discomfort of transport itself. It is easy to believe that transport by a helicopter represents a greater strain to the patient than ground transport does. In these authors' opinion it is not necessarily so. In fact, the strain of rough roads or a longer transport may more than offset any potential disadvantages of rotor-wing transports. Factors such as transport duration and the caregiver's ability to reduce pain, inform and comfort the patient, and eventually give sedative medication is probably more important than the mode of transportation.

1. Stress

Two studies published in 1988 [14,16], indicated that helicopter transport of acute cardiac patients may be associated with more untoward events than ground transport of equal duration. A number of published reports over the past 10 years [15,17] do not confirm the suggestion that air transport of cardiac and noncardiac patients represents an unacceptable risk due to stress.

The most important stressors of transportation are noise, vibration, and acceleration forces. Motion sickness may also be a problem.

2. Noise

Noise may be defined as a sound that is unpleasant, distracting, unwarranted, or in some other way undesirable. This definition is subjective, indicating that adverse effects on exposed persons depend on their subjective experience of noise. The psycological discomfort may affect patient morbidity. Moreover, depending on level and duration, noise results in hearing loss and may have detrimental effects on other body systems.

Noise (sound pressure level) is measured in decibels (dB), but is commonly reported in dBA, where A represents a weighting system used to relate the noise to the ear's hearing profile, de-emphasizing the lower frequencies. The sound pressure levels increase logarithmically (6 dB = twice, 12 dB = four times, etc.). A further interesting point is that two noise sources of a similar sound pressure level raise the level by 3 dB when measured together. In other words, any measure that reduces the measured sound pressure level by 3 dB signifies a reduction of no less than half in sound energy.

The major noise source in most vehicles is the engine. In ground ambulances, additional noise is generated by road friction (type of tire is an important factor), air movement, adjacent traffic, and of course the siren, when in use. In aircraft, major noise sources are engines, transmission systems, propellers/rotor blades, jet efflux, flow of air, and cabin conditioning and pressurizing systems. Helicopters have a different noise spectrum from fixed-wing aircraft. Gearbox and various transmission chains are major sources of inside noise. Typical maximum noise levels in EMS helicopters are 95 to 100 dBA, while ground ambulances have maximum levels of 70 to 75 dBA (when not using the siren). The new EMS helicopter generation, exemplified by the Eurocopter EC 135 and the MD 902 Explorer, are distinctively less noisy, as the level is reduced by approximately 10 dB. European standards (Comité Européen de Normalisation [CEN] inquiry, 1998; air, water, and difficult terrain ambulances) require that when noise exposure exceeds 85 dBA, relevant protection shall be established and available. This prospective standard is expected to require that babies inside transport incubators shall not be exposed to noise over 60 dBA, identical to the Canadian Standards Association's 1992 recommendation.

Macnab et al. measured noise and vibration levels inside and outside a neonatal transport incubator in seven transport vehicles (land, air, and water) [19] and found that the maximum and average unweighted noise levels inside the incubator in all but one vehicle (a fixed-wing air ambulance) were over 99 dB, far exceeding the recommended limits. The incubator was shown to amplify noise at the lower frequencies. The authors conclude that current noise and vibration levels could affect patient morbidity for neurologically immature and/or physiologically compromised infants and children. On the other hand, many clinicians report that infants tend to show few signs of stress during air ambulance incubator transport of limited duration as long as sudden noise is avoided.

Noise protection is an important issue in HEMS. During patient loading and unloading the engines should not be running. Thorough patient information about the hearing protection device and communication technique is important. Also, unconscious and anesthesized patients should be protected by headsets, as the acoustic reflex of the middle ear may be impaired in these situations, increasing the chance of hearing damage.

Ground ambulances should avoid using the siren while transporting awake patients. When the traffic situation necessitates use of this warning signal, the patient should be warned in advance.

Active noise reduction techniques may play an important role in the future. This is an electronic system that works by continuous sampling of noise inside the earshell of the headset with a small microphone. This signal is inverted in phase through the headset speaker, thus reducing noise levels by destructive interference of the acoustic field. The system provides good low-frequency noise attenuation, but mid- and high-frequency noise levels may be increased [20].

3. Vibration

Vibration is oscillatory motion. The extent of the oscillation determines the magnitude of the vibration, and the repetition rate of the cycles of oscillation determines the frequency of the vibration. There are many possible means by which the vibration magnitude can be measured. The severity of human vibration exposure is best expressed in terms of vibration acceleration (ms^{-2}). Frequency is expressed by hertz (Hz). Although we focus on potential adverse effects of human vibration during transport, one should not forget that vibration may be ''good,'' both pleasant and healthy.

The discomfort produced by whole-body vibration depends on vibration magnitude, frequency, direction, the position at which the vibration contacts the body, and the duration of the vibration. There is also a great individual variation of experienced discomfort. Whole-body vibration generally concerns frequencies between 0.5 and 100 Hz and acceleration magnitudes between about 0.01 and 10 ms^{-2} [21]. The ISO 2631 [23] weighting for the comfort of healthy adults is shown in Table 1. This standard indicates that the human body is most sensitive to vibration in the frequency range between 1 and 80 Hz. Vibration in the range of 4 to 8 Hz is tolerated least.

Table 1 Approximate Indications of the Likely Reactions to Various Magnitudes of Weighted Vibration According to ISO 2631

Comfort level	Acceleration (ms^{-2})
Not uncomfortable	<0.31
A little uncomfortable	0.315 to 0.63
Fairly uncomfortable	0.5 to 1.0
Uncomfortable	0.8 to 1.6
Very uncomfortable	1.25 to 2.5
Extremely uncomfortable	>2.0

Whole-body vibration causes a wide range of physiological effects [21]. Cardiovascular responses appear to be similar to the effects of moderate exercise (in the 2 to 20 Hz range), and there may be increased respiratory air flow and oxygen uptake. Vibration may contribute to motion sickness.

Exposure to whole-body vibration occurs during transport in vehicles of various sorts, and undesirably high levels can be encountered in helicopters, in fixed-wing aircraft during low-level flight, and in ground vehicles when traveling over rough roads. One very significant factor in helicopters is the main rotor speed and number of rotor blades. Macnab et al. [19] measured the weighted vibration levels in different vehicle types. The much-used EMS helicopter BK 117 (four-bladed) averaged a vibration level similar to the ground ambulance Ford Econoline 350, classified as "fairly uncomfortable," while the Bell 222A helicopter (two-bladed) averaged a vibration level classified as "very uncomfortable." (See Table 1.) The fixed-wing air ambulances had the best vibration records in this study. Obviously, vibration levels in ground ambulances depend very much on the road conditions. The level of vibration is also influenced by the mattress quality and the location within the ambulance [22].

4. Acceleration Forces

Acceleration forces during transport may affect the body. Linear acceleration is a change in the vehicle's speed, for instance during a fixed-wing aircraft takeoff or during braking of a car. Radial acceleration is a change in the direction of movement of the vehicle, like turning and looping. The physical impact of these forces on the body depends on the strength, duration, and direction of the force. One should have special focus on the cardiovascular system, blood perfusion, and intracranial pressure. If these functions are impaired due to disease or injury, the vulnerability of course increases.

Acceleration forces are named G units, where G expresses the relationship between the acceleration a and the acceleration due to the pull of gravity g (G = a/g). This means that when influenced by 2 G, a person weighing 70 kg "weights" 140 kg. Acceleration forces working transversely to the long axis of the body are tolerated better than forces working linearly. Positive (+) G means that the force works from head to feet, negative (−) G from feet to head. A positive G load brings blood to the lower extremities, decreases the blood pressure, and increases lung shunting. Healthy persons typically faint off after 15 sec when influenced by +5 G. Opposite forces (negative G) give elevated intracranial pressure and bradycardia. One faints off at −4 G after only a few seconds. These facts should always be considered when positioning patients in vehicles of different types for transport. For instance, when elevating the head end of the stretcher during the takeoff and landing of a fixed-wing air ambulance, the effect on the cardiovascular system and intracranial pressure is greatly reduced. Small jet-powered planes may experience a linear acceleration force of 0.5 G during takeoff. During helicopter transport, patients are normally not influenced by any significant acceleration force, unless flying in very turbulent air.

5. Motion Sickness

Motion sickness is a normal response to an abnormal environment. Decisive factors are the severity of the unfamiliar motion and the duration of the exposure. Susceptibility changes with age. It is rare below the age of 2 years, then the susceptibility rises sharply to a peak between the ages of 3 and 12 years. After that, there is an increase of tolerance with age. Females are more susceptible to motion sickness than males of the same age.

Patients under transport are often prone to nausea and vomiting as a result of their disorder, their mental state, or because they have been given opiats. Vibration of low frequencies (0.1 to 1 Hz) may contribute to motion sickness. When lying in a compartment without a view of the horizon or another stable visual reference outside the vehicle, susceptibility increases.

A supine position reduces the incidence of motion sickness. It may also help to close the eyes, unless it is possible to give the patient an outlook. Head movements should be reduced to a minimum. Fresh air causes symptomatic improvement. If not contraindicated, antiemetic drugs such as metclopramide or droperidol, should be given generously. The patient's attention should be drawn away from the state of her or his stomach. Reassurance, and when needed, sedative drugs, may help:

One should always keep in mind that nausea and vomiting may be caused by hypoxemia or low blood pressure.

D. Hypobar Environment Considerations

Two main concerns arise when exposing a human being to hypobar conditions: hypoxia and barotrauma. When transporting patients by air ambulance, these issues should be considered. Helicopters do not have pressurized cabins, while fixed-wing aircraft usually do. On the other hand, EMS helicopters seldom cruise at higher altitudes than about 3000 feet above the ground.

The atmospheric pressure is reduced by 20% at an altitude of 6000 feet above sea level. The alveolar oxygen partial pressure and therefore also the arterial oxygen partial pressure is reduced by no less than 29%, however. At impaired lung function, the effect may be even more dramatic. The ultimate consequences for tissue oxygenation are determined by the hemoglobin concentration, the profile of the oxygen dissociation curve, and the blood perfusion of the tissues. When exposing patients to hypobaric conditions, one should monitor hemoglobin oxygen saturation closely and give supplementary oxygen as needed. The oxygenation requirements should be assessed prior to departure. Since most oxygen delivery systems have limited oxygen concentration abilities and the oxygen resources onboard may be limited, one should consider the need of positive pressure ventilation during flight. Patients requiring 40% or more oxygen at ground level are in the danger zone.

According to the law of Boyle-Mariotte, at constant temperature the volume of a given mass of gas is inversely proportional to the pressure on it. This means that gases expand when exposed to reduced atmospheric pressure. The volume of entrapped gas increases by 20% at 5000 feet and 40% at 8000 feet altitude.

Expanding gas in closed body cavities, like gas in the gastrointestinal system or pathological gas introduced into tissue or potential cavities during trauma (pneumothorax), may cause serious problems. Drainage of such cavities is mandatory prior to flight unless the aircraft cabin pressure can be kept very close to sea level. Patients with air embolus should not be exposed to a cabin altitude above about 1000 feet.

Gas in medical equipment should also be kept in mind. Orthopedic air splints, vacuum splints, pneumatic antishock suits, balloon cuffs on tracheal airways, and so on should be monitored closely and the air pressure adjusted as needed.

Decompression sickness occurs if environmental air pressure is halved. This occurs at an altitude of about 18,000 feet. Since patients being transported by air ambulances never will be exposed to such an air pressure drop, unless an accident occurs the problem is of no significance. There is one important exception, however; persons who have sea dived within the past 24 hr. In fact, decompression sickness patients are often transported by air to a pressure chamber. In this case, fixed-wing aircraft should keep the cabin pressure at sea level, while helicopters should fly below 1000 feet.

E. Therapeutic Limitations During Transport

The transport situation is characterized by many kinds of limitations and restrictions. The patient compartment is small, access to the patient is reduced, and illumination often bad. Such medical resources as oxygen, pressurized air, and electrical power are limited. There are also weight limitations. The monitoring opportunities may be reduced. If complications occur, the attendants will have to deal with them alone. These aspects are quite similar, regardless of the mode of transport, and together with the patient influence factors are the main reasons for reducing transport time.

In this respect, there are some unique characteristics of air transport. One of them is that you cannot just stop the vehicle if, for instance, you need silence or the assistance of the driver. Air patient transport therefore generally requires more planning than ground transport.

Some procedures are best not carried out in noisy helicopters. After endotracheal intubation, confirmation of tube placement is of vital importance. It is impossible to assess breath sounds during helicopter transport [24]. Noise also compromises the ability to auscultate blood pressures. State-of-the-art capnographs and noninvasive, automated blood pressure monitors compensate for this problem to a great extent, however. It is nevertheless recommended to carry out intubation prior to takeoff if this intervention is expected to be required during transport.

Electrocardiography (ECG), oxygen saturation, and temperature monitoring are other vital parameters that are often monitored during transport [18]. High-quality portable multimodal monitors are available. Equipment for use onboard aircraft require national aviation authority approval specific to the type of aircraft in which it is to be used. Each item of equipment must be tested to exclude potential hazard, for example, interference with aircraft navigation systems. While the helicopter is thus unaffected by the equipment, the reverse is not necessarily the case. The accuracy and reliability may be affected adversely by the electromagnetic and vibratory environment. One should be skeptical to the monitor readings in flight and double check with clinical signs. Monitor alarm systems are not designed for the helicopter environment. Both audible and visual alarms are easily missed. The use of defibrillators in flight is considered to be safe, but must always be authorized by the pilot in command.

There have been published case reports of gravely affected pacemaker function during aeromedical transport.

The transport situation generally requires increased vigilance by the attendents.

IV. WHY USE A HELICOPTER FOR ANY RESPONSE (SCENE OR INTERFACILITY)?

A. Trauma Scene Responses

Emergency medical system studies published during the past 15 to 20 years have focused very much on the mode of transportation. Which benefits the patient more, ground or air transport? In fact, it has not been clearly demonstrated that the mode of transportation itself has any importance. What really counts is that the patient care is adequate and that the care is given early enough. A more relevant question, therefore, is what is proper acute care medicine and when is early enough. These issues are addressed in other parts of this volume.

In prehospital trauma care medicine, two more debates are ongoing: the debate of ''scoop and run'' versus ''stay and stabilize'' and the one of proper staffing of the prehospital trauma team. The crew does what has to be done at the scene for stabilization of critical life functions and then does the rest en route. The scene time optimally is about 10 min unless there is prolonged extrication. It is beyond the scope of this chapter to discuss these controversies in detail, so, we summarize here some conclusions that we suggest are *not* controversies.

1. In severe trauma, re-establishment of the airway, ventilation, and oxygenation should be carried out in the field without any delay.
2. Endotracheal intubation facilitates airway control, ventilation, and oxygenation.
3. In severe trauma, brain injury and hemorrhagic shock are the leading causes of death.
4. Hypoxia and hypotension following severe brain injury should be corrected as soon as possible.
5. The most important factor in uncontrolled hemorrhage patients is the time from injury to the provision of definitive surgery.
6. Severe trauma patients require definitive treatment within 60 min.

This leads to the assumption that the prehospital trauma team should be able to

Safely carry out endotracheal intubation in trauma patients. This procedure sometimes requires the administration of anesthetic drugs.

Carry out triage and bring the severe trauma patient to a trauma center within a maximum 60 min from the time of injury.

The EMS system, means of transport included, should be organized accordingly. A total system approach is needed.

We observe that EMS systems and HEMS systems in Europe are different from the systems in North America. The HEMS in most European countries are based on the philosophy of advanced trauma life support in the field. Most programs include qualified physicians (anesthesiologists, emergency medicine specialists, or trauma surgeons) (Fig. 1). Most American systems, on the other hand, are based on the scoop and run theory, and just 5% of the U.S. medical rotor-wing programs fly with a physician (Fig. 2). These system differences are hardly exclusively explained by disagreement regarding trauma care strategy. First, penetrating trauma patients contribute to a greater part of the urban trauma patient population in the United States. Blunt trauma injuries occur relatively more frequently in Europe and in the rural United States. Rural trauma patients in the United States have much longer transport times because of the great distances involved. Penetrating injury patients profit by rapid transport to a trauma center (using whatever means are readily available), while the management of blunt trauma seems to be more complex; for example, regarding fluid resuscitation [25,26]. The training of professional categories may also be different. A study from Montreal, Canada [29], showed significant prehospital delays and high rates of inappropriate on-site trauma care provided by physicians, while most European authors conclude that the inclusion of an emergency physician in the trauma team gives positive effects [27]. This is supported by a recent study from Australia,

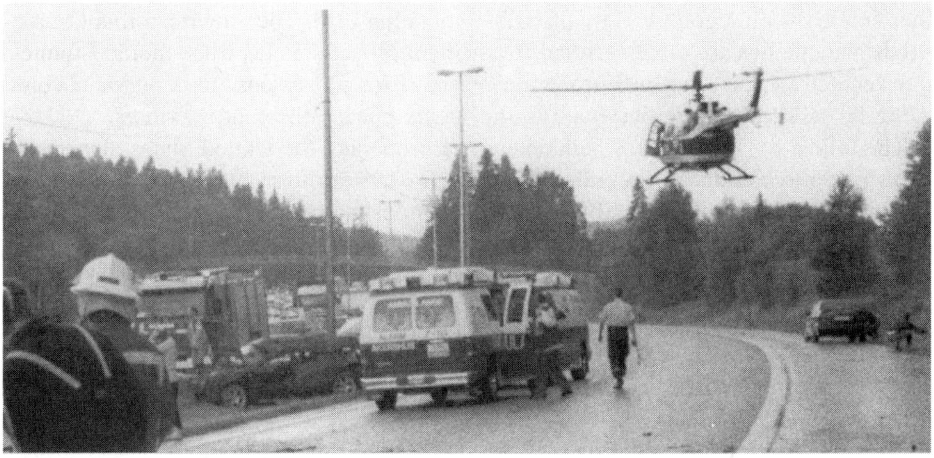

Figure 1 In Norway the helicopter brings an anesthesiologist to the trauma scene. (Photo courtesy of B. Eklund.)

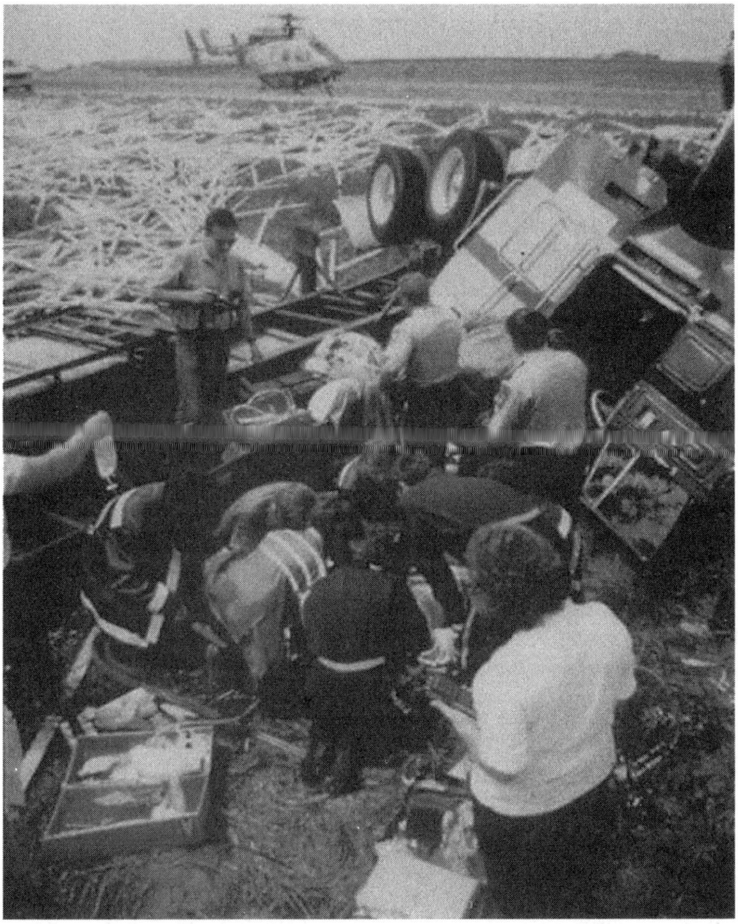

Figure 2 In the United States, the helicopter brings critical care flight nurses and paramedics to the severe trauma scene.

another country with a great variety of HEMS manning (28). The American flight nurses and flight paramedics are often certified for medical procedures [8] (tube thoracostomies, central veneous access) that in Europe are reserved for physicians. Both services could therefore be said to bring tertiary care to the scene, but by different providers.

The utilization of the EMS helicopters in Europe and the United States also shows different patterns. European programs typically fly 80% primary missions (scenes) and 20% secondary missions (interfacility). The exact opposite operational profile is the typical one in the United States. In Norway, 50% of the scene missions concern medical cases, also helping to explain the need for a physician on the team, whereas in the United States medical scenes are infrequent. Most medical patients in the United States receive interfacility transports.

It is reasonable to say that to fulfill the needs of trauma patients as to proper care and rapid transport to a trauma center the inclusion of a helicopter in the EMS system is of greater importance in rural areas than in urban ones. It is also reasonable to say that the longer the transport distances and the more medical cases, the greater the need for a physician in the team. An advanced trauma life support team covers a much wider area by a helicopter than it does with a ground vehicle. This is especially the case in remote areas with weak communications infrastructure, such as mountaineous regions. Helicopters usually travel two to three times as fast as a ground ambulance and can usually fly the most direct route. Ground resources should always be dispatched parallel to the helicopter, however, as the helicopter is more weather-dependent and may suspend the mission for the benefit of a more serious case.

In the trauma setting, for a helicopter team to be effective and useful at a scene it must be activated sooner rather than later. One simple criterion, indicating the need of such a tertiary resource at the site, is that the patient is not able to follow simple commands [30]. It has thus been demonstrated that first responders are as good at calling for the helicopter as hospital personnel are. An important major component in dispatching and coordinating ground and air response to trauma emergency is a well-run communications center with triage guidelines that tell the dispatchers what responses are appropriate for particular situations, based on time, distance, and mechanism of injury factors.

In the typical setting, which a region has many local hospitals and just one trauma center, the helicopter patient of course benefits from a direct transfer to the trauma center. It has been demonstrated that this policy gives a shorter and less costly hospital stay. In the case of a very unstable patient, (e.g., one suspected of internal bleeding), or if the helicopter team is not able to control the airway, go to the nearest hospital that has adequate human competence and equipment. In fact, some patients, for example, those critically injured from stabbing or gunfire, should be transported to a nearby hospital by vehicle that is immediately available, regardless if this is, for instance, a police car.

Consequently, the question of ground versus air scene response in trauma care is a complex issue. In fact, it is more an organizational issue than a medical one.

One should keep in mind that helicopters do not save lives. They do, however, make emergency medicine easily available to parts of the trauma patient population that otherwise would have been poorly served.

B. Interfacility Responses

As stated earlier, transport represents stress to the patient. One type of vehicle cannot generally be considered superior above others. It is often desirable, however, to reduce the transport time. The most appropriate mode of transport will be considered according to different operational factors (weather conditions, distances, resource availability), patient requirements, and the urged of time. Interfacility transports are most often a question of patient transport to a higher-level facility. Frequent trauma diagnosis are multisystem trauma, brain injury, burns, and amputations. Some of these patients, but not all, require the fastest available transport. At distances more than about 40 to 50 km a helicopter is the preferred mode of transport, and fixed-wing aircraft at distances more than 200 to 250 km. In the United States helicopter typically make transports up to 150 miles, while fixed-wing aircraft make transports over 150 miles. Obviously, there will be a great variation of these limits, according to helipad and airport positions relative to the hospitals as well as according to the road quality and the traffic situation [28].

In many EMS systems the air ambulance teams are more qualified than the ground ambulance teams are. Some hospitals will call an air ambulance because they do not have available medical personnel to escort the patient. Such a motive cannot be said to be medical. It may very well be warranted, however.

C. Air Medical Crew

Simply put, the helicopter brings critical care assessment and treatment modalities to a scene or hospital that would otherwise get basic or primary care. The air medical crew, whether nurse, paramedic, or physician, brings skills to stabilize critically injured patients. Table 2 indicates the differences among levels of care in the United States.

Table 2 Comparisons of Care in the Field

Basic	Advanced	Air Medical
CPR	CPR	CPR
Advanced first aid	Advanced first aid	Advanced first aid
MAST	MAST	MAST
HARE and other splints	HARE and other splints	HARE and other splints
Defibrillation	Monitoring, defibrillation, cardioversion	Monitoring, defibrillation, cardioversion
Some IVs	More sophisticated IVs, external jugular	Central lines, intraosseous, along with usual IV access
Fluid resuscitation, limited	Fluid resuscitation	Fluid resuscitation + blood
Minimal drugs	Limited drugs	Multiple cardiovascular and other emergency drugs by bolus and drip
Basic and semiadvanced airways (Combitube)	Endotracheal intubation, cricothyrotomies	ETI, oral and nasal, rapid sequence intubation, Cricothyrotomy
	Transcutaneous pacing	Transcutaneous pacing
	Needle chest decompression	Tube thoracostomies
	Glucose determination	Multiple lab determinations (e.g., i-Stat device)
		Arterial lines
		Intraaortic balloon pumps

V. ORGANIZATIONS

There are a number of national and international organizations that have developed guidelines for the safe and proper use of air medical helicopters. The Association of Air Medical Services (*AAMS*) is an organization of air medical providers, both rotor- and fixed-wing, that has served as a voice for the industry in the United States for the past 15 to 20 years. This organization has been a leader in air medical education conferences, developing standards and acting as an advocate for the air medical industry. The National Association of EMS Physicians (*NAEMSP*) also has had an active *air medical transport committee*, which has developed a number of guidelines pertinent to practice in the air medical environment.

In the United States and to some extent internationally, the Commission on Accreditation of Medical Transport Systems (*CAMTS*) has worked to improve air medical and ground out-of-hospital care by improving safety standards and medical care by a benchmarking accreditation process.

There are a number of other organizations that have worked hard to improve air medical care, including the Air and Surface Transport Nurses Association (*ASTNA*), the National Flight Paramedic Association (*NFPA*), the National EMS Pilots Association (*NEMSPA*), the American Association of Respiratory Care (*AARC*), which have also sought to make the industry safer and more effective. One further group deserves mention because it is the most international of all of these, and that is the Air Medical Physicians Association (*AMPA*), which brings together medical directors of air medical services for consensus building about the proper role of the air medical director and to help the new medical director learn the ropes using such resources as the *Air Medical Directors' Handbook*.

VI. SUMMARY

Helicopters do not work in a vacuum. The air medical component needs to be a part of an integrated out-of-hospital care system. Such an integrated system needs active medical direction to actively oversee the process to ensure that each part of the system is used appropriately. There are appropriate uses of ground ambulances and crew members and appropriate use of the critical care resources of the helicopter. Helicopters are expensive resources, but are cost-effective when used under the right circumstances. There is no question that when used at the right time helicopters, can make a difference in the most seriously injured patients. The complex factors that are weighed in calling for the helicopter include the time to the local hospital versus the time to the regional trauma center, mechanisms of injury, the stability of the patient and the need for critical care interventions to the patient at scene (e.g., aggressive advanced airway management or tube thoracostomy), and traffic and terrain considerations. Local guidelines need to be in place to help determine when first responders or ambulance personnel should activate the air medical component of the EMS system.

REFERENCES

1. Air Medical Committee, National Association of EMS Physicians. Air medical dispatch: Guidelines for trauma scene response. Prehosp Disas Med 7:77–78, 1992.
2. AJ Macnab. Air medical transport: ''Hot air'' and a French lesson. J Air Med Trans 11:15–18, 1992.

3. G Carter, R Couch. The evolution of air transport systems: A pictorial review. J Emerg Med 6:499–504, 1988.
4. SN Neel. Helicopter evacuation in Korea. US Armed Force Med J 6:681–702, 1955.
5. SN Neel. Army aeromedical evacuation procedures in Vietnam: Implications in rural America JAMA 204:309–313, 1968.
6. WG Baxt, P Moody. The impact of rotorcraft aeromedical emergency care services on trauma mortality. JAMA 249:3047–3051, 1983.
7. U Schmidt, SB Frame, ML Nerlich, et al. On scene helicopter transport of patients with multiple injuries—Comparison of a German and an American system. J Trauma 33:548–555, 1992.
8. RE Burney, L Passins, D Hubert, R Maio. Comparison of aeromedical crew performance by patient severity and outcome. Ann Emerg Med 21:375–378, 1992.
9. LF Eljaiek, R Norton, R Carmona. NAEMSP Position paper: Medical director for air medical transport programs. Prehosp Disas Med 10:283–284, 1995.
10. Safety Study—Commercial Emergency Medical Service Helicopter Operations. Washington, DC: National Transportation Safety Board, report no. NTSB/SS-88/01. 1988.
11. LJ Connell, WD Reynard. Emergency Medical Service Helicopter Incidents Reported to the Aviation Safety Reporting System. The Ohio State University 7th International Symposium on Aviation Psychology, 1993.
12. R Frazer. Air medical accidents: A 20-year search for information 1999. AirMed; Sept.–Oct. pp. 34–39.
13. P Frøyland. Accident Risk in Emergency Driving. project no. 0-871. Oslo; Institute of Transport Economics, 1982.
14. AA Tyson Jr, DK Sundberg, DG Sayers, KP Ober, RE Snow. Plasma catecholamine levels in patients transported by helicopter for acute myocardial infarction and unstable angina pectoris. Am J Emerg Med 6:435–438, 1988.
15. CT Bolliger, A Kiener, W Weber, M Reigner, R Ritz. Helikoptertransport: Stressbelastung für Patienten? Notfallmedizin 16:36–41, 1990.
16. S Schneider, Z Borok, M Heller, P Paris, R Stewart. Critical cardiac transport: Air versus ground? Am J Emerg Med 6:449–452, 1988.
17. CK Stone, SH Thomas. Interhospital transfer of cardiac patients by air. Am J Emerg Med 11: 651–652, 1993.
18. AP Morley. Prehospital monitoring of trauma patients: Experience of a helicopter emergency medical service. Brit J Anaesth 76:726–730, 1996.
19. A Macnab, Y Chen, F Gagnon, B Bora, C Laszlo. Vibration and noise in pediatric emergency transport vehicles: A potential cause of morbidity? Aviat Space Environ Med 66:212–219, 1995.
20. AS Wagstaff, OJ Woxen, HT Andersen. Effects of active noise reduction on noise levels at the tympanic membrane. Aviat Space Environ Med 69:539–544, 1998.
21. MJ Griffin. Handbook of Human Vibration. Academic, 1990.
22. HB Sherwood, A Donze, J Giebe. Mechanical vibration in ambulance transport. J Ob Gyn Neonat Nurs 23:457–463, 1994.
23. Guide to the Evaluation of Human Exposure to Whole-Body Mechanical Vibration. Revision of International Standards Organization (ISO 2631), ISO/TC 108/SC 4 N 190, Dec. 1, 1989.
24. RC Hunt, DM Bryan, VS Brinkley, TW Whitley, NH Benson. Inability to assess breath sounds during air medical transport by helicopter. JAMA 265:1982–1984, 1991.
25. W Bickell, MJ Wall Jr, PE Pepe, R Russell Martin, VF Ginger, MK Allen, KL Mattox. Immediate versus delayed fluid resuscitation for hypotensive patients with penetrating torso injuries. New Eng J Med 331:1105–1109, 1994.
26. T Matsuoka, J Hildreth, DH Wisner. Uncontrolled hemorrhage from parenchymal injury: Is resuscitation helpful? J Trauma 40:915–921, 1996.
27. BL Hübner. Evaluation of the immediate effects of preclinical treatment of severely injured

trauma patients by helicopter trauma team in the Netherlands. PhD thesis, Drukkerij Elinckwijk bv. Utrecht, 1999.

28. RA Bartolacci, BJ Munford, A Lee, PA McDougall. Air medical scene response to blunt trauma: Effect on early survival. MJA 169:612–616, 1998.
29. JS Sampalis, S Boukas, A Lavoie, A Nikolis, P Frechette, R Brown, D Fleiszer, D Mulder. Preventable death evaluation of the appropriateness of the on-site trauma care provided by Urgences-Santé Physicians. J Trauma 39:1029–1035, 1995.
30. W Meredith, R Rutledge, AR Hansen, DW Oller, M Thomason, P Cunningham, CC Baker. Field triage of trauma patients based upon the ability to follow command: A study in 29,573 injured patients. J Trauma 38:129–135, 1995.

36

Trauma in Rural and Remote Areas

LANCE SHEPHERD

University of Calgary and Shock Trauma Air Rescue Service, Calgary; Banff Prehospital EMS and Banff Emergency Department, Banff, Canada

TIM AUGER

Parks Canada, Banff National Park, Banff, Canada

TORBEN WISBORG

Hammerfest Hospital and Royal Norwegian Rescue Helicopter Service, Hammerfest, Norway

JANET WILLIAMS

West Virginia University, Morgantown, West Virginia

I. INTRODUCTION

The fact that rural populations differ from urban populations in demographic and health characteristics explains in part why there are unique demands and challenges associated with the provision of prehospital care in rural, mountainous, oceanic, and other remote areas. There are so many region-specific issues and varieties of services that a search for concrete guidelines is often futile. A brief tour of a few emergency medical services (EMS) that deal with rural and remote trauma may prove insightful, but in no way represent the spectrum of rural trauma or its management worldwide.

Regional variability is quite apparent to a traveler to rural locations. For a tourist who enjoys seeing different ways of life, traveling to smaller and more remote populations may be very rewarding. Evolutionary biologists have long felt that the uniqueness of small populations in harsh climactic or geographical areas provides the genetic heterogeneity a species requires to survive when changes become global [1]. Similarly, we may find many aspects of rural trauma care do not respond well to guidelines derived in the more homogeneous urban centers. Unique local solutions can be enlightening to us all.

II. WHAT IS "RURAL" OR "REMOTE?"

What is rural? Somewhere between 25–50% of the world's population live in rural communities. The definition of rural varies greatly between countries and even within regions in the same country. Rural may be defined by population density, distance from urban centers, ease of access to health care facilities, and so on. Further, the density of a population that is used to define an area as rural is relative to the population density of that geographical area as a whole. For example, the Yukon Territory of northern Canada reports 0.06 people per square km, of which only 4% are rural dwellers. The largest city is Whitehouse, with a population of approximately 20,000 [2]. India reports a population density of 305 per square km, of which 73% are rural dwellers. The largest city is Mumbai, with approximately 10 million people (1991 census). In most cases the definition of rural, then, seems to be an operational one. If a subset of a population is separated from higher standards of service by distance or other barriers it may be deemed rural.

III. RURAL MECHANISMS OF TRAUMA

Just as the very definition of rural is myriad, so too are the mechanisms of rural trauma, which often are not seen in urban settings. The literature is full of interesting injury patterns that relate to the local geography, industry, and cultures. Horrendous limb and vascular traumas are associated with use of heavy machinery in agricultural and mining communities around the world [3,4]. Agricultural communities can also see severe unintentional anticholinesterase poisonings, which are very rare elsewhere. Recreational and sports-related injuries are common, especially in small resort towns. A high number of unintentional gunshot wounds have been found in rural North American communities [5]. Devastating injuries result from stepping on undetected land mines in certain areas of rural Cambodia [6]. Avalanches take the lives of many backcountry skiers throughout the world. Falls or kicks from horses can be common and severe in the communities associated with equines for labor or recreation [7]. All of these injuries are comparable to other illnesses, which can have predictable demographic distributions, and epidemic outbreaks. The importance of looking for successful strategies for prevention cannot be underestimated.

IV. RURAL TRAUMA MORBIDITY AND MORTALITY

Rural populations are at higher risk for trauma morbidity and mortality than urban populations. This disparity may be explained by mechanisms of injury that result in higher severity of trauma, adverse geographic and climatic conditions, longer discovery and transport times and lack of medical command direction, as well as variable availability, accessibility, and skill levels of prehospital personnel in rural areas. A great deal of time can pass before a trauma victim in a remote site is discovered. Once discovered, victims may face long extrication and transport times. Pediatric trauma mortality is higher in rural centers than in urban pediatric and nonpediatric centers [8], and higher rates of death and morbidity specifically related to motor vehicle crashes, most notably in children and young adolescent males, is well documented [9–12]. Contributing factors may include notably higher speed limits and low use of occupant restraints, as well as passengers who ride in the back of pickup trucks. Adverse climatic conditions may predispose trauma victims to hyperthermia, hypothermia, or dehydration. In oceanic environments, strong winds and currents can make the use of nonrescue vessels difficult, leaving only dedicated rescue vessels and rescue helicopters as options for assisting trauma victims.

V. RURAL TRAUMA SYSTEMS

The final variable is treatment. Existing EMS to manage rural and remote trauma are as diverse as the entities they treat. In most regions it is difficult to show which of all the aforementioned variables are the most significant. Treatment is probably the most discussed, as it may be the most alterable. As would be expected, rural or remote trauma treatment strategies themselves are born out of an utterly immense series of factors. Population density, geography, climate, injury patterns, funding, culture, politics, available personnel, and available equipment are only a few. It is difficult to compare systems, not only because of their inherent variability in the above-mentioned factors, but also in the variability between study data elements. Attempts to unify definitions and the reporting of variables may improve the utility of future studies and allow comparisons. The development of an Utstein style for major trauma data reporting may prove to be as beneficial as it has been for cardiac arrest [13].

There are several phases of an EMS response system. The following discussions center on general elements of such systems, but this is not intended to be a template for an accurate analysis or data collection model of trauma systems. For a uniform approach to defining and analyzing variables in any particular trauma system the reader would be well advised to stay current with the International Trauma Anaesthesia and Critical Care Society (ITACCS) initiative on ''recommendations for uniform reporting of data following major trauma—The Utstein Style'' [13].

A. System Notification

A reasonable place to begin studying a rural or remote trauma management system would be *system notification*. When an injury occurs, how is EMS notified or called for? Many systems have tried to speed the timing and quality of information transfer that occurs in the original call for help. The medium of communication may vary immensely, and technology is rapidly changing the way EMS is accessed. Many affluent societies today have widespread cellular phone communications, including automatic crash notification systems. With multiple cell towers in an area, it may be possible for a call answering service to have the immediate global positioning system (GPS) position of the caller. In many areas 911 centers and similar call answering and dispatching services are well developed. The penetration of such technology into more remote locations is dependent on funding and infrastructure development. More remote locations, such as sparsely populated mountainous regions, may not have cell phone access or radio communication capabilities. Satellite communications technology may prove to be very beneficial in the future.

Even if communication capabilities are present, an effective prehospital response requires that the general public know how and when to access EMS. Call answering, emergency information delivery, and dispatch of rescue and medical services is ideally integrated into one seamless operation (such as 911 services in much of North America). Although most remote areas cannot afford such sophisticated services, they are increasingly available through nearby urban or nationally supported communication centers.

B. System Activation

Once a call for EMS assistance has been made, *system activation* occurs. System activation is often routine, simple, and efficient in higher-volume centers, in which similar responses are made on a daily basis. For example, EMS quality assurance studies may analyze how quickly various ready and waiting dedicated response vehicles can be moving with the appropriate personal and equipment on board from the "time of call" (the first call to the dispatcher from the public). This interval is often referred to as "chute time." System studies may focus on a variety of intervals. For example, a "call to response interval" is the time from the call to the time when the vehicle stops moving at the destination. The total time from call to actual arrival at the patient's side (rather than the closest curb) is the "call to patient arrival" interval. As populations become sparse and EMS calls rare, planning, organization, and quality outcome measurement may become more involved. Training of rural dispatchers is critical, since they must obtain accurate information in a timely fashion before or as EMS are responding. Dispatch centers need to be skilled in eliciting the medical information required to identify the critically injured from minimally trained or lay people. Urgency, form of transport, care given, and destinations may all hinge on this information. The reliability of this information may improve with the level of training the first responder has received. Centers that receive and coordinate responses to requests for help need to know not only what can be sent out from larger centers, but what is more closely available rurally. The first responder's capabilities and the patient's condition will determine what further resources are required.

If the call for EMS involves both difficult access to the patient as well as life- or limb-threatening trauma, a rarely used combination of EMS personnel and equipment may have to be summoned to provide optimal care. Careful planning, frequent practices and drills, personnel education, and efficient and ongoing communications between members of the response team may improve the efficiency and safety of the response personnel. Some common training issues may include helicopter safety, equipment weights, familiarity with environmental hazards, and identification of emergency medical treatment priorities. If all these issues have not been prepared for well in advance they will not come together well at a moment's notice.

C. The First Responder

A critical component of the EMS response is the "first responder." The training and equipment of the first person to care for the injured also varies infinitely. There may be only the moral support of a friend available or there may be a full medical team at the scene. For example, Norwegian search and rescue teams have encountered patients at fixed offshore oil installations, fishing vessels, military vessels, and leisure crafts. Even nuclear-powered submarines have been targets for rescue missions. The medical facilities on board vessels vary. There are highly equipped emergency rooms staffed by midlevel providers at oil installations with online medical direction through satellite communication to medical experts. There are also worn-out, single-handed trawlers that are considered "miracles" to still be afloat. There are millions of first responders worldwide. They may include local paramedics, ski patrol, firemen, the general public, hotel staff, guides, police, and so on. In all services, the first responder is not only important for the care that can be immediately given, but also for the information he or she relays.

D. The Mode of Transportation

The optimal mode of transportation is a central topic in rural EMS. Most rescue services have experienced controversies in geographic and medical guidelines on choosing one mode over another. For example, there are often gray zones as to what distances helicopters may be faster than ground transport in a given area. Where urban-based medical helicopter services respond to rural communities, the travel time to get there must be considered. Early launches with early recognition of critical injuries can increase the utility of the helicopter service. Also, at certain longer distances fixed-wing aircraft can be faster and more efficient than helicopters if both are available. When times are similar, can one system associated with a given mode of transport give a higher level of care for a critical illness or injury based on crew or equipment? There may be many factors to consider.

The helicopter has often been thought of as the panacea of transport to deliver rapid medical care to critical patients. Helicopters may indeed be the most rapid and direct form of transport as well as the fastest deliverer of care to the scene. Unfortunately helicopters may not be practical or feasible where the densities of populations are not sufficient to support the expense of such a service. For private EMS, this may be easily calculated based on the expected number of calls, billings per patient, and cost of operation. Partial or completely government-supported services usually have to justify their existence with some form of cost/benefit analysis. In the field of helicopter rescue, there are few studies that have reasonable methods for looking at changed outcomes due to such services. Usually such services are already in operation and it is not feasible or ethical to withdraw services for control group studies. Further, cost analysis studies continue to have inherent ethical difficulties in assigning reasonable prices to human life and disabilities.

A world tour of emergency medical aviation would be very interesting. In many European alpine countries, the conditions are generally such that a dedicated emergency helicopter is often based within 10 to 15 min flying time of even the farthest corner of the Alps. Here, every incident is in effect a mountain rescue. Besides skiers, climbers, and mountain walkers, workers and farmers are routinely hoisted or slung off steep slopes. The machine is most often dedicated to medical or rescue evacuations, and therefore fully equipped for whatever arises. The numerous bases in the Alps through France, Switzerland, and Austria often have crews made up of pilots, physicians, and rescue specialists who are on full standby to respond to mountain accidents or motor vehicle accidents. The service is essentially an air ambulance that covers all the terrain, whether flatland or mountainous, in a densely populated continent. Many such regions have come to expect helicopter support as a basic component of EMS.

Elsewhere helicopter-assisted prehospital care will vary, depending on a number of factors. In the Western Hemisphere, dedicated helicopters are becoming more common near major centers. Whether these are equipped to "short haul" (sling or winch rescue) is another matter. Many world areas with mountainous or oceanic rescue needs contain sparse populations.

Specialized rescue services in such areas usually depend on public funding (e.g., military services), if they exist at all. The most visible difference in services throughout the world lies in the choice of aircraft. Usually this is based on economics and the suitability of the machine to the most common missions encountered. There are advantages and disadvantages of various rotor-wing aircraft.

Medium helicopters (e.g., the Bell helicopter or the Westland Sea King) may carry 10 to 15 passengers, are extremely powerful, can carry heavy loads, and handle winch operations. They may be well suited to the evacuation of multiple casualties with multiple onboard specialized personnel at reasonably long ranges and under difficult environments. Examples may include rescues from ocean craft and downed aircraft. These machines may be the rescue instrument of choice for a variety of services, such as military or coast guard services, that frequently encounter relatively remote rescues of large groups of people in difficult conditions. It is important to note, however, the hiring rate for these helicopters is two to four times the rate for smaller helicopters. Also, the rotor size is huge, and downwash can be a problem for tight or close-in rescue work.

On the other hand, specialized light helicopters, which typically carry four to seven passengers, are often more readily available and may be preferred by rescue operations, depending on the type of rescue missions flown. Specialized twin-engine light helicopters may be specifically engineered for emergency evacuation as their main application. Examples include the MB 105 or Eurocopter EC 135. These machines have become the first choice in many dedicated rescue and medical operations. These machines may cost two to four times as much as the more common configurations of light helicopters, such as the Bell Jet Rangers, the Aerospatials, and the Hughes 500 series, however.

Similarly, the type of fixed-wing aircraft will vary with economics and missions. In the far reaches of North America, the population density is sparse and the distances to be covered are very large. Small jet aircraft such as the Citation or Lear jet are frequently used. In remote regions there may be no facilities to land a jet (or any fixed-wing aircraft). The only timely help possible is often a parachute drop of personnel and supplies from a long-range propeller-driven aircraft (such as the Hercules). Slower aircraft with shorter ranges that are capable of extracting the victims may then be brought into range by staging fuel depots. A variety of twin-engine propeller-driven aircraft are found in use for distances encountered between that of the jet or the helicopter. In the near future, vertical take-off and landing (VTOL) aircraft, such as the Bell/Boeing MV-22 Osprey, may become the ultimate long-range rescue and medical aircraft. These machines not only take off and land vertically, but also fly at the speeds and ranges of fixed wing aircraft.

In all aircraft, the more rural services often may be limited by a lack of ''instrument flight rule'' (IFR) navigational aids. These services are frequently at the mercy of weather conditions that do not allow ''visual flight rule'' (VFR) flying.

E. Personnel and Equipment

Perhaps less visible, but of equal importance, is the choice of personnel and equipment. Specialized, dedicated rescue machines are frequently loaded with medical equipment and personnel, which may be ideal for air transport of the patient, but often limits the aircraft's versatility to perform difficult evacuations and its range of operations. Variable configurations may be required, depending on the missions an EMS is expected to perform. The medical crew configuration may vary internationally. For example, North American services may utilize paramedics with advanced life support training more widely, while the model of anesthetist-assisted transport is more common in Europe.

At the opposite end of the spectrum from the specialized dedicated emergency medical helicopter is the use of nondedicated commercial aircraft that may be outfitted and crewed for a number of different operations. There are some key issues surrounding the use of emergency evacuation aircraft, both heavy and light and dedicated and nondedicated. Clearly, any risks of emergency response must be carefully analyzed.

Pilots and medical and rescue crews must be trained and experienced in the forms of missions they will be called on to perform. Ad hoc helicopter rescue is exceedingly dangerous, with the capability and history of killing whole crews of well-meaning rescuers. A chief controlling factor in the use of aircraft, helicopters especially, is power. The more power in reserve, the greater the margin of safety and stability for the helicopter. The power reserve is a function of the load weight. Every ounce counts, including the remaining fuel on board, the number of crew members and the size of crew, and the amount of equipment being carried. In difficult or dangerous operations, the weight of the removable seats or even the tool kit may be enough to affect the ability of the pilot to recover from a crucial change in flying conditions. For the thinner air of high altitudes or hot weather, weight becomes even more critical.

The most advanced rescue crews and equipment are only employed where a proportionate market exists to pay for them. Careful risk and cost analysis will prescribe a heli-rescue capability somewhere along a sliding scale of factors. A case in point to illustrate is the comparison of the dedicated rescue teams of the European Alps to the national mountain parks in North America. For example, Banff National Park contains over 1200 square miles, of which 98% is wilderness and is served only by a few roads and highways. A local commercial helicopter service is utilized by the park for rescue and medical flights. These helicopters are used in daily commercial duties, which comprise the majority of revenues earned by these machines. The pilots are flying continuously in the wilderness environment, resulting in maintenance of their expertise. When called for, they must be quickly outfitted for search and rescue or medical calls. Any one of the machines may be called into service, thereby ensuring a higher likelihood of a rapid response time without the severe expense of contracting a full-time standby machine. The key tools (i.e., the medical and/or the specialized sling gear) are quickly transferable between aircraft. In addition, the practical difficulties of the geographic setting are addressed by the versatility of these arrangements. Because of the size of the area covered, the ferry times to the sites of the incidents are routinely 15 min or greater and can be as much as 1 hr or more and cover over 100 miles. In this situation fuel caches are necessary, and part of what might be called ''the art'' of a rescue is in the selection of appropriate equipment and personnel in the first place, since return to the base is impractical. Fuel efficiency is a key factor. Minimizing externally mounted equipment such as winches is also important.

The arrangement of a rescue service requires close cooperation and teamwork between the various agencies and personnel involved. Depending on the anticipated difficulties, for mountain rescue missions the mission leader (a park warden who is usually a qualified professional mountain guide as well) assembles a two-to-three person team from rescuers and paramedics. The paramedics are capable of advanced life support procedures (e.g., rapid sequence intubations with the use of paralytic medications, electrocardiography, and thrombolytics). An arrangement of special attachment points facilitates rapid attachment of modular paramedic kits within the helicopter cabins to improve the medical working environment in flight (Fig. 1). The medical equipment may be heavy and bulky. In the most awkward and dangerous situations the primary objective may be to extract the patient and deliver him or her quickly to the nearest stable position, at which advanced life support can be commenced. Sling rescues are carried out with a fixed rescue line system that can be attached to the helicopter. The patients are usually immobilized in a vacuum mattress and slung horizontally in a basket to a staging area (Fig. 2). Here they receive further medical care and packaging for the rest of the journey to the primary hospital. The geography involved can include forested trails on steep terrain, canyons, rivers, massive icefalls, and high altitudes.

Rescues in the high arctic can be of an extremely remote nature, with severe geography and weather. The Canadian military search and rescue technicians (SAR Techs) have responded to survivors from downed aircraft 3200 km from base. Helicopters are too slow, and the local geography and weather exclude landing any form of medical jet aircraft. In this environment, rescue personnel parachute out of Hercules aircraft to the survivor's side with enough equipment to continue to survive for 72 hr in extreme conditions. Conditions are so harsh and transport times are so long that survival techniques outweigh complex medical treatments and equipment in importance. Hercules transport aircraft can fly disassembled helicopters to the nearest landing facility. The helicopters are then assem-

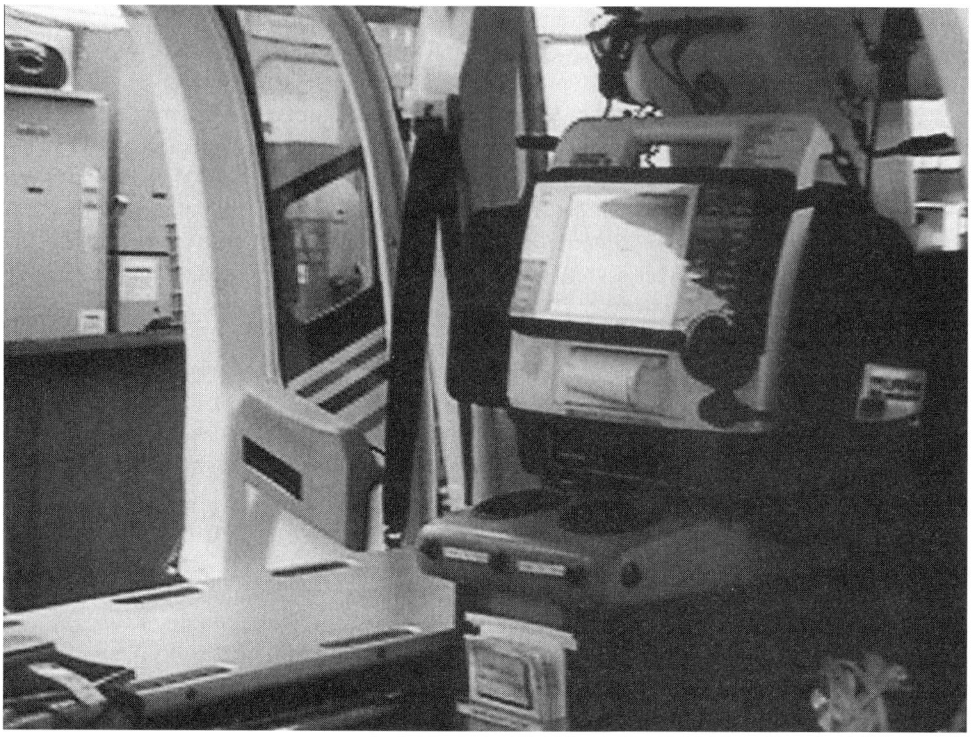

Figure 1 Rapid mounting of medical equipment in a nondedicated aircraft.

bled, and staged extraction may begin. Staged extraction may also be undertaken by local float plane or helicopter services, if they exist. Long-distance air medical evacuation is then undertaken from the closest airport that will accept large aircraft (A. Macauley, personal communications, 2000; Fig. 3).

Northern oceanic rescues are also a good example of services tailor made to their missions. For example, four rescue helicopter bases employing Westland Sea-King helicopters cover the coastal area of Norway. The helicopters are staffed with six persons: two pilots, one navigator, a mechanic, a rescuer, and finally a physician, usually a certified anesthesiologist. In addition to these heavy and relatively slow helicopters the 14 ambulance helicopter bases are able to perform coastal underslung rescues using a static long line. A standard procedure during trauma treatment at sea is that the rescuer is hoisted on board the vessel with the victim. The rescuer then guides hoisting of the physician if it is considered necessary to treat the patient on board the vessel. Depending on the distance to shore the team will either hoist the patient to the helicopter or remain on the vessel while steaming to shore.

Hoisting of patients may be a dangerous procedure for all the team, but for the patient especially. In hypothermia, hypotension, or cardiac failure, the vertical position may induce loss of consciousness due to cerebral hypoperfusion. There are three main techniques for hoisting patients: one sling (around the chest), two slings (around the chest and knees), and a stretcher on which the patient may lie. Even in normal subjects, one-half will faint in a stretcher placed at 50 degrees head-up position for 27 min [14]. Lung function is markedly reduced in the stretcher position as compared to a single or double

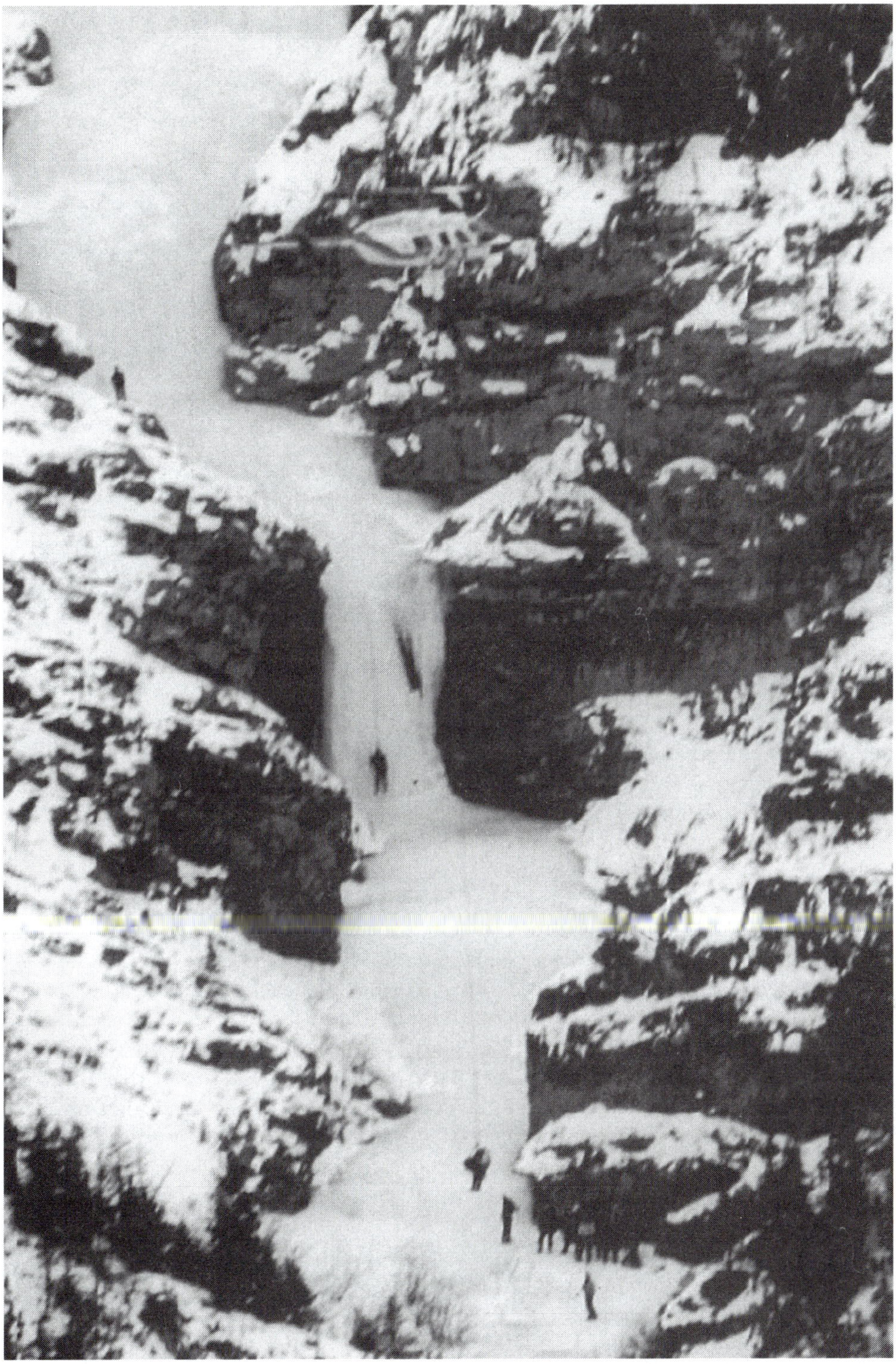

Figure 2 Fixed sling rescue. (Photo courtesy of Brad White, Canadian National Parks.)

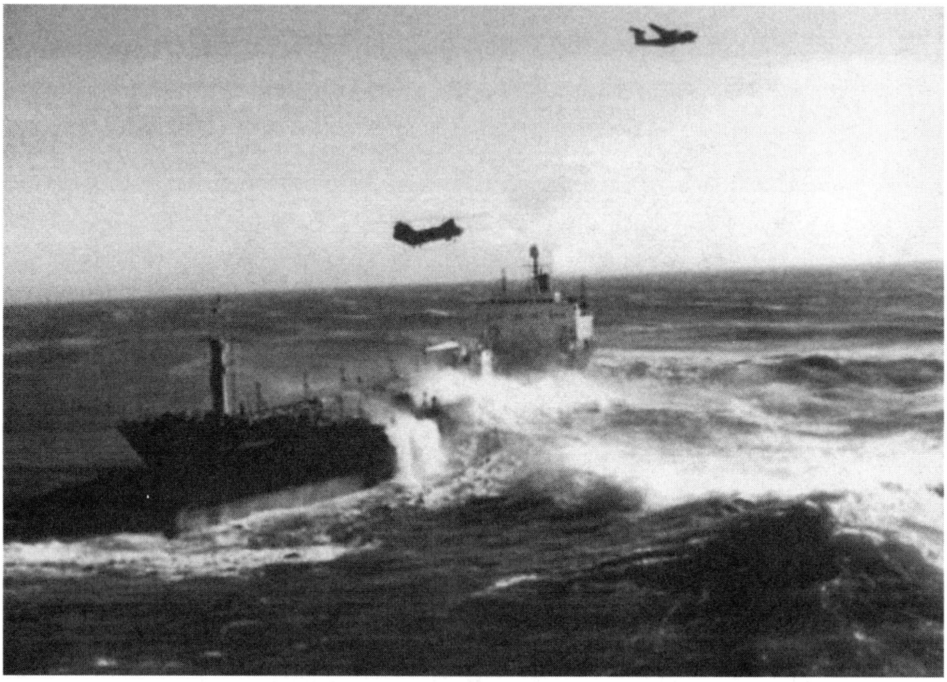

Figure 3 Canadian SAR Techs. (Photo courtesy of Canadian Coastguard.)

sling [15]. Offshore helicopter missions are also not without dangers to the rescue team. Thorough training of all team members in an emergency landing at sea (''ditching procedures''), an underwater helicopter evacuation, and the use of spare air has been shown to improve survival after helicopter crashes. Even exit routes for the crew in emergency sea surface landings have been evaluated [16].

As illustrated above, EMS must be tailored to the variety of circumstances in each site. The focus of EMS is the patient. Modern technology offers many options, but we are often reminded to consider the whole picture. Costs vary from major to prohibitive. Safety is often a more complex element than can be appreciated at the outset. Careful risk analysis is crucial to making the right decisions and evolving a balanced service that reflects the complex needs of each specific site.

In providing highly trained personnel and equipment there is a rural–urban paradox; that is to say, in rural environments the need for advanced care at the scene and in transport may be greater than in urban environments—but is seldom available. In theory, due to the long transport times, the treatment and transport methods of the prehospital personnel should have a greater effect on the outcome of patients than that in short-haul urban environments. Due to lower volumes, less funding, and sometimes less political power, however, high levels of rural care and transport can be hard to obtain. Due to lower call volumes it is hard to maintain the skills of first responders and prehospital personnel, but some solutions have been found.

One example is the rotation of staff between rural and urban environments or the rapid deployment of urban-based level I center transport teams. Another may be hospital-

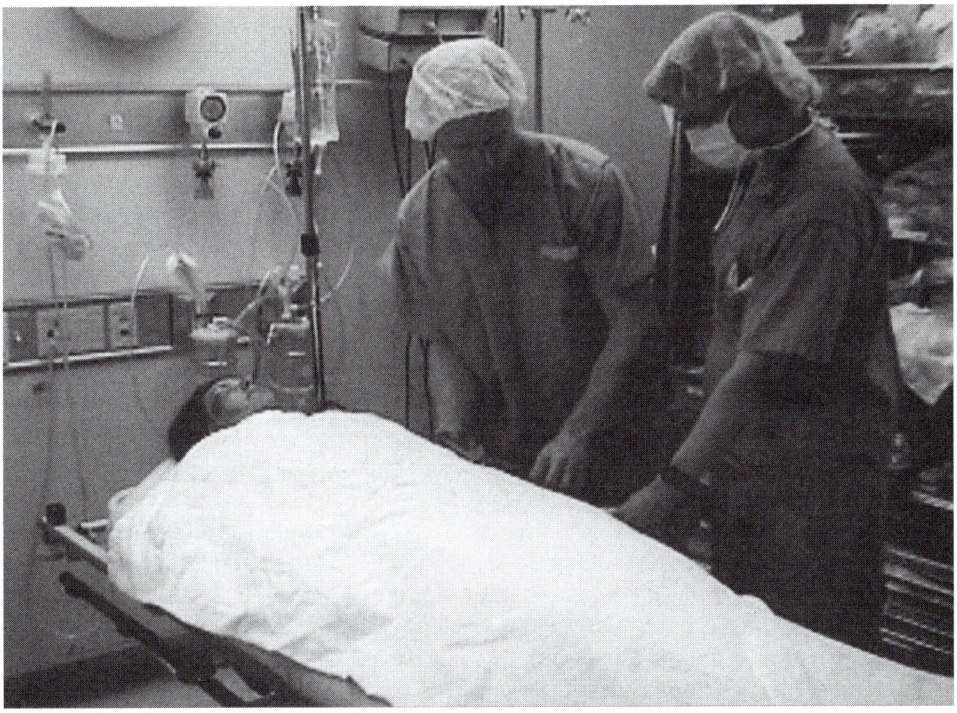

Figure 4 Hospital-based paramedics may function as anesthetic assistants, cast technicians, IV starters, and physician extenders. Hospital-based EMS can provide additional patient care in rural hospitals as well as maintain skills.

based service. In North America, EMS have been traditionally associated with fire departments instead of hospitals over the last 20 to 30 years. This generally occurred as the result of urban-based systems that simply realized there were more fire departments widely spread in a city than hospitals. Response times for fire-based ambulance services may thus be faster. In urban environments ambulance staff members may receive plenty of practice in their procedural skills with the many calls that they respond to in a day. In contrast, in a rural service the call volumes are generally less, and skills maintenance (IV starts or intubations, e.g.) may be more difficult. In a rural community, if a hospital exists, basing EMS out of the hospital may greatly improve medical skills through participation in hospital duties (IV starts prior to surgery, cardiac run team, cast technician's anesthetic assistant, and physician extender; Fig. 4).

F. The Role of the Rural Hospital

The role of rural hospitals in the care of rural and remote injuries is the next variable encountered. Few rural or remote hospitals can ever expect to have the resources and specialized personnel required to definitively and optimally manage severe trauma cases. Timely transport to level I trauma centers is a goal of care in all trauma systems. What about in rural areas, however, in which the time of event to the time of arrival at a level I trauma center is greater than 1 hr? The question arises as to whether EMS should stop for resuscitation and triage at level III rural hospitals or bypass them completely. Are there any possible negative outcomes associated with long-distance transfers from the scene by EMS? Would overall outcomes be improved? Is there a "cutoff point" beyond which direct transports have worse outcomes and within which they have improved outcomes? Would such systems be too costly, with the resulting "overtriage" and increased aeromedical flights? Are there things that can be done to improve trauma care in rural level III hospitals so that brief stops for stabilization and triage may improve outcomes? For the most part these questions remain unanswered, but the following is a summary of the literature that gives some insights.

When reviewing articles in this field it appears that the systems being studied vary so widely it is often difficult to compare or generalize results. Some rural stops in the studies are advanced trauma life support (ATLS) stabilization only. Some are open surgical procedures only in very unstable, selected cases (with varying diagnostic studies to try to rule out entities beyond an institution's capabilities [e.g., major vessel repairs]). Still others will aim to definitively manage the trauma patient right through to rehabilitation. The American College of Surgeons guidelines recommend direct transports to a level I trauma center if time of event to time of arrival at the center can be 1 hr or less. There is little to address the issues of more distant responses. A number of studies and trauma databases have recognized that there is an increased mortality in trauma patients who are treated at small rural hospitals [12,17,18]. In 1997 Sampalis et al. reviewed 1603 trauma cases. Sixty-three percent were transported directly to a level I trauma center, while 37% were first treated at the level III institutions and later transferred [19]. Those transported directly had less mortality and morbidity. (Judging by the length of time held at the level III centers prior to transport, however, these were not stops for stabilization but rather attempts at definitive care. Further, there was no mention of cases that did well rurally and were not transferred.)

Other studies have identified some factors that may contribute to trauma deaths in rural hospitals. For example, Aaland and Smith identified 68 (3%) delayed diagnoses (missed injuries) out of 1800 major trauma victims over a 2-year period. Most of these were nonspinal orthopedic injuries. Thirty-four percent required surgical intervention, however, and one patient died from the "missed injury." They noted these "misses" were more likely to occur in blunt (versus penetrating) trauma, altered mental status, those intubated in the field, and those requiring immediate operation [20]. Other studies have implicated failures to recognize injury severity, failure to institute standard resuscitation procedures, and slow times to surgical involvement [21–23]. Level II centers with a focused trauma service can provide good results [24,25]. Certo et al. in Vermont noted 10 preventable deaths in a series of 45 rural trauma mortalities. They felt only two of the 10 deaths could have been prevented by rural hospital bypass, however, and instead suggested stabilization at outlying rural facilities before transfer to a trauma center. Driscoll and Vincent showed that timely trauma resuscitation efforts affect outcomes [26]. Bickel et al. demonstrated a poorer outcome with fluid resuscitation prior to surgery for urban penetrating trauma [27]. They note that this outcome needs to be taken with caution, however, and cannot currently be generalized to rural systems facing long transport times to definitive surgery. From the neurotrauma literature, cases associated with a single episode of hypotension or hypoxia have dramatically poorer outcomes [28], therefore maintenance of blood pressure with crystalloids, blood products, and inotropes has remained as standard practice. Further, detailed neurological examinations have been shown to affect neurosurgical decisions at receiving centers [28]. Many of the "potentially preventable" trauma deaths in rural areas noted in the aforementioned studies specifically mention airway/respiratory events.

Priorities for rural hospitals include:

Recognition/triage of life-threatening conditions
Provision of advanced airway management (intubations, difficult airway techniques, chest tube insertion, blood gases if available, etc.)
Maintainence of spinal precautions and recognition of neurodeficits
Performance of a good neurological examination and documentation for brain injury
Minimization of length of stay in the emergency department

Instituting specific systems to deal with specific injuries in an area can result in improved outcomes. For example, instituting a statewide program for the prevention and treatment of burns in the state of Maine resulted in reduced mortality and morbidity [29]. Areas of North Carolina exposed to multivariate analysis found that the existence of trauma centers and advanced life support-certified EMS were two variables identified to reduce trauma death rates [30]. Emphasis on rural physician training in ATLS may improve rural trauma care. Both Martin et al. in 1990 and Hicks et al. in 1982 pointed out the wide deviations that can occur from standard trauma care [22,26]. Kearney et al. felt skilled rural stabilization before transfer was worth the delay in definitive care at a level I center [31]. Veenema and Rodewald demonstrated by retrospective review that stabilization and triage at their level III trauma center before a 40-min transfer to a level I trauma center resulted in outcomes comparable to national standards. They reviewed severe trauma patients (trauma triage score of 11 or less) who were treated at their level III rural centers prior to death, or transfered to the regional level I trauma center. With trauma injury severity score (TRISS) methodology, they calculated the probabilities of survival and death for each case and compared this to actual survival. Due to the numbers and resulting asymmetric power analysis, they felt they could conclude with confidence that first stabilizing at their rural center does not decrease survival. They could not comment on whether there was improved survivability [32], however. To date, this is the extent of outcome studies performed to answer the question of rural and remote center stops to stabilize and triage, as opposed to bypass. As more studies appear in this realm, they will have to be applied with caution due to the high variability in rural geography, hospital services, and prehospital services. A tightened definition of study variables may improve this topic in the future [13].

Level I center transport teams may be available for transport from rural hospitals or the scene of injury. Urban level I centers generally have the most advanced resources in personnel, funding, and equipment. Many urban centers have critical care teams that respond to rural areas by helicopter, fixed-wing aircraft, or other means. In rural or remote regions with no local medical services they may be the closest form of critical care available. The drawback to such services is usually the time required to travel the greater distance from the urban center to the scene. Usually rural areas with some form of first responder or prehospital services can get to the scene faster and administer initial care and transport sooner. The advantages of level I center teams are a generally higher level of care, better communications with the receiving center for a faster flow of procedures on arrival, and the freeing up of rural services to maintain service in their areas (rather than undergo long transports out of their regions). Such services depend on good communications and early launches for predetermined rendezvous sites (Fig. 5).

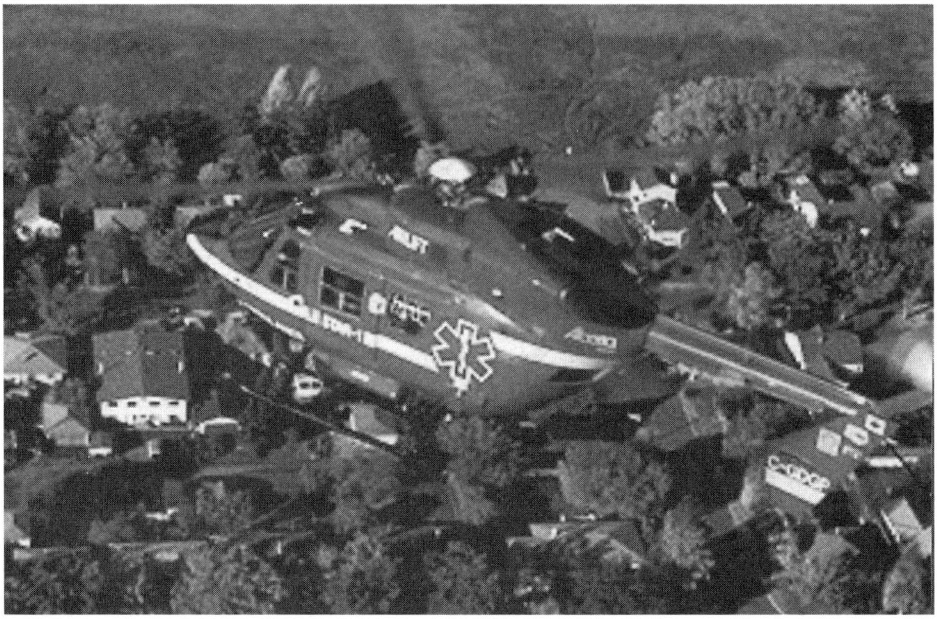

Figure 5 A level I center transport team rendezvous at a rural hospital. (Photo courtesy of Doyle R. Buehler, Aviationphoto.com.)

The care of trauma patients in remote and rural areas requires smooth integration of

Communication systems
Adequate number of skilled first responders
Local emergency medical services
Rural hospitals with appropriate infrastructure
Urban-based transport teams
Urban tertiary care hospitals

REFERENCES

1. S Gould. Hen's Teeth and Horses Toes. New York: Norton, 1983.
2. Microsoft Encarta, 1997.
3. P Baque, C Trojani, M Batt, R Hassen-Khodja, H Bariseel, P Pittaluga, S Declemy, B Prate, P Le Bas. Lower limb trauma caused by power-driven cultivators: Report of 23 cases. J Trauma 45:485–488, 1998.
4. TY Lee, SG Gerberich, RW Gibson, WP Carr, J Shutske, CM Renier. A population-based study of tractor-related injuries: Regional rural injury study-1 (RRIS-I). J Occup Environ Med 38:782–793, 1996.
5. RF Sing, CC Branas, EJ MacKenzie, CW Schwab. Geographic variation in serious nonfatal firearm injuries in Pennsylvania. J Trauma 43:825–830, 1997.
6. M Sharp. The Jaipur limb and foot. Med War 10:207–211, 1994.
7. GD Hobbs, DM Yealy, J Rivas. Equestrian injuries: A five-year review. J Emerg Med 12: 143–145, 1994.
8. DK Nakayama, WS Copes, W Sacco. Differences in trauma care among pediatric and non-pediatric trauma centers. J Pediat Surg 27:427–431, 1992.

9. SM Rock. Impact of the 65 mph speed limit on accidents, deaths and injuries in Illinois. Accid Anal Prev 27:207–214, 1995.
10. IM Jorgensen. The epidemiology of fatal unintentional child injuries in Denmark. Dan Med Bull 92:285–290, 1995.
11. CN Mock, E Adzotor, D Denno, E Conklin, F Rivara. Admissions for injury at a rural hospital in Ghana. Am J Public Health 85:927–931, 1995.
12. SB Baker, B O'Neil. Geographic variations in mortality from motor vehicle crashes. New Eng J Med 316:1384–1387, 1987.
13. WF Dick, PJ Baskett. Recommendations for Uniform Reporting of Data Following Major Trauma—The Utstein Style. A Report of the Working Party of the International Trauma Anaesthesia and Critical Care Society (ITACCS). Resuscitation 42:81–100 (B), 1999.
14. P Madsen, LB Svendsen, JG Jorgensen, et al. Tolerance to head-up tilt and suspension with elevated legs. Aviat Space Environ Med 69:781–784, 1998.
15. RE Haagensen, K-A Sjöborg, S Mjelstad, PA Steen. Lung function during hoist rescue operations. Prehosp Disas Med 13:73–76, 1998.
16. CJ Brooks, PL Potter, B Hognestad, J Baranski. Liferaft evacuation from a ditched helicopter: Dry shod vs. swim away method. Aviat Space Environ Med 68:35–40, 1997.
17. RH Cales, DD Trunkey. Preventable trauma deaths: A review of trauma care systems development. JAMA 254:1059–1063, 1985.
18. TF Certo, FB Rogers, DB Pilcher. Review of care of fatally injured patients in a rural state: 5 year followup. J Trauma 23:559–565, 1983.
19. JS Sampalis, R Denis, P Frechette, R Brown, D Fleiszer, D Mulder. Direct transport to tertiary trauma centers versus transfer from lower level facilities: Impact on mortality and morbidity among patients with major trauma. J Trauma 43:288–95 (discussion 295–296), 1997.
20. MO Aaland, K Smith. Delayed diagnosis in a rural trauma center. Surgery 120:774–779, 1996.
21. BA Houtchens. Major trauma in the rural mountain west. JACEP 6:343–350, 1977.
22. GD Martin, TH Cogbill, J Landercasper, PJ Strutt. Prospective analysis of rural interhospital transfer of injured patients to a referral trauma center. J Trauma 30:1014–1020, 1990.
23. TC Hicks, DF Danzl, DM Thomas, LM Flint. Resuscitation and transfer of trauma patients: A prospective study. Ann Emerg Med 11:296–299, 1982.
24. LC Zulick, PA Dietz, K Brooks. Trauma experience of a rural hospital. Arch Surg 126:1427–1430, 1991.
25. WW Wenneker, DH Murray, T Ledwich. Improved trauma care in a rural hospital after establishing a level II trauma center. Am J Surg 160:655–658, 1990.
26. PA Driscoll, CA Vincent. Variation in trauma resuscitation and its effect on patient outcome. Injury 23:111–115, 1992.
27. WH Bickell, MJ Wall Jr, PE Pepe, RR Martin, VF Ginger, MK Allen, KL Mattox. Immediate versus delayed fluid resuscitation for hypotensive patients with penetrating torso injuries. New Eng J Med 331:1105–1109, 1994.
28. The Brain Trauma Foundation. The integration of brain specific treatments into the initial resuscitation of the severe head injury patient. J Neurotrauma 13:653–659, 1996.
29. DE Clark, MS Katz, SM Campbell. Decreasing mortality and morbidity rates after the institution of a statewide burn program. J Burn Care Rehab 13:261–270, 1992.
30. R Rutledge, J Messick, CC Baker, S Rhyne, J Butts, A Meyer, T Rickets. Multivariate population-based analysis of the association of County Trauma Centers with per capita county trauma death rates. J Trauma 33:29–37 (discussion 37–38), 1992.
31. PA Kearney, L Terry, RE Burney. Outcomes of patients with blunt trauma transferred after diagnostic or treatment procedures of four-hour delay. Ann Emerg Med 20:882–886, 1991.
32. KR Veenema, LE Rodewald. Stabilization of rural multiple-trauma patients at level III emergency departments before transfer to a level I regional trauma center. Ann Emerg Med 25:175–181, 1995.

37

Trauma Care Support for Mass Events, Counterterrorism, and VIP Protection

RICHARD CARMONA

University of Arizona, Tucson, Arizona

CHRISTOPHER M. GRANDE

International Trauma Anesthesia and Critical Care Society (ITACCS), Baltimore, Maryland; Harvard Medical School and Brigham and Women's Hospital, Boston, Massachusetts; West Virginia University School of Medicine, Morgantown, West Virginia; and SUNY Buffalo School of Medicine, Buffalo, New York

DARIO GONZALEZ

Fire Department of the City of New York/Emergency Medical Services, New York, New York

I. INTRODUCTION

The concept of trauma (as well as medical) care support for special venues, events and actions such as mass gatherings, counterterrorism, and VIP/dignitary protection has grown in size and sophistication over the past two decades [1].

The literature in these areas was nearly nonexistent prior to this time. It should be noted and strongly stated that preparation for trauma care in any of these venues is part of the larger emergency medical system (EMS) plan and not an entity unto itself. In fact, except for some terrorist events, most chief complaints or requests for care in these areas are usually of a medical nature or for minor trauma [1,2].

Mass events are not limited to stadiums or concert halls; many take place over large geographic areas as well as indoors and outdoors. Examples would include (but not be limited to) sporting events, concerts, parades, marathons, and various demonstrations and rallies. Based on past events and reported experiences, it is safe to say that the EMS personnel should plan for the worst and hope for the best [3]. This is because although most encounters will be of a minor variety, mass casualties and/or catastrophic events can occur at any mass gathering [4,5].

In addition, it has been demonstrated that emergency providers and public health and public safety personnel must work together to plan for these events [6].

Terrorism—which may be defined as the planned threat or use of violence to attain one's political, ideological, or religious goals [7]—may be the predominant form of urban warfare worldwide in the future.

Where conventional warfare is relatively predictable, terrorism and terrorist acts can achieve monumental results in a given community by overwhelming its resources and physically and psychologically devastating the citizens [8,9].

In the past two decades we have seen the dramatic rise of international as well as domestic terrorist acts [7–9].

Counterterrorism refers to those actions that are aimed at preventing terrorist actions and/or responding to a terrorist act. The terrorist achieves his goals by many potential means, including threats and actual actions. Of the latter, only the terrorists' imagination and experience limits the potential options and subsequent devastation. In order to counter terrorism it is essential that we understand the mind set of the terrorist as well as the conventional and unconventional options that a terrorist may use.

VIP/dignitary protection has evolved into a science, largely due to the accumulated expertise of the U.S. Secret Service as well as a few other agencies, such as the U.S. Marshall's Service, that have a long history and experience in this area [10]. Trauma care support via tactical emergency medical support (TEMS) has also evolved [11]. Although the great majority of VIP/dignitary protection details nationally exist to protect high-profile prisoners, celebrities, and others by local law enforcement, the ultimate dignitary protection detail is that of the POTUS, or the president of the United States. Coverage for the health care needs of the traveling POTUS have been definitively and prospectively planned for many years [12,13].

II. TRAUMA CARE SUPPORT FOR MASS EVENTS

As with trauma centers, trauma care support at mass gatherings is part of a larger emergency medical service system (EMSS). At most mass gatherings what actually is created is a ''mini EMS'' that operates transiently for the duration of the event. This mini EMS is a reflection of the larger EMS within which it operates. That is because most if not all of the physical and personnel resources are drawn from the existing EMS. This would include but not be limited to emergency medical technicians (EMTs), ground and air transport resources, nurses, physicians, and medical directors. In addition, for those patients requiring transfer from the venue, they will enter the larger existing EMS and generally be transported to the nearest appropriate facility.

Mass gatherings are generally defined as events that have more than 1000 persons assembled [14]. It is estimated that over 200,000,000 people attend sporting events annually in the United States [14]. Estimates are that other mass gatherings account for even more attendees annually. It is interesting to note that although most mass gatherings are transient or episodic there are unique circumstances at some continuous mass gathering venues, such as airports [15] and larger cruise ships. In addition there are other unique assemblies of fewer than 1000 people that require special attention (e.g., large commercial aircraft) [16].

A. History

In the mid-1960s there began to emerge a body of literature that addressed care at mass gatherings [17]. Some of these reports and subsequent programs emerged out of the necessity to provide on-site emergency care in a timely fashion when external resources could not respond as quickly as needed. This may have been due to community demands or simply the difficulty in safely navigating through large crowds to find the patient.

Over the next three decades numerous publications emerged addressing various aspects of care at mass gatherings [18]. Most of the literature that has been published in this area is directed at general medical care and does not specifically address trauma issues. Based on reports of patient encounters in the literature, most trauma (when seen) is of a minor variety and non-life-threatening [2]. This is also the unpublished experience of the lead author (RC), who has been the special events medical director for mass gatherings at the University of Arizona since 1988.

Although the reported incidence of trauma in most venues is small, serious as well as life-threatening injuries do occasionally occur, as do catastrophic events with multiple casualties. A contingency plan to deal with single and multiple trauma scenarios is thus necessary [4,5].

B. Event Planning

Planning should begin with an assessment of the population expected to attend as well as the physical (geographic) setting and weather.

Needs and resources will vary considerably among the various combinations and permutations of variables. Examples would be (1) our (RC) preparation for the Senior Olympics (senior citizens competing in sports events of 1997) in Tucson, Arizona, in May, when the temperatures reached 100° with very low humidity, and (2) a football game at the University of Arizona on a December evening, when the temperature may drop to freezing [19].

Assessment of the expected participating and viewing population is extremely important. Population examples would be children competing at the Special Olympics (competitive sporting events for handicapped children) and adult senior citizens at the Senior Olympics. Each has significantly differing medical histories, comorbidities, and needs. The viewing audience would also be expected to be different. The Special Olympics would have a more general population distribution, whereas the Senior Olympics tends to attract a larger geriatric population of spectators. Various populations also have the propensity to consume lesser or larger amounts of alcohol and/or illicit drugs.

For example, at a teenage rock concert the use of various illicit substances would not be uncommon, and therefore preparing for these consequences (to include an increased incidence of trauma from accidents and/or fights) may be worthwhile. When alcohol was banned within the stadium at University of Arizona football games, there was a subsequent decrease in fights, injuries, and some types of medical calls [19]. After thorough consideration of the expected population demographics the event planners should be able to reasonably predict various scenarios (including "worst case") and plan accordingly.

C. Physical and Geographic Settings

The confines of the events are extremely important for many reasons. First, understanding the density of the population is necessary to determine how to distribute the medical resources within the venue. In addition, planning for ingress and egress of emergency vehicle traffic is essential, hence planning for gatherings such as Woodstock in 1970 versus a university football game would be very different. Certain venues provide unique challenges because of their huge geographic areas. An example would be a marathon, a triathalon, or the Olympic Games [20].

Certain geographic settings would also suggest that the planners consider the potential for increased injuries. An example would be an off-road dirt bike competition.

Other geographic considerations include the terrain for the spectators. For example, at an off-road dirt bike race, where viewers are scattered over uneven rocky surfaces, one would expect falls, strains, and sprains, as well as some fractures.

If held at altitude (say in the mountains above Denver) and attended by people who normally reside at sea level, this same event could cause further problems with altitude-related hypoxia, and everything from the usual medicine and pulmonary complaints to increased falls and auto accidents.

Geographic proximity to definitive care centers as well as modes of transportation are also important geographic considerations.

Finally, weather is an important factor, because of the potential for extremes of cold and heat as well as rain and snow, all of which can contribute to anticipated increased injuries. When planning the general approach to providing trauma or any other care at mass gatherings it is essential to review the previous experience of your own as well as others, along with reviewing the considerable literature on the subject.

D. Effective Utilization of Resources: Incident Command System

Careful prospective site, population, weather, and resource analysis is essential when planning for trauma care at any venue. Even though all the planning and individual resources are available, a preplanned method of working together in a seamless system is necessary. Multiple agencies, each with a significant contribution to the trauma care system at a given venue, must be able to effectively communicate in a timely manner. In general, at any venue the three areas contributing to the newly created system for trauma care support are law enforcement, EMS, and facilities management. In most states it is the senior law enforcement official who by statute is in charge of providing any response to or support at any mass gathering. Facilities management personnel are key in assuring expedient movement in and about any facility or venue. For example, they often can directly or remotely control all elevators, access to tunnels, and otherwise inaccessible areas needed to facilitate patient movement and transport. Each group has a particular significant contribution to make to the system. Each group normally has its own independent communication systems and methods of operation, however. These relationships must be decided beforehand in order to function smoothly during an event. Methods for dealing with these relationships have been around for three decades. They evolved out of necessity after a series of devastating wildfires in California. Local resources were rapidly depleted, and neighboring and distant firefighters and law enforcement and EMS personnel were forced to work together for the first time. This resulted in what became the Incident Command System (ICS) [21]. Most communities now have some form of ICS. Although each has its particular differences the underlying philosophy is a set of common policies, procedures, personnel, and resources that can be integrated into a common organizational structure to improve all types of emergency responses.

Utilizing this response approach, in Arizona [19] and elsewhere [1,14], we (RC) have developed a system termed ''unified command.'' In this model, a senior law enforcement officer, EMS person, and facilities manager are linked together at a central location at the venue to coordinate all necessary support that is required. For example, at University of Arizona football games, all three individuals are seated together in a sky box where they have a continuous visual assessment of the venue and can work together immediately and effectively to coordinate a resource request and movement. A requirement for each of these individuals is that he or she is an expert in his or her own area and is fully aware of all venue and local and community resources that are available should the need arise. Remember that any given response to provide trauma care will usually require security or law enforcement assistance, movement of personnel and equipment, and coordination with local law enforcement, EMS, and hospitals in the community.

Consideration should also be given to the level of care within the venue. Generally a two-tiered approach is the most cost-effective; that is, a first tier of basic EMTs to provide basic life support (BLS) support that is augmented by a second tier of paramedics who will provide advanced life support (ALS) support when needed.

There are many variations of community EMS configuration that may be applicable. However, distribution of EMS resources within the venue is determined by geography, population and population density, and other factors previously discussed. Generally, community EMS guidelines and law will govern the care dispensed at a given venue. On-site medical direction can often facilitate assessment and treatment decisions.

It should be noted that at many venues, especially larger ones, other trauma care providers may also be utilized at first aid stations or elsewhere. These would include first responders, nurses, and physicians' assistants. If utilized, all need to be incorporated into the plan to include communications.

Communication across disciplines at any given venue are often difficult. Emergency medical system, law enforcement, and facilities managers rarely have compatible radio systems, therefore aside from the ''unified command,'' provisions must be made for interdisciplinary communication. This may include but not be limited to common emergency frequencies and the use of programmable radios and cell phones.

E. Linkages with Local EMS

The local EMS must be aware of the plan at the mass gathering to include the nearest trauma center(s). Medical control on or away from the scene must be provided by a physician knowledgeable in emergency care as well as having expertise in prehospital procedures, policies, and protocols.

F. Triage

When an incident occurs that exceeds the immediate resources available a disaster is declared. Triage, the sorting of the injured and/or ill, allows scarce resources to be conserved and used efficiently. The triage system used at any mass gathering should be the same as or conform to local EMS expectations. This is because local EMS will be interfacing with the providers at the venue and their response should not be impeded by unknown systems. Triage has been used for nearly two centuries [22], and many systems are available for use. The system used in any given community (and venue), however, should be common and known and accepted by all [23].

G. Transportation

When needed, air resources should be used carefully, based on established prospective guidelines that are generally predicated on time and distance factors. Air resources during a disaster or multiple casualty incident are not only used for transport but also as an airborne platform to assess the entire venue and at times act as a command and control platform. Transportation for ground units needs to be coordinated by the unified command to include agreed-upon routes of ingress and egress. This is especially crucial in mass casualty and disaster responses, in which a transportation officer generally oversees this function as part of the ICS. The transportation officer will be coordinating their traffic according to the resources requested by the triage officer. It is therefore important to know the level of transport unit (BLS or ALS) and triage appropriate to the level of unit needed.

H. Spectrum of Expected Occurrences

As stated earlier, most requests for care and/or responses by prehospital providers will be of a minor or ambulatory nature. When involving trauma this usually consists of supportive care for minor cuts, abrasions, contusions, and musculoskeletal chief complaints [1,2]. Also, the types of problems encountered are strongly related to the venue type, attending population, weather, and geographic location [18].

Disasters and worst case scenarios at mass gatherings are relatively rare events. This contingency should always be incorporated into the operational plan for trauma care at mass gatherings. This is because unanticipated events such as a bleacher collapse, plane crashes at air shows, auto crashes at races, and more recently intentional acts can cause multiple casualty or catastrophic events [4,5,7,8]. One unanticipated consequence of our new and emerging global society is the realism of domestic terrorism. The terrorist who seeks to make a statement typically may do so by targeting a mass gathering at which widespread chaos and injury can be caused with little difficulty while at the same time depleting a community's resources and devastating it physically and psychologically [7,24].

By definition, a disaster or worst case scenario will be beyond the scope of the trauma care provided at any given venue. The operational plan should therefore provide for immediate linkages with local EMS via pre-existing protocols, policies, and procedures, including the ICS.

I. Special Situations

At venues at which there are existing health care staff (trainers, therapists, team physicians) it is important to ensure that they are all aware of and incorporated into the operational plan for two reasons. First, athletes or other types of participants at venues sometimes may require care outside that available from trainers and team physicians, and working together creates a seamless continuum of care that benefits the patient. An example would be when a university football player is severely injured (e.g., altered mental status, airway management problem, and breathing, circulatory, or neurologic impairment), a rapid assessment on the field is first done by the trainers and team physician who will then rapidly "hand signal" EMS staff who enter and assume care within seconds [19]. At the University of Arizona this relationship has been operational for over a decade and has worked exceptionally well [19].

J. Jurisdictional Issues: Command and Control

The mini EMS created in support of any mass gathering is part of a larger community EMS. Prospectively, various agencies, medical directors, and other stakeholders need to work out all command and control issues for a given venue. In more mature systems a given command and control template that has been previously agreed upon by all may be adaptable to most mass gathering venues [19].

Although jurisdictional issues between EMS agencies may initially require delicate negotiations and diplomacy, all issues need to and can be resolved prospectively.

Another area of jurisdiction is that of the athletes and/or venue participants, who may have their own trainers or physicians present. Although these primary care providers are responsible for keeping the athlete (or other participant) healthy, they often have little or no emergency care experience. Where trauma care at mass gatherings has not been thought through these providers will call 911, as they have for many years. Establishing linkages with the university or other venue primary care providers is therefore extremely important, since they often feel an ''ownership'' for the athlete or participant. The ensuing seamless system provides for a professional, efficient, and timely continuum of care.

K. Training Issues

Once an operational plan has been established and jurisdictional issues (if any) are resolved training should be scheduled to ensure a thorough understanding by all participants. Reviewing the operational interrelationships is important, as well as a discussion of the particular nuances of any venue. For example, for an injured university football player how and when should equipment be removed? How will movement and transfer be accomplished?

For race car venues, how do EMS and fire/rescue interface after a car crash in which extrication of an injured driver is required? These are only two of many possible scenarios that the providers at mass gatherings must face. All questions will not be addressed at the first or second training session; rather, this is a dynamic process that requires refinement as the experience grows over many years.

Understanding the literature and networking with peers with experience in this area can certainly shorten the learning curve of those with less experience entering this arena.

L. Summary

Trauma care for mass gatherings has progressed to a unique specialty area within EMS. Over the past two decades a general approach to care at mass gatherings has emerged in the literature and in practice. Administrative, operational, and care plans are now widely available in many communities. Although most requests for care are of a minor variety, prospective planning for potential catastrophic or multicasualty events is essential. This is not only because of natural or accidental disasters but also because of the new emerging threat of domestic terrorism.

III. COUNTERTERRORISM

Terrorism may simply be defined as the planned threat or actual use of violence to attain one's political, ideological, or religious goals. Counterterrorism refers to those activities aimed at preventing and/or responding to a terrorist act. As in health care, the best approach to counterterrorism is prevention via an intelligence network. The mere threat of a significant terrorist action is often enough to destabilize a community by inciting instability in its population while at the same time depleting its resources in preparation for an anticipated event [25].

Although requiring few personnel or logistical resources, an actual terrorist event can rapidly paralyze a community directly and/or indirectly: directly, with weapons (unconventional) of mass destruction (WMD; nuclear, chemical, or biological warfare), which may be extremely difficult to detect until the clinical exposure begins [25]; indirectly, by electronically or otherwise disabling essential communications and/or utilities in a given community. In addition, although unconventional terrorist acts are increasing in nature, conventional means of terrorism are still the predominant threat, as in the Oklahoma City bombing [7,8]. After a terrorist event, the physical repair of surviving persons and structures may take a considerable amount of time. The psychological devastation may last a lifetime, however.

A. Historical Perspective

History and the literature are full of conventional [8] and more recently unconventional terrorist acts [9]. Although most of the literature recounts acts of the past two decades [25], terrorism has been used as a tool for centuries. Counterterrorism as formally practiced today by federal, state, and local law enforcement is a relatively new science predicated on intelligence gathering electronically and via human interaction. When the intelligence systems in place fail to detect and prevent a potential terrorist event in a timely fashion the community must then respond to the consequences of that event. Due to the increased incidence of domestic terrorism and the ever-increasing threat of WMD a heightened awareness and state of preparedness has emerged in the past decade [7,25].

Trauma care as part of counterterrorist activities has two components. First is to prepare for the consequences of a potential threat or threats as detected via intelligence, and second is to actually be able to provide the care should the threat be carried out. In the past, preparing for trauma care for a potential conventional terrorist threat was similar to preparing for any catastrophic event, such as an earthquake or hurricane [5]. The new, insidious unconventional threats of WMD, however, make our planning extremely difficult because of many unique circumstances, such as an inability to detect the threat(s) early on, as well as the very different and difficult clinical sequelae of the unconventional terrorist act.

B. Trauma Care Support for Counterterrorist Activities

All trauma care support for counterterrorist activity begins within a local EMS. Local EMS planning for counterterrorism first involves a threat assessment followed by a needs and resource assessment. The threat assessment is largely determined by a given community's geographic location, targets of opportunity, and intelligence gathered by various law enforcement agencies. Examples would be large cities that are centers of commerce and information and communities with military installations and various industries, especially those related to defense. Once potential threats are identified a resource and needs assessment can be conducted to determine what resources are available and what may be needed for a given worst case scenario. In general, most communities with an integrated EMS with policies, procedures, and protocols to include mutual aid and intergovernmental agreements have the capacity to respond to most any conventional terrorist threat, the most common still being various explosive devices [7].

Where most communities are deficient, however, is in their planning and actual ability to respond to the newer domestic terrorist threat of WMD. A unique set of problems arises here, in part characterized by a poor ability to anticipate or identify most WMD threats as well as having specific antidotes or treatment for various agents [1]. What we cannot see, hear, or smell may ultimately prove to be the most devastating consequences of unconventional terrorist acts [1]. Since local EMS is generally going to be the first responder and care giver during the first 24 to 72 hr after any disaster it is absolutely essential that EMS and law enforcement work together to attain maximum efficiency and efficacy in developing the community trauma care/EMS plan for potential terrorist-type activity. As with the local EMS plans the counterterrorist portion should be tested and evaluated on a routine basis.

State resources in support of trauma care for counterterrorist activities vary widely. Funds may be available via law enforcement, EMS, and other state agencies, such as transportation, education, and the National Guard. These funds (when available) are often for training, but occasionally may be used for equipment purchases to enhance response capability.

The federal government has a large number of agencies that may be activated in support of local and state disasters. These agencies are also active in the planning and training areas by providing guidance and sometimes support to local agencies [26].

In the United States, the National Disaster Medical System (NDMS) was formed in the early 1980s to meet the medical needs of a civilian population affected by disaster [26]. An offshoot of NDMS was the creation of disaster medical assistance teams (DMAT). These are multidisciplinary regional teams that may be deployed to a disaster or function as a local asset receiving large amounts of casualties. These are locally sponsored teams that are available at the state level [26].

It is interesting to note that not until 1974 with the Disaster Relief Act (allowing state government to request federal emergency assistance) and the creation of the Federal Emergency Management Agency (FEMA) in 1979 did the United States have the ability to provide a coordinated disaster response on a national level [26]. The creation of FEMA allowed the consolidation of several federal programs while giving them more responsibility as lead agencies to coordinate a multidisciplinary response consisting of many federal agencies [26]. The military response to a given disaster is largely at the discretion of state government and the governor via the National Guard. These troops can be activated and mobilized on short notice to respond to a myriad of events.

C. Tactical Issues

During a disaster, local, state, and federal agencies must work together. This is a very complex task, since these groups are often culturally and logistically incompatible. The ICS is one method to facilitate these necessary linkages [21]. In addition, in the event of a terrorist-caused disaster law enforcement and EMS must have a plan to function cooperatively. Although many terrorist events may be characterized by a single action such as an explosion [8], it is not uncommon to have ongoing threat exposure [9], as in the Columbine High School shooting, where there were also numerous ‘‘booby trap’’ explosive devices. Threat analysis, preferably prospectively, is extremely important in that it allows planners and responders to be prepared and thus reduce morbidity and mortality by their approach and use of equipment, such as protective gear, self-contained breathing apparatus, or WMD precautions.

D. Tactical Emergency Medical Support

Tactical emergency medical support is a program that officially began over a decade ago [11,27]. The purpose of TEMS is to educate EMS providers as to how they may support and interact with law enforcement special operations teams (e.g., SWAT) prior to and during high-risk operations, including counterterrorist-type activities. The spectrum of TEMS is wide, and includes civilian EMS personnel who support tactical teams as well as tactical teams that have fully qualified tactical operators who are also medically trained. This is similar to the military model of the U.S. Army Special Forces, (Green Berets), the Naval Special Warfare Group (SEALS), and the Air Forces Para-Rescue Program (PJs).

Very often in responding to a terrorist action and its consequences it is unknown if the threat is over (tactically stable) or still evolving. Personnel trained in TEMS have an advantage in (at a minimum) being tactically familiar, sometimes proficient, or even expert in these areas. In addition, responding to and providing care in a potential crime scene presents unique challenges [28]. The TEMS program is now standardized nationally and provided through several venues, including the Counter Narcotics Tactical Operations Medical Support Course (CONTOMS) of the Department of Defense and the Uniformed Services University of the Health Sciences [24], as well as the National Tactical Officers Association (NTOA) and Heckler & Koch (H&K).

E. Weapons of Mass Destruction

The concept of WMD emerged as we ended the twentieth century, to encompass what we previously called chemical, nuclear, and biological weapons (NBC). Weapons of mass destruction have in common the potential for mass destruction and a high number of victims with relatively small amounts of substance or effort utilized [29].

Those of us who were in grade school in the 1950s remember participating in civil defense drills, building home shelters, and hiding under our desks in school to prepare for the possible threat of a nuclear attack during the Cold War. Most experts agree that the biggest threat to our national security today is in the area of ''bioterrorism.'' Chemical and nuclear threats are still possible, but are more difficult to obtain and disseminate than bioactive agents, which are cheap and easy to obtain and spread. Not only are WMDs a threat to us from our international adversaries (many of whom could not hope to advance their agendas via conventional means), but they also present a formidable challenge for domestic terrorism from radical groups in the United States. Trauma care from WMD is expected to be small if any because most of the clinical consequences of WMD are medical and result in incapacitation primarily by cardiopulmonary, GI, and/or CNS dysfunction.

In the last several years there has been a plethora of publications regarding WMD [24,25,29–31] that attempt to deal with administrative, system, clinical, and care issues. When they occur, physical injuries will most likely be secondary to the primary terrorist event and may be due to panic and flight-related accidents.

F. Spectrum of Possible Threats and Clinical Consequences

The spectrum of threats and subsequent clinical challenges is only limited by the imagination and experience of the terrorist. The consequences of unconventional terrorist acts such as WMD are potentially devastating, but are generally medically and not trauma related. The conventional weapons threat is the one in which significant physical injury and property damage may be incurred, and is the most likely to occur (compared to WMD).

Terrorist attacks are most commonly manifested in large urban centers that contain targets of opportunity [8]. These may include large gatherings, such as professional or collegiate athletic events, airports, and businesses that the community or government are dependent upon.

Interestingly, although WMD is a growing concern, the most obscure and newly emerging threat is cyberterrorism. This is because via cyberterrorism one can remotely or directly unleash conventional and unconventional terrorist acts while also paralyzing the infrastructure (communications, logistics, health care, etc.) of a given community.

Dealing with all of the components of WMD (chemical, biological, and nuclear threats) is beyond the scope of this review. Planning and caring for victims secondary to a WMD event is distinctly different from the conventional threats that most EMSs are structured to deal with. The closest model we now have operationally is that of dealing with hazardous materials (hazmat) exposure. This may be used as a template, but the WMD threats require significantly more planning and complex response.

When faced with a terrorist attack and multiple casualties, the goal of the EMS is to identify the total number of casualties and rapidly sort (triage) them in various categories of salvageability and nonsalvageability in order to utilize scarce resources efficiently. After a conventional terrorist action (e.g., bomb) this is relatively simple. For most communities a disaster (i.e., casualties exceeding immediately available resources) would be declared and various previously adopted plans would be initiated. In an unconventional terrorist act you may not know the agent, degree, or method of dissemination or the amount of casualties for some time. For example, persons who now appear normal may themselves already be infected (if a bioagent), become vectors, and not be symptomatic for some time, depending on the incubation period for the agent. Chemical and nuclear agents will present similar dilemmas.

As previously stated, most current terrorist acts, whether domestic or international, are of a conventional variety, with the most common vehicle being an explosive device. Blast-type injuries have been reported and characterized since the invention of gunpowder and the advent of war [7].

In the past, however, that experience in the United States has been during wartime, and consequently it was military surgeons and their hospitals that had this experience. Since the end of the Vietnam conflict there has been no concentrated experience in the military, or in military hospitals, for that matter [32]. In fact, since the late 1970s the greatest concentration of experience in caring for wounds and blast injuries has been in our urban trauma centers and not in the military, as in previous decades [32].

The effects of blast injuries have been categorized [7]. Primary blast injures are those caused to air-filled organs and are very often occult. Examples of commonly affected organs and systems are the auditory, respiratory, and GI tract. In secondary blast injuries, the most commonly occurring mechanism is due to the impact of debris striking the patient and penetrating or causing blunt trauma.

A tertiary injury is when the body itself is displaced by the blast. Expected injuries resulting from acceleration and deceleration would be similar to ejection from a high-speed auto accident. Burns and inhalation injuries are also common after blasts.

Prehospital and hospital providers must therefore be familiar with the insidious nature and delayed manifestations of some blast injuries. Triage and early care of blast victims is remarkably similar to that of all trauma patients, however.

After a terrorist bombing chaos ensues [1,7]. Arriving law enforcement and EMS units must first ensure (as best as possible) that there is no further or ongoing threat. A secondary blast or event sniper fire has occurred in some instances. After the scene is secured (remember it is a crime scene) [28], the processes that take place would be those that occur after any catastrophic event in any given community.

G. Training, Equipment, and Supply Issues

Most EMS agencies in the United States are trained and capable of responding to a wide variety of conventional multicasualty or catastrophic events. This would include the worst case scenario of multiple trauma and medical casualties at a hazardous materials release-related event. Mutual aid agreements generally exist in order to link scarce but available resources via an ICS.

These systems form the backbone or infrastructure of EMSs today. They also provide the template and strong base to add on the additional training and equipment needed to have an effective counterterrorist program.

In general, training regarding terrorism, the terrorist mind-set, and the unique methods of terrorism are needed. In addition, education regarding the clinical consequences of both conventional and unconventional (WMD) acts are needed. Specifically, intense training is also needed in all aspects of WMD. Finally, unique equipment (currently in development) is needed for the early detection and mitigation of WMD events.

H. Summary

Terrorism, once only something we read about in the international arena, is alive and predictably occurring with greater frequency in the United States. If we continue to build on the strong EMSSs we have developed over the past three decades our capabilities will be maximally and efficiently enhanced.

IV. VIP/DIGNITARY PROTECTION

VIP/dignitary protection details are formed for the purpose of protecting the ''principal'' or protectee. The principal(s) or protectee(s) range from high-profile prisoners to movie stars, dignitaries, and the POTUS. The agencies responsible for providing these details range from local law enforcement to federal agencies such as the Secret Service. Jurisdiction for the detail is generally determined by the local law enforcement agency except when a higher governmental agency has legal jurisdiction, such as the state police protecting a governor and federal agencies such as the U.S. Secret Service protecting the president and vice president. When a higher governmental agency assumes primary responsibility for the principal the local agency often provides secondary support as directed by the lead or primary agency. Another exception is when the lead agency is a nongovernmental or private agency that is hired to provide protection for a celebrity or other person.

Although a wide variety of protective details exist they all have in common the need to plan for trauma (and medical) care for the principal [33].

A. Options for Trauma Support

Trauma care support for protective details may be provided internally or externally. Internal refers to those agencies that have dually trained officers (or protectors) who are also prehospital providers or professionals of other levels of health care. When the agency has this capacity it still must have linkages with local EMSs in the event that they need support or the principal needs definitive care in a local hospital [10,12,13]. Except for select agencies that have the mission volume and budget to recruit and retain dual certified (law enforcement/protection and EMS) individuals, most agencies have external trauma (and medical) support [10].

This is typically accomplished via linkages with local EMS agencies, which are staged at a convenient nearby location. Agencies utilizing external support as the main primary provider need to be aware of operational security (OPSEC) issues in some protection details. Certain principals' movements are purposely kept confidential to make it more difficult for a terrorist, assassin, or other perpetrator to successfully engage the principal. VIP/dignitary protection details at the local level are often provided by police special operations units, such as special weapons and tactics (SWAT) teams and similar units. Many of these details provide their trauma and medical care for these details via their TEMS program [10,11,27].

B. Interfacing with Local EMS

Local protection details are generally aware of the health care resources in the community [34]. This would include EMS configuration, response times, and the location of trauma and other specialty centers. Dependent on OPSEC issues, these details should make every effort to prospectively develop a plan with local EMS, whether or not they have internal or external TEMS capacity. The difficulty arises when a traveling dignitary or celebrity is protected by a federal or other national agency when the protectee may travel nationwide or internationally. An interesting example is the U.S. Secret Service protecting the POTUS and his immediate family. The U.S. Secret Service has links (via its local offices) with most trauma centers nationally and in some cases internationally. These linkages were established many years ago [12,13]. Although the president routinely travels with his own medical entourage they realize that it is essential to have relationships with local trauma directors and centers should definitive care be needed. This may take the form of unanticipated injury or illness, as when President Reagan fell off his horse in northern Mexico and suffered a closed head injury [13], to actual assassination attempts, again as when President Reagan was shot in Washington, D.C.

Depending on the perceived risk to the principal, the notoriety of the principal, and the lead agency, advance teams may be deployed to review every aspect of the principal's movements, including contingency routes for travel to trauma centers [34]. These centers are also routinely canvassed, and tentatively have plans for everything from the command post location to specific personnel who may be involved with the care of the POTUS and the rooms to be used. Although most protective details do not require this detail, some preplanning is strongly suggested for all.

C. The Medical Plan as Part of the Overall Tactical Plan

A medical plan as part of an overall tactical plan is essential for protective details. The degree of detail of the plan is dependent on multiple factors, including the policy of the lead agency, the principal's visibility, notoriety, and personal history, which includes his or her health and overall risk and threat assessment. Medical threat analysis as part of the medical plan generally refers to evaluation of all factors internally (protectee's history) and externally (e.g., geography, weather, specific activities that may impact the protectee and therefore also the protective detail). Examples would be when President Bush decided to go skydiving in Yuma, Arizona. Other presidents have gone skiing and scuba diving or participated in other risk activities.

The medical history of the principal is extremely important in assessing risk in any given protective detail for a myriad of activities of the protectee [34]. Once again, using the example of the POTUS or former POTUSs (the POTUS has Secret Service protection for life), the range of health status is from extremely healthy and physically active to relatively sedentary with significant medical problems, including endocrine, metabolic, and/or cardiac, with an implantable automatic defibrillator in one protectee.

These details became extremely important in assessing risk and developing a prospective plan for all contingencies, internally or externally, when the local EMS and community resources must be accessed.

Weather is also important in that protectees are traveling and active in desert climates at sea level to mountain snowstorms at significant altitude. Weather coupled with geography frequently are significant factors in risk assessment when developing the medical plan. They also directly relate to the tactical plan because of movement considerations, choice of transportation, and positioning of the protectee within the protective detail.

When internal support (TEMS) is available to the detail these personnel are typically positioned near the principal in the entourage but not with primary protective responsibility. When coupled with internal support or alone, external support (TEMS) may be placed at strategic locations along a route or ''trail'' behind a motorcade, for example. There is a great deal of variability in providing TEMS that is dependent on many of these variables [10].

D. Transportation

The person in charge of the detail (along with the protectee) will determine the protectee's mode(s) of transportation as well as the transportation of the TEMS portion of the detail. In many details when internal TEMS is available they are indistinguishable from the remainder of the protective detail in dress or mode of transportation. External TEMS, usually from local EMS, frequently dress and travel in their own ambulances as part of an entourage or when moving from location to location.

Transportation routes for the protectee are often predetermined (with contingency alternatives available). In high-profile protective details these routes are often kept secret, therefore those protective details with internal TEMS will be aware of the preplanning while external TEMS support elements may only find out at the time of deployment and then only incrementally as the protectee advances from location to location.

These decisions are meant to increase OPSEC. Depending on the protective detail, routes may be random or best available at the time of day to those that are meticulously checked prospectively, as with the travels of the POTUS. Advance teams of Secret Service, local law enforcement, explosive ordinance disposal (EOD) teams, and others will study the routes, seal manhole covers, remove mailboxes, and perform other activities to decrease risk to the POTUS. Again this is probably the most labor-intensive of all planning for any protective detail; most protective details do not need nearly this much scrutiny in route selection or other areas.

Tactical emergency medical support providers working with a protective detail should be aware that transportation and routing issues will impact their medical plan and must be considered, if possible, especially when determining the nearest appropriate definitive care, including trauma centers.

E. Communications

Communication during the provision of TEMS for protective details must take place on many levels. When the detail has the capacity for the internal provision of trauma care via TEMS the communication issues are simplified. This is because those officers and providers are used to working with one another and speaking the same radio language (e.g., 10 codes) and are aware of primary and alternate frequencies. When TEMS is provided externally (or when internal TEMS interfaces with community EMS) they must establish radio linkages with the protective detail as well as community EMS. This is usually accomplished by the external EMS detail being given a radio by the protective detail or assigning a protective detail person to the external TEMS support.

Depending on the notoriety of the protectee as well as the size of the community and the number of stops during a given protective detail the plan may very well contain more than one hospital being selected for definitive care, depending also on the time and distance requirements during the duration of the detail. Air transport assets may also be incorporated into the plan, also depending on the time and distance requirements.

F. Equipment Issues

Depending on the type of protective detail as well as the medical history of the protectee a wide variety of TEMS support and equipment are available on or near protective details. Again using the POTUS as an example, the POTUS travels with his own medical team, which has a detailed history and knowledge of any unique medical requirements. These are generally primary care providers, although President Reagan's chief physician was a surgeon [13].

Any emergent ALS-level care will therefore most likely be provided or complemented by local ALS providers. With high-risk protective details such as the POTUS, ALS equipment is readily available in relatively close proximity to the POTUS. Protective details with a lesser degree of threat and/or very healthy individuals may choose only to have BLS capability immediately accessible, with ALS capability available on demand with a reasonable response time.

Occasionally unique situations arise in some high-risk protective details, as when the POTUS (or high-profile dignitary or official) decides to go skydiving, scuba diving, or rock climbing or rappelling. These venues all require special equipment availability as well as specially trained individuals, such as a flight surgeon, a dive medical officer with hyperbaric chamber capability, and TEMS providers skilled in rope work and high-angle rescue.

Equipment and specialized personnel may require extra planning and coordination, depending on the uniqueness of the protective detail and the health status, risk assessment, and notoriety of the protectee.

G. Postmission Debriefing

Just as the protective detail tactically debriefs each protective detail mission the TEMS component must also review its entire preplanning, planning, and performance during the mission. Even the most successful missions can be improved and/or become more efficient by careful objective and impartial review. Whether TEMS is provided internally (TEMS providers are usually part of tactical debriefing) or externally, the protective detail team and leader should carefully assess the TEMS component performance and seek input as to any problem that occurred or opportunities for improvement.

H. Summary

Trauma care (and medical) support via TEMS for VIP/dignitary protection details is a growing and complex subset of the provision of EMS. This care may be provided internally or externally, depending on the resources available to a given agency. Careful planning and attention to detail is essential for the successful provision of trauma care support to these protective details [33,34].

REFERENCES

1. C Morres, F Burkle, S Lillibridge, eds. Disaster medicine. Emerg Clin North Am 14:2, 1996.
2. D Spaite, L Criss, T Valenzuela. A new model for providing pre-hospital medical care in large stadiums. Ann Emerg Med 17:825, 1988.
3. JT Kerr, EC Weiman, A Kuehl. Liberty weekend: ''Plan for the Worst and Hope for the Best.'' JEMS 11:40, 1986.
4. GP Lilja, M Madsen, J Overton. Multiple casualty incidents. In: A Kuehl, ed. Pre-Hospital Systems and Medical Oversight. 2nd ed. St. Louis: NAEMSP. Mosby-Lifeline, 1994, pp. 441–445.
5. L Bosner, E Pretto, R Carmona, J Leanning. Catastrophic events. In: A Kuehl, ed. Pre-Hospital Systems and Medical Oversight. 2nd ed. St. Louis: NAEMSP. Mosby-Lifeline, 1994, pp. 447–453.
6. GD Mears, AH Yancey. Mass Gatherings. In: J Tintinalli, ed. Emergency Medicine: A Comprehensive Study Guide. New York: McGraw-Hill, 2000.
7. M Stein, A Hirschberg. Medical consequences of terrorism: The conventional weapon threat. In: A Rodriguez, K Maull, D Feliciano, eds. Surgical Clinics of North America: Trauma Care in the New Millennium. vol. 79. no. 6. Philadelphia: Saunders, Dec. 1999, pp. 1537–1552.
8. S Mallonee, S Shariat, G Stennies. Physical injuries and fatalities resulting from the Oklahoma City bombing. JAMA 276:382, 1996.
9. T Okumyra, K Suzuki, H Fukuda, A Kohama, N Takasu, S Ishimatsu, S Hinohara. The Tokyo Subway Sarin attack: Disaster management. Part I and part II. Acad Emerg Med 5:613–617, 1998.
10. R Carmona, D Rasumoff. TEMS support for VIP/dignitary protection details. Tact Edge 17: 60–61, 1999.
11. L Heiskill, R Carmona. Tactical emergency medical support, an emerging specialized area of pre-hospital care. Ann Emerg Med 23:778–785, 1994.
12. G Strauch. Ensuring the care of the president. Bull Amer Coll Surg 84:15–18, 1999.
13. R Carmona. Unpublished Communications with the White House, Secret Service, Presidential Physicians, and R Carmona, 1985–1993.
14. G Mears, A Yancy. Mass Gatherings. In: J Tintinalli, ed. Emergency Medicine: A Comprehensive Study Guide. McGraw-Hill, 2000.
15. AA Cwinn, N Dinnerman, PT Pons, et al. Pre-Hospital care at a major international airport. Ann Emerg Med 17:1042, 1988.
16. C Speizer, DJ Rennie, H Brenton. Prevalence of in-flight medical emergencies on commercial airlines. Ann Emerg Med 18:26, 1989.

17. SW Carveth. Cardiac resuscitation program at the Nebraska football stadium. Dis Chest 53: 8–11, 1968.
18. R Leonard. Medical support for mass gatherings in emergency clinics of North America. Disas Med 14:383–397, 1996.
19. R Carmona. University of Arizona and Rural Metro Corporation. Unpublished EMS call data from University of Arizona special events (mass gatherings), 1987–2001.
20. SF Wetterhall, DM Coulombier, J Herndon, et al. Medical care delivery at the 1996 Olympic Games. JAMA 279:1463, 1998.
21. E Auf Der Heide. Disaster Response: Principles of Preparation and Coordination. St. Louis: Mosby, 1989.
22. DJ Larre. Surgical Memoirs of the Campaigns of Russia, Germany and France. Philadelphia: Carey, Lea, 1832 (translated).
23. L Gans, T Kennedy. Management of unique clinical entities in disaster medicine. Emerg Clin North Am 14:301–326, 1996.
24. K Yeskev, C Llewellyn, J Vayer. Operational medicine in disasters in emergency clinics of North America. Disas Med 14:429–438, 1996.
25. T Inglesby, D Henderson, J Bartlett, et al. Anthrax as a biological weapon: Medical and public health management. JAMA 281:1735, 1999.
26. P Roth, J Gaffney. The federal response plan and disaster medical assistance teams in domestic disasters in emergency clinics of North America. Emerg Clin North Am 14:371–382, 1996.
27. R Carmona, D Rasumoff. Essentials of tactical emergency medical support. Tact Edge 8:54–56, 1990.
28. R Carmona, D Rasumoff. Forensic aspects of tactical emergency medical support: TEMS. Tact Edge 10:54–55, 1992.
29. G Benjamin. Chemical and biological terrorism: Planning for the worst. Physician Exec 80–82, Jan–Feb. 2000.
30. J Waeckerle. Domestic preparedness for events involving weapons of mass destruction. JAMA 283:252–254, 2000.
31. Arizona Department of Health Services Prevention Bulletin. 14:2000.
32. R Carmona. The paradox of military trauma and emergency medical care. JAMA 266:217, 1991.
33. D LaCombe, C Grande. EMS Support of Executive Protection and Counter-Terrorism Operations. In: J DeBoer, M Duboulz, eds. Handbook of Disaster Medicine: Emergency Medicine in Mass Casualty Situations. International Society of Disaster Medicine. Utrecht: Van der Wees Uitgeverij, 1999, pp. 359–382.
34. D Carrison, C Grande. In sickness and in health. Secur Mgt 65–69, March 2000.

38

Patient Turnover: Arriving and Interacting in the Emergency Department

STEPHEN R. HAYDEN and GARY M. VILKE

University of California San Diego Medical Center, San Diego, California

ANDREAS THIERBACH

University Hospital, Mainz, Germany

MICHAEL SUGRUE

The Liverpool Hospital, Sydney, Australia

I. PREHOSPITAL COMMUNICATION WITH TRAUMA TEAM

A. Prearrival

Communication between prehospital providers and hospital-based trauma teams is essential to optimize care in the critically injured trauma patient. Clearly, long, drawn-out reports take precious time away from patient management, therefore radio reports in the field and patient turnover reports at the hospital must be succinct and contain the key elements needed to facilitate continued patient care and further evaluation.

Prehospital systems employ many different guidelines for hospital contact. With major trauma patients, however, most fall into the category of requesting a prehospital report. This will offer the opportunity to mobilize appropriate resources early, often before the patient arrives at the hospital.

Modes of making contact vary, often depending on terrain and distances. Radio frequencies are the most utilized resource. With areas of irregular terrain, radio repeaters are usually in place to offer adequate transmission in most areas. Some agencies will use cellular or digital phone systems for contact. These systems have the drawback that they will often be zoned or have ''dead areas'' in which contact cannot be made or continued. This is particularly a problem in mountainous regions. Additionally, most are not designed to be rugged enough for the prehospital setting. The advantage to cellular phones is that they can be used to send prehospital electrocardiograms via fax-modem, not often useful in trauma, but often a reason they are the contact modality of choice in some systems. Many prehospital providers have both, usually implementing radio as the primary communication source and having a cellular or digital phone as a backup modality. Some systems will have centralized medical control systems, which offer online control and will forward prehospital patient information to the appropriate trauma receiving facility. These systems typically implement radio frequencies as the communication modality. Other systems require the prehospital care providers to call the receiving trauma center directly to give the prehospital report.

1. Mechanism-Injury-Vitals Treatment (MIVT)

With these communication systems in place, reports can be received by the trauma team prior to patient arrival. This can allow for earlier preparation. If the patient has evidence of head trauma and a low Glasgow coma scale (GCS) score, then the neurosurgeon can be forewarned and the CT scanner prepared. If there is an unstable, challenging airway, then the receiving physician has the opportunity to prepare for a difficult intubation.

The content of the report is therefore paramount. Too abbreviated a report can leave out certain key features, and too long a report delays care to the patient. The mechanism-injury-vitals treatment (MIVT) (see Table 1) format offers a simple yet complete way to give a prehospital report.

Under *mechanism*, a single sentence should suffice to give the trauma team a clear picture of what happened to the patient. For example: ''29-year-old male unrestrained driver in a compact car head-on into a tractor-trailer truck at freeway speeds with deployment of airbag and significant space intrusion.'' This offers to the listener a fairly vivid image as to what happened to the patient. Occasionally an additional phrase can be added if the situation dictates to describe the presence of alcohol or drugs, deaths of others in the same accident, or confounding variables, such as smoke inhalation or seizure or hypoglycemia as an inciting event.

The next part of the report succinctly describes the *injuries* of the patient. An example would be: ''Positive head trauma with blood from right ear and GCS = 8, right flail chest, distended abdomen and deformity of right ankle with distal neurovascular intact.'' This gives the listener an impression of what is found in a primary survey. If the patient is conscious, then the report will reflect the patient's complaints (e.g., ''the patient complains of neck pain, abdominal pain, back pain and left wrist pain'').

The third part of the report gives the patient's *vital signs*, including pulse, blood pressure, respiratory rate, and oxygen saturation if available.

The final part of the report is prehospital *treatment*. The hospital should be given a report that reflects if spinal precautions have been placed, but the specifics need not be given in detail. Placement of the IV, including size and location in addition to fluid type and flow rate, should be given. The use and flow of O_2 should be stated as well. The hospital should be aware if medications have been used or if procedures have been performed. If the patient is intubated and is being monitored on a quantitative end-tidal CO_2 detector, then the value should be relayed at this time. The estimated time of arrival (ETA) should be given at the end of report and it should be confirmed that the hospital received the report and has no questions. A typical report would be given as follows: ''The patient

Table 1 Mechanism-Injury-Vitals Treatment (MIVT)

Mechanism (M)
How did injury/accident occur?
Describe vehicle(s)
Presence of alcohol/drugs
Deaths at scene
Confounding variables
Injuries (I) of patient
Primary survey
Level of consciousness
Glasgow coma scale
Vital signs (V)
Pulse
Blood pressure
Respiration
Temperature
Oxygen saturation
Treatment (T)
Airway management and oxygen administered
Spine precautions
Intravenous placement (size and placement) and fluids given
Medications administered
Procedure performed
Estimated time of arrival
Confirmation that receiving hospital has received information

is in full spinal precautions, O_2 15 liters by nonrebreather face mask, 16-gauge IVs placed in bilateral antecubital fossas with normal saline running wide open. The left leg has been splinted, and our ETA is 10 minutes. Do you copy?''

2. Updates

If the patient has a long transport time and the condition changes or significant interventions had to be performed, the prehospital provider should update the trauma team before arrival. Worsening status or specific findings may cause a change in the disposition of the patient in the hospital. In some systems the patient will be taken directly to the operating room (OR) if specific predetermined criteria are met. For example, persistent hypotension despite fluid resuscitation or penetrating chest trauma with hypotension will dictate an automatic OR resuscitation in some systems. This can only be done, however, if there is reliable and timely communication between the prehospital providers and the trauma service. Updates should only be called in to the hospital if it directly affects patient care or disposition. For example, if the patient worsens or remains hypotensive despite fluid resuscitation, then the paramedics might update the receiving facility about the patient's status and request an OR resuscitation if the trauma system has that option in place. Routine updates or reports should be held until patient turnover at the hospital.

B. At Arrival

The prehospital report mimics the report to be given upon turnover to the trauma or emergency department team. The whole report should take less than 30 sec. If a full report has already been received, some services only request an update of the patient status from the time of the report, including interventions, response to therapy, and recent vital signs.

Some systems will advocate that if the patient is a minor trauma victim only a minimal report needs to be given over the radio. This would basically be: 30-year-old male in low-speed motor vehicle accident, only complaining of neck pain with stable vital signs with an ETA of 5 min. Then a full MIVT report can be given at patient turnover at the hospital. This avoids tying up the radio for prehospital providers who may need it for more seriously ill patients. If there is a multiple victim incident (MVI), radio reports should be kept to a minimum, as multiple reports will need to be given by the field medical commander.

Communications between the prehospital providers and the hospital staff must be brief and efficient, as the information relayed is key in maintaining a smooth transition from the field to the hospital team and optimizing patient care.

II. ROLES AND RESPONSIBILITIES OF THE EMERGENCY MEDICAL SERVICES (EMS) AND TRAUMA TEAM

A. EMS Personnel

Upon arriving to the emergency department (ED), it is imperative that EMS personnel communicate essential information to the receiving team in a concise yet complete manner. This should follow a standardized format, such as the MIVT format above. Prehospital providers are the eyes and ears in the field. They must succinctly describe the scene, mechanism of injury, damage to vehicles, and special environmental considerations (temperature, prolonged exposure to water, sun, etc.), as well as other persons involved in the same accident and what injuries they sustained. All these factors will help the trauma team to understand what forces acted on the patient and may suggest certain characteristic injury or disease patterns when assessing the patient.

EMS personnel must also attempt to ascertain eyewitness reports and historical information, such as prior medical/psychiatric history, medications, allergies, evidence of drug use or alcohol consumption, and any advanced directives or living will provisions, if they are shown to exist.

Finally, a detailed account of interventions that occurred in the field as well as the corresponding response to these interventions is crucial. What were the initial vital signs, GCS, cardiac rhythm, and other appropriate physiologic parameters? What procedures were performed and how did the patient respond? How much IV fluid was administered or autologous blood transfused? What medications were given and what response did they produce? All this information must be communicated in a concise and efficient manner.

B. Trauma Team

The trauma or ED team leader must allow prehospital providers to deliver their report without interruption to ensure all necessary information is communicated. Prior to arrival, the team leader will have assigned ED and trauma personnel to various roles in the resuscitation (e.g., airway management, vascular access, chest procedures, medication delivery, runner, scribe). After the report has been given, the current patient condition must be confirmed. Airway, chest, and vascular devices will need confirmation of function. Subsequent systematic patient evaluation and stabilization can then occur as per local trauma protocols.

III. CONTINUOUS PATIENT TREATMENT

The overall strategy of trauma patient treatment and management of the early phase can be defined as a continuously repeated, priority-driven process of patient assessment, resuscitation, and reassessment. This overall strategy differs only in available resources, if pre- and intrahospital parts of the strategy are compared.

The general approach to evaluation of an acute trauma victim differs from that of patients with diseases. It usually has the following three sequential components:

Rapid overview of the situation (especially on scene)
Primary survey of the vital functions
Secondary survey; that is, the comprehensive evaluation from head to toe

Resuscitation is initiated, if needed, at any time during this continuum (e.g., in the field, during transport, or at ED arrival). A rapid overview in any phase of patient care should take only a few seconds and is used to determine whether the patient is in stable condition or not. The primary survey involves rapid evaluation of the so-called vital functions (i.e., those that are crucial to survival). The ABCs of airway patency, breathing, and circulation are assessed, then a brief neurologic examination is performed. The secondary survey involves a more extensive and elaborate systematic examination of the entire body to identify additional injuries.

Within this general framework, the members of the trauma team identify injuries, pre-existing conditions, and the resulting functional abnormalities that require either immediate treatment or provision for resuscitative and anesthetic management [1]. Optimal trauma care usually requires the coordination of multiple specialists into one concerted effort. Such EMS personnel as emergency physicians (in central European countries, usually an anesthesiologist) or paramedics, trauma surgeons, and anesthesiologists, as well as other surgical subspecialties, have to be integrated into treatment.

As brief as the turnover period may be, it is a crucial period during which the primary concern must be the continuation of patient care. The coordination is the team leader's responsibility. In Germany, leadership may be divided into the so-called trauma coordinator (performed by an anesthesiologist) and the trauma surgeon. The trauma coordinator is responsible for the primary survey and all measures or therapeutic interventions connected to it. The trauma surgeon's responsibility covers the secondary survey and all necessary diagnostic and surgical interventions. Standards of care in any local system have to be expressed concisely as an algorithm of care and followed by anyone involved in the trauma victim's treatment.

A. Measures of EMS Personnel and Trauma Team Members

Most important at patient turnover in the ED, therapeutic measures such as ventilation or oxygenation and application of infusions or drugs have to be continued without suspension or delay. The same rules are to be applied for a continuing monitoring of vital parameters such as overall neurologic, respiratory, and cardiocirculatory status.

Table 2 Standardized Patient Turnover

Arrival in the ED
Trauma team members start monitoring vital functions
The team leader receives the report of the EMS unit
Patient monitoring is established
EMS monitors may be removed
The patient is moved to the ED stretcher
From this time on, responsibility is transferred to the trauma team
Before leaving the ED
EMS crew and the trauma team leader have to check turnover
It must be determined whether or not there are any more questions
Documentation has been completed

A standardized patient turnover has been proven advantageous in many trauma centers (see Table 2).

Such EMS equipment that cannot be removed from the patient (e.g., rigid collars, splints) should be returned to the EMS unit as soon as possible.

B. Standardized Report to the Trauma Team

When the EMS personnel arrives in the ED, it is important to present the essential patient information in an orderly, concise fashion so that communication with the trauma team is facilitated and important information is not inadvertently omitted. The MIVT format described earlier also facilitates a structured oral turnover report to the receiving trauma team.

IV. DOCUMENTATION

A thorough and accurate medical record is—not only for legal reasons—essential for the documentation of both findings and the treatment rendered. It also ensures the standardization and completion of information at patient turnover and guarantees the continuity of patient treatment. The documentation has to be as precise and detailed as possible.

In some cases, especially in unstable, multiple-injured patients, it may be necessary to complete the documentation after patient turnover to the trauma team because of the ''lack of hands'' for recordkeeping beforehand. These exceptions to proper recordkeeping have to be kept to a minimum. Alternately, a ''scribe'' can be assigned to document the trauma resuscitation as a specific duty of a trauma team member.

A. Forms and Contents

Proper documentation of all findings, observations, and treatment is of great importance not only to the patient, but also to the EMS and the receiving units. It should be completed during treatment on self-copying forms, providing up to three copies for the receiving unit, the EMS, and the emergency physician or paramedic in charge. The design may vary according to local needs, but it is essential that the key elements described below be understood easily by different observers.

A vast amount of paperwork is generated for each trauma victim, and it is essential that each can be individually identified. One method is to prepare specially designated

Table 3 EMS Medical Records

Date and times
Time call was received
Response time
Time at beginning of transport
Time the patient arrived at the trauma center
Gender and, if available, precise patient information (full name, date of birth, address, social security number)
Chief complaint
Present problems (more detailed description of complaints)
Past medical history (e.g., significant other injury, illness, medications, or allergies)
Observations of the scene (e.g., mechanism of injury)
Vital signs and findings of complete physical examination
Parameters of monitoring
Precise recordings of any treatment rendered
Condition during transport
Patient position
Changes in vital signs or monitor readings
Continued therapy
Changes in the patient's status prior to arrival in the ED

medical record numbers, eventually including bar codes, for the EMS units as well as for the receiving trauma center. These record numbers may be placed on blood tubes, documentation forms, and patient belongings. Any medical records of the EMS (provided by emergency physicians or paramedics, depending on the type of EMS) have to cover a number of aspects [2] (see Table 3).

Any further intrahospital documentation is usually done on anesthesia and surgery records. These may vary from different sheets of paper to some kind of computerized online recording.

V. REPLACEMENT OF DEVICES PLACED IN THE FIELD

A. Vascular Catheters

1. Peripheral Intravenous (IV) Catheters

It has long been held as dogma that the field is a dirty environment and that IVs placed in the prehospital setting must be changed upon arrival or admission to the hospital (Table 4). Many intensive care units (ICUs) have a standing policy to replace all IVs started elsewhere (field, ED, hospital ward) [3,4]. While numerous authors have questioned the need for routine placement of IV catheters in the prehospital setting [5], the first major report of whether IVs started in the field by paramedics or emergency medical technicians (EMTs) were associated with higher complication rates came from Lawrence and Lauro in 1988 [4]. They studied a series of 82 patients with IVs placed in the prehospital setting and 109 patients with IVs placed in the ED. They found a 34% incidence of phlebitis and a 22% rate of fever in the field IV group, compared to 7% phlebitis and 4% fever in the ED IV group. Both differences were statistically significant. This study has been referred to by many authorities as proof that there is an increased infection rate for IVs placed in

Table 4 Replacement of Devices Placed in Prehospital Setting

Device	Replace on arrival to ED
Peripheral IV	No
Central line	
Subclavian	No
Femoral	No
Basilic	No
Intraosseus line	Yes
Chest tube	No
EOA/EGTA	Yes
PTLA/Combitube	No[a]
Endotracheal tube	No
Urinary catheters	No
Gastric catheters	No

[a] The PTLA/Combitube does not need immediate replacement on arrival. After the patient has been stabilized, however, it should be replaced electively with an ETT.

the field, and therefore that catheters should be replaced upon arrival in the ED or upon hospital admission.

There were several important limitations to this study, however, that make the results less relevant today. First, while the specific numbers were not reported, the authors state that more effective handwashing techniques and a greater use of gloves in the field might decrease the infection rate. Today, with the routine use of universal precautions, aseptic technique in the field has clearly improved. Second, this was a small study in which a group of only 17 paramedics placed the prehospital IVs, therefore the results may not be applicable to all EMS systems.

A more recent study published in 1995 by Levine et al. [3] reported only one infectious complication in 859 IV lines begun in the field (0.12%) compared to four of 2326 lines placed in the hospital (0.17%) $p = 0.59$. The authors of this study used the Centers for Disease Control (CDC) criteria for a clinically significant skin and soft tissue infection [6]. Neither of these studies included patients admitted to an ICU, because standard policy in their institutions was for all IVs started elsewhere to be replaced upon admission to the ICU.

Although the data are sparse, based on the available evidence there is no indication for replacing IVs started in the field upon arrival at an ED or trauma unit. Careful monitoring of IV sites for infection, infiltration, or malfunction should be performed and catheters replaced when any of these complications occurs. Even in the Lawrence and Lauro study only 31% of field IVs ultimately needed to be replaced, compared to 11% of IVs started in the hospital [4]. It would seem prudent to monitor for the development of such complications before replacing the catheter.

2. Central Venous Catheters

There are few studies that report complications of central venous catheters placed in the prehospital setting. In fact, there are few circumstances in the field in which a central line would provide significant benefit over a peripheral IV. There have been a number of studies reporting the complication rates of central venous catheters placed in the ED without full barrier protection (gowns, masks, etc.) using standard sterile technique only [7–9]. Complications (including infectious complications), success rates, malposition rates, and pneumothorax are comparable to catheters placed in the ICU or ward environments with full barrier and sterile technique. These studies do not differentiate among femoral, subclavian, or long-line basilic central line sites. If peripheral IV access is not possible or practical, it is reasonable to believe that properly trained personnel using an appropriate sterile technique (aseptic skin preparation, sterile gloves, and catheter kits) can place central lines in a prehospital setting with acceptable complication rates and therefore obviate the need for immediate replacement upon ED arrival.

3. Intraosseous (IO) Lines

When peripheral IV access cannot be successfully performed on pediatric patients, intraosseous (IO) placement of a rigid catheter/needle can be performed to administer fluids, medications, or even blood. These IO lines, however, are by their nature temporary access, and whether placed in the field, ED, or ICU setting should be replaced once the patient is stabilized and other vascular access can be achieved.

B. Tube Thoracostomy

Decompression of traumatic pneumothorax or hemothorax with emergent tube thoracostomy is accepted as definitive treatment for many patients with thoracic trauma [10,11]. Controversy exists whether or not tube thoracostomy should be performed in the prehospital setting due to the potential for certain complications and because of alternatives that exist (principally needle aspiration of the chest, or simple thoracostomy).

In 1995, Barton et al. reported on a series of patients with severe thoracic trauma treated by an aeromedical service [12]. One hundred and twenty-three patients received 169 needle aspirations (NA); 39 bilateral aspirations. Eighty-four patients had 106 chest tubes (CT) placed. Thirty-two patients received needle aspiration prior to CT placement. Fifty-four percent of the NA group and 61% of the CT group had clinical improvement in their condition (p = NS), and there was no difference in overall mortality between groups. No cases of subsequent infection, lung damage, or bleeding were reported in the CT group. In 1998 Schmidt et al. reported a series of 76 prehospital CT placed by third-year surgical residents flying on an aeromedical service [13]. No infections or lung injury occurred in this group, and only four required replacement for malposition. Interestingly, only half of these patients received any prophylactic antibiotics.

Special mention should be made of a technique suggested by Deakin et al. in 1995 of ''simple thoracostomy''[14]. This method is reserved for a subset of thoracic trauma patients that have been intubated and are receiving positive pressure ventilation. The technique is identical to tube thoracostomy, with an opening created through the chest wall and pleura in the fifth intercostal space, midaxillary line, but no tube is inserted. Pneumothorax and hemothorax can be decompressed, and a dressing is placed over the wound. Intubation of the trachea and positive pressure ventilation prevent air from entering the pleural space through the open wound.

Based on current evidence, there is no indication to routinely replace CT from the field unless they are found to be malpositioned. Needle aspiration should be attempted first and may be all that is necessary in the field if improvement in the clinical condition occurs. An alternative for intubated patients is simple thoracostomy.

C. Airway Devices

Endotracheal intubation (ETI) is considered the definitive method of securing an airway in the prehospital, ED, and hospital settings. With a properly placed endotracheal tube (ETT) the airway is theoretically sealed from the bag to the lungs, and nearly the entire tidal volume can be delivered to the pulmonary system, maximizing both oxygenation and ventilation. Despite this, some EMS systems have restricted ETI due to a lack of training, a lack of ongoing experience with ETI, or concern over possible complications. Alternative airway devices have therefore been developed that presumably require less operator skill to place them. These devices include the esophageal obturator airway (EOA), esophageal gastric tube airway (EGTA), the pharyngeotracheal lumen airway (PTLA), and most recently the esophageal–tracheal Combitube. The EOA and EGTA have been extensively studied and are found to provide inadequate ventilation and have a high incidence of complications [15–17]. The EOA is never more effective than ETT, and often significantly inferior. If a patient arrives in the ED or trauma unit, the EOA should therefore quickly be replaced with an ETT.

The PTLA and Combitube are more recent devices that are inserted blindly into either the trachea or esophagus. These tubes have 2 lumens, and once the position is confirmed as tracheal or esophageal the patient can be ventilated through the proper lumen.

Numerous studies have been performed comparing these airways to ETT [18–20]. Oxygenation and ventilation are comparable, although there are numerous cases reported in which the PTLA or Combitube is less effective than ETT, and since an ETT can reliably be used to deliver drugs in the prehospital setting it will likely continue to be recommended as the initial prehospital airway of choice [20]. The PTLA or Combitube should be used as an alternative airway if ETI is unsuccessful. If a patient arrives in the ED with a PTLA or Combitube and appears to be adequately ventilated and oxygenated then the device does not need immediate replacement. The patient should be otherwise stabilized, and then can be definitively intubated with an ETT in a more controlled fashion.

D. Urinary Catheters

The issue of replacing an indwelling urinary catheter placed in the field is rarely confronted or reported in the literature, as there are few reasons to place a urinary catheter in the prehospital setting. Transport times to the ED or trauma unit for definitive care increase, and little added benefit is achieved. In fact, urinary catheterization is contraindicated in the presence of urethral trauma, and this may not be immediately apparent in the field. Blood at the urethral meatus or penile/scrotal hematoma may be present, but pelvic fracture or a high-riding prostate may not be identified in a field examination.

Decompression of a large, distended bladder may be necessary if a patient is extremely agitated due to this, but decompression could be performed by either suprapubic aspiration (in the case of suspected urethral trauma) or by in-and-out bladder catheterization. Indwelling urinary catheters might be placed to monitor urine output for prolonged transport times. If this is deemed necessary, careful insertion using aseptic technique should be performed and the catheter assessed regularly for any signs of complications while in the hospital.

E. Gastric Catheters

Nasogastric (NG) or orogastric (OG) tubes are often placed in a prehospital setting to decompress the stomach and thus facilitate ventilation, prevent aspiration of stomach contents, or to deliver therapy such as activated charcoal. Obtunded patients should have their airway protected prior to NG or OG tube placement. It is not necessary to routinely replace these devices if they are placed in the field unless they are malpositioned. Proper tube position can be assessed by instilling a 40 to 60 cc bolus of air into the NG or OG tube and listening for an appropriate rush of air over the stomach with a stethoscope. Alternately, tube placement can be confirmed radiographically after ED arrival.

VI. DEBRIEFING

A. EMS Personnel

A short debriefing of the EMS personnel should be conducted if the patient is in stable condition immediately after the trauma team takes over the responsibility. In other cases, it may be necessary to gather again and discuss problems (e.g., rising from prehospital treatments or measures not in accordance with the standards in hospital).

B. Trauma Team Members

Usually trauma team members have sufficient experience in working together in critical situations. The debriefing should be part of the continuous process of quality improvement. A meeting is usually held only if problems in a specific case occurred within a fixed interval of some months. These meetings should be chaired by the people responsible for the treatment of the patients in the ED (e.g., anesthesiologist or emergency physician as multiple-trauma coordinator, and trauma surgeon as responsible for the surgical therapy).

C. Videotape or Audiotape Review

Videotaping and audiotaping of the treatment in an ED poses some remarkable advantages as well as serious problems. Video cameras aimed at the trauma victim allow all resuscitations to be recorded. This footage is very useful to optimize measurements and overall patient management in the ED. Furthermore, a videotape is an excellent teaching tool when used to highlight correct resuscitation techniques or demonstrate shortcomings in a resuscitative effort. Specific measures (e.g., resuscitation) may easily be tape-recorded and evaluated after the case ends. Problems may arise, however, from legal implications in cases of inadvertent outcome and possible malpractice.

VII. DIFFERENCES BETWEEN PARAMEDIC-BASED AND PHYSICIAN-BASED EMS SYSTEMS

Emergency medical services systems can be configured in a variety of different ways, each with its own advantages and disadvantages. In the United States, for example, most systems are paramedic- or EMT-based. In Europe and other parts of the world many prehospital services are physician-staffed. Aeromedical systems can employ physicians, nurses, and paramedics. Many different factors contribute to the development of one system or another. Local geography, capabilities of the receiving hospitals, costs and what entities (public or private) sponsor such services, applicable statutes, equipment, and resources all play a role in planning and implementing EMS systems.

Most paramedic-based systems are limited in scope and practice by government regulations. Standardized protocols are established for specific medical/traumatic conditions, and a series of standard orders are created that detail the initial interventions a paramedic may do without a physician order. Therapy beyond standing orders can only occur after consulting a designated physician (base station MD) by radio or other form of telecommunication. Generally speaking, properly trained paramedics practicing within the scope of their training and standard protocols do a good job of stabilizing and transporting a wide variety of conditions. Paramedics can be trained to provide advanced airway management, including rapid sequence intubation (RSI), peripheral vascular access, medication delivery, and certain limited advanced cardiac life support (ACLS) and advanced trauma life support (ATLS) procedures. Studies on success rates of intubation, for example, have shown success rates of 90–97% [15,21,22]. The main difficulty with such systems comes from fitting an individual patient into standardized protocols instead of conforming interventions and treatments to the needs of an individual patient.

Physician-based systems, on the other hand, typically provide more advanced and comprehensive care in the prehospital environment if appropriate resources and medical equipment are available. Properly trained physicians can perform advanced procedures in the field, such as cricothyroidotomy, tube thoracostomy, pericardiocentesis, and even open thoracotomy, if necessary. Numerous studies have confirmed that such procedures can be successfully performed in the field [12,13,21,23,24]. Very few studies have evaluated *if* providing such advanced procedures results in better patient outcomes compared to systems in which more limited procedures are performed by paramedics, however. One study by Baxt and Moody demonstrated that patient outcome was improved when the prehospital aeromedical crew, was made up of a physician–flight nurse combination, compared to a flight nurse–paramedic team [25].

There remains a great deal of controversy as to what prehospital care strategy results in better patient outcome: definitive care/intervention provided on the scene (i.e., advanced procedures or other management provided by physician-staffed units) or rapid stabilization and transport to an appropriate receiving hospital for definitive care (scoop-and-run approach). There is not an easy answer to this question; each individual medical/traumatic condition must be evaluated and the potential benefits of early intervention and advanced management in the field balanced against an increase in scene time and the potential delay in arrival to the receiving hospital such interventions will produce.

VIII. TYPICAL COMPLAINTS AND PROBLEMS

A. EMS Personnel

Paramedics and emergency physicians often complain that members of the trauma team do not allow them to finish the report of their diagnosis and treatment but start to manipulate the patient, IV catheters, and so on. Another problem is how to identify the trauma team leader (i.e., the one in command of further diagnostics and therapy). A short introductory ''meeting'' of the arriving and receiving team leader facilitates communication and demonstrates professionalism.

B. Trauma Team Members

The most frequent complaints of the receiving team are related to inaccurate and over- or underestimated reports from the scene. A brief but complete standardized report enables the trauma team to prepare properly for the individual patient. The facilities and resources needed include special personnel (e.g., thoracic surgeons), diagnostic and therapeutic equipment such as ultrasonography, or the immediate availability of packed red blood cells at the time of patient arrival in the ED.

C. Patients

Patients are the weakest part of the three groups of people involved. Many conscious patients complain about the careless and ''businesslike'' behavior of EMS personnel and trauma team members. Observation of trauma team management of patients by someone not involved in the actual treatment reveals sometimes astonishing truths: conscious patients are often not informed about the extent of their injuries and individual diagnoses, therapeutic plans are not explained, and communication is only directed to other members of the trauma team, not toward the patient.

The patient's relatives may pose another problem. Since trauma occurs unexpectedly, often in young and otherwise healthy people, significant psychologic trauma may be present. All too often trauma team members do not recognize when patients or relatives need help to cope with the psychological impact of their injuries. Furthermore, physicians are often incapable of providing this help. Social and other support services are thus a critical part of the immediate care of trauma patients [26].

IX. SUMMARY

- Communication between prehospital providers and hospital-based trauma teams is essential to optimize care in the critically injured trauma patient.
- Radio frequencies are the most utilized resource; however, the advantage to cellular phones is that they can be used to send prehospital electrocardiograms via fax-modem.
- The MIVT format offers a simple yet complete way to give a prehospital report.
- If the patient has a long transport time and the condition changes or significant interventions have to be performed, the prehospital provider should update the trauma team before arrival.
- Upon arriving to the ED, it is imperative that EMS personnel communicate essential information to the receiving team in a concise yet complete manner.
- The trauma or ED team leader must allow prehospital providers to deliver their report without interruption to ensure all necessary information is communicated.
- The general approach to evaluation of an acute trauma victim differs from that of patients with diseases. It usually has three sequential components.
  - Rapid overview of the situation (especially on scene).
  - Primary survey of the vital functions.
  - Secondary survey (i.e., the comprehensive evaluation from head to toe).
- A thorough and accurate medical record is essential for the documentation of findings and treatment rendered, and not only for legal reasons.
- Peripheral IV lines and central lines started in the field do not need to be changed on ED arrival.
- Chest tubes, endotracheal tubes, PTLA/Combitubes, and urinary and gastric catheters placed in a prehospital setting do not need immediate replacement upon ED arrival.
- Intraosseus lines or EOA/EGTA should be replaced when the patient arrives at the ED.

Both EMS personnel and ED/trauma team personnel should debrief after patients are brought to the hospital.

Differences exist in EMS systems, ranging from all-volunteer EMS personnel to physicians and highly trained nurses and paramedics responding to the scene of a major trauma.

REFERENCES

1. L Capan, SM Miller. Trauma and burns: Initial evaluation and resuscitation. In: PG Barash, BF Cullen, RK Stoelting, eds. Clinical Anesthesia. Philadelphia: Lippincott-Raven, 1997.
2. N Caroline. Emergency care in the streets. In: N Caroline, ed. Boston: Little, Brown, 1995, pp. 72–90.
3. R Levine, DW Spaite, TD Valenzuela, EA Criss, AL Wright, HW Meislin. Comparison of clinically significant infection rates among prehospital- versus in-hospital-initiated i.v. lines. Ann Emerg Med 25:502–506, 1995.
4. DW Lawrence, AJ Lauro. Complications from i.v. therapy: Results from field-started and emergency department-started i.v.'s compared. Ann Emerg Med 17:314–317, 1988.
5. F Lederle, C Parenti, L Berskow. The idle intravenous catheter. Ann Int Med 16:737–738, 1992.
6. J Gamer, W Jarvis, T Emori. CDC definitions for nosocomial infections. Am J Inf Contr 16: 128–140, 1988.
7. D Cook, A Randolph, P Kernerman, C Cupido, D King, C Soukup, C Brun-Buisson. Central venous catheter replacement strategies: A systematic review of the literature. Crit Care Med 25:1417–1424, 1997.
8. M Ferguson, MH Max, W Marshall. Emergency department infraclavicular subclavian vein catheterization in patients with multiple injuries and burns. South Med J 81:433–435, 1988.
9. P Pappas, CE Brathwaite, SE Ross. Emergency central venous catheterization during resuscitation of trauma patients. Am Surg 58:108–111, 1992.
10. P Kulshrestha, K Iyer, B Das. Chest injuries: A clinical and autopsy profile. J Trauma 28: 844–847, 1988.
11. K Mattox. Thoracic injury requiring surgery. World J Surg 7:49–55, 1983.
12. ED Barton, M Epperson, DB Hoyt, D Fortlage, P Rosen. Prehospital needle aspiration and tube thoracostomy in trauma victims: A six-year experience with aeromedical crews. J Emerg Med 13:155–163, 1995.
13. U Schmidt, M Stalp, T Gerich, M Blauth, KI Maull, H Tscherne. Chest tube decompression of blunt chest injuries by physicians in the field: Effectiveness and complications [see comments]. J Trauma 44:98–101, 1998.
14. CD Deakin, G Davies, A Wilson. Simple thoracostomy avoids chest drain insertion in prehospital trauma. J Trauma 39:373–374, 1995.
15. P Pepe, M Copass, T Joyce. Prehospital endotracheal intubation. Ann Emerg Med 14:1085–1092, 1985.
16. T Michael. Comparison of the esophageal obdurator airway and endotracheal intubation in prehospital ventilation during CPR. Chest 87:814–819, 1985.
17. P Auerbach, E Geehr. Inadequate oxygenation and ventilation using the esophageal gastric tube airway in the prehospital setting. JAMA 250:3067–3071, 1983.
18. M Frass, R Frenzer, F Rausche. Evaluation of the esophageal tracheal Combitube in CPR. Crit Care Med 15:609–611, 1986.
19. M Frass, R Frenzer, G Mayer. The esophageal tracheal Combitube: Preliminary results with a new airway for CPR. Ann Emerg Med 16:768–772, 1987.
20. PE Pepe, BS Zachariah, NC Chandra. Invasive airway techniques in resuscitation. Ann Emerg Med 22:393–403, 1993.

21. CD Deakin. Prehospital management of the traumatized airway. Eur J Emerg Med 3:233–243, 1996.
22. EA Slater, SJ Weiss, AA Ernst, M Haynes. Preflight versus en route success and complications of rapid sequence intubation in an air medical service. J Trauma 45:588–592, 1998.
23. G DeLaurier, M Hawkins, R Treat, A Mansberger. Acute airway management: Role of cricothyroidotomy. Am Surg 56:12–15, 1990.
24. T Hatley, OJ Ma, N Weaver, D Strong. Flight paramedic scope of practice: Current level and breadth. J Emerg Med 16:731–735, 1998.
25. WG Baxt, P Moody. The impact of a rotorcraft aeromedical emergency care service on trauma mortality. JAMA 249:3047–3051, 1983.
26. S Tisherman. Interface of anesthesiology and surgery in the management of trauma. In: C Grande, ed. Textbook of Trauma Anesthesia and Critical Care. St. Louis: Mosby, 1993.

39

Psychological Aspects, Debriefing

BIRGIT SCHOBER

Rogaland Central and University Hospital, Stavanger, Norway

I. INTRODUCTION

A. Emotions? Psychology?

Why have such subjects been included in a textbook of trauma care? Are we not professionals with suitable control over our feelings? Is such discussion actually necessary? The answer is most definitely yes—it is exactly because we are professionals that it is important that we know and understand the emotions that both we and our patients experience during major trauma.

The victim of an accident will always have the experience of crisis or disaster. Physical trauma with pain releases a multiplicity of strong emotions from fear, anxiety, and desperation to complete apathy. Such emotions represent great psychological stress. Much research has been done on survivors from concentration camps and victims of war, disasters, and accidents. This research has shown that emotional strain can lead to actual psychological and physical morbidity [1]. Knowledge of normal and pathological reactions to traumatic crisis undoubtedly enables medical professionals to provide better emotional care for victims, their families, and even witnesses, and improves the outcome of the patient. It also helps to ensure the continued mental well-being of the health care professionals.

B. Case Report

The rescue helicopter comes to an accident in which a car left the road and overturned. A passenger in the front seat is seriously injured, unconscious, and hanging with her head down and an amputated thigh sticking out of the wreck. While the doctor is trying to establish an airway, he recognizes a young ambulance driver standing nearby in total

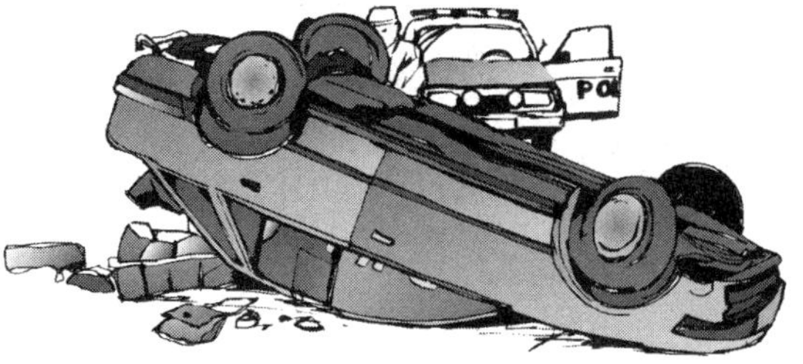

Figure 1 Accidents are a cause for psychological stress in victims and trauma teams. (Drawing courtesy of Ellen Jepson, 1996.)

apathy. The patient dies some minutes later. Somebody tells the doctor that this was the mother of the young driver. The doctor does not ask after the boy and leaves with the helicopter soon afterwards. Over the next few days he thinks as much about the young man as about the mutilated, dying patient. He feels bad at not having spoken to the boy.

This case demonstrates how complex emotional reactions can be. The subjective feeling of having failed the young man increases the stress of the doctor, who already has to cope with the death of the patient (Fig. 1).

Medical professionals themselves are prone to psychological stress, both while experiencing the accident event itself and with summation of strong impressions over time. Usually prehospital trauma care providers will experience feelings of satisfaction and other appropriate emotions, after having arrived at the scene of the event as competent professionals, taken care of the patient, and finally bringing him safely to the hospital. But what happens when the prehospital trauma team arrives too late or the situation requires too much? The professionals may become emotionally stressed, and in the long run there is a risk of "burn-out," which can have an adverse effect on both their health and their efficiency in the job.

The intention of this chapter is to provide some insight into the variety of emotional reactions connected with prehospital trauma care and to discuss strategies that can be used to deal more successfully with these emotions.

II. THE VICTIM

Man tends to have a sense of inviolability ("accidents happen to others, but not to me") [2]. This is, of course, an illusion, but also an appropriate psychological mechanism making it possible to live a normal life without the continuous feeling of threat and danger. When one is suddenly involved in an accident or disaster and one's own life or that of a loved one is threatened, however, one cannot maintain this mechanism. The psychological reactions that follow are often independent of the nature of the trauma, but to a large extent reflect the personal meaning of the accident to the victim [3]. These acute stress reactions (ASR) are quite similar in most people and should be regarded as normal.

A. Acute Stress Reactions (ASR)

The International Statistical Classification of Diseases, 10th review defines an acute stress reaction "as a transient disorder of significant severity which develops in an individual without any other apparent mental disorder in response to exceptional physical and/or mental stress'' [4]. It is considered to occur only when the person involved perceives that an external demand exceeds his or her capability to deal with it [5].

Acute stress reactions are rapid-onset responses (without minutes or hours) to sudden and severe stressful events. They are self-limiting, usually resolved in a month, and are found in all mentally healthy persons. A predisposition to psychiatric illness may aggravate the reactions. The incidence rate of ASR is reported to be up to 75% [5]. (Table 1). The symptoms include mental, emotional, behavioral, and physical changes [5].

Mental symptoms: absence of emotional responsiveness with reduction in awareness and consciousness. In extreme cases there may be total apathy. The victim is often disoriented and does not react appropriately to extrinsic stimuli. The lack of emotions may be falsely interpreted as coping well with the situation. Subjectively, the victim has a sense of disturbance of time (e.g., time stands still or flies away), or a sense of numbing. Partial or complete amnesia may occur. The victim may also experience an increased vigilance with a detailed memory of the accident (Fig. 2).

Emotional symptoms: intense anxiety and panic, fear, feeling lost and abandoned, rapid swinging of moods with emotional outbursts. The helper observes the behavior of the patient to be totally inappropriate to the trauma.

Behavioral changes: the inner chaos is often expressed in motor restlessness or hyperactivity. Some show a tendency to withdraw. An increased startle reaction is typical. These disturbances may hinder the rescue work, and it can be necessary to have someone independent of the rescue team (e.g., a spectator) take care of the person.

Physical symptoms: related to the enhanced activity of the endocrine system and consist of tachycardia, chest pains, difficulty in breathing, tremor, sweating, nausea and vomiting, and involuntary urination and defecation (Fig. 3).

Table 1 Acute Stress Reactions (ASR)

Acute stress reactions
Rapid onset
Self-limiting
In mentally healthy persons
Symptoms
Disoriented
Numbing
Intense anxiety
Increased startle reactions
Motor restlessness
Withdrawal
Autonomic arousal
Management
Mental first aid
Acceptance
Reassurance
Practical support

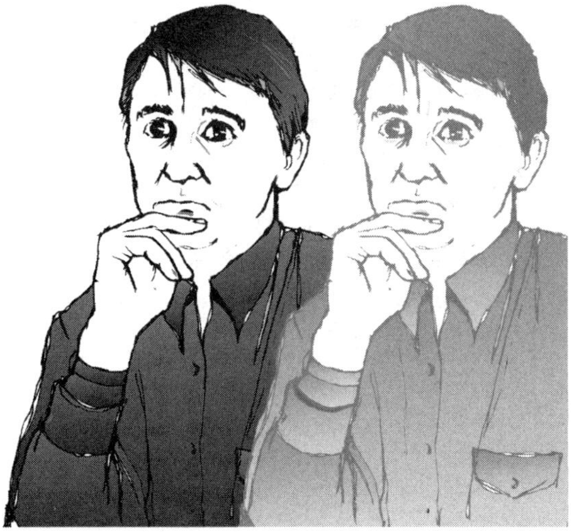

Figure 2 Feeling ''beside one's self'' is normal in an acute stress situation. (Drawing courtesy of Ellen Jepson, 1996.)

Which pattern of reaction predominates depends on the individual psychological structure of the victim. The same applies to the severity of the symptoms. If the victim experienced especially strong sensory input (e.g., loud noise, strong smells) or perceives the situation to be life-threatening, then the ASR may be more severe. A complicated life situation, low level of stress tolerance, and lack of social support can also aggravate the symptoms.

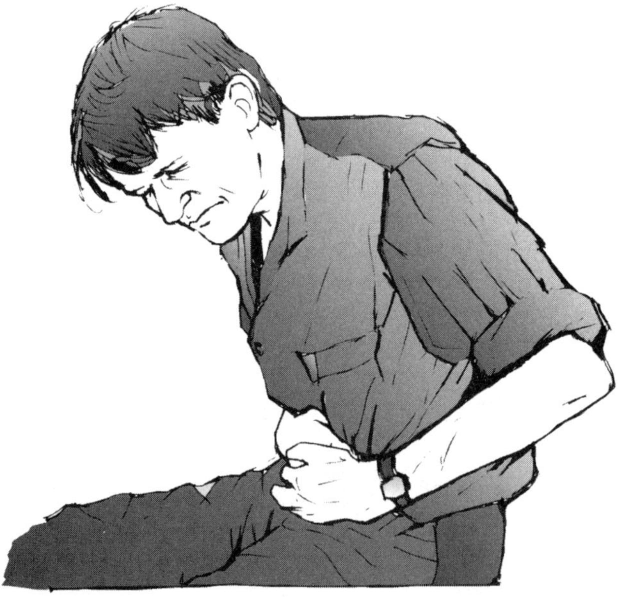

Figure 3 Psychological stress can include physical symptoms. (Drawing courtesy of Ellen Jepson, 1996.)

B. Management

The management of ASR consists of mental first aid. That means basic crisis intervention involving the expression of empathy and the acceptance of feelings and behavior, and giving hope. The victims should be encouraged to talk about their feelings and experiences related to the accident. Knowledge and information gives people a sense of control and helps them to cope with the reality of their situation at the time of the trauma. Those persons with minor injuries should be advised as to how they can assist with the rescue process. Nonverbal and practical support is the base of psychological stability and helps to relieve the emotional pressure. Mental first aid can be described with three Cs (closeness, concern, contact) [5] (Fig. 4).

Medication is indicated only when the patient remains excited or excessively anxious. Anxiolytics might be used, but studies have shown none or poor beneficial effect of early administration of benzodiazepines in trauma victims for the prevention of mental illness [7]. If medication is deemed necessary, it should only be given for a few days.

C. Psychiatric Intervention

About 1–3% of those who exhibit ASR develop an acute psychosis that needs psychiatric intervention and possible admission to a special ward. Factors that are described to be predictors of post traumatic stress disorder (PTSD) are the pretrauma vulnerability, the magnitude of the stressor, the preparation for the event, and the individual immediate and short-term responses [8].

D. Posttraumatic Stress Disorder

Posttraumatic stress disorder describes the development of psychological symptoms after a traumatic event beyond normal human experiences, such as a serious threat toward one's life and the physical integrity of oneself or one's relatives, a sudden disaster with destruction of the environment, or as a witness to others being seriously injured in an accident or by violence. The onset of symptoms is delayed—occurring during weeks or months after the event. Like ASR, anyone is susceptible to developing PTSD, but again people who already have psychiatric problems are more vulnerable. Children are also at increased

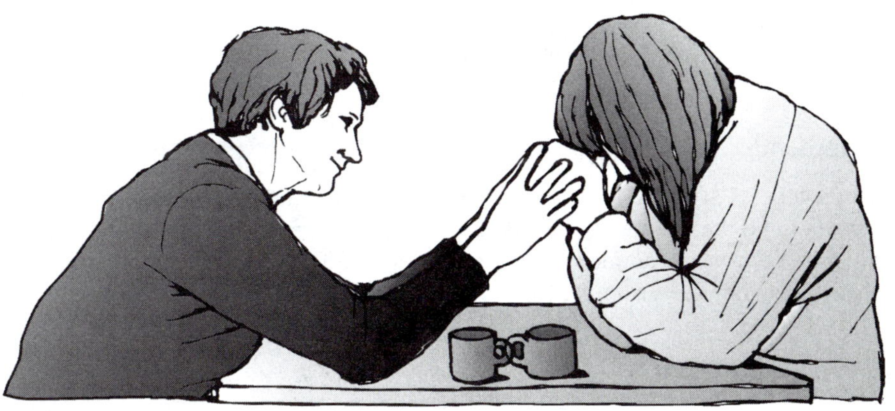

Figure 4 Mental first aid. (Drawing courtesy of Ellen Jepson, 1996.)

Table 2 Post Traumatic Stress Disorder (PTSD)

Post traumatic stress disorder
Overwhelming stressor
Delayed onset (after weeks or months)
Symptoms
Intensive recollections
Irritability
Sleep disturbances
Anxiety
Avoidance
Persistent physical reactions
Prognosis
Variable
Treatment
Psychotherapy
Antidepressants

risk, as their coping mechanisms are still relatively immature. The child's response to disaster depends on his or her own perception of the trauma, which in turn is influenced by his or her cognitive and physical development [9].

As much as 30% of patients with ASR can develop PTSD after a period of 3 to 12 months after a traumatic event. The symptoms are as follows [10] (see Table 2.)

- Persistently intrusive recollections of the traumatic event, such as waking flashbacks and nightmares.
- Persistent avoidance associated with the trauma. The patient tries to avoid feelings, thoughts, and activities that remind him of the event. He feels numb and loses interest in everyday activities and even loving relationships.
- Persistent symptoms of anxiety and increased arousal manifest themselves as hypervigilance, sleep disturbances, irritability, and poor concentration.
- Persisting physical reactions.

The prognosis of PTSD is variable. The symptoms may resolve themselves or may persist throughout the patient's life. Posttraumatic stress disorder is a psychiatric diagnosis that often occurs in combination with other disorders such as anxiety or panic disorder, substance abuse, and/or depression. Patients suffering from PTSD are also more susceptible to somatical illness.

E. Management

The management of PTSD includes different forms of psychotherapy, of which behavioral therapy appears to be the most effective. Where depressive symptoms are prominent the patient may benefit from an antidepressant drug therapy. The role of debriefing in this context is controversial (see also Sec. IV.D, Table 2) [8].

III. THE PROFESSIONALS

Health care personnel are exposed to the same stress as the victims. Working in prehospital trauma care demands a certain adaptation to stress. During education and practical experience we learn to achieve the necessary emotional distance from the patient that protects us from identification and enables us to act professionally. There is an individual variation in this adaptation, and this ability to cope in itself may change over time. To maintain control and be effective when on duty, it is necessary to know one's own emotional reactions and limits.

A. Factors Aggravating Stress in Prehospital Trauma Care

It is inevitable that rescue teams experience long periods of waiting while on duty. These intervals can also be a time of stress. The professionals are constantly on alert, often with little to do except dwell on their performances at former turnouts. The emergency call then comes and activates the prehospital personnel both physically and mentally. Often there is little information about the accident. This creates an element of uncertainty until arrival at the patient. Now the rescue teams become exposed to a multitude of impressions, demands, and expectations, which differ from one situation to the other. They are expected to assume leadership. They have to make decisions on their own, and with fewer resources than in the hospital. Sometimes it is necessary to expose the patient to high-risk procedures, and sometimes they are too late or fail.

1. Case Report

An experienced rescue team is called to a patient who has been involved in an explosion accident. The patient has burns over nearly his whole body. His head, neck, and upper extremities have third degree burns. The patient is awake and complains of pain. His oxygenation is poor. The mucous membranes in his mouth are also burnt. Transport time to the next hospital is about 40 min. The emergency physician decides to intubate the patient, although conditions for intubation are extremely poor because of the burn damage of the neck, mouth, and upper airway. The procedure becomes complicated by aspiration and the patient dies at the scene. The physican accuses himself during the next week of having failed. He thinks that if he had brought the patient to the hospital there would have been better conditions for handling the difficult intubation and the patient might be alive. He senses the smell of burned skin for several days after the accident.

This example demonstrates some of the stress for the medical professionals, such as difficult decisions, the death of the patient under a high-risk procedure, and strong sensual impressions.

B. Factors That Influence Coping with Stress

There are two main factors that influence coping with stress. The individual situation of the professional, and the environmental factors under which he has to work. The individual factors include, for example, poor experience and training in the work situation, a complicated life situation, and a bad social network. Former psychiatric problems and unresolved grief also have a negative impact on coping with stress. Such negative feelings as guilt, inadequacy, and loss of self-confidence may lead to such psychological avoidance mechanisms as suppression, projection, or rationalizing. The people concerned usually deny these phenomena, but try to find a scapegoat for mishaps or become cold and arrogant toward patients and co-workers.

The most important environmental factor is work stress, including being both undercharged and overcharged, or when the situation at work is neither predictable nor controllable.

Table 3 Burnout Syndrome

Burnout syndrome
Emotional exhaustion
Detachment
Loss of empathy
Physical exhaustion
Prevention and management
Realistic attitude toward own capability
Good social relations
Optimistic attitude
Individual strategies
Organizational strategies

1. Case Report

The helicopter team has a patient with a severe head injury onboard who needs neurosurgical intervention. There are two suitable hospitals nearby, but both refuse the patient because of lack of capacity. Precious minutes go by while discussions continue on the radio. Finally the rescue team just delivers the patient at one of the hospitals. The incident is reported to the responsible department without any consequences. The members of the rescue team are frustrated in not having any influence and feel their efforts to save the patient's life in the field to be meaningless.

This case reflects a grave system failure that can adversely affect the patient's outcome and diminish the motivation of the professionals. Individual and environmental factors interlink with each other. This may result in an unfavorable cycle and may lead to burnout.

C. Burnout Syndrome

Professional burnout is quite common. Studies have found that up to 60% of emergency physicians have moderate to high burnout rates [11]. Burnout is caused by disproportionally high efforts and poor satisfaction in addition to stressful working conditions. It often occurs in people who expect a lot of themselves (perfectionism) or who feel that others expect a lot of them (hero complex) and who have not clearly defined their limits to others (poor communication). Burnout often doesn't surface for years (Table 3).

The main symptoms [12] are as follows:

- Emotional exhaustion with sleeping difficulties, reduced concentration, emotional lability, and irritability
- Physical exhaustion
- Detachment from other staff members and especially from patients (loss of empathy)
- Loss of satisfaction and a sense of decreased accomplishment

D. Prevention and Management

There are many stress management strategies, all of which approach the problem differently. They can be divided into individual stress management strategies and organizational strategies. The first group includes educative interventions, such as workshops, different relaxation techniques such as biofeedback, meditation, or relaxation training, and most promising, cognitive–behavioral methods.

Organizational strategies include modifying work conditions, such as distributing ''dirty work'' evenly and building in time-outs. These strategies are more effective in reducing stress than the individual methods [13].

IV. DEBRIEFING

Debriefing has its origins in the military and was used to clarify the facts of combat. It was observed that debriefing appeared to have a positive effect on maintaining group morale and on reducing psychological stress immediately after combat. In the 1980s debriefing was transferred to civilian life by Mitchell as critical incident stress debriefing (CISD) [14]. Since than it has become a widely used method of stress reduction.

A. Critical Incident Stress Debriefing

Primarily CISD (Table 4) is a group meeting that takes place in the first 24 to 72 hr after the distressing incident. It is one session, and may last 1 to 3 hr. It should be led by one, preferably two, mental health professionals.

B. Purpose

The purpose of CISD is to clarify the sequence of events and to clear up any misunderstandings. Emotions related to the trauma should be examined and explained. The feeling of solidarity in the group should be strengthened, and the group should learn from mishaps. Critical incident stress debriefing is thought to be a support for people through normal reactions to an abnormal event. It also provides an opening for identifying those at a risk of developing psychological problems. Finally, it is meant to prevent the development of PTSD [15].

C. Carrying Out CISD

In carrying out CISD, all people involved should participate, but nobody must be pushed to speak. Since the meeting is designed to reduce stress, one should establish a comfortable

Table 4 Critical Incident Stress Debriefing (CISD)

Purpose
Clarify
Inform
Strengthen group feeling
Draw conclusions
Discover people at risk for developing problems
Implementation
Introduction
Facts
Reactions and emotions
Practical advice
Conclusions

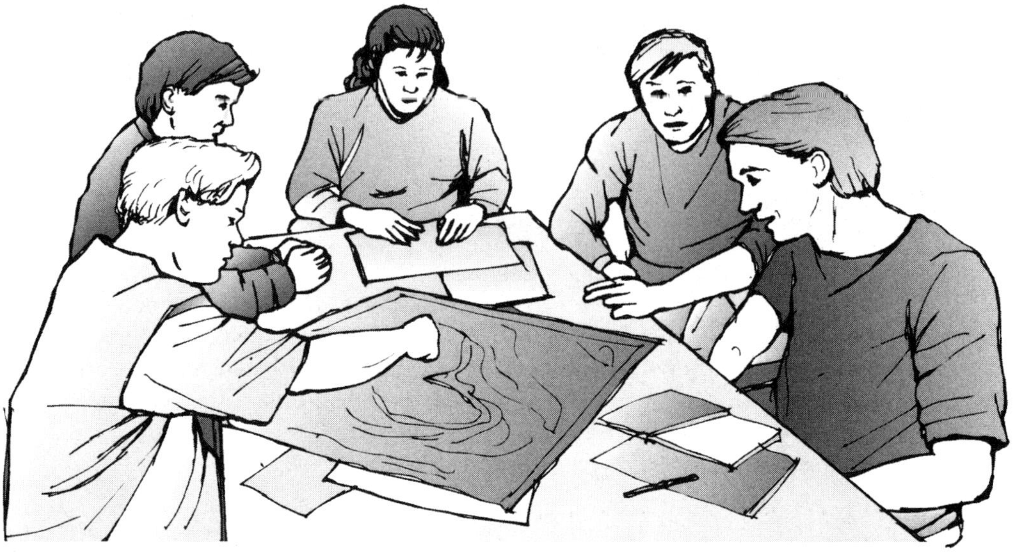

Figure 5 CISD is a group process. (Drawing courtesy of Ellen Jepson, 1996.)

and safe atmosphere (Fig. 5). Critical incident stress debriefing is formalized in terms of the following processes and stages [5]:

Introduction: the leader informs the group about the intention of the meeting and explains the schedule. It is emphasized that everything that is said must remain confidential and that no one is looking for a scapegoat.

The facts: brief review of the traumatic event.

Thoughts and impressions: everyone should be given the opportunity to place his or her own efforts in the context as a whole. Enhance different impressions of the trauma; give room for talking about misunderstandings.

Emotional reactions: in this part of othe debriefing, everyone should have the chance to express the individual emotions that were experienced, such as having failed in one's role, fear of being injured under a risky rescue procedure, and identification with the victim. The leader should ask how the group members are doing now. Are there sleeping disturbances, nightmares, and so on?

Normalization and planning for the future: here the leader should reassure that the emotions experienced are quite normal. Practical advice should be given. Is there anybody who requires further psychological support or who wants to speak more privately with a doctor or a priest? If insufficient equipment or inadequate procedures have caused feelings of failure or guilt, one has an opportunity to initiate the correcting steps.

Disengagement: summary of the meeting. If necessary, fix a date for a second meeting.

D. Evaluation of CISD

Debriefing has been used in a considerable range of circumstances including rescue workers involved in natural disasters, soldiers exposed to combat, children who were taken hostage in their school, victims of acute burn trauma and road accidents, bystanders in cardiopulmonary resuscitation, and rape victims or women who had undergone abortion. There are many studies that have shown debriefing to be helpful [15,16], but in more recent years criticism has been raised against it. Some studies found no positive effect on psychological outcome, and some studies even showed an adverse effect [15].

In 1998, the Cochrane depression, anxiety, and neurosis group reviewed brief psychological interventions for the treatment of immediate trauma-related symptoms and the prevention of PTSD [15]. Overall, they found that the quality of the studies was poor and only six fulfilled the inclusion criteria (early intervention, one single session, some form of emotional airing). There was no evidence that debriefing reduced general psychological morbidity or prevented development of PTSD.

E. Comments and Conclusions

These findings raise many questions. Why is the research into this topic of such bad quality? Generally, it is accepted that the traditional design of research is a problem in psychiatry. To hold back intervention could be ethically irresponsible [16]. In most of the studies the term debriefing is not clearly defined. Debriefing is, as the word says, a concept to help a briefed group (e.g., a rescue team). The mostly voluntary participation in debriefing may lead to self-selection of the groups in that, people with more distress seek debriefing. Debriefing has also been used for individuals and for totally different groups of traumatized people. A group intervention cannot automatically be transfered to crisis intervention for the individual, however. What else can explain the negative findings? Were the interventions too short, was follow-up too short, or was the timing of the intervention wrong? Can the debriefing session trigger a ''secondary trauma'' [15]?

In several studies the participants of a briefing group experienced the meeting as positive even if the results of the studies did not show a positive effect. In some cases the debriefing groups expressed a negative attitude toward mental health personnel. Some authors remark on the symbolic meaning of debriefing (at least someone—the employer, the society—cares) [16].

The conclusions that can be drawn out of this are the following:

At present there is no evidence that the routine use of individual debriefing is helpful.
No recommendations can be made concerning group debriefing and debriefing used in children.
More research, including more extensive intervention, has to be done [15].

It is desirable to spread the knowledge about stress reactions and coping strategies as widely as possible, as has already been done for mouth-to-mouth resuscitation among the lay population. The more people know, the better they cope. Exposed groups such as rescue teams can profit especially from pre-existing stress management strategies [17].

It may be that CISD becomes just one part of a more extensive intervention management that is more flexible and can be better adapted to suit the situation. Necessary knowledge about traumatic stress management should be obtained on the following four different levels [18]:

Basic level: those who come into contact with people exposed to trauma, such as policemen a firefighter, etc. in order to provide preventive measures
Second level: primary health services, such as nurses and doctors of somatical specialties or rescue teams, in order that they can serve as ''gatekeeper''

Mental health services: psychiatrists have to be able to treat almost all of the psychological reactions after trauma

Expert level: psychiatrists with specialist experience in treating people with extremely complicated mental states

V. SUMMARY

An accident or disaster initiates many psychological reactions and emotions in all enveloped people. Most of these reactions have to be considered as normal.

Victims of traumatic events show in a high degree of acute stress reaction immediately after the trauma. This usually disappears after days or weeks.

Persistent stress reactions may lead to psychological disorders such as PTSD.

In the health care providers, the acute reactions will not be as marked as in the victims. The accumulation of stress over time may lead to symptoms of burnout, however.

Knowledge about stress reactions enables rescue teams to provide mental first aid to the patient and take care of him in a more holistic way. This may help to prevent psychiatric morbidity in the patient (Fig. 6).

Debriefing is one strategy to cope with acute traumatic stress. Its benefit to reduce psychiatric morbidity in both victims of accidents and disasters and rescue teams is considered controversial. The quality of research generally is poor.

At present there is no evidence that the routine use of debriefing is helpful to prevent psychiatric disorders. More research has to be done, however. More flexible strategies of stress management after trauma have to be included in the research.

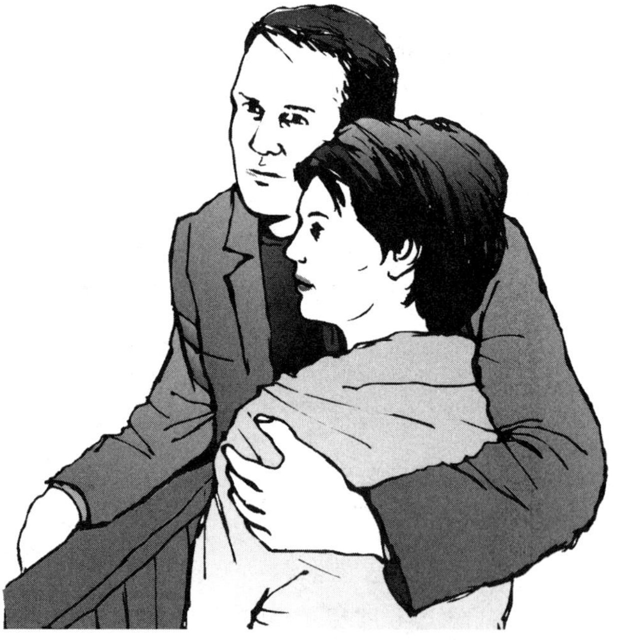

Figure 6 Closeness, concern, and conduct are all part of mental first aid in trauma care. (Drawing courtesy of Ellen Jepson, 1996.)

REFERENCES

1. L Eitinger. Late psychological problems after concentration camp incarceration. Nord Med 106(4):132–133, 136, 1991.
2. UF Malt. Når kroppen blir wyk eller skades. In: L Weisæth, L Mehlum, eds. Mennesker, traumer og kriser. Oslo: Universitetsforlaget, 1993, pp. 162–175.
3. UF Malt, OM Olafssen. Psychological appraisal and emotional response to physical injury: A classical, phenomenological study of 109 adults. Psychiatric Med 10:117–134, 1992.
4. International Statistical Classification of Diseases. 10th rev. Geneva: World Health Organization, 1992, pp. 146–149.
5. J Haslerud, GR Bloch-Thorsen, E Waldenstrøm. Mental first aid in disasters, accidents and crises. Stavanger, Norway: Psychiatric Educational Fund, 1998.
6. A Sund, in cooperation with L Weisæth, A Holen, UF Malt. Ulykker, katastrofer og stress. Oslo: Gyldendal Norsk Forlag, 1985, pp. 33–45, 69–71.
7. E Gelpin, O Bonne, D Brandes, AY Shalev. Treatment of recent trauma survivors with benzodiazepines: A prospective study. J Clin Psychiatry 57:390–394, 1996.
8. BA Van der Kolk, A McFarlane, L Weisæth. Traumatic Stress. New York: Guilford, 1996.
9. Work Group on Disasters: Federal Center for Mental Health Services, American Academy of Pediatrics. Psychological Issues for Children and Families in Disasters. Elk Grove Village, Illinois, 1994.
10. L Weisæth. Traumateriseringsprosessen de psykiatriske følgetilstander. In: L Weisæth, L Mehlum. Mennesker traumer og kriser. Oslo: Universitetesforlag, 1993.
11. R Goldberg, RW Boss, L Chan, J Goldberg, WK Mallon, D Moradzadeh, EA Goodman, ML McConkie. Burnout and its correlates in emergency physicians: Four years experience with a wellness booth. Acad Emerg Med 3:1156–1164, 1996.
12. P Keel. Psychological stress caused by work: Burnout syndrome. Soz Praventivmed 38(suppl. 2):131–132, 1993.
13. C Cherniss, S Dantzig. In RR Kilburg, PF Nathan, RW Thoreson, eds. Professionals in Distress. Washington, DC: American Psychological Association, 1986, pp. 255–273.
14. JT Mitchell. When disaster strikes . . . The critical incident stress debriefing procedure. J Emerg Med Serv 8:36–39, 1983.
15. S Wessely, S Rose, JI Bisson. A systematic review of brief psychological interventions (''debriefing'') for the treatment of immediate trauma related symptoms and the prevention of the post traumatic stress disorder. In: The Cochrane Database of Systematic Reviews. vol. 4. Oxford: Cochrane Library, 1998.
16. A Dyregrov. A Psykologisk debriefing—en virksom metode? Tidskrift for Norsk Psykologforening 36:99–106, 1999.
17. AJ Macnab, JA Russel, JP Lowe, F Gagnon. Critical incident stress intervention after loss of an air-ambulance: Two year follow up. Prehosp Disast Med 14:8–12, 1999.
18. L Weisæth. Nivåer av nødvendig kompetanse innen traumatisk stress. Consultation-liaison-Psychiatry. Annual Conference, Oslo, April 12–13, 1999.

40

Enhancing Patient Safety and Reducing Medical Error: The Role of Human Factors in Improving Trauma Care

PAUL BARACH

University of Chicago, Chicago, Illinois

> The value of history lies in the fact that we learn by it from the mistakes of others, as opposed to learning from our own which is a slow process.
>
> —W. Stanley Sykes (1894–1961)
> dedication, *Essays on the First Hundred Years of Anesthesia, Vol. 1, 1960.*

I. INTRODUCTION: THE NEGLECTED DISEASE

Trauma injuries are among the most serious and neglected public health problems facing developed societies. Although various types of injury deaths—motor vehicle fatalities, homicides, suicides, falls, poisonings, drownings—have been listed in mortality statistics for decades, they have been ignored by all but a few epidemiologists and public health researchers. Influential and important discussions of the future direction of epidemiological and public health research make no mention of injury and therefore do not allow the proper learning for prevention [1,2].

Each year approximately one out of four Americans is injured seriously enough to require medical attention. Injuries account for 25% of all emergency department visits and are the leading cause of death among Americans aged 1 to 44 years [3]. Throughout the world, trauma is now the leading cause of death during half of the human life span [4]. They account for more years of potential life lost before age 65 than result from cancer, heart disease, and stroke combined.

Injuries and the events preceding them are generally more obvious and closer together in time than are diseases and the events that precede them. The role of human behavior is often erroneously assumed to be more important to injury causation than to disease causation [5]. We now know that injuries, like diseases, affect identifiable ''high-risk'' groups, follow an often predictable chain of events, and are therefore preventable. Furthermore, the impact of injuries that do occur can be minimized by the optimal provision of acute care and the rehabilitation of injured persons. The combination of prevention, acute care, and rehabilitation has come to be called *injury control* [6].

II. THE EMERGING ISSUE OF PATIENT SAFETY

Modern medical care is complex, expensive, and at times dangerous. Hospitals are a vital part of our health care system, routinely providing valuable services, but they are also places in which poor care can lead to preventable harm. Medical injuries are adverse events attributable to the medical management of patients. Many stakeholders in health care have begun to struggle together to resolve the moral, scientific, legal, and practical dilemmas around this epidemic. To achieve this goal, an environment fostering a rich reporting culture must be created to capture accurate and detailed data about the nuances of care.

In November 1999, the Institute of Medicine (IOM) published a landmark report entitled *To Err Is Human: Building a Safer Health System* [8]. Produced by the IOM's Committee on Quality of Health Care in America, the report estimated that between 44,000 and 98,000 patients die preventable deaths annually in hospitals in the United States, with many times more suffering injuries. The IOM report estimated that total national costs for adverse events (lost income, lost household production, disability, health care costs) are between $38 billion and $50 billion annually [9]. The annual toll of these errors exceeds the combined number of injuries due to motor vehicle and aviation crashes, suicides, falls, poisonings, and drownings [5,7]. Medical errors are adverse events that are preventable with our current state of medical knowledge. The IOM report concluded that a 50% reduction in medical errors is achievable over the next 5 yeasr and should be a minimum goal for national action.

During the past 25 years, three large-scale studies have examined the incidence of adverse events in hospitals. Adverse events were defined as injuries caused by medical management rather than by the disease or condition of the patient. The first, an analysis of approximately 20,000 records of patients hospitalized in California in 1974, found that adverse events occurred in 4.5% of hospitalizations and negligent adverse events in almost 1% of the case [10]. The second study, in which researchers reviewed approximately 30,000 records of patients hospitalized in New York State in 1984, revealed 3.7% of hospitalization involved serious adverse events [9].

The study team concluded that among the 2.8 million admissions to New York hospitals, there were about 98,000 adverse events, of which approximately 37,000 involved substandard care. More recently similar results were reported in a two-stage medical record review in Utah and Colorado [11]. Finally, a large Australian study using a similar methodology of the New York study found similar results [12]. There have also been more narrowly focused studies using different methodologies that indicate that medical injury continues to be a serious problem. These data can and have been challenged, but experts nevertheless agree that it is the best information available. The term patient safety encompasses preventing errors of action and judgment, making errors visible, and mitigating the effects of errors. It is critical to recognize that not all bad patient outcomes for patients are due to medical errors.

A. Human Error and Performance Limitations

Although there was virtually no research in the field of safety problems in medicine until the mid-1980s, in other fields (e.g., aviation, road and rail travel, nuclear power, chemical processing) safety science, human error, and the intense study of accidents have been well developed for several decades [13]. While any doctor or nurse could provide examples of occasions on which patients were injured during treatment or had narrowly avoided serious injury, very few studies had been published. Several factors have contributed to the growing interest in human errors and medical accidents. The rapidly rising rate of litigation in the 1980s and increasing interest from the media brought medical accidents to the attention of both doctors and the general public. Systems of complaint and compensation have been widely criticized, leading to calls for reform from lawyers, doctors, and organizations representing patients.

In parallel with these changes, researchers from several disciplines have developed methods for the analysis of accidents of all kinds [14,15]. Theories of error and accident causation have evolved that are applicable across many human activities, although they have not as yet been widely used in medicine. These developments have led to a much broader understanding of accident causation, with less focus on the individual who makes an error and more on pre-existing organizational factors that provide the context in which errors occur. An important consequence of this has been the realization that an accident analysis may reveal deep-rooted, unsafe features of organizations.

The most obvious impetus of the renewed interest in human error beyond health care has been the growing concern over the terrible cost of human error: the Tenerife runway collision in 1977 (leaving 540 killed), Three Mile Island in 1979, the Bhopal methyl isocyante tragedy in 1984, and the *Challenger* and Chernobyl disasters in 1986 [16]. There is nothing new about tragic accidents caused by human error, but in the past the injurious consequences were usually confined to the immediate vicinity of the disaster. Today the nature and scale of potentially hazardous technologies in society and hospitals means that human error can have adverse effects way beyond the confines of the hospital.

Over the past few years there has been a noticeable spirit of *glasnost* within the medical profession concerning the role played by human error in the causation of medical adverse events [17]. The involvement of human factor specialists in this inquiry has brought two benefits. First, it has introduced techniques such as the critical incident analysis and event reporting systems. Initially developed in the field of aviation, these can be applied to the medical accident process. Second, these investigations have clearly shown that medical mishaps share many important causal similarities with the breakdown of other social-technical systems [16]. Third, it has allowed us to understand error-producing conditions and performance-shaping factors so that we may design systems that are error-tolerant and systems-robust (see Table 1).

Table 1 Error-Producing Conditions

Error-Producing Conditions
Unfamiliarity with task
Time shortage
Poor signal: noise ratio
Poor human–system interface
Designer–user mismatch
Information overload
Risk misperception
Poor feedback from system
Inexperience
Poor instructions or procedures
Inadequate checking
Educational mismatch of person with task
Disturbed sleep patterns
Hostile environment
Boredom

Source: Adapted from Ref. 16.

III. INJURY CONTROL AND PREVENTION OF MEDICAL ERRORS

In 1985, the National Research Council report went on to point to the fact that injuries are highly patterned—subject to study and targeting of interventions, that many interventions are known to be effective but are unused, and that modest increases in funding would have large payoffs in cost savings [18]. The reduction of injuries is justifiable on humane grounds, particularly since they disproportionately affect the health of the young. In times of cost constraints, injury reduction is also an economic necessity. Injury control is one of the most promising ways to reduce large health costs in the immediate future.

During the past few decades, injury control has emerged as a distinct discipline within public health [5]. There are many parallels between injury control and the prevention of medical errors. A key tenet of injury control is that injuries are not "accidents" or random, uncontrollable acts of fate; rather, many injuries are predictable and preventable [16]. By the same token, medical adverse events are predictable and preventable. As the IOM report notes, "errors can be prevented by designing systems that make it hard for people to do the wrong thing and easy for people to do the right thing" [8]. In the absence of such systems, medical adverse events will predictably continue to occur.

The IOM published a report on injury control 14 years before the release of its report on patient safety [18]. In its 1985 report the IOM identified the following general approaches to injury prevention: education (behavior change), legislation and regulation, product design, and environmental design. Examples include boat operator safety classes (education), safety belt laws (legislation and regulation), insulated electric hand tools (product design), and light reflectors and rumble strips along highways (environmental design). The 1999 report, using similar tenets, recommended similar strategies to enhance patient safety, including: (1) communication of information on safety to professional and lay audiences (education); (2) action by Congress to require reporting of adverse events that result in death or serious harm (legislation and regulation); (3) action by the Food and Drug Administration to enhance the safe use of pharmaceuticals through drug packaging and labeling and the choice of drug names (product design); and (4) removal of concentrated solutions of hazardous medications, such as potassium chloride, from patient care units (environmental design) [8].

A. Designing Reporting Systems for Adverse Events in Health Care

Medical errors can occur in the delivery of clinical preventive services, conceivably with serious or even fatal consequences. These errors might include inaccurate measurement in screening tests (e.g., blood pressure), inaccurate reading of screening X-rays (e.g., mammograms) or biological specimens (e.g., Pap smears), failure to contact patients promptly regarding abnormal or indeterminate results of screening tests and procedures (e.g., mammograms and Pap smears), and failure to identify or act on contraindications for biological or pharmaceutical agents (e.g., vaccines, bupropion for smoking cessation). Preventive medicine specialists must familiarize themselves with strategies aimed at avoiding medical errors in order to reduce their occurrence within their own sphere of work.

We recommend that state governments collect the data submitted as part of a mandatory reporting of adverse events resulting in death or serious harm. We also recommend a voluntary reporting system for less serious injuries or noninjuries events (''near misses''). In most cases state health agencies would be given the responsibility for administering these new surveillance systems, hence public health officials responsible for collecting data on widely accepted ''reportable conditions'' (e.g., HIV, tuberculosis, and influenza) would be in charge of collecting data on medical errors. Public health officials might be able to use existing surveillance systems for collecting and reporting information on adverse medical events.

Reporting adverse events in health care thus provides two reasons for preventive medicine to address patient safety. First, surveillance—a core tool of epidemiology and preventive medicine—will be an integral component of efforts to enhance patient safety. Second, officials in preventive medicine and public health will be involved in operating the reporting systems for adverse medical events. Lessons learned from traditional public health reporting systems would help guide the development of effective reporting systems for medical errors [19].

B. Systems Change

Many preventive medicine practitioners are responsible for protecting and improving the health of populations. These include public health officiers responsible for the health of a state or community, occupational medicine physicians responsible for the health of a workforce, aerospace medicine physicians responsible for the health of operating crews and passengers of air and space vehicles and the support personnel required to operate such vehicles, and preventive medicine physicians employed by health plans, medical group practices, or integrated health care systems who are responsible for the health of a population of patients or health plan members. These practitioners are often in charge of systems of care, and they are familiar with system improvement as a key component of quality assurance. Indeed, one of the seven basic components of preventive medicine is ''planning, administration, and evaluation of health and medical programs and the evaluation of outcomes of health behavior and medical care'' [5]. System change is an essential ingredient of efforts to reduce medical errors, and thus trauma care and preventive medicine specialists are uniquely positioned to help achieve those changes.

Table 2 Haddon's Matrix Applied to Motor Vehicle-Related Injuries

Phase factor	Preevent	Event	Postevent
Host	Driver education, alcohol avoidance, fatigue	Age, hemophilia	First aid training
Vehicle	Antilock brakes, motor vehicle inspection	Tempered glass, safety belts, air bags	Flame-retardant fabric, puncture-resistant gas tanks
Environment	Speed limits, pedestrian overpasses	Breakaway poles, impact barriers	911 emergency number, trauma care systems, regional spine and rehab centers

Source: Ref. 22.

IV. ACCIDENTS AND INJURIES

The evolution in thought about injuries is reflected in their classification. Injuries often are classified as accidental or intentional [20]. The word accidents encompasses a very large and fuzzy set of events. Only a small proportion of these are injurious. Any unintended, incidental event that interferes in one's daily pursuits is an accident. The term is intertwined with the notion that some human error or behavior is responsible for most injuries. This focus of attention on the human factors involved tends to detract from an examination of the full range of factors that contribute to injuries, particularly to their severity [5].

Although the word accident had various meanings historically, it is now primarily a euphemism for lack of intent or unpreventable occurence, as though intent were a primary consideration in injury prevention [20]. Here the term injury or a specific type of injury (e.g., amputation, burn, laceration) is used to indicate the phemonenon of interest.

A. Epidemiological Model

Based on the experience of scientific investigation of infectious diseases, injury epidemiologists have applied the epidemiological model of infectious disease to injuries. The core concepts are the *host* (person injured), the *agent* that injures, and the *vector or vehicle* that may acutely convey the exposure agent as well as other environmental agents [21]. Injury epidemiology identifies the various forms of energy—mechanical, thermal, chemical, electrical, ionizing radiation—needed to cause injury.

B. Factors and Phases of Injury

The transfer of energy to human begins at rates and in amounts above or below the tolerance level of human tissue is the necessary and specific cause of injury. The amount of energy concentration outside the bands of tolerance of tissue determines the severity of the injury. To alert researchers to the factors contributing to injury incidence as well as the severity and the timing of involvement of those factors, William Haddon devised the scientific basis of injury control by creating matrix of broad categories of factors and phases of injury. This *Haddon matrix*, along with some examples of factors important in each cell, is shown in Table 2 [22].

The factors that contribute to incidence and severity of injury are of relevance if these factors can be modified. It is important to know how many potential years of life are affected by injury, and whether or not subsets in the population are disproportionately involved. The major modifiable factors that contribute to injury are energy and the characteristics of the energy vehicles.

C. Injury Control Model—the Nature of Energy

Mechanical or kinetic energy is most commonly responsible for injuries. When a person must stop suddenly, as in a crash of a vehicle, energy must be dissipated in the vehicle, environment, or in the tissues of the individual. The shape and elasticity of the materials struck will determine the damage to the tissue. Inflexible, protruding, or pointed objects on dashboards, for example, will penetrate the human anatomy. Devices such as child restraints, lap and shoulder belts, land air bags reduce the severity of injury by reducing the contact with a less flexible surface, the so-called second collision. They also increase the uniformity of the deceleration of the occupant and vehicle and they spread the load over dozens of square inches. Helmets and other energy-absorbing materials can also dissipate energy.

V. PREVENTION STRATEGIES

1. *Active vs. passive countermeasures.* Injury countermeasures can be grouped into active measures requiring conscious cooperation of the individual in order to be protective on every occasion on which they are used. Examples include safety belts and motorcycle helmets. Passive countermeasures include air bags and automatic sprinkler systems.
2. *Education, enforcement, and engineering.* These are the cornerstones of any effective intervention.
3. *Strategies to control hazards* (Table 3). William Haddon defined 10 logically distinct technical strategies for injury prevention [23]. Table 3 lists strategies, with examples relevant to some of the more common injuries. The adoption of any one strategy is dependent on financial, regulatory and political considerations. Injury prevention costs can be minimized by targeting strategies to agents, vehicle or vectors, hosts, and environments.

A. Practicing Injury Control

The *first step* in developing effective programs to control injuries is understanding the magnitude and scope of the problem [24]. Population-based data and surveillance data are needed to monitor patterns and trends and to evaluate the impact of injury countermeasures.

The second step is to identify the causes and factors that modify the risk of the individual at risk. This can be done with descriptive studies or quasi-experimental designs while controlling for the effects of confounding variables.

The third step is to develop and test interventions and countermeasures. One must consider the target population, the feasibility of the countermeasures and their acceptability to this population, and their cost.

The final critical step is implementing effective interventions and then evaluating

Table 3 Options Analysis: Strategies and Examples of Injury Control

1.	Prevent the creation of the hazard → ban production and sale of assault weapons to civilians.
2.	Reduce the amount of the hazard → require that all passenger vehicles have lower centers of gravity or wider track width.
3.	Prevent the release of the hazard that already exists → provide canes and walkers to the elderly and handrails in their environments.
4.	Modify the rare or spatial distribution of the release of the hazard from its source → use child restraints and seat belts in motor vehicles.
5.	Separate by time or space the hazard and that which is to be protected → remove trees and poles from near roadsides. Separate pedestrian pathways.
6.	Separate the hazard and that which is to be protected by interposition of a material barrier → install air bags in cars.
7.	Modify surfaces and structures to minimize injury → use breakaway designs for utility poles and light poles along roadsides.
8.	Make what is to be protected more resistant to damage → issue bulletproof vests to police officers and security guards.
9.	Begin to counter the damage already done by the environmental hazard → use smoke and carbon dioxide detectors.
10.	Stabilize, repair, and rehabilitate the object of the damage → implement trauma care systems throughout the world.

Source: Ref. 23.

their impact. Measures of cost-effectiveness such as dollars spent per life saved or per injury prevented are particularly important.

B. Trauma Prevention in the Future

1. *Data collection and registry*. Cost-containment managed care should increase the incentive of health care personnel to prevent illness and injury. Trauma registries and other databases will play a key role in monitoring the performance of health systems, identifying high-risk groups, and evaluating the impact of injury prevention programs.
2. *Research*. Injury control must demonstrate its value in successfully competing for a shrinking pool of health care dollars [see Table 4].
3. *Advocacy*. Evaluation of data may indicate that a countermeasure is effective but rarely used. Passage of mandatory laws will have a major impact. The results can be impressive, particularly when coupled with ongoing education efforts and visible enforcement. States with mandatory motorcycle helmet laws report compliance rates as high as 98%. The building of coalitions is essential to assembling a broad base of support for legislative action [25]. Population-based data are important, but the testimony of disabled patients, surviving family members, and health care providers is needed to give the emotional context.

VI. SIMULATION IN TRAUMA EDUCATION AND IMPROVED CARE

Simulation has been used in teaching medicine for hundreds of years. In the sixteenth century, manikins (or ''phantoms,'' as they were called) were developed to teach obstetri-

Table 4 Objectives of Injury Research and Control and Data Needs

Objective	Data needed
1. Select most important injuries for study	E-coded fatalities and hospitalizations, develop common taxonomy
2. Apply countermeasures	Surveillance of who, where, when, and how injured
3. Find modifiable factors that will reduce injury and quantify injury reduction	Reliable and valid measures of factors and research designs to control for confounding factors
4. Develop causal models	Measure risk factors
5. Evaluate effectiveness of intervention	Injury rates or risk-related behavior
6. Evaluate cost-effectiveness of interventions	Cost of each intervention

Source: Adapted from Ref. 5, p. 19.

cal skills in order to reduce perceived high maternal/infant mortality rates [26]. Simulation has also been used effectively in the education of those involved in emergency care and trauma management [27]. The care for trauma victims and the education of their caregivers are costly in time and personnel. The role of simulation here is crucial. It allows for training and assessment of one's capacity to perform the right actions in difficult physical and often ethically complex situations.

The ability to develop comeptence in high-fidelity simulators has been demonstrated in such diverse fields as aviation, disaster management, and complex military environments. Over the past 10 years, realistic trauma simulation has undergone rapid development and utilization worldwide. The issues facing educators and clinicians treating trauma patients who incorporate simulation into training curricula include standardization of training, validation of performance outcome measures, and improved methodology of clinical studies. In order to validate simulation assessment, benchmarking across many levels of skill expertise is a necessary first step. Another challenge the simulator movement will face is the justification for its existence in the current highly cost-sensitive health care environment. In addition, in trauma and high-risk medicine disciplines, there is a need to conduct controlled outcome studies of simulator training. This will be required prior to setting standards for licensure and recertification. Ensuring participant safety and confidentiality surrounding the simulation experience will help guarantee its success as a respected and reliable method for teaching and learning.

VII. CONCLUSIONS

Prevention of trauma injuries and enhancing patient safety is linked in many ways. Prevention specialists must ensure safety in the confines of the delivery of trauma care. In addition, preventive medicine specialists can bring the tools of their trade to safety improvement efforts in other specialties of medicine and at the level of "the system." We recommend that organizations devoted to trauma care join the burgeoning campaign to enhance patient safety.

Trauma is a public health problem that is neglected relative to its importance in lost life and disability. Injury prevention has more immediate health and economic benefits than chronic disease control. Interventions reduce injuries, their severity, and their consequences by modifying these factors at specific phases of the injury: before, during, and after the acute phase. Research that focuses on modification of the means of exposure to the agent will contribute most to injury prevention. Modifying systems and products is often more feasible than altering the behavior of an individual. Failure to recognize the difficulty of ''improving'' behavior has often led to the failure to apply more effective alternative countermeasures to the injury problem. The leadership of physicians and other health care professionals is essential to the success of these efforts.

We need to standardize information about adverse events in trauma care that result in death or serious harm. Professional societies must make a visible commitment to patient safety by establishing a permanent committee dedicated to safety improvement in trauma care. The committee would: (1) develop a curriculum on patient safety and encourage its adoption in training and certification requirements of trauma care health care professionals; (2) disseminate information on patient safety to members at conferences and through the society's publications and Web site; (3) recognize patient safety in practice guidelines and in standards related to the introduction and diffusion of new technologies, therapies, and drugs in trauma care; and (4) collaborate with other professional societies and disciplines in a national summit on the professional's role in patient safety.

REFERENCES

1. N Pearce. Traditional epidemiology, modern epidemiology, and public health. Am J Pub Health 86:678–683, 1996.
2. M Susser, E Susser. Choosing a future for epidemiology: I. Eras and paradigms. Am J Pub Health 86:668–673, 1996.
3. SP Baker. Injury science comes of age. JAMA 262:2284–2285, 1989.
4. P Barass et al. Injuries to Adults in Developing Counties: Epidemiology and Policy. Washington, DC: World Bank, 1991, pp. 1–132.
5. L Robertson. Injury Epidemiology: Research and Control Strategies. 2nd ed. New York: Oxford University Press, 1998.
6. W Haddon Jr. Advances in the epidemiology of injuries as a basis for public policy. Pub Health Rep 95:411–421, 1980.
7. DP Rice, EJ Mackenzie, eds. Cost of Injury in the United States: A Report to Congress. San Francisco Institute for Health and Aging, University of California, and Baltimore; Injury Prevention Center, Johns Hopkins University, 1989.
8. Committee on Quality of Health Care in America, Institute of Medicine. To Err Is Human: Building a Safer Health System. Washington, DC: National Academy Press, 1999.
9. LL Leape, TA Brennan, N Laird, D Cullen. Incidence of adverse events and negligence in hospitalized patients: Results of the Harvard Medical Practice Study I. New Eng J Med 324: 370–376, 1991.
10. DH Mills. Report on the medical insurance feasibility study. West J Med 128:360–376, 1978.
11. MJ Thomas, DM Studdert, H Burtsin. Incidents and types of adverse events and negligent care in Utah and Colorado. Med Care 38:261–271, 2000.
12. RM Wilson, WB Runciman, RW Gibberd. The Quality in Australian Healthcare Study. Med J Austr 163:458–471, 1995.
13. SD Sagan. The Limits of Safety: Organizations, Accidents, and Nuclear Weapons. Princeton, NJ: Princeton University Press, 1994.
14. BA Turner, NF Pidgeon. Man-Made Disasters. London: Butterworth and Heinemann, 1997.
15. J Senders, N Moray. Human Error: Cause, Prediction, and Reduction. Hillsdale, NJ: Lawrence Erlbaum, 1994.

16. J Reason. Managing the Risks of Organizational Accidents. Hawts: Ashgate, Aldershot, 1997.
17. M Millenson. Demanding Medical Excellence: Doctors and Accountability in the Information Age. Chicago: University of Chicago, 1997.
18. Committee on Trauma Research. Injury in America: A Continuing Public Health Problem. Washington, DC: National Academy Press, 1985.
19. C Vincent, M Ennis, RJ Audley. Medical Accidents. Oxford, England: Oxford University Press, 1993.
20. H Loimer, M Druir, M Guarnieri. Accidents and acts of God: A history of the terms. Am J Pub Health 86:101–107, 1996.
21. W Haddon Jr. On the escape of tigers: An ecologic note. Tech Rev 72:44, 1970.
22. W Haddon Jr. A logical framework for categorizing highway safety phenomena and activity. J Trauma 12:197, 1972.
23. W Haddon Jr. Energy damage and the ten countermeasure strategies. J Trauma 13:321, 1973.
24. JA Waller. Injury Control: A Guide to the Causes and Prevention of Trauma. Lexington, MA: Heath, 1985.
25. JA Waller. Reflections on a half century of injury control. Am J Pub Health 84:664, 1994.
26. GH Buck. Development of simulators in medical education. Gesnerus 48:7, 1991.
27. S Small, R Wuerz, R Simon, N Shapiro, A Conn, G Setnik. Demonstration of high fidelity simulation team training for emergency medicine. Acad Emerg Med 6:312–323, 1999.

Index